D0792992

OXFORD MEDICAL PUBLICATIONS

Oxford Handbook of
Acute Medicine

Published and forthcoming Oxford Handbooks

Oxford Handbook for the Foundation Programme 2e
Oxford Handbook of Acute Medicine 3e
Oxford Handbook of Anaesthesia 2e
Oxford Handbook of Applied Dental Sciences
Oxford Handbook of Cardiology
Oxford Handbook of Clinical and Laboratory Investigation 2e
Oxford Handbook of Clinical Dentistry 4e
Oxford Handbook of Clinical Diagnosis 2e
Oxford Handbook of Clinical Examination and Practical Skills
Oxford Handbook of Clinical Haematology 3e
Oxford Handbook of Clinical Immunology and Allergy 2e
Oxford Handbook of Clinical Medicine—Mini Edition 7e
Oxford Handbook of Clinical Medicine 7e
Oxford Handbook of Clinical Pharmacy
Oxford Handbook of Clinical Rehabilitation 2e
Oxford Handbook of Clinical Specialties 8e
Oxford Handbook of Clinical Surgery 3e
Oxford Handbook of Complementary Medicine
Oxford Handbook of Critical Care 3e
Oxford Handbook of Dental Patient Care 2e
Oxford Handbook of Dialysis 3e
Oxford Handbook of Emergency Medicine 3e
Oxford Handbook of Endocrinology and Diabetes 2e
Oxford Handbook of ENT and Head and Neck Surgery
Oxford Handbook of Expedition and Wilderness Medicine
Oxford Handbook of Gastroenterology & Hepatology
Oxford Handbook of General Practice 3e
Oxford Handbook of Genitourinary Medicine, HIV and AIDS
Oxford Handbook of Geriatric Medicine
Oxford Handbook of Infectious Diseases and Microbiology
Oxford Handbook of Key Clinical Evidence
Oxford Handbook of Medical Sciences
Oxford Handbook of Nephrology and Hypertension
Oxford Handbook of Neurology
Oxford Handbook of Nutrition and Dietetics
Oxford Handbook of Obstetrics and Gynaecology 2e
Oxford Handbook of Occupational Health
Oxford Handbook of Oncology 2e
Oxford Handbook of Ophthalmology
Oxford Handbook of Paediatrics
Oxford Handbook of Palliative Care 2e
Oxford Handbook of Practical Drug Therapy
Oxford Handbook of Pre-Hospital Care
Oxford Handbook of Psychiatry 2e
Oxford Handbook of Public Health Practice 2e
Oxford Handbook of Reproductive Medicine & Family Planning
Oxford Handbook of Respiratory Medicine 2e
Oxford Handbook of Rheumatology 2e
Oxford Handbook of Sport and Exercise Medicine
Oxford Handbook of Tropical Medicine 3e
Oxford Handbook of Urology 2e

Oxford Handbook of Acute Medicine

THIRD EDITION

Punit S. Ramrakha

Consultant Cardiologist
Stoke Mandeville Hospital, Aylesbury
and Hammersmith Hospital
London, UK

Kevin P. Moore

Professor of Hepatology
University College London Medical School
University College London, UK

Amir Sam

Wellcome Trust Clinical Research Fellow and SpR in
Endocrinology and Diabetes
Hammersmith Hospital
Imperial College London, UK

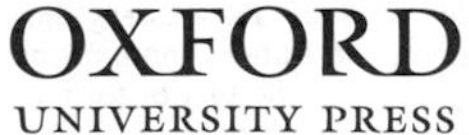

OXFORD
UNIVERSITY PRESS

Great Clarendon Street, Oxford OX2 6DP

Oxford University Press is a department of the University of Oxford. It furthers the University's objective of excellence in research, scholarship, and education by publishing worldwide in

Oxford New York

Auckland Cape Town Dar es Salaam Hong Kong Karachi Kuala Lumpur Madrid Melbourne Mexico City Nairobi New Delhi Shanghai Taipei Toronto

With offices in

Argentina Austria Brazil Chile Czech Republic France Greece Guatemala Hungary Italy Japan Poland Portugal Singapore South Korea Switzerland Thailand Turkey Ukraine Vietnam

Published in the United States
by Oxford University Press Inc., New York

First edition published 1997
Second edition published 2004
Third edition published 2010
Reprinted 2011,2013,2014,2015,2016,2017

British Library Cataloguing in Publication Data
Data available

Library of Congress Cataloging-in-Publication Data
Data available

Typeset by Glyph International Ltd., Bangalore, India
Printed in China
on acid-free paper by
C&C offset printing Co.,Ltd

ISBN 978–0–19–923092–1

11

Oxford University Press makes no representation, express or implied, that the drug dosages in this book are correct. Readers must therefore always check the product information and clinical procedures with the most up-to-date published product information and data sheets provided by the manufacturers and the most recent codes of conduct and safety regulations. The authors and publishers do not accept responsibility or legal liability for any errors in the text or for the misuse or misapplication of material in this work. Except where otherwise stated, drug dosages and recommendations are for the non-pregnant adult who is not breastfeeding.

Foreword

The first edition of the *Oxford Handbook of Acute Medicine* was published in 1997. Since then acute medicine has evolved as a fully established speciality within the UK and over 95% of hospitals now have an acute medical unit. Patients presenting as a medical emergency who need to be seen and assessed within an in-patient hospital environment now constitute the largest group of patients occupying in-patient hospital beds. It is imperative, therefore, that all staff are trained in the management of acute medical emergencies and importantly have easy access to information to support management of this acutely unwell sub group of patients. This text book is clearly structured and is supported by useful diagrams and algorithms and hence the information is readily accessible. The practical procedure section is comprehensive. While many practising clinicians will not be required to undertake all these procedures they will be involved in discussion on these issues with patients and relatives and this text will be an invaluable guide.

The handbook series from Oxford University Press already provides useful information to many clinicians working in clinical practice. Irrespective of age or seniority for clinicians directly involved in the early diagnosis and management of patients who present acutely this book will provide a concise aid. The clear and up-to-date content of this text reflects the experience of the authors and I am personally delighted to provide a foreword to a book which will undoubtedly help support the growing number of trainees' working in the field of acute medicine.

Derek Bell
Professor of Acute Medicine
Imperial College London

Preface

The management of acute medical emergencies is the most demanding and stressful aspect of medical training. The aim of this handbook is to give confidence to doctors to manage acute medical problems effectively, safely, and in line with current clinical guidelines. This edition has been radically revised by Dr Amir Sam, and we have tried to update and ensure that every aspect of the care recommended is in line with current clinical guidelines. The third edition of the *Oxford Handbook of Acute Medicine* includes summary boxes for the key points in the management of common medical emergencies. These concise and practical 'management key points' can be a useful guide to junior doctors in the casualty. The layout of the book reflects clinical practice: assessment, differential diagnosis, immediate management, and some aspects of long-term therapy. We have included an extensive section on practical procedure, since we believe it is important that all doctors are aware of how and why certain procedures are undertaken (e.g. insertion of a TIPS). Throughout the book the text commonly exceeds that required for the management of specialist problems by the generalist. We make no apology for this. This is intended to provide the doctor with an understanding of specialist interventions so that they are more conversant with what is possible and what is happening to their patient. Finally we have included a new section on differential diagnosis of common presentations.

Acknowledgements

We would like to thank all of the contributors who provided initial drafts of chapters which have evolved over time, as well as friends and colleagues who gave up their time to read a chapter and verify its accuracy. We would also like to thank OUP for their encouragement during the re-writing of this book. PSR is indebted to Vandana and his parents for their support and motivation. KPM is indebted to Janet, Alice, and Thomas for their continued patience when the portable computer accompanied family holidays. Finally, we would like to acknowledge the environment at the Hammersmith Hospital where we trained, and learnt that acute medicine is both interesting and fun.

Advice on chapter revisions was also given by the following:

Mike Beckles, Consultant Physician, Royal Free Hampstead NHS Trust
Sanjay Bhagani, Consultant Physician, Royal Free Hampstead NHS Trust
David Collas, Consultant Physician, Watford General Hospital
Jenny Cross, Consultant Physician, Royal Free Hampstead NHS Trust
Daniel Darko, Consultant Physician and Endocrinologist, Central Middlesex Hospital
Andrew Davenport, Consultant Physician, Royal Free Hampstead NHS Trust
Seyed Hamidreza Naghavi, Specialist Registrar in Occupational Medicine, Imperial College Healthcare NHS Trust
Wing May Kong, Consultant Physician and Endocrinologist and Honorary Senior Lecturer, Central Middlesex Hospital
Victoria Salem, Academic Clinical Fellow, Hammersmith Hospital
Richard Stratton, Consultant Physician, Royal Free Hampstead NHS Trust

Contents

Detailed contents

3 Gastroenterological emergencies 223

11 Rheumatological emergencies 621

12 Dermatological emergencies 653

13 Psychiatric emergencies 669

Symbols and abbreviations

📖	cross reference
↑	increased
↓	decreased
→	leading to
~	approximately
1°	primary
2°	secondary
♂	male
♀	female
A&E	accident and emergency
AAA	abdominal aortic aneurysm
Ab	antibody
ABC	airway, breathing, and circulation
ABG	arterial blood gas
ACE	angiotensin-converting enzyme
ACEI	angiotensin-converting enzyme inhibitor
AChR	acetylcholine receptor
ACLS	advanced cardiac life support
ACS	acute coronary syndrome
ACTH	adrenocortico stimulating hormone
AD	adrenaline
ADH	anti-diuretic hormone
AF	atrial fibrillation
AIDS	acquired immunodeficiency syndrome
AKI	acute kidney injury
ALI	acute lung injury
ALL	acute lymphoblastic leukaemia
ALP	alkaline phosphatase
ALT	alanine transaminase
AMA	anti-mitochondrial antibody
AMI	acute myocardial infarction
AML	acute myeloid leukaemia
ANA	anti-nuclear antibody
ANCA	anti-neutrophil cytoplasmic antibody
AP	anteroposterior
aPC	activated protein C
APSA	C anistreplase

APTT	activated partial thromboplastin time
AR	aortic regurgitation
ARDS	adult respiratory distress syndrome
ARF	acute renal failure
AS	aortic stenosis
ASA	acetyl salicylic acid
ASD	atrial septal defect
ASOT	anti-streptococcal titre
AST	aspartate transaminase
ATN	acute tubular necrosis
ATP	adenosine triphosphate
AV	atrioventricular
AVNRT	atrioventricular-nodal re-entry tachycardia
AVR	aortic valve replacement
AVRT	accessory pathway tachycardia
AXR	abdominal X-ray
AZT	zidovudine
BAL	bronchoalveolar lavage
BBB	bundle branch block
BC	blood cultures
bd	twice a day
BIH	benign intracranial hypertension
BLS	basic life support
BM	bone marrow
BMT	bone marrow transplant
BNF	*British National Formulary*
BOOP	bronchiolitis obliterans organizing pneumonia
BP	blood pressure
Ca	carcinoma
CABG	coronary artery bypass graft
CAD	coronary artery disease
cAMP	cyclic AMP
CAVH	continuous arteriovenous haemofiltration
CAVHD	continuous arteriovenous haemodiafiltration
CBD	common bile duct
CCDC	Consultant in Communicable Disease Control
CCF	congestive cardiac failure
CCHF	Crimean-Congo haemorrhagic fever
CCU	coronary care unit
CEA	carcinoembryonic antigen

CHB	complete heart block
CI	cardiac index
CK	creatine phosphokinase
CMV	cytomegalovirus or continuous mandatory ventilation
CNS	central nervous system
CO	cardiac output
COAD	chronic obstructive airways disease
COP	cryptogenic organizing pneumonia
COPD	chronic obstructive pulmonary disease
CPAP	continuous positive airways pressure
CPK	creatinine phosphokinase
CPR	cardiopulmonary resuscitation
CrAg	cryptococcal antigen
CRF	chronic renal failure
CRP	C-reactive protein
CSF	cerebrospinal fluid
CSM	carotid sinus massage
CT	computed tomography
CTPA	CT pulmonary angiography
CVA	cerebrovascular accident
CVP	central venous pressure
CVVH	continuous venovenous haemofiltration
CVVHD	continuous venovenous haemodiafiltration
CVS	cardiovascular system
CXR	chest X-ray
D&V	diarrhoea and vomiting
DA	dopamine
DAT	direct antigen test
DBP	diastolic blood pressure
DC	direct current
DDAVP	desmopressin
DI	diabetes insipidus
DIC	disseminated intravascular coagulation
DKA	diabetic ketoacidosis
DM	diabetes mellitus
DNA	deoxyribonucleic acid
DSH	deliberate self-harm
DT	delerium tremens
DTPA	diethylenetriaminepentaacetic acid
DU	duodenal ulcer

DVT	deep vein thrombosis
E	ecstasy
EBV	Epstein-Barr virus
EC	extracellular
ECG	electrocardiogram
Echo	echocardiogram
ECV	extracellular volume
EEG	electroencephalogram
EF	ejection fraction
EG	ethylene glycol
EM	electron microscopy
EMD	electromechanical dissociation
EMG	electromyogram
ENT	ear nose and throat
EP	electrophysiological
EPS	electrophysiological studies
ERCP	endoscopic retrograde cholangiopancreatography
ESR	erythrocyte sedimentation rate
ET	endotracheal
ETT	endotracheal tube
FBC	full blood count
FDP	fibrinogen degradation products
FEIBA	Factor VIII inhibitor bypassing activity
FEV1	forced expiratory volume (1 minute)
FFP	fresh frozen plasma
FH	family history
FNAB	fine needle aspiration biopsy
FRC	functional residual capacity
FSH	Follicle stimulating hormone
FVC	forced vital capacity
G6PD	glucose-6-phosphate dehydrogenase
G&S	group and save
GB	gall bladder
GBM	glomerular basement membrane
GBS	Guillain–Barré syndrome
GCS	Glasgow Coma Scale
GCSF	granulocyte colony-stimulating factor
GFR	glomerular filtration rate
GH	growth hormone
GHB	gammahydroxybutyric acid

GI	gastrointestinal
GIT	gastrointestinal tract
glc	glucose
GP	general practitioner
GP	glycoprotein
GTN	glyceryl trinitrate
GU	genitourinary
GUM	genitourinary medicine
GVHD	graft-versus-host disease
HAAR	T highly active anti-retroviral therapy
HACEK	*Haemophilus, Acintobacillus, Cardiobacterium, Eikenella* and *Kingella* spp. (causes of culture negative endocarditis)
HAIgM	hepatitis A Ig M
HAPO	high-altitude pulmonary oedema
HAV	hepatitis A virus
HBc	hepatitis B core
HbS	hepatitis B surface
HBsAG	hepatitis B surface antigen
HBV	hepatitis B virus
HCG	Human chorionic gonadotropin
HCV	hepatitis C virus
HDL	high-density lipoprotein
HDU	high dependency unit
HIV	Human immunodeficiency virus
HLA	human lymphocyte antigen
HMG-CoA	hydroxy methyl glutaryl-coenzyme A
HOCM	hypertrophic obstructive cardiomyopathy
HONC	hyperosmolar non-ketotic coma
HR	heart rate
HRS	hepatorenal syndrome
HRT	Hormone replacement therapy
HSV	herpes simplex virus
HT	hypertension
HTLV	human-T-lymphotropic virus
HUS	haemolytic–uraemic syndrome
I:E	inspiratory:expiratory ratio
IABP	intra-aortic balloon pump
IBD	inflammatory bowel disease
ICD	implantable cardioverter defibrillator
ICP	intracranial pressure

ICU	intensive care unit
ID	Infectious disease
IE	Infective endocarditis
IgA	immunoglobulin A
IgE	immunoglobulin E
IgG	immunoglobulin G
IgM	immunoglobulin M
IHD	ischaemic heart disease
IJV	internal jugular vein
IM	intramuscular
INR	international normalized ratio (prothrombin ratio)
IPPV	intermittent positive pressure ventilation
ITP	idiopathic thrombocytopanic purpura
ITU	intensive therapy unit
IV	intravenous
IVC	inferior vena cava
IVI	intravenous infusion
IVIG	intravenous immunoglobulin
IVU	intravenous urogram
JPS	joint position sense
JVP	jugular venous pressure
KS	Kaposi's sarcoma
LA	left atrium
LAD	left anterior descending coronary artery
LBBB	left bundle branch block
LDH	lactate dehydrogenase
LDL	low-density lipoprotein
LFT	liver function test
LH	luteinizing hormone
LHRH	luteinizing hormone releasing hormone
LMN	lower motor neuron
LMS	left main stem
LMWH	low-molecular-weight heparin
LP	lumbar puncture
LSD	lysergic acid diethylamide
LV	left ventricular
LVEDP	left ventricular end diastolic pressure
LVF	left ventricular failure
LVH	left ventricular hypertrophy
MACE	major cardiac events

MAI	*Mycobacterium avium intracellulare*
MAOI	monoamine oxidase-inhibitor
MAP	mean arterial pressure
MAT	multifocal atrial tachycardia
MC&S	microscopy, culture, and sensitivity
MCA	middle cerebral artery
mcg	microgram/s
MCTD	mixed connective tissue disease
MCV	mean corpuscular volume
MDMA	'ecstasy'
MI	myocardial infarction
MOF	multiple organ failure
MR	magnetic resonance or mitral regurgitation
MRA	magnetic resonance angiography
MRCP	magnetic resonance cholangio-pancreatography
MRI	magnetic resonance imaging
MRSA	meticillin-resistant *Staphylococcus aureus*
MS	multiple sclerosis
MSU	midstream urine
MV	mitral valve
MVP	mitral valve prolapse
MVR	mitral valve replacement
MVT	monomorphic ventricular tachycardia
N&V	nausea and vomiting
NA	noradrenaline
NABQ	*N*-acetyl-benzoquinoneimine
NAC	*N*-acetyl-cysteine
NANB	non-A, non-B
NBM	nil by mouth
NBTV	non-bacterial thrombotic vegetation
NCS	nerve conduction studies
NG	nasogastric
NIPPV	nasal intermittent positive pressure ventilation
NIV	non-invasive ventilation
NPV	negative pressure ventilation
NQ-MI	non-Q-wave MI
NR	normal range
NSAID	non-steroidal anti-inflammatory drug
NSTEMI/UA	non-ST elevation myocardial infarction
OCP	oral contraceptive pill

od	once a day
OD	overdose
OER	oxygen extraction ratio
OI	opportunistic infection
OPG	orthopentamogram
OSA	obstructive sleep apnoea
PA	pulmonary artery
PACI	partial anterior circulation infarct
PAN	polyarteritis nodosa
Panca	antineutrophil cytoplasmic antibody type-p
PaO2	partial pressure of oxygen in arterial blood
PAWP	pulmonary artery wedge pressure
PBC	primary biliary cirrhosis
PCA	patient-controlled analgesia
PCI	percutaneous coronary intervention
PCP	*Pneumocystitis jirovecii (carinii)* pneumonia
PCR	polymerase chain reaction
PCV	packed cell volume
PCWP	pulmonary capillary wedge pressure
PDA	peritoneal dialysis or patent ductus arteriosus
PE	pulmonary embolism or phenytoin equivalent
PEA	pulseless electrical activity
PEEP	positive end-expiratory pressure
PEF	peak expiratory flow
PEFR	peak expiratory flow rate
PEG	percutaneous endoscopic gastrostony
PEP	post-exposure prophylaxis
PET	positron emission tomography
PFO	patent foramen ovele
PHI	primary HIV infection
PiCCO	pulse contour cardiac output
PMH	past medical history
PML	progressive multi-focal leucoencephalopathy
PMN	polymorphonuclear cells (neutrophils)
PMR	polymyalgia rheumatica
PO	per os (by mouth)
PPI	proton pump inhibitor
PR	per rectum
PSA	prostate-specific antigen
PSC	primary sclerosing cholargitis

PT	prothrombin time
PTH	parathyroid harmone
PUO	pyrexia of unknown origin
PVE	prosthetic valve endocarditis
PVR	pulmonary vascular resistance
PVT	polymorphic ventricular tachycardia
qds	four times a day
Qw-MI	Q-wave MI
RA	right atrium or rheumatoid arthritis
RAD	right axis deviation
rAPC	recombinant activated protein C
RAS	renin angiotensin system
RBBB	right bundle branch block
RBC	red blood cell
RCA	right coronary artery
RCP	Royal College of Physicians
RF	rheumatic fever
RNA	ribose nucleic acid
RNP	ribo nucleic protein
RR	respiratory rate
RS	respiratory system
RSV	respiratory syncytial virus
rt-PA	recombinant tissue plasminogen activator
RTA	road traffic accident
RUQ	right upper quadrant
RV	right ventricular
RVDP	right ventricular end-diastolic pressure
RVF	right ventricular failure
RVOT	right ventricular outflow tract
SAH	sub arachnoid haemorrhage
SARS	severe acute respiratory syndrome
SBE	subacute bacterial endocarditis
SBP	systolic blood pressure
SCU	subclavian vein
SIADH	syndrome of inappropriate ADH secretion
SIMV	synchronized intermittent mandatory ventilation
SK	streptokinase
SL	sublingual
SLE	systemic lupus erythematosus
SOB	short of breath

SOL	space-occupying lesion
SR	slow release
SSRI	selective serotonin reuptake inhibitor
SSS	staphylococcal scalded skin syndrome
STEMI	ST elevation myocardial infarction
STS	serological tests for syphilis
SVC	superior vena cava
SVR	systemic vascular resistance
SVT	supraventricular tachycardia
SXR	skull X-ray
TB	tuberculosis
TBG	thyroid-binding
tds	three times a day
TEN	toxic epidermal necrolysis
TFT	thyroid function test
TIA	transient ischaemic attack
TIBC	total iron binding capacity
TIPS	transvenous intrahepatic portosystemic shunting
TnI	troponin I
TnT	troponin T
TOE	transoesophageal echocardiogram
tPA	tissue plasminogen activator
TPHA	*Treponema pallidum* haemagglutination
TPN	total parentral nutrition
TPR	temperature, pulse and respirations
TR	tricuspid regurgitation
TRALI	transfusion-related acute lung injury
TRH	thyrotropin releasing hormone
TSH	thyroid stimulating hormone
TT	thrombin time
TTP	thrombotic thrombocytopenic purpura
TURBT	transurethral resection of bladder tumour
TURP	transurethral resection of prostate
U&Es	urea and electrolytes
U	units
UA	unstable angina
UC	ulcerative colitis
UFH	unfractionated heparin
UMN	upper motor neuron
URTI	upper respiratory tract injection

US	ultrasound
USS	ultrasound scan
UTI	urinary tract infection
UV	ultraviolet
VC	vital capacity
VE	ventricular extrasystole
VF	ventricular fibrillation
VMA	vanillyl mandellic acid
VOR	vestibulo-ocular reflex
VPB	ventricular premature beats
VQ	ventilation (v)-perfusion (Q)
VSD	ventriculo-septal defect
VT	ventricular tachycardia
vW	von Willebrand
VZIG	varicella zoster immunoglobulin
VZV	varicella zoster virus
WBC	white blood cell
WCC	white cell count
WPW	Wolff–Parkinson–White
XR	X-ray
ZN	Ziehl–Nieelson syndrome

Chapter 1

Cardiac emergencies

Adult basic life support

Basic life support is the backbone of effective resuscitation following a cardiorespiratory arrest. The aim is to maintain adequate ventilation and circulation until the underlying cause for the arrest can be reversed. 3–4min without adequate perfusion (less if the patient is hypoxic) will lead to irreversible cerebral damage. The usual scenario is an unresponsive patient found by staff who alert the cardiac arrest team. The initial assessment described next should have already been performed by the person finding the patient. The same person should have also started CPR. Occasionally you will be the first to discover the patient and it is important to rapidly assess the patient and begin CPR. The various stages in basic life support are described here and summarized in Fig. 1.1.

1. Assessment of the patient

- ***Ensure safety of rescuer and victim.***
- ***Check whether the patient is responsive***. Gently shake victim and ask loudly 'are you all right?'
  - If victim responds place them in the recovery position and get help.
  - If victim is unresponsive shout for help and move on to assess airway.

2. Airway assessment

- ***Open the airway***. With two fingertips under the point of the chin, tilt the head up. If this fails, place your fingers behind the angles of the lower jaw and apply steady pressure upwards and forwards. Remove ill-fitting dentures and any obvious obstruction. If the patient starts breathing, roll the patient over into the recovery position and try to keep the airway open until an orophyrangeal airway can be inserted (see 🕮 Fig. 1.2, p.7).
- ***Keep airway open, look, listen, and feel for breathing.*** Look for chest movements, listen at the victim's mouth for breathing sounds, and feel for air on your cheek (for no more than 10sec).
  - If patient is breathing turn patient into the recovery position, check for continued breathing, and get help.
  - If patient is not breathing or making occasional gasps or weak attempts at breathing send someone for help. Start rescue breaths by giving two slow effective breaths, each resulting in a visible rise and fall in the chest wall.

3. Assessment of circulation

- Assess signs of circulation by feeling the carotid pulse for no more than 10sec.
  - If there are signs of circulation but no breathing continue rescue breaths and check for a circulation every 10 breaths (approximately every minute).
  - If there are no signs of circulation start chest compression at a rate of 100 times per minute. Combine rescue breaths and compression at a rate of 30 compressions to two effective breaths.
- The ratio of compressions to lung inflation remains the same for resuscitation with two persons.

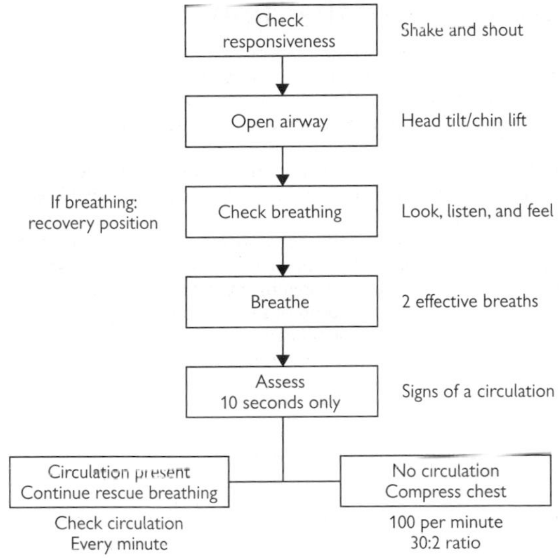

Fig. 1.1 Adult basic life support. Send or go for help as soon as possible according to guidelines. For further information see the Resuscitation Council (UK) website http://www.resus.org.uk/

Adult advanced life support

- It is unlikely that an effective spontaneous cardiac activity will be restored by basic life support without more advanced techniques (intubation for effective ventilation, drugs, defibrillation, etc.). Do not waste time. As soon as help arrives, delegate CPR to someone less experienced in ALS, so that you are able to continue.
- Attach the patient to a cardiac monitor as soon as possible to determine the cardiac rhythm and treat appropriately (see Universal treatment algorithm, 🕮 p.8).
- Oropharyngeal (Guedel) or nasopharyngeal airways help maintain the patency of the airway by keeping the tongue out of the way (see Fig. 1.2). They can cause vomiting if the patient is not comatose. ET intubation is the best method of securing the airway. Do not attempt this if you are inexperienced.
- Establish venous access. Central vein cannulation (internal jugular or subclavian) is ideal but requires more training and practice and is not for the inexperienced. If venous access fails, drugs may be given via an ET tube into the lungs (except for bicarbonate and calcium salts). Double the doses of drugs if using this route, as absorption is less efficient than IV.

Post-resuscitation care

- ***Try to establish the events*** that precipitated the arrest from the history, staff, witnesses, and the hospital notes of the patient. Is there an obvious cause (MI, hypoxia, hypoglycaemia, stroke, drug overdose or interaction, electrolyte abnormality, etc.)? Record the duration of the arrest in the notes with the interventions and drugs (and doses) in chronological order.
- ***Examine the patient*** to check both lung fields are being ventilated. Check for ribs that may have broken during CPR. Listen for any cardiac murmurs. Check the neck veins. Examine the abdomen for an aneurysm or signs of peritonism. Insert a urinary catheter. Consider an NG-tube if the patient remains unconscious. Record the Glasgow Coma Score (see 🕮 p.432) and perform a brief neurological assessment (see 🕮 p.332).
- ***Investigations: ECG***—looking for MI, ischaemia, tall T-waves (↑K+); ***ABG***—mixed metabolic and respiratory acidosis is common and usually responds to adequate oxygenation and ventilation once the circulation is restored. If severe, consider bicarbonate; ***CXR***—check position of ET-tube, look for pneumothorax; ***U&Es***; and ***glucose***.
- After early and successful resuscitation from a 1° cardiac arrest, the patient may rapidly recover completely. The patient must be transferred to HDU or CCU for monitoring for 12–24h. Commonly the patient is unconscious post arrest and should be transferred to ITU for ventilation and haemodynamic monitoring and support for ≥24h.
- Change any venous lines that were inserted at the time of arrest for central lines inserted with sterile technique. Insert an arterial line and consider PA catheter (Swan–Ganz) if requiring inotropes.
- ***Remember to talk to the relatives***. Keep them informed of events and give a realistic (if bleak) picture of the arrest and possible outcomes.
- When appropriate consider the possibility of organ donation and do not be frightened to discuss this with the relatives. Even if discussion

with the relatives is delayed, remember corneas and heart valves may be used up to 24h after death (see 📖 p.442).

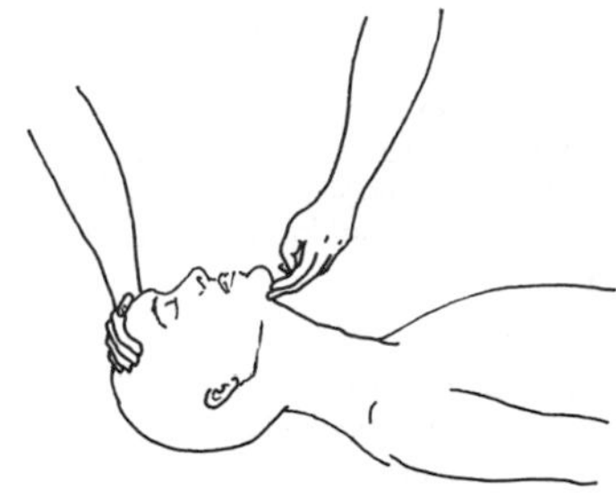

Jaw lift to open the airway

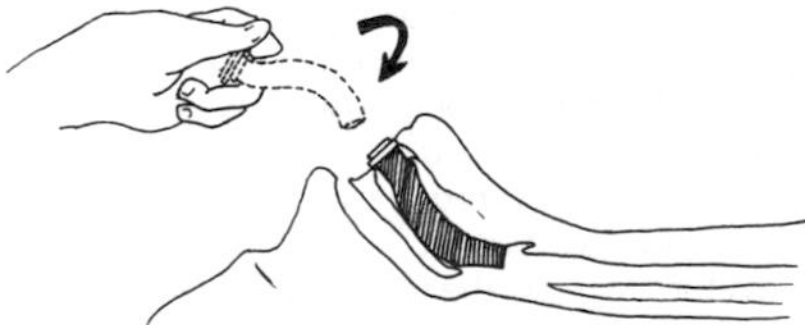

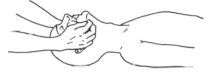

Jaw thrust (thrust the angle of the mandible upwards)

Insertion of oropharyngeal airway (start with the tip pointing cranially (towards nose) and rotate 180° as you insert so that it finally points into larynx as shown)

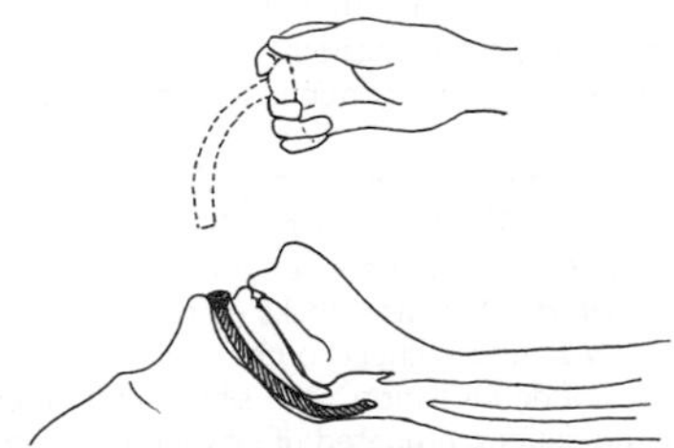

Insertion of nasopharyngeal airway (follow the curve of the nasal passage to introduce into the larynx)

Fig. 1.2 Insertion of oropharyngeal and nasopharyngeal airway.

Universal treatment algorithm

- Cardiac rhythms of cardiac arrest can be divided into two groups (see Fig. 1.3):
  - VF/VT
  - Non-VF/VT (asystole and PEA).
- The principle difference in treatment of the two groups of arrhythmias is the need for attempted defibrillation in the VF/VT group of patients.
- Fig. 1.3 summarizes the algorithm for management of both groups of patients.

VF/VT

- VF/VT are the most common rhythms at the time of cardiac arrest.
- *Precordial thump*. If arrest is witnessed or monitored, a sharp blow with a closed fist on the patient's sternum may convert VF/VT back to a perfusing rhythm. It is particularly effective if delivered within 30sec after cardiac arrest.
- Success in treatment of VF/VT is dependent on *prompt defibrillation*. With each passing minute in VF, the chance of successful defibrillation declines by 7–10%.
- Defibrillation in the current guidelines involves a single shock of 150–200J biphasic (or 360J monophasic).
- Each shock should be immediately followed by CPR without reassessing the rhythm or feeling for a pulse. This is because if a perfusing rhythm has not been restored, delay in trying to palpate the pulse will further compromise the myocardium. If a perfusing rhythm has been restored, the pulse is rarely palpable immediately after defibrillation and giving compressions does not enhance the chance of VF recurring. In the event of post-shock asystole, compressions may induce VF.
- Current guidelines suggest a ratio of 30 chest compressions to 2 breaths. When airway is secured, chest compressions can be continued *without* pausing during ventilation.
- Continue CPR for 2min and then pause briefly to check the monitor.
- If VF/VT persists give a futher (2nd shock) of 150–360J biphasic (or 360J monophasic).
- Resume CPR immediately and continue for 2min, then pause briefly to check the monitor.
- If VF/VT persists give adrenaline 1mg IV followed by a 3rd shock of 150–360J biphasic (360J monophasic).
- Resume CPR immediately and continue for 2min, then pause briefly to check the monitor.
- If VF/VT persists give amiodarone 300mg IV followed immediately by a 4th shock of 150–360J biphasic (or 360J monophasic).
- Resume CPR immediately and continue for 2min.
- Give adrenaline before alternate shocks (approximately every 3–5min): 1mg IV or 2–3mg via endotracheal route.
- In between cycles of defibrillation, reversible factors must be identified and corrected, the patient intubated (if possible), and venous access obtained. If organized electrical activity is seen (when the monitor is checked at points suggested earlier in this algorithm), check for a pulse:
  - If present: start post-resuscitation care.
  - If pulse absent: switch to the non-VF/VT side of the algorithm.

Non-VF/VT (asystole and PEA)

- The outcome from these rhythms is generally worse than for VF/VT unless a reversible cause can be identified and treated promptly.
- Chest compressions and ventilation (30:2) should be undertaken for 2min with each loop of the algorithm. When airway is secured, chest compressions can be continued without pausing during ventilation.
- Recheck the rhythm after 2min. If organized electrical activity is seen: check for a pulse.
  - If present: start post-resuscitation care.
  - If absent: continue CPR.
  - If VF/VT: change to the VF/VT side of the algorithm.
- Give adrenaline 1mg IV as soon as intravascular access is achieved and with alternate loops (every 3–5min).
- Give atropine 3mg IV if there is asystole or if PEA is slow (<60/min).
- In asystole, if P waves are present on the strip/monitor, pacing (external or transvenous) must be considered.
- Identification of the underlying cause (Fig. 1.3) and its correction are both vital for successful resuscitation. Resuscitation must be continued whilst reversible causes are being sought.

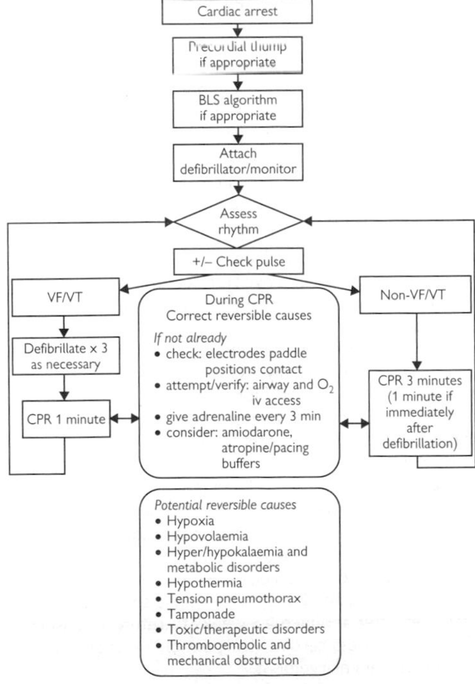

Fig. 1.3 Universal treatment algorithm (for further details see the Resuscitation Council (UK) website http://www.resus.org.uk)

Acute coronary syndrome (ACS)

ACS is an operational term used to describe a constellation of symptoms resulting from acute myocardial ischaemia. An ACS resulting in myocardial injury is termed MI. ACS includes the diagnosis of UA, NSTEMI, and STEMI. The term ACS is generally assigned by ancillary/triage personnel on initial contact with the patient. Guidelines for identification of ACS are summarized on 📖 p.44.

Definition

The current nomenclature divides ACS into two major groups, on the basis of delivered treatment modalities (see Fig. 1.4).

- STEMI: an ACS where patients present with ischaemic chest discomfort and ST-segment elevation on ECG. This group of patients must undergo reperfusion therapy on presentation.
- NSTEMI and UA: ACS where patients present with ischaemic chest discomfort associated with transient or permanent non-ST elevation ischaemic ECG changes. If there is biochemical evidence of myocardial injury the condition is termed NSTEMI and in the absence if biochemical myocardial injury the condition is termed UA (Fig. 1.4). This group of patients is not treated with thrombolysis.

Initial management of ACS

- All patients with suspected ACS should be placed in an environment with continuous ECG monitoring and defibrillation capacity.
- Give aspirin and clopidogrel (300mg PO of each if no contraindications) and do not give any IM injections (causes a rise in total CK and risk of bleeding with thrombolysis/anticoagulation). There is some evidence that a loading dose of 600mg of clopidogrel achieves quicker platelet inhibition and should be considered for patients going to the cardiac cathlab for immediate PCI.

Immediate assessment should include:

- Rapid examination to exclude hypotension and note the presence of murmurs and to identify and treat acute pulmonary oedema.
- Secure IV access.
- 12-lead ECG should be obtained and reported within 10min.
- Give high-flow O_2 (initially only 28% if history of COPD).
- Diamorphine 2.5–10mg IV PRN for pain relief.
- Metoclopramide 10mg IV for nausea.
- GTN spray 2 puffs (unless hypotensive).
- Take blood for:
  - FBC/U&Es: supplement K^+ to keep it at 4–5mmol/L.
  - Glucose: may be ↑acutely post MI, even in non-diabetics, and reflects a stress-catecholamine response, which may resolve without treatment.
  - Biochemical markers of cardiac injury.
  - Lipid profile: total cholesterol, LDL, HDL, triglycerides.
  - Serum cholesterol and HDL remain close to baseline for 24–48h but fall thereafter and take ≥8 weeks to return to baseline.
- Portable CXR to assess cardiac size, pulmonary oedema, and to exclude mediastinal enlargement.

- General examination should include peripheral pulses, fundoscopy, abdominal examination for organomegaly, and aortic aneurysm.
- Consider alternative diagnoses (see Box 1.1)

Box 1.1 Conditions mimicking pain in ACS

- Pericarditis
- Dissecting aortic aneurysm
- Pulmonary embolism
- Oesophageal reflux, spasm, or rupture
- Biliary tract disease
- Perforated peptic ulcer
- Pancreatitis.

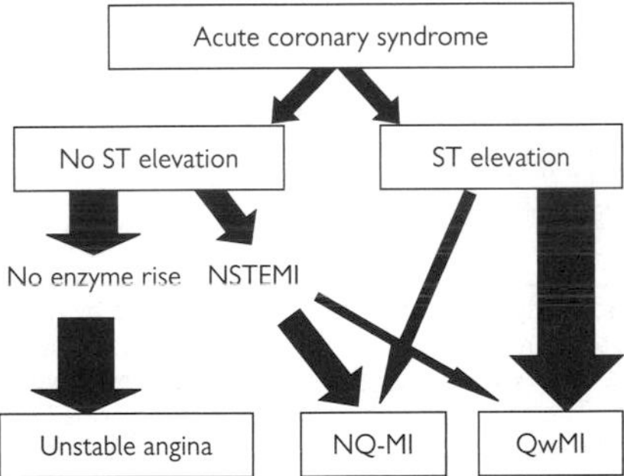

Fig. 1.4 Nomenclature of ACS. Patients with ACS may present with or without ST elevation on the ECG. The majority of patients with ST elevation (large arrows) ultimately develop QwMI whereas a minority (small arrow) develop a NQ-MI. Patients without ST elevation are experiencing either UA or an NSTEMI depending on the absence or presence of cardiac enzymes (e.g. troponin) detected in the blood. Adapted from Antman EM (1997). Acute myocardial infarction. In Braunwald EB (ed) *Heart Disease: A Textbook of Cardiovascular Medicine*. Saunders, Philadelphia, PA.

ST elevation myocardial infarction (STEMI)

Patients with an ACS who have ST-segment elevation/LBBB on their presenting ECG benefit significantly from immediate reperfusion and are treated as one group under the term STEMI.

Presentation

- Chest pain usually similar in nature to angina, but of greater severity, longer duration, and not relieved by SL GTN. Associated features include nausea and vomiting, sweating, breathlessness, and extreme distress.
- The pains may be atypical such as epigastric or radiate through to the back.
- Diabetics, the elderly, and hypertensives may suffer painless ('silent') infarcts and/or atypical infarction. Presenting features include breathlessness from acute pulmonary oedema, syncope or coma from arrhythmias, acute confusional states (mania/psychosis), diabetic hyperglycaemic crises, hypotension/cardiogenic shock, CNS manifestations resembling stroke 2° to sudden reduction in cardiac output, and peripheral embolization.

Management

Diagnosis is normally made on presentation followed by rapid stabilization to ensure institution of reperfusion therapy without delay. This is in contrast to NSTEMI/UA where diagnosis may evolve over period of 24–72h (see 🕮 p.44). The management principles of the various stages are outlined here and expanded on subsequently (also see Box 1.2).

- Stabilizing measures are generally similar for all ACS patients (see 🕮 p.10)
  - All patients with suspected STEMI should have *continuous ECG monitoring* in an area with full resuscitation facilities.
  - Patients should receive immediate *aspirin* 300mg PO and *clopidogrel* 300mg PO (if no contraindications), *analgesia*, and O_2.
  - Rapid examination to exclude hypotension and note the presence of murmurs and to identify and treat acute pulmonary oedema. Examine for signs of aortic dissection (e.g. aortic regurgitation murmur, unequal BP in the arms). RVF out of proportion to LVF suggests RV infarction (see 🕮 p.28).
  - Blood for FBC, biochemical profile, markers of cardiac injury, lipid profile, glucose and portable CXR.
- *Diagnosis* must be made on the basis of history, ECG (ST elevation/ new LBBB), and biochemical markers of myocardial injury (NB if ECG changes diagnostic, reperfusion must not be delayed to wait for biochemical markers) (see 🕮 p.16).
- *Treatment:*
  - General medical measures (see 🕮 p.18)
  - Reperfusion (see 🕮 p.20).
- *All patients with STEMI should be admitted to CCU.*
- *Discharge and risk prevention* (see 🕮 p.30).

Box 1.2 Factors associated with a poor prognosis

- Age >70 years
- Previous MI or chronic stable angina
- Anterior MI or RV infarction
- LV failure at presentation
- Hypotension (and sinus tachycardia) at presentation
- Diabetes mellitus
- Mitral regurgitation (acute)
- Ventricular septal defect

STEMI: diagnosis 1

This is based on a combination of history, ECG, and biochemical markers of cardiac injury. In practice, history and ECG changes are normally diagnostic, resulting in immediate reperfusion/medical treatment. Biochemical markers of cardiac injury usually become available later and help reconfirm diagnosis as well as provide prognostic information (magnitude of rise).

ECG changes (also see Box 1.3)

- ***ST-segment elevation*** occurs within minutes and may last for up to 2 weeks. ST elevation of ≥2mm in adjacent chest leads and ≥1mm in adjacent limb leads is necessary to fulfil thrombolysis criteria. Persisting ST elevation after 1 month suggests formation of LV aneurysm. Infarction site can be localized from ECG changes as indicated in Table 1.1.
- ***Pathological Q waves*** indicate significant abnormal electrical conduction, but are not synonymous with irreversible myocardial damage. In the context of a 'transmural infarction' they may take hours or days to develop and usually remain indefinitely. In the standard leads the Q wave should be ≥25% of the R wave, 0.04s in duration, with negative T waves. In the precordial leads, Q waves in V4 should be >0.4mV (4 small squares) and in V6 >0.2mV (2 small squares), in the absence of LBBB (QRS width <0.1sec or 3 small squares).
- ***ST-segment depression*** (ischaemia at distance) in a 2nd territory (in patients with ST-segment elevation) is 2° to ischaemia in a territory other than the area of infarction (often indicative of multivessel disease) or reciprocal electrical phenomena. Overall it implies a poorer prognosis.
- ***PR-segment elevation/depression*** and alterations in the contour of the P wave are generally indicative of atrial infarction. Most patients will also have abnormal atrial rhythms such as AF/flutter and wandering atrial pacemaker and AV nodal rhythms.
- ***T-wave inversion*** may be immediate or delayed and generally persists after the ST elevation has resolved.
- ***Non-diagnostic changes***, but ones that may be ischaemic, include new LBBB or RBBB, tachyarrhythmias, transient tall peaked T waves or T-wave inversion, axis shift (extreme left or right), or AV block.

Box 1.3 Conditions that may mimic ECG changes of a STEMI

- Left or right ventricular hypertrophy
- LBBB or left anterior fasciculatar block
- Wolff–Parkinson–White syndrome
- Pericarditis or myocarditis
- Cardiomyopathy (hypertrophic or dilated)
- Trauma to myocardium
- Cardiac tumours (1° and metastatic)
- Pulmonary embolus
- Pneumothorax
- Intracranial haemorrhage
- Hyperkalaemia
- Cardiac sarcoid or amyloid
- Pancreatitis.

Table 1.1 Localization of infarcts from ECG changes

Anterior	ST elevation and/or Q-waves in V1–V4/V5
Anteroseptal	ST elevation and/or Q-waves in V1–V3
Anterolateral	ST elevation and/or Q-waves in V1–V6, I, and aVL
Lateral	ST elevation and/or Q-waves in V5–V6 and T-wave inversion/ ST elevation/Q-waves in I and aVL
Inferolateral	ST elevation and/or Q-waves in II, III, aVF, and V5–V6 (sometimes I and aVL)
Inferior	ST elevation and/or Q-waves in II, III, and aVF
Inferoseptal	ST elevation and/or Q-waves in II, III, aVF, and V1–V3
True posterior	Tall R-waves in V1–V2 with ST depression in V1–V3
	T-waves remain upright in V1–V2
	This can be confirmed with electrodes on the back for a posterior ECG. Usually occurs in conjunction with an inferior or lateral infarct
RV infarction	ST-segment elevation in the right precordial leads (V3R–V4R)
	Usually found in conjunction with inferior infarction. This may only be present in the early hours of infarction

STEMI: diagnosis 2

Biochemical markers of cardiac injury

Serial measurements evaluating a temporal rise and fall should be obtained to allow a more accurate diagnosis. CK and CK-MB from a skeletal muscle source tend to remain elevated for a greater time period in comparison to a cardiac source.

CK

- Levels twice upper limit of normal are taken as being abnormal.
- Serum levels rise within 4–8h post STEMI and fall to normal within 3–4 days. The peak level occurs at about 24h but may be earlier (12h) and higher in patients who have had reperfusion (thrombolysis or PCI); the enzymes from the damaged muscle are 'washed out' of the infarcted area with restored circulation.
- False positive rates of ~15% occur in patients with alcohol intoxication, muscle disease or trauma, vigorous exercise, convulsions, IM injections, hypothyroidism, PE, and thoracic outlet syndrome.

CK-MB isoenzyme is more specific for myocardial disease. Levels may be elevated despite a normal total CK. However, CK-MB is also present in small quantities in other tissues (skeletal muscle, tongue, diaphragm, uterus, and prostate) and trauma or surgery may lead to false positive results. If there is doubt about myocardial injury with CK-MB levels obtained, a cardiac troponin must be measured.

Cardiac troponins (TnT, TnI)

- Both TnI and TnT are highly sensitive and specific markers of cardiac injury.
- Serum levels start to rise by 3h post MI and elevation may persist up to 7–14 days. This is advantageous for diagnosis of late MI.
- In most STEMI cases the diagnosis can be made using a combination of the clinical picture and serial CK/CK-MB levels. In the event of normal CK-MB levels and suspected non-cardiac sources of CK, troponins can be used.
- Troponins can also be elevated in non-ischaemic myocyte damage such as myocarditis, cardiomyopathy, and pericarditis.

Other markers

There are multiple other markers, but with increasing clinical availability of troponins, measurements are not recommended. These include AST (rise 18–36h post MI) and LDH (rise 24–36h post MI).

The time course of the various markers is seen in Fig. 1.5.

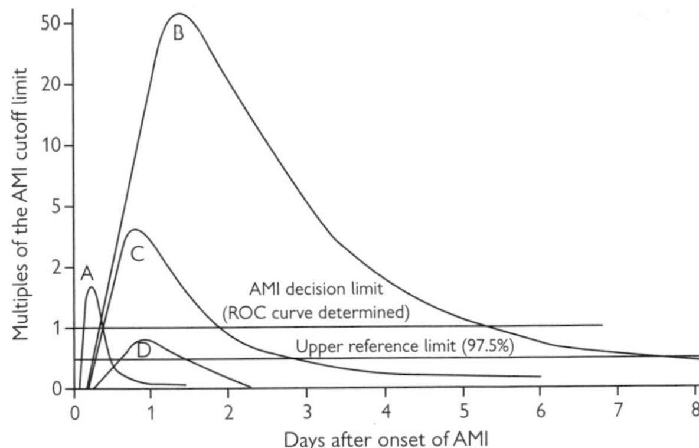

Fig. 1.5 Graph of the appearance of cardiac markers in the blood versus time of onset of symptoms. Peak A: early release of myoglobin or CK-MB isoforms after AMI. Peak B: cardiac troponin after AMI. Peak C: CK-MB after AMI. Peak D: cardiac troponin after unstable angina. Adapted from Wu AH *et al.* (1999). *Clin Chem* **45**: 1104–21.

Box 1.4 Key points: non-ACS causes of raised troponin

- Troponin is a sensitive marker of myocyte damage.
- Raised troponin is not specific to thrombotic coronary artery occlusion.
- Measurement of troponin levels in broad populations with low pretest probability of thrombotic disease greatly reduces its positive predictive value for NSTEMI.
- Causes of elevated troponin other than acute thrombotic coronary artery occlusion include:
  - Sepsis
  - Myocarditis/pericarditis
  - PE
  - Cardiac failure
  - Renal failure
  - Stroke
  - Cardiac contusion
  - Tachycardia
- In patients with raised troponin, determine the pretest probability of coronary artery disease (chest pain, risk factors for ischaemic heart disease, ischaemic ECG changes, wall-motion abnormalities on echocardiography).
- Patients with a low pretest probability of CHD/ACS are unlikely to benefit from a treatment aimed at coronary artery thrombosis (i.e. antithrombotic/antiplatelet therapy, coronary angiography and revascularization). In these patients identify and treat the underlying cause of raised troponin (see earlier list).

STEMI: general measures

Immediate stabilizing measures

These are as outlined on 📖 p.10.

Control of cardiac pain

- ***Diamorphine 2.5–10mg IV*** is the drug of choice and may be repeated to ensure adequate pain relief, unless evidence of emerging toxicity (hypotension, respiratory depression). Nausea and vomiting should be treated with metoclopramide (10mg IV) or a phenothiazine.
- ***Oxygen*** to be administered at 2–5L/minute for at least 2–3h. Hypoxaemia is frequently seen post MI due to ventilation–perfusion abnormalities 2° to LVF. In patients with refractory pulmonary oedema, CPAP, or via formal endotracheal intubation may be necessary. Beware of CO_2 retention in patients with COPD.
- ***Nitrates*** may lessen pain and can be given providing that patient is not hypotensive (SL or IV). They need to be used cautiously in inferior STEMI, especially with RV infarction, as venodilation may impair RV filling and precipitate hypotension. Nitrate therapy has no effect on mortality (ISIS-4).

Correction of electrolytes

Both low potassium and magnesium may be arrhythmogenic and must be supplemented especially in the context of arrhythmias.

Strategies to limit infarct size

β-blockade, ACEI, and reperfusion.

β-blockade

- Early β-blockade in limiting infarct size, reducing mortality, and early malignant arrhythmias. All patients (including primary PCI and thrombolysis patients) should have early β-blockade, but those with the following features will benefit most:
  - Hyperdynamic state (sinus tachycardia, ↑BP)
  - Ongoing or recurrent pain/reinfarction
  - Tachyarrhythmias such as AF.
- Absolute contraindications: HR <60bpm, SBP <100mmHg, moderate to severe heart failure, AV conduction defect, severe airways disease.
- Relative contraindications: asthma, current use of calcium channel-blocker and/or β-blocker, severe peripheral vascular disease with critical limb ishaemia, large inferior MI involving the right ventricle.
- Use short-acting agent IV initially (metoprolol 1–2mg at a time repeated at 1–2-minute intervals to a maximum dose of 15–20mg) under continuous ECG and BP monitoring. Aim for a pulse rate of 60bpm and SBP of 100–110mmHg. If haemodynamic stability continues 15–30min after last IV dose start metoprolol 50mg tds. Esmolol is an ultra-short-acting IV β-blocker, which may be tried if there is concern whether the patient will tolerate β-blockers.

ACEIs

After receiving aspirin, β-blockade (if appropriate), and reperfusion, all patients with STEMI/LBBB infarction should receive an ACEI within the first 24h of presentation.

- Patients with high-risk/large infarcts particularly with an anterior STEMI, a previous MI, heart failure, or impaired LV function on imaging (ECHO) or those who are elderly will benefit most.
- The effect of ACEIs appears to be a class effect: use the drug you are familiar with (e.g. ramipril 1.25mg od).

STEMI: reperfusion therapy (thrombolysis) 1

Reperfusion occurs in 50–70% of patients who receive thrombolysis within 4h of onset of pain (cf. ~20% of controls). As with primary PCI, thrombolysis also results in reduction in mortality, LV dysfunction, heart failure, cardiogenic shock, and arrhythmias. However, the magnitude of the benefits obtained is smaller. Furthermore, patients must undergo cardiac catheterization to delineate their coronary anatomy before revascularization (achieved at the same time with primary PCI). Time is once again of paramount importance and thrombolysis should be administered as soon as possible. (See Box 1.5.)

Indications for thrombolysis

- Typical cardiac pain within previous 12h and ST elevation in two contiguous ECG leads (>1mm in limb leads or >2mm in V1–V6).
- Cardiac pain with new/presumed new LBBB on ECG.
- If ECG is equivocal on arrival, repeat at 15–30-min intervals to monitor progression.
- Thrombolysis should not be given if the ECG is normal, or if there is isolated ST depression (must exclude true posterior infarct).
- Remember patients with diabetes may present with dyspnoea or collapse without chest pain. Look for new ST elevation on the ECG.
- True posterior infarction presents with ST depression in anterior chest leads (V1–V3) often with ST changes in inferior leads as well. If suspected, administer thrombolysis.

Timing of thrombolysis

- Greatest benefit is achieved with early thrombolysis (especially if given within 4h of onset of first pain).
- Patients presenting between 12–24h from onset of pain should be thrombolysed if there are any persisting symptoms and/or ST-segment elevation on the ECGs.
- Patients presenting within 12–24h from the onset of pain whose clinical picture and ECGs appears to have settled should be managed initially as a NSTEMI followed by early catheterization.

Choice of thrombolytic agent

- This is partly determined by local thrombolysis strategy.
- Allergic reactions and episodes of hypotension are greater with SK.
- Bolus agents are easier and quicker to administer with a decrease in drug errors in comparison to first-generation infusions.
- rtPA has a greater reperfusion capacity and a marginally higher 30-day survival benefit than SK, but an ↑ risk of haemorrhage.
- More recent rPA derivatives have a higher 90-min TIMI-III flow rate, but similar 30-day mortality benefit to rtPA.
- An rtPA derivative should be considered for any patient with:
  - Large anterior MI, especially if within 4h of onset.
  - Previous SK therapy or recent streptococcal infection.
  - Hypotension (SBP <100mmHg).

- Low risk of stroke (age <55 years, SBP <144mmHg).
- Reinfarction where immediate PCI facilities are not available.

The characteristics of the major thrombolytic agents are given in Box 1.6.

Patients who gain greatest benefit from thrombolysis

- Anterior infarct
- Marked ST elevation
- Age >75 years
- Impaired LV function or LBBB, hypotensive
- SBP <100mmHg
- Patients presenting within 1h of onset of pain.

Box 1.5 Key points: STEMI

- Rapid reperfusion is the cornerstone of management of STEMI.
- Reperfusion is marked by normalization of ST segments on ECG.
- primary PCI and thrombolysis are the main reperfusion modalities.
- The best long-term outcome is achieved with primary PCI.

Box 1.6 Doses and administration of thrombolytic agents

SK

- Give as 1.5MUin 100mL normal saline IV over 1h.
- There is no indication for routine heparinization after SK as there is no clear mortality benefit and there is a small increase in risk of haemorrhage.

Alteplase (rtPA)

- The GUSTO trial suggested that 'front-loaded' or accelerated rtPA is the most effective dosage regimen.
- Give 15-mg bolus IV then 0.75mg/kg over 30min (not to exceed 50mg), then 0.5mg/kg over 60min (not to exceed 35mg).
- This should be followed by IV heparin (see text).

Reteplase

- Give two IV bolus doses of 10 units 10min apart.

Tenecteplase

- Give as injection over 10sec at 30–50mg according to bodyweight (500–600mcg/kg).
- Maximum dose is 50mg.

APSAC (anistreplase)

- Give as an IV bolus of 30mg over 2–5min.

STEMI: thrombolysis 2

Complications of thrombolysis

- Bleeding is seen in up to 10% of patients. Most are minor at sites of vascular puncture. Local pressure is sufficient but occasionally transfusion may be required. In extreme cases, SK may be reversed by tranexamic acid (10mg/kg slow IV infusion).
- Hypotension during the infusion is common with SK. Lay patient supine and slow/stop infusion until the BP rises. Treatment with cautious (100–500mL) fluid challenges may be required especially in inferior/ RV infarction. Hypotension is not an allergic reaction and does not warrant treatment as such.
- Allergic reactions are common with SK and include a low-grade fever, rash, nausea, headaches, and flushing. Give hydrocortisone 100mg IV with chlorphenamine 10mg IV.
- Intracranial haemorrhage is seen in ~0.3% of patients treated with SK and ~0.6% of those with rt-PA.
- Reperfusion arrhythmias (most commonly a short, self-limiting run of idioventricular rhythm) may occur as the metabolites are washed out of the ischaemia tissue. See 🕮 pp.38–39.
- Systemic embolization may occur from lysis of thrombus within the left atrium, left ventricle, or aortic aneurysm.

Absolute contraindications to thrombolysis

- Active internal bleeding
- Suspected aortic dissection
- Recent head trauma and/or intracranial neoplasm
- Previous haemorrhagic stroke at any time
- Previous ischaemic stroke within the past 1 year
- Previous allergic reaction to fibrinolytic agent
- Trauma and/or surgery within past 2 weeks at risk of bleeding.

Relative contraindications to thrombolysis

- Trauma and/or surgery more than 2 weeks previously
- Severe uncontrolled hypertension (BP>180/110) with/without treatment
- Non-haemorrhagic stroke over 1 year ago
- Known bleeding diathesis or current use of anticoagulation within therapeutic range (INR 2 or over)
- Significant liver or renal dysfunction
- Prolonged (>10min) of cardiopulmonary resuscitation
- Prior exposure to SK (especially previous 6–9 months)
- Pregnancy or postpartum
- Lumbar puncture within previous 1 month
- Menstrual bleeding or lactation
- History of chronic severe hypertension
- Non-compressible vascular punctures (e.g. subclavian central venous lines)
- Proliferative diabetic retinopathy (risk of intraocular bleed).

Box 1.7 Management key points: STEMI

- Aspirin, clopidogrel, O_2, continuous ECG monitoring.
- Analgesia: diamorphine (+ metoclopramide), GTN (monitor BP).
- Reperfusion therapy without delay: primary PCI (gold standard) or thrombolysis.
- If primary PCI not available: carefully and rapidly assess indications and contraindications to thrombolysis.
- IV heparin should be used with rtPA (and its derivatives) but not with streptokinase.
- Early short-acting β-blockers e.g. metoprolol (if not contraindicated).
- Correct low potassium and magnesium.
- ACEI within the first 24h of presentation.

STEMI: reperfusion by primary percutaneous coronary intervention (PCI)

Time is of the essence for reperfusion and each institution should have its recommended protocol. It is imperative that there are no delays in both the decision-making and implementation processes for reperfusion. If primary PCI is chosen one telephone call should ensure a rapid response.

Primary PCI

- Primary PCI is the current gold standard reperfusion strategy for treatment of STEMI.
- Primary PCI requires significant coordination between the emergency services, community hospitals, and invasive centres. It must only be performed if:
  - A primary PCI programme is available *and*
  - The patient presents to an invasive centre and can undergo catheterization without delay.

Indications for primary PCI

- All patients with chest pain and ST-segment elevation or new LBBB fulfil primary PCI criteria (compare with indications for thrombolysis).
- This will include a group of patients where ST-segment elevation may not fulfil thrombolysis criteria.
- In general, patients in whom thrombolysis is contraindicated should be managed by primary PCI. Cases where there is significant risk of bleeding must be managed individually.

Outcome in primary PCI

- Data from >10 large randomized trials demonstrate a superior outcome in patients with STEMI who are treated with primary PCI in comparison to thrombolysis.
- There is a significant short-term, as well as long-term reduction in mortality and major cardiac events (MACE) (death, non-fatal reinfarction, and non-fatal stroke) in STEMI patients treated with primary PCI. Furthermore, primary PCI patients have overall better LV function, a higher vessel patency rate, and less recurrent myocardial ischaemia.
- Multiple studies (including PRAGUE-2 and DANAMI-2) have also demonstrated that interhospital transportation for primary PCI (community hospital to invasive centre) is safe and primary PCI continues to remain superior to thrombolysis despite the time delays involved.

Complications

- These include bleeding from arterial puncture site, stroke, recurrent infarction, need for emergency CABG, and death, which are similar to high-risk PCI cases (1%).
- The best results are obtained from high-volume centres with experience of primary PCI.

- Each primary PCI centre will have its own policy for management of cases including the use of LMWH/UFH, and antiplatelet agents (e.g. IIb/IIIa). It is generally accepted that in the acute phase only the 'culprit' lesion(s)/vessel(s) will be treated. The pattern of disease in the remainder of the vessels will determine whether total revascularization should be performed as an inpatient or as an elective case, at some stage in the future.
- STEMI patients treated with primary PCI can be discharged safely within 72h of admission without the need for further risk stratification.
- Primary PCI is more cost-effective in the long term with significant savings from fewer days in hospital, a lower need for readmission, and less heart failure.
- Post-discharge care, 2° prevention, and rehabilitation remain identical to other MI cases.

Rescue PCI

As an adjunct to thrombolysis, PCI should be reserved for patients who remain symptomatic post thrombolysis (failure to reperfuse) or develop cardiogenic shock (see 📖 p.42). We recommend all patients who do not settle post thrombolysis (ongoing symptoms and ongoing ST elevation with/without symptoms (<50% resolution of ST elevation at 90min post-lysis)) should be discussed with the local cardiac centre for urgent catheterization and revascularization.

Surgery for acute STEMI

Emergency surgical revascularization (CABG) cannot be widely applied to patients who suffer a MI outside of the hospital. CABG in uncomplicated STEMI patients after 6h from presentation is contraindicated 2° to significant haemorrhage into areas of infarction. Unstable patients have a very high perioperative mortality.

CABG in the context of an acute STEMI is of value in the following situations:

- Persistent or recurrent chest pain despite thrombolysis/primary PCI.
- High-risk coronary anatomy on catheterization (LMS, LAD ostial disease).
- Complicated STEMI (acute MR, VSD).
- Patients who have undergone successful thrombolysis but with surgical coronary anatomy on catheterization.
- Patients known to have surgical coronary anatomy on catheterization performed prior to admission with STEMI.

STEMI: additional measures

Low molecular weight and unfractionated heparin

LMWH

- There are trial data for the use of LMWH and thrombolysis (e.g. enoxaparin 30mg IV bolus, then 1mg/kg SC q12h).
- LMWH can be used at a prophylactic dose to prevent thromboembolic events in patients slow to mobilize as an alternative to UFH.

UFH

- There is no indication for 'routine' IV heparin following SK.
- IV heparin (4000U/max. IV bolus followed by 1000U/hour max. adjusted for an aPTT ratio of 1.5–2.0 × control) should be used routinely following rt-PA and its derivatives for 24–48h.

Clopidogrel

- The addition of clopidogrel to aspirin and fibrinolytics has been shown to reduce the incidence of death or major adverse cardiac event by 20% at 30 days. Longer-term therapy is under investigation.
- If coronary stents are deployed, patient should remain on clopidogrel ideally for 12 months as for patients with NSTEMI.

Glycoprotein IIb/IIIa inhibitors

- There does not appear to be any benefit of GP IIb/IIIa in combination with full or reduced dose thrombolytics in STEMI.
- GP IIb/IIIa inhibitors are recommended routinely in the context of STEMI patients treated with primary PCI. Best data is with abciximab.
- They can also be used in the context of rescue PCI subsequent to failed thrombolysis although there is a greater risk of bleeding. Each case must be judged on its merits.

Magnesium

- Earlier trials giving Mg^{2+} before or with thrombolytics showed some benefit in mortality. ISIS-4 showed no benefit from the routine use of IV magnesium post MI. However Mg^{2+} was given late (6h) after thrombolysis by which time the protective effect of Mg^{2+} on reperfusion injury may have been lost. Trials are ongoing.
- Current accepted role for Mg^{2+} is confined to Mg^{2+}-deplete patients and patients with reperfusion, supraventricular, and ventricular arrhythmias
- Dose: 8mmol in 20mL 5% glucose over 20min followed by 65mmol in 100mL 5% dextrose over 24h (contraindications: serum Cr>300μmol/L, 3° AV block).

Calcium antagonists

- Best avoided, especially in the presence of LV impairment.
- Diltiazem and verapamil started after day 4–5 in post-MI patients with normal LV function have a small beneficial effect.
- Amlodipine is safe to be used in patients with poor LV post MI.
- Nifedipine has been shown to increase mortality and should be avoided.

Digoxin

- Has little role in management of an acute STEMI and heart failure, complicating an acute MI.
- Can be used safely in management of arrhythmias and heart rate.

Right ventricular (RV) infarction

- RV infarction results in elevated right-sided pressures (RA, RVEDP) and low left-sided pressures (BP, CO).
- It is common in inferior STEMI.

Diagnosis

- *Clinical*: signs of right heart failure (↑JVP, Kussmaul's sign, pulsus paradoxus) with absence of pulmonary oedema in the context of a low output state (↓BP, cold peripheries).
- *ECG*: in patients with inferior STEMI a 0.1mV (>1mm) ST-segment elevation in any one of leads V4R–V6R is highly sensitive and specific for RV infarction. See Fig. 1.6 for different ECG patterns identified in right-sided precordial leads. Changes may be transient and present in the early stages only.
- *Echo*: looking for RV dilation and wall-motion abnormalities.

Management

- Aim to maintain a high RV preload:
  - Initially give 1–2L of colloid rapidly.
  - Avoid use of nitrates and diuretics as they reduce pre-load and can worsen hypotension.
  - In patients requiring pacing, AV synchrony must be maintained to ensure maximal CO (atrial and ventricular wires).
  - Cardiovert any arrhythmias (SVT, AF/flutter, or ventricular rhythms).
- Reduce afterload:
  - This is particularly important if there is concomitant LV dysfunction.
  - Insert IABP.
  - Arterial vasodilators (Na nitroprusside, hydralazine) or ACEIs can be used with caution.
- Inotropic support should ideally be avoided and used only if all other measures fail to restore haemodynamic status.
- Reperfusion of the RCA (PCI or thrombolysis) has been demonstrated to improve RV function and reduce mortality.

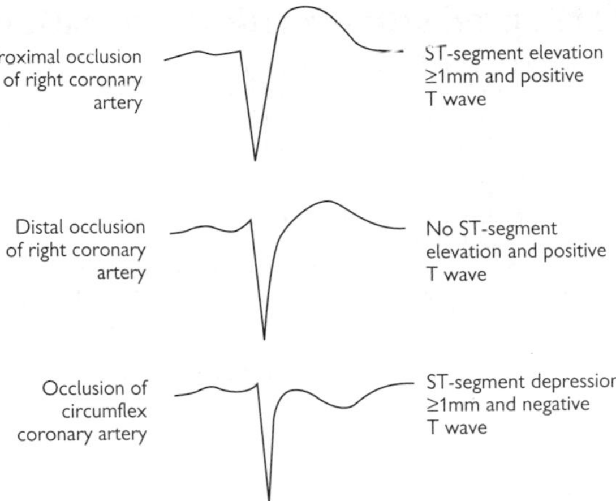

Fig. 1.6 ST elevation and T-wave configuration in lead V4R in inferoposterior AMI. Proximal occlusion of the RCA produces ST elevation ≥1mm and a positive T wave. Distal occlusion is characterized by a positive T wave but no ST elevation. Occlusion of the circumflex artery produces a negative T wave and ST depression of at least 1mm. Adapted from Wellens HJ (1999). *N Engl J Med* **340:** 381–383.

STEMI: predischarge risk stratification

It is important to identify the subgroup of patients who have a high risk of reinfarction or sudden death. They should undergo coronary angiography with a view to revascularization prior to discharge (if not treated with primary PCI) and/or electrophysiological investigations as necessary.

Primary PCI group

- STEMI patients treated with primary PCI are at a much lower risk of developing post-MI complications.
- There is ongoing debate whether patients treated with primary PCI should have total revascularization as an inpatient or whether this can be achieved after functional testing on an outpatient basis. Follow your local policy.
- Patients who should have electrophysiological assessment prior to discharge are listed below.

Thrombolysis group

Patients treated with thrombolysis should be risk stratified prior to discharge and high-risk patients should have inpatient (or early outpatient) angiography. High-risk patients include those with:

- Significant post-infarct angina or unstable angina.
- Positive exercise test (modified Bruce protocol) with angina, >1mm ST depression or fall in BP.
- Cardiomegaly on CXR, poor LV function on Echo (EF <40%).
- Documented episodes of regular VEs and VT 24h post infarction.
- Frequent episodes of silent ischaemia on Holter monitoring.

Electrophysiological study

All STEMI patients with (1) non-sustained VT and documented EF <40% or (2) sustained/pulseless VT/VF (regardless of EF) should undergo electrophysiological testing prior to discharge (MADIT and MUSTT trials) with a view to defibrillator implantation.

Discharge and secondary prevention

- Length of hospital stays in uncomplicated patients. The thrombolysis group need to undergo risk stratification prior to discharge and tend to have a mean hospital stay of 5–7 days. The primary PCI group have a shorter hospital stay between 3–4 days.
- Prior to discharge an agreed plan between patient (and patient's family) and physician is necessary to address modifiable risk factors, beneficial medication, and rehabilitation programme.
- Modifiable risk factors include:
  - Management of lipids and use of statins
  - Detection and treatment of diabetes
  - Ensuring BP is adequately controlled
  - Counselling to discontinue smoking
  - Advice on a healthy diet and weight loss.
- It is vital patients understand the medical regimen and, in particular, the importance of long-term 'prognostic medication'. Unless there are contraindications all patients should be on a minimum of:
  - Aspirin 75mg od (if true allergy, use clopidogrel 75mg od alone)

- Clopidogrel 75mg od (for 12 months)
- ACEI at the recommended dosage
- Statin at the recommended dosage
- The role of long-term formal anticoagulation is controversial.

- All patients must be offered a cardiac rehabilitation programme.

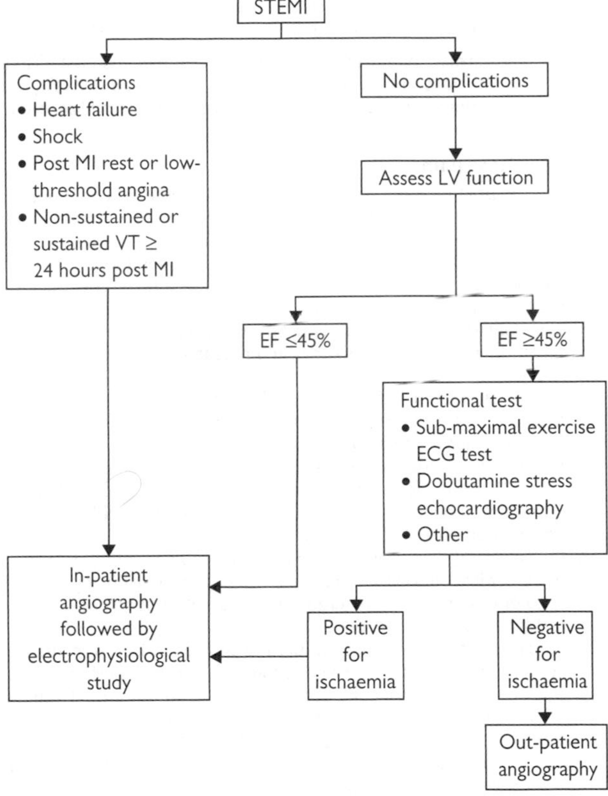

Fig. 1.7 Suggested strategy post STEMI in patients who have undergone thrombolysis to determine the need for inpatient angiography/EPS. Adapted from Antman EM (2000). *Cardiovascular Therapeutics*, 2nd edn. Saunders, Philadelphia, PA.

STEMI: complications

Complications include:

- Continuing chest pain
- Fever
- A new systolic murmur: VSD, acute MR, or pericarditis
- Arrhythmia: VT, AV block ectopics, and bradycardia
- Pump failure: hypotension, cardiac failure, and cardiogenic shock.

Complications are encountered more commonly in patients post STEMI, but can also be found in NSTEMI patients (see 📖 p.44). In NSTEMI patients, complications are more common where multiple cardiac events have occurred.

Further chest pain

- Chest pain post MI is not necessarily angina. A careful history is needed to characterize pain. If there is doubt about the aetiology of pain in the absence of ECG changes, stress/thallium imaging may aid diagnosis.
- A bruised sensation and musculoskeletal pains are common in the first 24–48h, especially in patients who have received CPR or repeated DC shock. Use topical agents for skin burns.
- *Recurrent infarction* is an umbrella term including both extension of infarction in the original territory and repeated infarct in a 2nd territory.
  - Usually associated with recurrent ST elevation.
  - If cardiac enzymes not yet back to normal a significant change is a 2-fold rise above the previous nadir.
  - Patients should ideally undergo immediate PCI. Thrombolysis is an alternative, but a less attractive approach. Standard thrombolysis criteria must be met (see 📖 p.20). Bleeding is a risk (NB: SK should not be used on a 2nd occasion).
- *Post infarction angina* (angina developing within 10 days of MI) should be treated with standard medical therapy. All patients with angina prior to discharge should undergo cardiac catheterization and revascularization as an inpatient.
- *Pericarditis presents* as sharp, pleuritic, and positional chest pain, usually 1–3 days post infarct. It is more common with STEMI. A pericardial friction rub may be audible. ECG changes are rarely seen. Treat with high-dose aspirin (600mg qds PO) covering with a proton pump inhibitor (e.g. lansoprazole 30mg od PO). Other NSAIDs have been associated with higher incidence of LV rupture and ↑ coronary vascular resistance and are probably best avoided.
- *Pericardial effusion* is more common with anterior MI especially if complicated by cardiac failure. Tamponade is rare and the result of ventricular rupture and/or haemorrhagic effusions. Detection is with a combination of clinical features and echocardiography. Most small effusions resolve gradually over a few months with no active intervention.
- *Pulmonary thromboembolism* can occur in patients with heart failure and prolonged bed rest. Routine use of prophylactic LMWH and

UFH combined with early mobilization have reduced incidence of PE. Sources include lower limb veins and/or RV (see 📖 p.120).

- *Fever:* often seen and peaks 3–4 days post MI. It is associated with elevated WCC and raised CRP. Other causes of fever should be considered—infection, thrombophlebitis, venous thrombosis, drug reaction, pericarditis.

Ventricular septal defect post myocardial infarction (MI)

- Classically seen 24h (highest risk) to 10 days post MI and affects 2–4% of cases.
- *Clinical features* include rapid deterioration with a harsh pan-systolic murmur (maximal at the lower left sternal edge), poor perfusion, and pulmonary oedema. The absence of a murmur in the context of a low output state does not rule out a VSD.

Diagnosis

- Echocardiography: the defect may be visualized on 2D-Echo and colour flow Doppler shows the presence of left-to-right shunt. Anterior infarction is associated with apical VSD and inferior MI with basal VSD. Failure to demonstrate a shunt on Echo does not exclude a VSD.
- PA catheter (especially in absence of Echo or inconclusive Echo results): a step-up in O_2 saturation from RA to RV confirms the presence of a shunt, which may be calculated by:

$$\text{Qp: Qs} = \frac{(\text{Art sat} - \text{RA sat})}{(\text{Art sat} - \text{PA sat})}$$

where Qp = pulmonary blood flow; Qs = systemic blood flow

Management

Stabilization measures are all temporizing until definitive repair can take place. Hypotension (see 🕮 p.40) and pulmonary oedema (see 🕮 p.40) should be managed as described elsewhere. Important principles are given here:

- Invasive monitoring (PA catheter and arterial line) to dictate haemodynamic management. RA and PCWP dictate fluid administration or diuretic use. CO, mean arterial pressure, and arterial resistance determine the need for vasodilator therapy.
- If SBP >100mmHg, cautious use of vasodilator therapy, generally with nitroprusside, will lower the systemic vascular resistance and reduce the magnitude of the shunt. Nitrates will cause venodilatation and increase the shunt and should be avoided. Not be used with renal impairment.
- Inotropes if severely hypotensive (initially dobutamine but adrenaline may be required depending on haemodynamic response). Increasing systemic pressure will worsen shunt.
- Consider intra-aortic balloon pumping in most cases.
- Liaise with surgeons early for possible repair. Operative mortality is high (20–70%) especially in the context of perioperative shock, inferoposterior MI, and RV infarction. Current recommendations are for high-risk early surgical repair combined with CABG ± MV repair/replacement.
- If patient has been weaned off pharmacological and/or mechanical support it may be possible to postpone surgery for 2–4 weeks to allow for some level of infarct healing. Patients should ideally undergo catheterization prior to surgical repair to ensure culprit vessel(s) are grafted.
- Closure of the VSD with catheter placement of an umbrella-shaped device (Amplatzer™) has been reported to stabilize critically ill patients until definitive repair is possible.

Acute mitral regurgitation post MI

- MR due to ischaemic papillary muscle dysfunction or partial rupture is seen 2–10 days post MI. Complete rupture causes torrential MR and is usually fatal.
- Presentation is acute onset severe breathlessness with hypoxia, acute pulmonary oedema, diaphoresis, and with rapid deterioration.
- More commonly associated with inferior MI (posteromedial papillary muscle) than anterior MI (anterolateral papillary muscle).
- 'Silent MR' is quite frequent and must be suspected in any post-MI patient with unexplained haemodynamic deterioration.
- Diagnosis is by Echo. In severe MR, PA catheterization will show a raised pressure with a large *v* wave on the PCWP.

Management

(See 🕮 p.114.)

- Treatment with vasodilators, generally nitroprusside, should be started as early as possible once haemodynamic monitoring is available.
- Mechanical ventilation may be necessary.
- Liaise with surgeons early for possible repair.

Pseudoaneurysm and free wall rupture

- Demonstrated in up to 6% of STEMI patients and leads to sudden death in two-thirds.
- A proportion present subacutely with cardiogenic shock allowing time for intervention.
- Diagnosis of subacute cases can be made on a combination of clinical features of pericardial effusion, tamponade, and Echo.
- Patients who have undergone early thrombolysis have a lower chance of wall rupture.
- Stabilization of the patient follows similar lines to cardiogenic shock (see 🕮 p.42). Case must be discussed with surgeons immediately with view to repair.

Cocaine-induced MI

- The incidence of cocaine-induced MI, LV dysfunction, and arrhythmias are on the increase.
- It has been estimated that 14–25% of young patients presenting to urban emergency departments with non-traumatic chest pain may have detectable levels of cocaine and its metabolites in their circulation. Of this group, 6% have enzymatic evidence of MI (figures are from the USA).
- Most patients are young, non-white, male cigarette smokers without other risk factors for ischaemic heart disease.

Diagnosis

- Can be difficult and must be suspected in any young individual with chest discomfort at low risk of developing ischaemic heart disease.
- Chest pain occurs most commonly within 12h of cocaine use. Effects can return up to 24–36h later 2° to long-lasting active metabolites.
- *ECG* is abnormal with multiple non-specific repolarization changes in up to 80% of cases and approximately 40% may have diagnostic changes of STEMI qualifying for reperfusion therapy (see 🕮 p.14).
- *Biochemical markers of cardiac injury* can be misleading, as most patients will have elevated CK levels 2° to rhabdomyolysis. TnT and TnI are vital to confirm myocardial injury.

Management

General measures

- These are the same as for anyone presenting with an MI. O_2: high-flow 5–10L unless there is a contraindication; analgesia; aspirin 75mg od.
- GTN: to be given at high doses as IV infusion (>10mg/hour final levels) and dose titrated to symptoms and haemodynamic response (see 🕮 p.18).
- Benzodiazepines: are critical to reduce anxiety and tachycardia.

Second-line agents

- *Verapamil* is given in high doses and has the dual function of reducing cardiac workload, hence restoring O_2 supply and demand, as well as reversing coronary vasoconstriction. Should be given cautiously as 1–2-mg IV bolus at a time (up to 10mg total) with continuous haemodynamic monitoring. This should be followed by a high-dose oral preparation to cover the 24-hour period for at least 72h after last dose of cocaine (80–120mg PO tds).
- *Phentolamine* is an α-adrenergic antagonist and readily reverses cocaine-induced vasoconstriction (2–5mg IV and repeated if necessary). It can be used in conjunction with verapamil.
- *Labetalol* has both α- and β-adrenergic activity and can be used after verapamil and phentolamine if patient remains hypertensive. It is effective in lowering cocaine-induced hypertension, but has no effect on coronary vasoconstriction.
- *Reperfusion therapy* evidence for use of thrombolysis is limited and generally associated with poor outcome 2° to hypertension-induced haemorrhagic complications. If patient fails to settle after implementing

first-line measures, verapamil, and phentolamine they should undergo immediate coronary angiography followed by PCI if appropriate (evidence of thrombus/vessel occlusion). In the event that angiography is not available thrombolytic therapy can be considered.

Caution

β-blockers must be avoided (e.g. propranolol). They exacerbate coronary vasoconstriction by allowing unopposed action of the adrenergic receptors.

Box 1.8 Pathogenesis and other complications of cocaine-induced MI

Pathogenesis

- The cause of myocardial injury is multifactorial, including an increase in O_2 demand (↑HR, ↑BP, ↑contractility) in the context of decrease in supply caused by a combination of inappropriate vasoconstriction (in areas of minor atheroma), enhanced platelet aggregation, and thrombus formation
- The effects can be delayed as the metabolites of cocaine are potent active vasoconstrictors and can remain in the circulation for up to 36h (or longer) resulting in a recurrent wave of symptoms

Other complications

- *Cocaine-induced myocardial dysfunction* is multifactorial and includes MI, chronic damage 2° to repetitive sympathetic stimulation (as in Pheochromocytoma), myocarditis 2° to cocaine impurities/infection, and unfavourable changes in myocardial/endothelial gene expression.
- *Cocaine-induced arrhythmias include* both atrial and ventricular tachyarrhythmias, as well as asystole and heart block—see post-MI arrhythmias (📖 p.38) and cardiopulmonary resuscitation (📖 p.6)
- *Aortic dissection*—see 📖 142.

Ventricular tachyarrhythmia post MI

Accelerated idioventricular rhythm

- Common (up to 20%) in patients with early reperfusion in first 48h.
- Usually self-limiting and short lasting with no haemodynamic effects.
- If symptomatic, accelerating sinus rate with atrial pacing or atropine may be of value. Suppressive antiarrhythmic therapy (lidocaine, amiodarone) is only recommended with degeneration into malignant ventricular tachyarrhythmias.

VPB

- Common and not related to incidence of sustained VT/VF.
- Generally treated conservatively. Aim to correct acid–base and electrolyte abnormalities (aim K^+ >4.0mmol/L and Mg^{2+} >1.0mmol/L).
- Peri-infarction β-blockade reduces VPB.

Non-sustained and monomorphic VT

- Associated with a worse clinical outcome.
- Correct reversible features such as electrolyte abnormalities and acid–base balance.
- DC cardioversion for haemodynamic instability.
- Non-sustained VT and haemodynamically stable VT (slow HR <100bpm) can be treated with amiodarone (300mg bolus IV over 30min, followed by 1.2g infusion over 24h). Lidocaine is no longer recommended as first line. Procainamide is an effective alternative, but is arrhythmogenic.
- For incessant VT on amiodarone consider overdrive pacing.

Ventricular fibrillation and polymorphic VT

- A medical emergency and requires immediate defibrillation.
- In refractory VF consider vasopressin 40U IV bolus.
- Amiodarone 300mg IV bolus to be continued as an infusion (see previous section) if output restored.
- Manage as cardiac arrest with usual ALS protocol (see 📖 p.6).

Atrial tachyarrhythmia post MI

- Includes SVT, AF, and atrial flutter.
- If patient is haemodynamically unstable, they must undergo immediate synchronized DC cardioversion.
- Haemodynamically stable patients can be treated with digoxin, β-blockers, and/or calcium channel blockers—see 📖 Table 1.8, p.71.
- Amiodarone can be used to restore sinus rhythm. However, it is not very effective in controlling rate. Class I agents should generally be avoided as they increase mortality.
- In AF and atrial flutter patients should undergo anticoagulation to reduce embolic complications if there are no contraindications.

Bradyarrhythmias and indications for pacing

Alternating or isolated RBBB/LBBB do not need pacing (unless haemodynamically unstable or progression to higher levels of block). New bifasicular block (RBBB with either LAD or RAD) or BBB with first-degree AV block may require prophylactic pacing depending on the clinical picture. Indications for pacing should not delay reperfusion therapy. Venous access (femoral or internal jugular vein) should be obtained first and pacing wire inserted later. External temporary cardiac pacing, atropine (300mcg to 3mg IV bolus), and isoprenaline can be used to buy time.

Bradyarrhythmias post MI

First-degree AV block

- Common and no treatment required.
- Significant PR prolongation (>0.20sec) is a contraindication to β-blockade.

Second-degree AV block

- This indicates a large infarction affecting conducting systems and mortality is generally ↑ in this group of patients.
    - Mobitz type I is self-limiting with no symptoms. Generally, requires no specific treatment. If symptomatic or progression to complete heart block will need temporary pacing.
    - Mobitz type II, 2:1, 3:1 should be treated with temporary pacing regardless of whether it progresses to complete heart block.

Third-degree AV block

- In the context of an inferior MI can be transient and does not require temporary pacing unless there is haemodynamic instability or an escape rhythm of <40bpm.
- Temporary pacing is required with anterior MI and unstable inferior MI.

Hypotension and shock post MI

(See 📖 p.42.)

The important principles in managing hypotensive patients with MI are:

- If the patient is well perfused peripherally, no pharmacological intervention is required. Consider lying the patient flat with legs elevated if necessary, provided there is no pulmonary oedema.
- Try to correct any arrhythmia, hypoxia, or acidosis.
- Arrange for an urgent Echo to exclude a mechanical cause for hypotension (e.g. MR, VSD, ventricular aneurysm) that may require urgent surgery.

Patients may be divided into two sub-groups:

Hypotension with pulmonary oedema (also see 📖 p.87)

- Secure central venous access: internal jugular lines are preferable if the patient may have received thrombolytic therapy.
- Commence *inotropes* (see 📖 p.42).
- Further invasive haemodynamic monitoring as available (PA pressures and wedge pressure monitoring, arterial line).
- Ensure optimal filling pressures, guided by physical signs and PA diastolic or wedge pressure. Significant MR will produce large v waves on the wedge trace and give spuriously high estimates of LVEDP.
- Ensure rapid coronary reperfusion (if not already done), either with thrombolytic therapy or primary PCI where available.
- Intra-aortic balloon counterpulsation (see 📖 p.774) may allow stabilization until PCI can be performed.

Hypotension without pulmonary oedema

This may be due either to RV infarction or hypovolaemia.

Diagnosis

- Check the JVP and right atrial pressure. This will be low in hypovolaemia and high in RV infarction.
- RV infarction on ECG is seen in the setting of inferior MI and ST elevation in right-sided chest leads (V3R–V4R).

Management

- In either case CO will be improved by cautious plasma expansion. Give 100–200mL of colloid over 10min and reassess.
- Repeat once if there is some improvement in BP and the patient has not developed pulmonary oedema.
- Invasive haemodynamic monitoring with a PA catheter (Swan–Ganz) is necessary to ensure hypotension is not due to low left-sided filling pressures. Aim to keep PCWP 12–15mmHg.
- Start inotropes if BP remains low despite adequate filling pressures.
- Use IV nitrates and diuretics with caution as venodilatation will compromise RV and LV filling and exacerbate hypotension.
- See 📖 p.28 for management of RV infarction.

Cardiogenic shock

- Affects between 5–20% of patients and up to 15% of MI patients can present with cardiogenic shock.
- Management involves a complex interaction between many medical, surgical, and intensive care teams with multiple invasive and non-invasive measures. Despite significant advances prognosis remains poor. Therefore, the absolute wishes of the patient with regard to such an invasive strategy should be respected from the outset.

Diagnosis

A combination of clinical and physiological measures:
- *Clinical:* marked, persistent (>30min) hypotension with SBP <80–90mmHg.
- *Physiological:* low cardiac index (<1.8L/mm/m^2) with elevated LV filling pressure (PCWP >18mmHg).

Management

- Complex and must be quick.
- Correct reversible factors including:
    - Arrhythmias and aim to restore sinus rhythm
    - Acid–base, electrolyte abnormalities
    - Ventilation abnormalities: intubate if necessary.
- Rapid haemodynamic, echocardiographic, and angiographic evaluation:
    - Haemodynamic: to ensure adequate monitoring and access including central venous lines, Swan–Ganz, arterial line insertion, urinary catheter.
    - Echocardiographic: to assess ventricular systolic function and exclude mechanical lesions, which may need to be dealt with by emergency cardiac surgery including MR (NB: tall v waves on PCWP trace), VSD, and ventricular aneurysm/pseudoaneurysm.
    - Angiographic: with a view to PCI or CABG if appropriate.
- Aim to improve haemodynamic status achieving a SBP ≥90mmHg guided by physical signs and LV filling pressures. As a general guide:
    - PCWP <15mmHg: cautious of IV fluids (colloids) in 100–200mL aliquots.
    - PCWP >15mmHg: inotropic support ± diuretics (if pulmonary oedema).
- Inotropes should be avoided if at all possible in acutely ischaemic patients. The aim should be to rapidly restore/maximize coronary flow and off-load LV. Early revascularization is vital and has been shown to decrease mortality. IABP will partially help achieve improved coronary perfusion, reduced LVEDP and improve BP.
- If haemodynamic status does not improve post revascularization and IABP insertion, inotropes should be used. Choice of agent can be difficult and should partly be guided by local protocols and expertise. Generally accepted choices depend on the clinical picture and include
    - If patient is hypotensive (± pulmonary oedema): start with dopamine (up to 5mcg/kg/min) and if ineffective substitute with adrenaline and/or noradrenaline.

- If patient has adequate BP (± pulmonary oedema): dobutamine to increase CO (starting at 2.5–5mcg/kg/min and increasing to 10mcg/kg/min) titrating to HR and haemodynamics. Phosphodiesterase inhibitors can be used as an alternative. If hypotension and tachycardia complicate dobutamine/PDI inhibitor treatment, (nor)adrenaline can be added as a 2nd agent to achieve desired haemodynamic effect.

- Use of diuretics, thrombolysis, GP IIb/IIIa antagonists, and LMWH/UFH should follow normal principles and be based on the clinical picture.

Non-ST elevation myocardial infarction (NSTEMI)/unstable angina (UA)

UA and NSTEMI are closely related conditions with similar clinical presentation, treatment, and pathogenesis but of varying severity. If there is biochemical evidence of myocardial damage the condition is termed NSTEMI and in the absence of damage, UA.

Unlike patients with a STEMI where diagnosis is generally made on presentation in the emergency department, diagnosis of NSTEMI/UA may not be definitive on presentation and evolves over the subsequent hours to days. Therefore, management of patients with NSTEMI/UA is a progression through a number of risk-stratification processes dependent on history, clinical features, and investigative results, which in turn determine choice and timing of a number of medical and/or invasive treatment strategies.

Fig. 1.8 is a summary of a recommended integrated care pathway illustrating a management plan for diagnosis and risk-directed treatment of a patient with STEMI/UA.

Clinical presentation

There are 3 distinct presentations:

- Rest angina—angina when patient is at rest.
- New-onset severe angina.
- Increasing angina—previously diagnosed angina which has become more frequent, longer in duration, or lower in threshold.

General examination (as indicated for all ACS—see 🕮 p.10) must be undertaken in particular to rule out pulmonary oedema, and assess haemodynamic stability, cardiac valve abnormalities, and diaphoresis.

Integrated management plan

We recommend that all patients follow a local integrated care pathway on presentation. The various stages are broadly outlined here. See relevant pages for further information.

- ***Initial stabilization*** (see also 🕮 p,10):
  - Transfer patient to area with continuous ECG monitoring and defibrillator facility.
  - Strict bed rest.
  - Give O_2, aspirin 300mg PO, SL nitrate and mild sedation if required.
  - If pain persists give diamorphine 2.5–5mg IV PRN with metoclopramide 10mg IV.
- ***General investigations:*** similar to STEMI patients (see 🕮 pp.12–6 including blood for FBC, biochemical profile and markers of myocardial injury, lipid profile, as well as CRP and TFT (if persistent tachycardia). Arrange portable CXR (rule out LVF, mediastinal abnormalities).
- ***Confirm diagnosis*** (see 🕮 p.46).
- ***Risk stratification*** (see 🕮 p.48) in order to determine appropriate medical and invasive treatment strategies. High-risk patients should be admitted to CCU and low/intermediate-risk patients to monitored beds in step-down unit.

- ***Treatment*** is based on patient's risk and includes:
  - Medical strategies:
    —anti-ischaemic (see 📖 p.51)
    —antiplatelet (see 📖 p.52)
    —antithrombic (see 📖 p.52).
  - Invasive strategies (see 📖 p.54).
- ***Secondary prevention and discharge.***

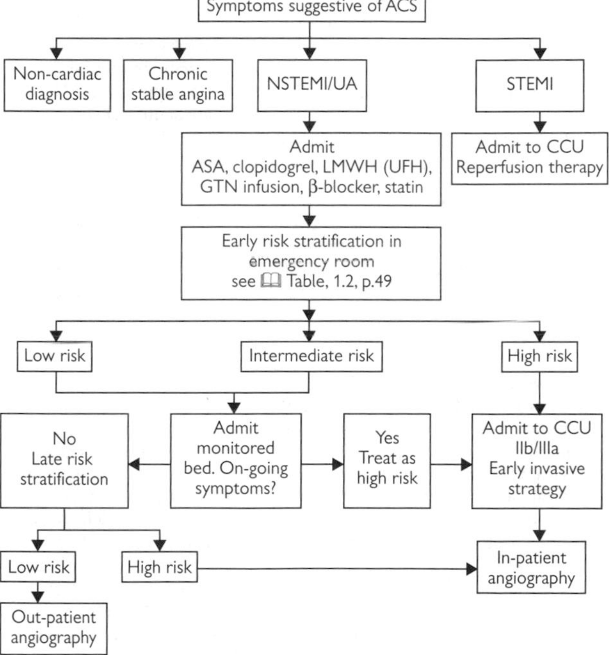

Fig. 1.8 NSTEMI/UA—integrated care pathway.

NSTEMI/UA: diagnosis

Diagnosis in NSTEMI/UA is an evolving process and may not be clear on presentation. A combination of history, serial changes in ECG, and biochemical markers of myocardial injury (usually over a 24–48-hour period) determine the diagnosis. Once a patient has been designated a diagnosis of ACS with probable/possible NSTEMI/UA they will require the following:

Serial ECGs

Changes can be transient and/or fixed especially if a diagnosis of NSTEMI is made. See 📖 Table 1.1, p.15 for localization of infarcts from ECG changes.

- ST-segment depression of ≥0.05mV is highly specific of myocardial ischaemia (unless isolated in V1–V3 suggesting a posterior STEMI).
- T-wave inversion is sensitive but non-specific for acute ischaemia unless very deep (≥0.3mV).
- Rarely Q-waves may evolve or there may be transient/new LBBB.

Serial biochemical markers of cardiac injury

These are used to differentiate between NSTEMI and UA, as well as determine prognosis. We recommend levels at 6, 12, 24, and 48h after last episode of pain. A positive biochemical marker (CK, CK-MB, or troponin) in the context of one or more of the aforementioned ECG changes is diagnostic of NSTEMI. If serial markers over a 24–72-hour period from the last episode of chest pain remain negative, UA is diagnosed.

- Cardiac troponin T and I: are both highly cardiac specific and sensitive, can detect 'microinfarction' in the presence of normal CK-MB, are not affected by skeletal muscle injury, and convey prognostic information (worse prognosis if positive). Troponins can be raised in non-atherosclerotic myocardial damage (cardiomyopathy, myocarditis, pericarditis) and should therefore be interpreted in the context of the clinical picture. Both TnT and TnI rise within 3h of infarction. TnT may persist up to 10–14 days and TnI up to 7–10 days. Results must be interpreted with caution in patients with chronic renal failure. See 📖 Fig. 1.5, p.17.
- CK levels do not always reach the diagnostic twice upper limit of normal and generally have little value in diagnosis of NSTEMI.
- CK-MB has low sensitivity and specificity CK-MB isoforms improve sensitivity (CK-MB2 >1U/L or CK-MB2/CK-MB1 ratio >1.5), but isoform assays are not widely available clinically.
- Myoglobin is non-cardiac specific, but levels can be detected as early as 2h after onset of symptoms. A negative test is useful in ruling out myocardial necrosis.

Continuous ECG monitoring

Can detect episodes of silent ischaemia and arrhythmia. Both have been shown to be more prolonged in NSTEMI than in UA.

NSTEMI/UA: risk stratification

NSTEMI/UA are a heterogeneous group of conditions with variable outcomes. An assessment of risk for adverse outcome is vital to ensure formation of an adequate management plan.

Risk stratification should begin on initial evaluation and continue throughout the hospital stay. At each stage patients with a high chance of a poor outcome should be identified and managed appropriately.

We recommend at least two formal risk-stratification processes:

Early risk stratification

(See 📖 Table 1.2, p.49) This should take place on presentation and forms part of the initial assessment used to make a diagnosis. It involves a combination of clinical features, ECG changes, and biochemical markers of cardiac injury as demonstrated in Table 1.2. Patients are divided into high risk and intermediate/low risk.

- *High-risk* patients should be admitted to CCU, follow an early invasive strategy, and be managed with a combination of:
  - ASA, clopidogrel, LMWH (UFH), IIb/IIIa
  - Anti-ischaemic therapy (first-line β-blocker, GTN)
  - Early invasive strategy (inpatient catheterization and PCI within 48h of admission).
- *Intermediate/low-risk* patients should be admitted to a monitored bed on a step-down unit and undergo a 2nd inpatient risk stratification once their symptoms have settled to determine timing of invasive investigations. Initial management should include:
  - ASA, clopidogrel, LMWH (UFH)
  - Anti-ischaemic therapy (first-line β-blocker, GTN)
  - Undergoing a late risk stratification in 48–72h from admission.

Late risk stratification

(See 📖 p.20.) This involves a number of non-invasive tests to determine the optimal timing for invasive investigations in intermediate/low-risk patients. Suggested guidelines are summarized on 📖 p.50. It is generally performed if there have been no further episodes of pain/ischaemia at 24–48h after admission.

- *Intermediate/low-risk* patients who develop recurrent pain and/or ischaemic ECG changes at any point during their admission, heart failure, or haemodynamic instability in the absence of a non-cardiac cause should be managed as a high-risk patient (IIb/IIIa and early invasive strategy).
- 📖 Fig. 1.8, p.45 is a summary of a recommended integrated care pathway combining diagnosis, risk stratification, and treatment.
- There are other risk-stratification assessment scores including Braunwald and TIMI. As recommended earlier, high-risk patients from these assessments should also follow an early invasive strategy and intermediate/low-risk patients a more conservative strategy.

Table 1.2 Short-term risk of death non-fatal MI in patients with UA*

Feature	High risk (at least 1 of the following features must be present)	Intermediate risk (no high-risk feature but must have 1 of the following features)	Low risk (no high- or intermediate-risk feature but may have any of the following features)
History	Accelerating tempo of ischaemic symptoms in preceding 48h	Prior MI, peripheral or cerebrovascular disease, or CABG, prior aspirin use	
Character of pain	Prolonged ongoing (>20min) rest pain	Prolonged (>20min) rest angina, now resolved, with moderate or high likelihood of CAD Rest angina (<20min) or relieved with rest or sublingual GTN	New-onset or progressive CCS Class III or IV angina the past 2 weeks without prolonged (>20min) rest pain but with moderate or high likelihood of CAD
Clinical findings	Pulmonary oedema, most likely due to ischaemia New or worsening MR murmur S_3 or new/worsening rales Hypotension, bradycardia, tachycardia Age >75 years	Age >70 years	
ECG	Angina at rest with transient ST-segment changes >0.05mV Bundle-branch block, new or presumed new Sustained ventricular tachycardia	T-wave inversions >0.2mV Pathological Q-waves	Normal or unchanged ECG during an episode of chest discomfort
Cardiac markers	Elevated (e.g. TnT or TnI >0.1ng/mL)	Slightly elevated (e.g. TnT >0.01 but <0.1ng/mL)	Normal

*Adapted from American College of Cardiology Practice Guidelines. Anderson JL, *et al.* (2007). *J Am Coll Cardiol* 2007; **50:** 1–157, doi : 10.1016/j. jacc.2007.02.013 (published online 6 August 2007)

NSTEMI/UA: late risk stratification

The highest risk of adverse outcome in patients who are designated as intermediate/low risk on presentation is during the early phase of admission. Therefore, it is important that the 2nd risk-stratification process occurs within 24–48h of admission if the patient is stable.

Late risk stratification is based on one of the following non-invasive investigations.

A patient is regarded as being at high risk of adverse outcome if they fulfil one of the features listed here. These patients should have inpatient cardiac catheterization.

Exercise ECG test

- ***Horizontal/down-sloping ST depression with:***
  - Onset at HR <120bpm or <6.5 METS
  - Magnitude of >2.0mm
  - Post-exercise duration of changes >6min
  - Depression in multiple leads reflecting multivessel disease.
- ***Abnormal SBP response:*** sustained decrease of >10mmHg or flat BP response with abnormal ECG.
- ***Other:***
  - Exercise induced ST-segment elevation
  - VT
  - Prolonged elevation of HR.

Stress radionuclide myocardial perfusion imaging

- Abnormal tracer distribution in more than one territory
- Cardiac enlargement.

LV imaging

- ***Stress echocardiography:***
  - Rest EF <35%
  - Wall motion score index >1.
- ***Stress radionuclide ventriculography:***
  - Rest EF <35%
  - Fall in EF >10%.

NSTEMI/UA: medical management 1

Anti-ischaemic therapy

All patients should be treated with a combination of the listed agents to ensure adequate symptom control and a favourable haemodynamic status (SBP ≈100–110mmHg, PR ≈60). All patients should be treated with adequate analgesia, IV nitrates, β-blockers, and statins (if no contraindications). Other agents can also be added depending on the clinical picture.

- ***Analgesia:*** diamorphine 2.5–5mg IV (with metoclopramide 10mg IV). Acts as anxiolytic. Reduces pain and SBP through venodilatation and reduction in sympathetic arteriolar constriction. Can result in hypotension (responsive to volume therapy) and respiratory depression (reversal with naloxone 400mcg 2mg IV).
- ***Nitrates:*** GTN infusion (50mg in 50mL nitrate saline at 1–10mL/hour) titrated to pain and keeping SBP >100mmHg. Tolerance to continuous infusion develops within 24h and the lowest efficacious dose should be used. Common side effects are headache and hypotension, both of which are reversible on withdrawal of medication. Absolute contraindication is use of sildenafil in the previous 24h. This can result in exaggerated and prolonged hypotension.
- ***ß-blockers:*** should be started on presentation. Initially use a short-acting agent (e.g. metoprolol 12.5–100mg PO tds), which if tolerated, may be converted to a longer-acting agent (e.g. atenolol 25–1000mg od). Rapid β-blockade may be achieved using short-acting IV agents such as metoprolol (see 📖 p.699). Aim for HR of ~50–60bpm. Mild LVF is not an absolute contraindication to β-blocker therapy. Pulmonary congestion may be 2° to ischaemic LV systolic dysfunction and/or reduced compliance. If there is overt heart failure β-blockade is contraindicated and a calcium antagonist (amlodipine 5–10mg od) can be used. By reducing HR and BP, β-blockers reduce myocardial O_2 demand and thus angina. When either used alone or in combination with nitrates and/or calcium antagonists, β-blockers are effective in reducing the frequency and duration of both symptomatic and silent ischaemic episodes.
- ***Calcium antagonists:*** diltiazem 60–360mg PO, verapamil 40–120mg PO tds. Their use aims to reduce HR and BP and is a useful adjunct to treatments with analgesia/nitrates/β-blockers. Amlodipine/felodipine 5–10mg PO od can be used with pulmonary oedema and in poor LV function. Calcium antagonists alone do not appear to reduce mortality or risk of MI in patients with UA. However when combined with nitrates and/or β-blockers they are effective in reducing symptomatic and silent ischaemic episodes, non-fatal MI, and the need for revascularization.
- ***Statins (HMG-CoA reductase inhibitors):*** high-dose statins (atorvastatin 80mg od) have been shown to reduce mortality and recurrent MI in the acute setting. The role of statins in 1° and 2° prevention of culture cardiovascular events is well documented.
- ***ACEIs:*** unlike patients with STEMI where early introduction of an ACEI has significant prognostic benefits, specific trails in the NSTEMI/UA setting are lacking. However, there is good evidence that both patients with low and high risk of cardiovascular disease will benefit from long-term ACE inhibition (HOPE and EUROPA Trials).

NSTEMI/UA: medical management 2

Antiplatelet therapy

All patients should be given aspirin and clopidogrel (unless contraindications). IIb/IIIa antagonists to high-risk patients only.

- ***Aspirin*** (300mg PO) should be administered immediately in the emergency department and continued indefinitely (unless contraindications). It has been shown to consistently reduce mortality and recurrent ischaemic events in many trials. In patients with aspirin hypersensitivity or major gastrointestinal intolerance clopidogrel 75mg od should be used.
- ***Thienopyridines***: clopidogrel (300mg od) should be given on admission to all patients with proven NSTEMI/UA, regardless of risk and be continued (75mg od) for at least 12 months. Clopidogrel should be withheld in patients requiring CABG for 5–7 days to reduce haemorrhagic complications. Clopidogrel is preferred over ticlopidine because of its rapid onset of action and better safety profile.
- ***Glycoprotein IIb/IIIa antagonists***: there are multiple short- and long-acting commercially available molecules. These agents should be used in conjunction with aspirin, clopidogrel, and LMWH (or UFH). Eptifibatide and tirofiban should be used in high-risk patients with ongoing ischaemia and elevated troponin in whom an early invasive management strategy is not planned/available (<24h). In patients with an early invasive strategy, all IIb/IIIa antagonists can be used. Infusion is generally continued for 12h post PCI. Taken as a group these agents protect NSTEMI/UA patients from death and non-fatal MI during the acute phase of their presentation and 24h post intervention. See Box 1.9 for doses and administration regimen.

Antithrombotic therapy

All patients should be given a LMWH (UFH).

- ***LMWHs*** have been shown to be as good as or superior to UFH in short-term reduction of death, MI, and revascularization in patients with NSTEMI/UA. They should be used in conjunction with aspirin and clopidogrel in all patients on presentation and be continued for 2–5 days after the last episode of pain and ischaemic ECG changes. Other advantages over UFH include SC administration, lack of monitoring, and reduced resistance and thrombocytopaenia. Box 1.9 lists the doses of various agents in use for treating NSTEMI/UA.
- ***UFH:*** multiple trials have demonstrated the reduction of risk of death and MI in patients with UA/NSTEMI. UFH should be started on presentation as an alternative to LMWH in conjunction with aspirin and clopidogrel. Infusion should be continued for 2–5 days subsequent to the last episode of pain and/or ischaemic ECG changes. An initial bolus of 60–70U/kg (maximum 5000U) should be followed by an infusion of 12–15U/kg/hour (≈1000U/hour). The infusion rate should be altered to achieve an aPTT value of 1.5–2.0 × control. Coagulation should be checked initially every 6h followed by once every 24h after 2 consistent values have been obtained.

Thrombolysis

There is no evidence to suggest that combing thrombolytic agents with aspirin, LMWH, and conventional anti-ischaemic therapy is of benefit. In the TIMI IIIB trial, the rt-PA group had a worse outcome at 6 weeks and risk of bleeding was also greater with the thrombolysis group.

Box 1.9 Doses of LMWH and GP IIb/IIIa antagonists for treating NSTEMI/UA

LMWH

- Dalteparin: 120U/kg bd (max. 10,000U twice daily).
- Enoxaparin: 1mg/kg bd (100U/kg twice daily).

GP IIa/IIIa antagonists

- Abciximab: bolus 250mcg/kg over 1min followed by IV infusion 125ng/kg/min.
- Tirofiban: 400ng/kg/min for 30min followed by IV infusion 100ng/kg/min.
- Eptifibatide: bolus 180mcg/kg followed by IV infusion 2mcg/kg/min.

Box 1.10 Management key points: NSTEMI

- Continuous ECG monitoring
- O_2
- Analgesia: diamorphine (+ metoclopramide), GTN (monitor BP)
- Aspirin, clopidogrel, LMWH
- β-blockers: initially short-acting agent, e.g. metoprolol (if no contraindications)
- High-dose statins
- Glycoprotein IIb/IIIa antagonists for high-risk patients only.

NSTEMI/UA: invasive versus non-invasive strategies

The current evidence supports early angiography and revascularization in patients who present with either high-risk features or intermediate/low-risk features with ongoing symptoms. Furthermore, low- and intermediate-risk patients who settle on medical therapy should undergo symptom-limited, non-invasive stress testing to identify a cohort of patients with an ↑risk of adverse outcome. This 2nd group will also benefit from an early invasive management.

Patients managed with an early conservative strategy tend to have an ↑need for antianginal therapy and rehospitalization for angina and many undergo coronary angiography within the year.

The following groups are recommended to benefit from an early invasive strategy (inpatient cardiac catheterization and PCI).

- Patients with high-risk features of NSTEMI/UA:
  - Recurrent angina/ischaemic ECG changes despite optimal medical therapy
  - Elevated troponin
  - New/presumed new ST-segment depression
  - Chest pain with clinical features of heart failure (pulmonary oedema, new/worsening MR, S_3 gallop)
  - Haemodynamic instability
  - Sustained ventricular tachycardia.
- Poor LV systolic function (EF <40%).
- Patients allocated to low/medium risk in whom subsequent non-invasive testing demonstrates high-risk features.
- PCI in previous 6 months.
- Previous CABG.
- Patients with other comorbidities (e.g. malignancy, liver failure, renal disease) in whom risks of revascularization are not likely to outweigh benefits.

NSTEMI/UA: discharge and secondary prevention

- ***Length of hospital stay*** will be determined by symptoms and the rate of progression through the NSTEMI/UA pathway. Generally patients are hospitalized for 3–7 days.
- ***2° prevention*** remains of paramount importance and is similar in principle to STEMI patients (see 📖 p.30).

Arrhythmias: general approach

Both tachyarrhythmias and bradyarrhythmias may present with significant symptoms and haemodynamic compromise. The approach to patients with arrhythmias depends upon:

- The effects of the rhythm on the patient
- The diagnosis from the ECG and the rhythm
- Any underlying cardiac abnormality or identifiable precipitant.

Effects of the rhythm on the patient

Patients with signs of severe haemodynamic compromise:

- Impending cardiac arrest
- Severe pulmonary oedema
- Shock: SBP <90mmHg
- Depressed consciousness.

Treat immediately with unsynchronized external defibrillation for tachyarrhythmia and temporary pacing for bradyarrhythmia (see 📖 p.82).

Patients with mild–moderate compromise:

- Mild pulmonary oedema
- Low cardiac output with cool peripheries and oliguria
- Angina at rest.

Try to record an ECG and long rhythm strip before giving any pharmacological agents and/or defibrillation. This will be invaluable for long-term management. If they deteriorate, treat as for severe haemodynamic compromise.

Diagnosing the arrhythmia

The main distinctions to make are:

- Tachy- (>120/min) versus brady- (<60/min) arrhythmia
- Narrow (≤120ms or 3 small squares) versus broad QRS complex
- Regular versus irregular rhythm.

Box 1.11 Multiple, common precipitating factors

Underlying cardiac disease

- Ischaemic heart disease
- Acute or recent MI
- Angina
- Mitral valve disease
- LV aneurysm
- Congenital heart disease
- Abnormalities of resting ECG
- Pre-excitation (short PR interval)
- Long QT (congenital or acquired).

Drugs

- Antiarrhythmics
- Sympathomimetics (β2 agonists, cocaine)
- Antidepressants (tricyclic)
- Adenylate cyclase inhibitors aminophylline, caffeine)
- Alcohol.

Metabolic abnormalities

- ↓ or ↑K^+
- ↓ or ↑Ca^{2+}
- ↓Mg^{2+}
- ↓PaO_2
- ↑$PaCO_2$
- Acidosis.

Endocrine abnormalities

- Thyrotoxicosis
- Pheochromocytoma.

Miscellaneous

- Febrile illness
- Emotional stress
- Smoking
- Fatigue.

Tachyarrhythmias heart rate (HR) >120bpm

History

Previous cardiac disease, palpitations, dizziness, chest pain, symptoms of heart failure and recent medication. Ask specifically about conditions known to be associated with certain cardiac arrhythmias (e.g. AF: alcohol, thyrotoxicosis, mitral valve disease, IHD, pericarditis; VT: previous MI, LV aneurysm).

Examination

BP, heart sounds and murmurs, signs of heart failure, carotid bruits.

Investigations

If patient is haemodynamically stable, before treatment in unstable patients, after restoration of a stable rhythm:

- 12 lead ECG and rhythm strip:
  - Regular versus irregular rhythm
  - Narrow versus broad QRS complex.
- Blood tests:
  - FBC, biochemistry, glucose (urgently)
  - Ca^{2+}, Mg^{2+} (especially if on diuretics)
  - Biochemical markers of myocardial injury.
- Where appropriate:
  - Blood cultures, CRP, ESR
  - Thyroid function tests
  - Drug levels
  - Arterial blood gases.
- CXR:
  - Heart size
  - Evidence of pulmonary oedema
  - Other pathology (e.g. Ca bronchus → AF, pericardial effusion →sinus tachycardia, hypotension ± AF).

Management

Haemodynamically unstable patients

- Arrhythmias causing severe haemodynamic compromise (cardiac arrest, SBP <90mmHg, severe pulmonary oedema, evidence of cerebral hypoperfusion) require urgent correction, usually with external defibrillation. Drug therapy requires time and haemodynamic stability.
- The only exception is a patient in chronic AF with an uncontrolled ventricular rate: defibrillation is unlikely to cardiovert to SR. Rate control and treatment of precipitant is first line.
- Sedate awake patients with midazolam (2.5–10mg IV) ± diamorphine (2.5–5mg IV + metoclopramide 10mg IV) for analgesia. Beware respiratory depression and have an anaesthetist, flumazenil, and naloxone to hand.
- Formal anaesthesia with propofol is preferred, but remember the patient may not have an empty stomach and precautions should be taken to prevent aspiration (e.g. cricoid pressure, ET intubation).

- Start at 200J synchronized shock and increase as required.
- If tachyarrhythmia recurs or is unresponsive try to correct ↓P_aO_2, ↑P_aCO_2, acidosis, or ↓K^+. Give Mg^{2+} (8mmol IV stat) and shock again. Amiodarone 150–300mg bolus IV may also be used.
- Give specific antiarrhythmic therapy (see 🕮 Table 1.3, p.58).

Haemodynamically stable patients

- Admit and arrange for continuous ECG monitoring and 12-lead ECG.
- Try vagotonic manoeuvres (e.g. Valsalva or carotid sinus massage see 🕮 p.68).
- If diagnosis is clear introduce appropriate treatment.
- If there is doubt regarding diagnosis, give adenosine 6mg as fast IV bolus followed by 5mL saline flush. If no response, try 9, 12, and 18mg in succession with continuous ECG rhythm strip.
- Definitive treatment should start as soon as diagnosis is known (🕮 pp.58–81).

Box 1.12 General principles

- *Narrow complex tachycardias* originate in the atria or AV node (i.e. SVT; see 🕮 Fig. 1.9, p.69).
- *Irregular, narrow-complex tachycardia* is most commonly AF or atrial flutter with varying AV block.
- *Broad complex tachyarrhythmias* may originate from either the ventricles (VT) or from the atria or AV node (SVT) with aberrant conduction to the ventricles (RBBB or LBBB configuration).
- If the patient has previous documented arrhythmias, compare the morphology of the current arrhythmia to old ECGs. The diagnosis of VT versus SVT and therapy may be evident from the last admission.

Treatment options in tachyarrhythmias

Table 1.3 Treatment options in tachyarrhythmias

Sinus tachycardia	Look for cause. β-blockade if anxious		
Atrial fibrillation **Atrial flutter** **SVT** (📖 p.68)	**Rate control (AV node)** • Digoxin • β-blockade • Calcium blocker (e.g. verapamil)	**Version to SR** • Flecainide • Amiodarone • Sotalol • Disopyramide • Synchronized DC shock	**Prevention** • Amiodarone • Sotalol • Quinidine • Procainamide
Junctional tachycardias (AVNRT) (📖 p.81)	• Adenosine • β-blockade • Verapamil • (Vagal stimulation)	• Digoxin • Flecainide • Synchronized DC shock	
Accessory pathway tachycardias (i.e. AVRT) (📖 p.80)	**At AV node** • Adenosine • β-blockade	**At accessory pathway** • Sotalol • Flecainide • Disopyramide • Quinidine • Amiodarone	**Termination only** • Synchronized DC shock
Ventricular tachycardia (📖 p.66)	**Termination and prevention** • Lidocaine • Procainamide • Amiodarone • Magnesium • DC shock	• Flecainide • Disopyramide • Propafenone • β-blockade	

Broad complex tachycardia: diagnosis

(QRS width >120ms or >3 small squares.)

Diagnostic approach

The following principles can be used to distinguish between different forms of broad complex tachyarrhythmia.

1 Examine the rhythm strip. Is it regular or irregular?

Regular
- VT (mono/polymorphic)
- SVT or atrial flutter with bundle branch block
- Atrial flutter or SVT with pre-excitation (e.g. WPW).

Irregular
- AF, atrial flutter, or multifocal atrial tachycardia with bundle branch block
- Pre-excited AF (e.g. WPW)
- Torsades de pointes (PVT).

2 Are there any features on the 12-lead ECG that help distinguish VT from SVT with aberrancy?

Factors favouring SVT
- A grossly irregular broad complex tachycardia with rates ≥200/min suggests AF with conduction over an accessory pathway.
- Slowing or termination by vagotonic manoeuvres.
- Evidence of atrial and ventricular coupling (e.g. with 1:2 AV block).

Factors favouring or diagnostic of VT
- Cycle length stability (<40ms R–R variation).
- QRS >140ms (3.5 small squares) especially with normal duration when compared with previous ECG in sinus rhythm.
- Marked left axis deviation (negative in lead II).
- QRS concordance in chest leads. If the predominant deflection of the QRS is positive this is highly suggestive of VT.
- In patients with previous LBBB or RBBB, it is difficult to distinguish VT from SVT with aberrancy. A different QRS morphology in tachycardia suggests VT (other clues are given in Table 1.4).
- Fusion or capture beats.
- Independent atrial activity (seen in ~25%).

3 What are the effects of adenosine?

The transient AV block produces one of three results:
- *The tachycardia terminates.* This suggests an SVT with aberrancy or RVOT tachycardia (technically a form of VT).
- *The ventricular rate slows unmasking atrial activity.* Either 'flutter' waves (atrial flutter with block or intra-atrial tachycardia) or AF. The tachycardia typically continues after a few seconds once the adenosine wears off.
- *No effect on the rhythm.* Check that the patient received a therapeutic dose of adenosine (and experienced chest tightness with the injection). Higher doses are required in patients on theophyllines. The diagnosis is most likely to be VT.

If there is any doubt about diagnosis in the acute setting the patient must be treated as VT until proven otherwise.

Morphologic rules

For any broad complex tachycardia with 'bundle branch block' morphology, assume it is VT unless (see Table 1.4):

Table 1.4 Differentiating broad complex tachyarrhythmias

	RBBB	LBBB
Lead V1	rSR' with R' >r RS with R >S	rS or QS with time to S-wave nadir <70ms
Lead V6	If a Q-wave is present, it must be 40ms and <0.2mV	R-wave with no Q-wave

Sensitivity 90%; specificity 67–85%.[1]

Reference

1 Griffith MJ *et al.* (1994). Ventricular tachycardia as default diagnosis in broad complex tachycardia. *Lancet* **343:** 386–8.

Monomorphic ventricular tachycardia (MVT)

Management (Box 1.13)

1. *Assess airway, breathing, and circulation immediately.*
2. *If patient is haemodynamically unstable:*

- Deliver precordial thump: this can induce a mechanical premature ventricular complex interrupting VT circuit and terminating arrhythmia.
- Immediate unsynchronized external defibrillation (200J, 200J, 360J). Patient is often unconscious and if so, no sedation is required.

3. *If patient is haemodynamically stable:*

- Patient should initially be treated with IV pharmacological agents. If this is unsuccessful they can be electrically cardioverted under sedation/ anaesthesia.
- Chemical cardioversion is empiric and the choice of agent depends on local policy and expertise. We recommend IV amiodarone, sotalol, or procainamide as first-line agents. Amiodarone is the agent of choice in the context of poor LV function. Second-line agents include lignocaine and β-blockers (the latter is particularly valuable in the setting of MI/acute ischaemia).
- Give IV magnesium (8-mmol bolus over 2–5min followed by 60mmol in 50mL glucose over 24h) for all patients, especially if there is a risk of hypomagnesaemia (e.g. diuretics, excessive ethanol intake). With recurrent VT bolus dose can be repeated safely. Save a serum sample for analysis later.

4. *Correct reversible factors:*

- Ischaemia must be treated especially in the context of post-infarction VT. This can initially be achieved with β-blockers. Patients should undergo revascularization at the earliest opportunity (see 📖 p.24).
- Electrolyte abnormalities must be corrected (aim K^+ ≥4.0–4.5, Mg^{2+} ≥1.0).
- Acidosis: if severe (pH ≤7.1) give bicarbonate (8.4% sodium–bicarbonate 50mL via a central line over 20min).

5. *If there is recurrent or persistent VT:*

- Synchronized DC shock under sedation or anaesthesia, with an anaesthetist present in case of sudden deterioration.
- Overdrive pacing using a temporary transvenous wire may be used to terminate VT. The combination of prolonged temporary pacing and antiarrhythmics for recurrent VT is particularly effective in situations where the VT is provoked by bradycardia. If possible, rhythm strips of onset of runs of VT must be analysed looking for bradycardia, heart block, or sick sinus syndrome. Dual-chamber temporary pacing may improve cardiac output by restoring AV synchrony.

6. ***Maintenance therapy*** is usually oral and depends on aetiology of VT. Patient must be discussed with cardiac electrophysiologist early and options for electrophysiological study, radiofrequency ablation of VT focus, and/or ICD implantation explored. Patient will need ambulatory ECG

monitor, exercise testing, or more invasive stimulation tests to monitor effectiveness of therapy.

Box 1.13 Key points: monomorphic VT

- Defined as ≥3 consecutive ventricular ectopics at a rate ≥100/min.
- Common early post MI (up to 40%). If self-limiting, without haemodynamic compromise, does not require treatment.
- Sustained VT in the setting of acute MI (LV dysfunction) is associated with a poor prognosis (short and long term) and requires urgent treatment. Patients should undergo electrophysiological assessment for ICD insertion.
- Accelerated idioventricular rhythm or 'slow VT' (rate 50–100/min) requires treatment if hypotensive (from loss of atrial contribution).

Investigations

- ECG: Acute MI, prolonged QT interval
- CXR: Cardiomegaly, pulmonaryoedema
- U&Es: Hypokalaemia, renal impairment
- Mg^{2+}, Ca^{2+}: ?deficiency
- Cardiac enzymes: Small rises common after DC shock
- ABG: ?hypoxia, acidosis
- Echo: For LV function and to exclude structural abnormality (e.g. aneurysm)

Once acute episode is over, consider referral to cardiologist for

- Holter monitoring
- Exercise testing
- Coronary angiography
- VT stimulation (provocation) testing.

Polymorphic ventricular tachycardia (PVT)

General management principles are identical to those for monomorphic VT. Most patients will be haemodynamically unstable and must undergo external defibrillation. PVT occurring in the following circumstances requires specific therapy:

- Ischaemic PVT in the context of MI
- Non-ischaemic PVT with QT prolongation (torsades de pointes)
- PVT associated with Brugada syndrome.

Ischaemic PVT

- Occurs in conjunction with acute MI and chronic myocardial ischaemia.
- MVT in the context of MI can convert to PVT.
- 1° treatment is complete revascularization. This must be followed by Holter, exercise ECG, and EP evaluation to determine arrhythmia threshold.
- A subset of patients especially with poor LV function, or where MVT degenerates into PVT, may require ICD implantation.

Non-ischaemic PVT with prolonged QT interval (torsades de pointes)

This is an irregular polymorphic VT (often self-limiting), which appears to 'twist' about the isoelectric line. It occurs in the setting of prolongation of the QT interval (QTc >500ms) but the relationship between degree of prolongation and risk of serious arrhythmias is unpredictable. It may present as recurrent syncope or dizziness. Quite often patients are mistaken as having seizures.

Brugada syndrome[1]

- Brugada syndrome is characterized by the triad of:
  - ST elevation in V1–V3
  - RBBB
  - Sudden death (or family history of sudden death) from VF.
- It is common in Japan and in SE Asia. Men are affected more than women.
- The inheritance pattern is autosomal dominant and some families have a mutation in the cardiac sodium channel SCN5A.
- Must obtain specialist advice from cardiac electrophysiologist. Patients will require EP studies with view to ICD implantation.
- Diagnosis is made by serial ECGs after administration of flecainide 2mg/kg body weight IV in 10min or procainamide 10mg/kg IV in 10min. The test is positive if an additional 1mm ST elevation appears in leads V1, V2, and V3. All positive individuals should undergo EP studies and further specialist evaluation.

Box 1.14 Causes of prolonged QT interval

Acquired

- Drugs
  - Antiarrhythmics (quinidine, procainamide, disopyramide amiodarone, sotalol)
  - Antipsychotics (pimozide, thioridazine)
  - Antihistamines (terfenadine, astemizole, especially if other prescribed drugs interact with them (e.g. ketoconazole, erythromycin)
  - Antimalarials (especially halofantrine)
  - Organophosphate poisoning
- Electrolyte abnormalities (↓K^+, ↓Mg^{2+}, and ↓Ca^{2+})
- Severe bradycardia (complete heart block or sinus bradycardia)
- Intrinsic heart disease (IHD, myocarditis)
- Intracranial haemorrhage (especially sub-arachnoid)

Congenital long QT syndromes

- Jervell–Lange-Neilsen syndrome (AR, with deafness)
- Romano–Ward syndrome (AD, normal hearing)

NB: Although amiodarone and sotalol prolong QT interval, polymorphic VT from these drugs is rare.

$$\text{Normal Qtc} = \frac{\text{QT}}{\sqrt{(\text{RR interval})}} = 0.38\text{–}0.46\text{sec (9–11 small squares)}$$

Management

Congenital long QT

- PVT in congenital QT prolongation is adrenergically driven and treatment must include long-term β-blockade (e.g. propranolol).
- Other adjunctive treatment includes pacemaker implantation and left stellate ganglionectomy.
- Patients should be considered for ICD therapy. On occasions decisions may be difficult because of the young age of patients.

Acquired long QT

- The 1° principle is to correct QT prolongation.
- Offending agent(s) must be identified and discontinued immediately.
- PVT in acquired QT prolongation is often 2° to prolonged pauses, which must be avoided.
- All patients should receive IV magnesium (8mmol as a bolus over 2–5min followed by a 60-mmol infusion over 24h)
- Overdrive temporary pacing (either ventricular or atria) terminates the arrhythmia. Continued pacing prevents recurrence of PVT.
- Isoprenaline may be used while preparations are being made for pacing. This accelerates the atrial rate and captures the ventricles. Aim for rate of 110–120bpm.

Reference

1. http://www.brugada.org/

Ventricular tachycardia: drugs

Table 1.5 Dosages of selected antiarrhythmics for the acute treatment of VT

Drug	Loading dose	Maintenance dose
Magnesium sulphate	8mmol (2g) IV over 2–15min (repeat once if necessary)	60mmol/48mL saline at 2–3 mL/hour
Lidocaine	100mg IV over 2min (repeat once if necessary)	4mg/min for 30min 2mg/min for 2h 1–2mg/min for 12–24h
Procainamide	100mg IV over 2min. Repeat every 5min to max. of 1g	2–4mg/min IV infusion 250mg q6h PO
Amiodarone	300mg IV over 60min via central line followed by 900mg IV over 23h, 200mg PO tds × 1 week, then 200mg PO bd × 1 week	200–400mg od IV or PO
Disopyramide	50mg IV over 5min repeated up to max. of 150mg IV 200mg PO	2–5mg/min IV infusion 100–200mg q6h PO
Flecainide	2mg/kg IV over 10min (max. 150mg)	1.5mg/kg IV over 1h then 100–250mcg/kg/h IV for 24h or 100–200mg PO bd
Bretylium	5–10mg/kg (7500mg) IV over 10–15min	1–2mg/min IV infusion

Narrow complex tachyarrhythmias (SVT)

These originate within the atrium or the conduction system above the bundle of His (Fig. 1.9). The important distinction to make is between regular and irregular tachyarrhythmias (see Table 1.6). Features of the different arrhythmias are shown in Table 1.7. The diagnosis not to miss is AVRT (tachycardias involving an accessory pathway) as digoxin and verapamil are contraindicated.

Making the diagnosis

This can be done by careful examination of the 12-lead tachycardia ECG rhythm strip and the effect of inducing AV block.

Examination of ECG: important features to demonstrate are whether rhythm is regular or irregular and to examine for presence/absence and morphology of P waves.

Irregular rhythm:

- No P waves visible:
  - Irregular rhythm with no discernible P-wave (chaotic base line with f-waves): treat as *atrial fibrillation* (see 🕮 p.72).
  - Irregular rhythm with no discernible P wave and 'saw-tooth' flutter waves (especially in inferior leads and V1): treat as *atrial flutter with variable block* (see 🕮 p.78).
- P waves visible:
  - Irregular rhythm with multiple P-wave morphologies (>3) and varying PR intervals: treat as multifocal atrial tachycardia (see 🕮 p.79).

Regular rhythm:

- No P waves visible:
  - No discernible P wave and 'saw-tooth' flutter waves (especially in inferior leads and V1): treat as *atrial flutter with block* (see 🕮 p.78).
- P waves visible:
  - P waves with normal morphology: treat as sinus tachycardia or sinus node re-entry tachycardia.
  - P waves within or distorting the start or end of QRS complex: treat as *AVNRT* (see 🕮 p.81).
  - QRS complex may/may not be followed by P waves with different morphology to sinus P waves: treat as AVRT (see 🕮 p.80).

Induce AV block by vagotonic manoeuvres (e.g. Valsalva, carotid sinus massage) and if unsuccessful, with adenosine. (Adenosine 6mg fast IV bolus (3mg if via central line) followed by 5mL saline flush. If no response try 9mg, 12mg, and then 18mg). Check that the patient has received a therapeutic dose of adenosine (and experienced chest tightness with the injection). Higher doses are required in patients on theophyllines.

- AVNRT and AVRT may terminate with adenosine.
- Transient AV block will unmask AF, flutter, and atrial tachycardia, but will not terminate.

- The exact diagnosis may be left to an experienced cardiologist.
- If there is degeneration of the rhythm into a broad complex tachyarrhythmia and/or haemodynamic compromise, the patient must be electrically cardioverted immediately.

It is important to remember that SVT with previous BBB/aberrancy or AVRT with pre-excitation can present with a broad complex tachycardia. Differentiation from VT may be difficult and if in doubt the patient must be treated as VT until proven otherwise. ECG features to distinguish between the two are outlined on 📖 p.60.

Table 1.6 Features of regular versus irregular tachycardia

Regular tachycardia	Irregular tachycardia
• Sinus tachycardia	• AF
• Atrial flutter (with 2:1 or greater block)	• Atrial flutter with variable block
• AVRT (i.e. with accessory path, e.g. WPW)	• Multi-focal atrial tachycardia
• AVNRT	
• Intra-atrial re-entry tachycardia	

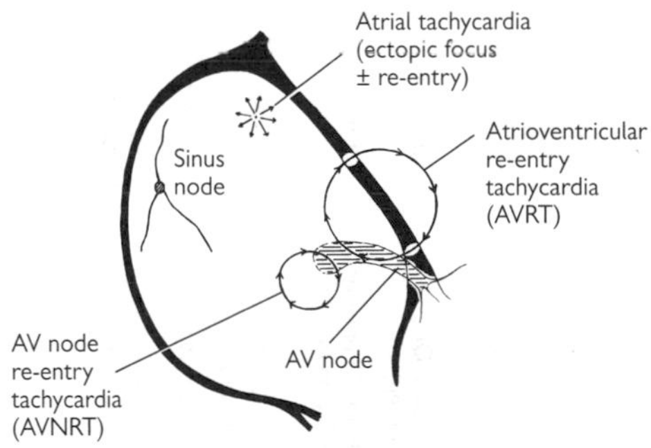

Fig. 1.9 Types of supraventricular tachycardia.

Table 1.7 Differential diagnosis of SVT

Arrhythmia	P wave configuration	Effect of adenosine	Comment
Sinus tachycardia (100–200/minute)	Normal P waves	Transient AV block	
Atrial fibrillation (<200/minute)	*f*-waves. Chaotic	Transient AV block	Irregular rhythm. Adenosine causes rate to slow briefly. Fast AF with broad QRS seen in AVRT (e.g. WPW)
Atrial flutter (75–175/minute)	Flutter waves (saw-tooth) (II,III,aVF and VI)	Transient AV block	Adenosine may convert to AF
AVNRT (140–200/minute)	Inverted buried in QRS (usually not seen)	Terminates	Most common recurrent SVT in adults
AVRT (e.g. WPW or accessory pathway) (150–250/minute)	Inverted after QRS (inferior leads, RP > PR interval)	Terminates	Normal QRS if antegrade down AV node; broad QRS if antegrade down pathway
Atrial tachycardia (Intraatrial re-entry) (100–200/minute)	Abnormal P wave (PR < RP) 2:1 AV block may be seen	Transient AV block	Dig toxicity, lung disease organic heart disease
Multifocal atrial tachycardia (100–130/minute)	Multiple P morphologies P	Transient AV block	Assoc. with lung disease and hypoxaemia

Note: Any of these may be associated with broad QRS complexes either from pre-existing bundle branch block, or rate-related intraventricular conduction abnormality.

Dosages of selected antiarrhythmics for SVT

Table 1.8 Dosages of selected antiarrhythmics for treatment of SVT

Drug	Loading dose	Maintenance dose
Digoxin	IV 0.75–1mg in 50mL saline over 1–2h PO 0.5mg q12h for 2 doses then 0.25mg q12h for 2 days	0.0625–0.25mg od (IV or PO)
Amiodarone	IV 300mg over 60min via central line followed by 900mg IV over 23h *or* PO 200mg tds x 1 week then 200mg PO bd x 1 week	200–400mg od (IV or PO)

Drug	Dosage
Propranolol	IV 1mg over 1min, repeated every 2min up to max. 10mg PO 10–40mg 3–4 times a day
Atenolol	IV 5–10mg by slow injection PO 25–100mg daily
Sotalol	IV 20–60mg by slow injection PO 80–160mg bd
Verapamil	IV 5mg over 2min; repeated every 5min up to max. 20mg PO 40–120mg tds
Procainamide	IV 100mg over 2min; repeated every 5min up to max. 1g PO 250mg q6h
Disopyramide	IV 50mg over 5min; repeated every 5min up to max. 150mg PO 100–200mg q6h
Flecainide	IV 2mg/kg over 10min (max. 150mg) *or* PO 100–200mg bd

Atrial fibrillation (AF): assessment

Presentation

- AF may present with palpitations, chest pain, breathlessness, collapse, or hypotension. Less commonly, it may present with an embolic event (stroke, peripheral embolus) or be asymptomatic. It occurs in 10–15% of patients post MI.
- Look for signs of an underlying cause (see Box 1.15).
- Try to establish the duration of the AF: this will determine the subsequent management (see later sections).

Investigations

These should be directed at looking for a precipitant and underlying heart disease. All patients should have

- ECG:
  - Broad QRS if aberrant conduction
  - ST-T-wave changes may be due to rapid rate, digoxin, or underlying cardiac disease.
- CXR: cardiomegaly, pulmonary oedema, intrathoracic precipitant, valve calcification (MS).
- U&Es: hypokalaemia, renal impairment.
- Cardiac enzymes: ?MI. Small rise after DC shock.
- Thyroid function: thyrotoxicosis may present as AF only.
- Drug levels: especially if taking digoxin.
- Mg^{2+}, Ca^{2+}.
- ABG: if hypoxic, shocked, or ?acidotic.
- Echo ±TOE: for LV function and valve lesions and to exclude intracardiac thrombus prior to version to SR.
- Other investigations depend on suspected precipitant.

Immediate management

Stabilize the patient

- General measures (see 📖 p.56) are as for any patient with an arrhythmia. Obtain venous access. Send bloods (see 📖 p.56) and if possible check the K^+ immediately on an ITU machine.
- Correct any electrolyte abnormality.
- If severe acidosis (pH ≤7.1) give sodium bicarbonate 50mL of 8.4% slowly IV over 20min.
- CSM or IV adenosine may help confirm the diagnosis, revealing chaotic atrial activity. This is particularly helpful in patients with a rate of 150/minute where atrial flutter should always be considered. CSM or adenosine will slow the ventricular rate and reveal flutter waves.
- Does the ECG in AF show intermittent or constant delta waves? This suggests WPW and digoxin and verapamil are contraindicated.

Further management

- Cardiovert to sinus rhythm if appropriate.
- Control the ventricular response rate.
- Try to prevent further episodes of AF.

Box 1.15 Causes of atrial fibrillation

Underlying cardiac disease

- Ischaemic heart disease
- Mitral valve disease
- Hypertension
- Heart failure
- Cardiomyopathy
- Pericarditis
- Endocarditis
- Myocarditis
- Atrial myxoma
- Post-cardiac surgery

Separate intrathoracic pathology

- Pneumonia
- Malignancy (1° or 2°)
- Pulmonary embolus
- Trauma

Metabolic disturbance

- Electrolytes (↓K^+, ↓Mg^{2+})
- Acidosis
- Thyrotoxicosis
- Drugs (alcohol, sympathomimetics)

AF: management

Rate control versus cardioversion

- Important principles required to make a decision are:
  - Are there advantages in immediate cardioversion? (e.g. ongoing ischaemia with fast ventricular rhythm, pulmonary oedema, haemodynamic instability).
  - If the patient is cardioverted will they remain in sinus rhythm? (e.g. underlying sepsis/thyroid disease, large LA, poor LV, MV disease).
  - What are the risks of thromboembolic complications and is anticoagulation required?
- Cardioversion can be achieved chemically or with external defibrillation.

Haemodynamically unstable patients

- All hypotensive patients should undergo external defibrillation using a synchronized shock of initially 200J (see 🕮 p.770).
- Do not attempt to defibrillate hypotensive patients with known chronic AF or a known underlying cause driving a fast ventricular response. Chances of success are very low (e.g. mitral stenosis, severe LV dysfunction, hyperthyroid, septic).
- Relative contraindications to defibrillation need to be weighed against the patient's clinical condition. If possible, aim to optimize clinical picture before cardioversion:
  - Hypokalaemia may be quickly corrected by giving 20mmol over 1h in 100mL normal saline via a central line.
  - If digitoxicity is a possibility, ensure K^+ is 4.5–5mmol/L and give magnesium sulphate 8mmol in 50mL normal saline over 15min, before attempting defibrillation at low energies initially (e.g. 20–50J).
  - AF >48h' duration carries a significant risk of thromboembolic complications unless patient is on long-term anticoagulation and INR has been therapeutic. Consider performing a TOE first.
- The procedure is detailed on 🕮 p.770.
- If DC shock fails initially:
  - Give IV amiodarone 300mg over 60min via a central line (followed by IV infusion of 900–1200mg over 24h).
  - Correct hypokalaemia (aim for K^+ 4.5–5.0mmol/L).
  - Attempt further DC shock.

Haemodynamically stable patients

- The initial aim should be rapid pharmacological rate control followed by a decision regarding restoration of sinus rhythm if appropriate.
- When making a decision regarding restoration of sinus rhythm, current evidence must be taken into account:
  - Management of AF with a rhythm-control strategy alone has no survival benefit over a rate-control strategy as long as high-risk patients are anticoagulated.
  - Rate control is not inferior to rhythm control for prevention of death and cardiovascular morbidity in patients with persistent AF after electrical cardioversion.
  - Patients in sinus rhythm are more likely to report a better 'quality of life' than those in AF.

AF >2 days' duration

- Control ventricular rate using one of, or a combination of, digoxin and class II, III, and IV agents (including: β-blocker, verapamil, diltiazem, or amiodarone). Can be given as IV preparation to achieve rapid rate control followed by oral preparations (see 📖 Table 1.8, p.71 for doses).
- If patient not anticoagulated start LMWH/UFH (UFH: give bolus of 5000U followed by infusion aiming for an aPTT ratio of 2–3) until warfarinization is adequate (aim for an INR of 2–3).
- Sinus rhythm may be restored by class Ia, Ic, and III agents (we recommend amiodarone, sotalol, quinidine, disopyramide, and flecainide).
- If patient needs to be electrically cardioverted, a TOE must be performed to look for intracardiac thrombus or spontaneous contrast (a marker of very sluggish flow). If negative, DC cardioversion may be performed safely. Give bolus of LMWH/UFH before cardioversion if not already on LMWH/UFH.
- Discharge when stable. Consider readmission following 4–6 weeks of warfarin for DC cardioversion.

AF <2 days' duration

- Although risk of embolism in new onset AF is low, we recommend anticoagulation at presentation with LMWH/UFH and subsequently warfarin (see previous section).
- Attempt chemical cardioversion if there are no contraindications to potential agents. Chances of success are much higher with shorter duration of AF. Possible agents include:
  - Flecainide 2mg/kg IV over 10min (max. dose 150mg). Must be avoided in patients with known IHD and/or poor LV function.
  - Disopyramide 50–100mg IV. Ventricular rate may increase and fibrillatory waves coarsen before reverting to sinus rhythm, so load with digoxin/β-blocker/verapamil before giving this.
  - Amiodarone may be used IV/PO. Dosing requires central line and it may take 24–48h for sinus rhythm to be achieved. Amiodarone has relatively poor rate-control properties and may need to be combined with β-blocker or verapamil initially.
- If cardioversion inappropriate or unsuccessful, achieve rate control as indicated in the previous section.
- DC cardioversion can be attempted if rate control is difficult.
  - Discharge when stable. Anticoagulation may be achieved on an outpatient basis if appropriate.

Box 1.16 Management key points: AF

All patients: treat reversible causes (e.g. thyrotoxicosis, chest infection), correct hypokalaemia, hypomagnesaemia.

Haemodynamically unstable patients

DC cardioversion (under GA or sedation).

Haemodynamically stable patients

- *AF >48h duration:*
  - Control ventricular rate (digoxin, β-blockers, verapamil, diltiazem).
  - Consider anticoagulation.
- *AF <48h' duration:*
  - Consider 'pill-in-pocket' strategy for cardioversion.
  - Chemical (e.g. flecainide or amiodarone) or DC cardioversion .
  - If cardioversion is inappropriate or unsuccessful: rate control.
  - Consider anticoagulation.

AF: rate control

Controlling the ventricular response rate

- Check that there is no history of WPW and that no delta waves are visible on the ECG.
- We recommend β-blockers and calcium channel blockers (verapamil and diltiazem) as first-line agents for rate control. They both have the advantage of maintaining ventricular rate during exertion. If single agent is not adequate either (1) combine β-blockers and calcium channel blockers (if BP adequate) or (2) add digoxin or amiodarone.
- Digoxin is an alternative drug and can equally be used as first-line agent. Patients should initially be given a full loading dose. The maintenance dose varies (0.0625–0.25mg od) depending on body mass, renal function, age, etc. Digoxin is poor at controlling ventricular rate during exertion.
- In patients with poor LV function, β-blockers and calcium channel blockers may not be appropriate, inducing heart failure and hypotension. Digoxin with or without amiodarone is a good combination (amiodarone will increase the plasma digoxin level so halve the maintenance digoxin dose).
- Other drugs that may be tried to control the ventricular rate are listed in 📖 Table 1.8, p.71.
- If controlling ventricular rate is difficult, consider alternative diagnosis, in particular MAT. Digoxin may make the arrhythmia worse (see 📖 p.79).

Long-term management

- Look for causes (see 📖 Box 1.14, p.65) and arrange an Echo.
- Patients successfully cardioverted acutely should be commenced on a prophylaxis regimen using class Ia, Ic, or III agents (e.g. sotalol, amiodarone, flecainide, propafenone). The choice of agent must be individualized:
  - Lone AF: use class Ic agents first, followed by class III or Ia if it fails.
  - Poor LV function: amiodarone is the agent of choice.
  - IHD: class III agents and β-blockers (prevent ischaemia and as a result ischaemia-driven AF) are agents of choice.
- If subsequently considered to be at low risk, treatment may be stopped at 1 month. Seek cardiac opinion if in doubt.
- Patients cardioverted electively should remain on warfarin and rhythm prophylaxis for 1 month pending outpatient review.
- Patients with paroxysmal AF require long-term therapy to try to maintain sinus rhythm (class III, class Ic, and class Ia). Digoxin only controls the ventricular rate and does not prevent AF. These patients may need long-term anticoagulation depending on:
  - Frequency and length of AF paroxysms
  - Presence of underlying structural, cardiac abnormalities, and
  - Other systemic risk factors of thromboembolic complications.

Atrial flutter

- This is rarely seen in the absence of underlying coronary disease, valve disease, 1° myocardial disease, pericarditis, or thyrotoxicosis.
- The atrial rate is 280–320/minute and atrial activity is seen as flutter waves in the inferior leads and V1 on the ECG.
- The AV node conduction is slower (most commonly 2:1 block, sometimes 3:1 or 4:1) and this determines the ventricular rate.
- Vagotonic manoeuvres and adenosine increase the AV block and reveal the flutter waves but only very rarely terminate the arrhythmia.

Management

- DC cardioversion is the therapy of choice as flutter can be resistant to pharmacological therapy.
  - Lower energies are needed (20–100J).
  - If flutter has been present >48h perform TOE and then cardiovert with LMWH/UFH cover (as for AF).
- Medical management:
  - Pharmacological agents recommended are similar to AF. Rate control and reversion rates can be low.
  - Digoxin, verapamil, and β-blockers can all be used to slow ventricular response. IV preparations can be used for more rapid action. The overall response can be poor. IV verapamil (2.5–5mg over 1–2min repeated every 5min to a maximum dose of 20mg) will slow the response rate and occasionally restore sinus rhythm in 15–20% of patients.
  - Ibutilide and dofetilide have been reported to have reversion rates of 50% and 70% respectively. Alternative agents are amiodarone, flecainide, quinidine, and procainamide.
  - NB: Class Ia drugs can enhance AV conduction and must always be used after rate control has been achieved.
- Flutter ablation can be performed in resistant and/or recurrent atrial flutter. Discuss with cardiac electrophysiologist.

Multifocal atrial tachycardia (MAT)

- Commonly occurs in critically ill patients especially with obstructive airways disease who may be hypoxaemic and hypercapnic. Theophylline toxicity is an important factor.
- Characterized by at least three different P-wave morphologies with varying PP and PR intervals. Atrial nodal rate is 120–180 with 1:1 conduction.
- Rapid regular rhythm may be difficult to differentiate from AF. However, differentiation is very important as MAT is not responsive to DC cardioversion and is exacerbated by digoxin.

Management

- The only true effective *treatment is to treat the underlying illness*. If associated with lung disease aim to improve P_aO_2 and P_aCO_2.
- Electrolyte abnormalities must be corrected. High-dose Mg^{2+} IV may restore sinus rhythm (15g over 5h).
- There is increasing evidence from small trials that metoprolol is the most effective therapy. Use cautiously IV. However, most patients with MAT and COPD may not tolerate even a cardioselective β-blocker.
- Verapamil is an alternative agent (5mg IV over 2min and repeated every 5min up to a maximum of 20mg; then 40–120mg PO tds) if the ventricular rate is consistently over >100/minute and the patient is symptomatic.
- DC shock and digoxin are ineffective.

Accessory pathway tachycardia (AV re-entrant tachycardia, AVRT)

- The three most common accessory pathways that produce paroxysmal tachycardias are described in 'Types of accessory pathways'.
- During re-entry tachycardia, the delta wave is lost as the accessory pathway is only conducting retrogradely.
- AF may produce very rapid ventricular rates as the accessory path has rapid antegrade conduction (unlike the AV node). The ECG will show the delta wave in some or all of the QRS complexes.

Management

- DC cardioversion should be used early if the tachycardia is poorly tolerated.
- Class Ia, Ic, and II agents are suitable for chemical cardioversion. We recommend IV flecainide or disopyramide. β-blocker may also be given especially if other agents are contraindicated (see 📖 Table 1.8, p.71.).
- Digoxin and verapamil should be avoided as they may accelerate conduction down the accessory pathway. Amiodarone is dangerous unless given very slowly (e.g. 300mg IV over 2–4h).
- If recurrent symptoms, patient should be referred for electrophysiological assessment and RF ablation. Seek specialist advice for long-term medical management.

Types of accessory pathways

Kent bundle (Wolff–Parkinson–White syndrome)

- ECG: short PR interval and delta wave:
  - Type A — Positive δ-wave in V1–V6
Negative in lead I
(Posterior left atrial pathway)
  - Type B — Biphasic or negative δ wave in V1–V3
Positive in lead I
(Lateral right atrial pathway)
  - Concealed — No δ-wave visible as pathway only, conducts retrogradely.
- Associated with Ebstein's, HOCM, mitral valve prolapse.

Mahaim pathway (rare)

Pathway connects AV node to right bundle resulting in a tachycardia with LBBB morphology.

James pathway (Lown–Ganong–Levine syndrome) (rare)

- Short PR interval but no delta wave.
- Pathway connects atria to AV node, His, or fascicles.

Atrioventricular-nodal re-entry tachycardia (AVNRT)

- AVNRT occurs 2° to a micro re-entrant circuit in the AV node.
- General principles are as outlined on 📖 p.56 (HR) >120bpm apply.
- Rate control can be achieved with (IV and PO) digoxin, β-blockers, and calcium channel blockers. β-blockers and calcium channel blockers can also promote reversion into sinus rhythm.
- Class Ic and Ia agents (we recommend flecainide) can also be used for chemical cardioversion and maintenance of sinus rhythm long term.
- If arrhythmia is resistant to treatment consider electrical cardioversion.
- Patients with recurrent symptoms should be referred for electrophysiological assessment and possible RF ablation.

Bradyarrhythmias: general approach

- Ask specifically about previous cardiac disease, palpitations, blackouts, dizziness, chest pain, symptoms of heart failure, and recent drugs.
- Examine carefully, noting the BP, JVP waveform (?cannon waves), heart sounds and murmurs, and signs of heart failure.

Investigations

• 12-lead ECG and rhythm strip:	Look specifically for the relationship between P-waves and QRS complex. A long rhythm strip is sometimes necessary to detect complete heart block if atrial and ventricular rates are similar
• Blood tests:	FBC, biochemistry, glucose (urgently) Ca^{2+}, Mg^{2+} (especially if on diuretics) Biochemical markers of cardiac injury
• Where appropriate:	Blood cultures, CRP, ESR Thyroid function tests Drug levels Arterial blood gases
• CXR:	Heart size ?signs of pulmonary oedema

Management

Haemodynamically unstable patients

- Give O_2 via facemask if the patient is hypoxic on air.
- Keep NBM until definitive therapy has been started to reduce the risk of aspiration in case of cardiac arrest or when the patient lies supine for temporary wire insertion.
- Secure peripheral venous access.
- Bradyarrhythmias causing severe *haemodynamic compromise* (cardiac arrest, asystole, SBP <90mmHg, severe pulmonary oedema, evidence of cerebral hypoperfusion) require immediate treatment and temporary pacing (the technique is described on 🕮 p.758).
  - Give atropine 1mg IV (Min-I-Jet®) bolus; repeat if necessary up to a maximum of 3mg.
  - Give isoprenaline 0.2mg IV (Min-I-Jet®) if there is a delay in pacing and the patient remains unstable. Set up an infusion (1mg in 100mL bag normal saline starting at 1mL/minute titrating to HR).
  - Set up external pacing system if available and arrange for transfer to a screening room for transvenous pacing. If fluoroscopy is not available, 'blind' transvenous pacing using a balloon-tipped pacing wire may be attempted.
- Bradycardia in shock is a poor prognostic sign. Look for a source of blood loss and begin aggressive resuscitation with fluids and inotropes.

Haemodynamically stable patients

- Admit to CCU with continuous ECG monitoring.
- Keep atropine drawn up and ready in case of acute deterioration.
- Does the patient require a temporary wire immediately? It may be of value to have appropriate central venous access (femoral or internal

jugular vein) in place in case of the need for emergency temporary wire insertion.
- Refer the patient to a cardiologist.

Box 1.17 External cardiac pacing

- In emergencies, external cardiac pacing may be used first but this is painful for the patient and is only a temporary measure until more 'definitive' transvenous pacing wire can be inserted.
- External cardiac pacing is useful as a standby in patients post MI when the risks of prophylactic transvenous pacing after thrombolysis are high.
- Haemodynamically stable patients with anterior MI and bifasicular block may be managed simply by application of the external pacing electrodes and having the pulse generator ready if necessary.
- Familiarize yourself with the machine in your hospital when you have some time: a cardiac arrest is not the time to read the manual for the apparatus!

Sinus bradycardia or junctional rhythm

(Heart rate <50/minute.)

Causes

- Young athletic individual
- Drugs (β-blockers, morphine)
- Hypothyroidism
- Hypothermia
- ↑vagal tone:
  - Vasovagal attack
  - Nausea or vomiting
  - Carotid sinus hypersensitivity
  - Acute MI (especially inferior)
- Ischaemia or infarction of the sinus node
- Chronic degeneration of sinus or AV nodes or atria
- Cholestatic jaundice
- Raised intracranial pressure.

Management

- If hypotensive or pre-syncopal treat as on 📖 p.82:
  - Atropine 600mcg–3mg IV bolus repeating as necessary.
  - Isoprenaline 0.5–10mcg/min IV infusion.
  - Temporary pacing.
  - Avoid and take steps to correct precipitants (see 'Causes').
  - Stop any drugs that may suppress the sinus or AV nodes.
- Long-term treatment:
  - If all possible underlying causes removed and if symptomatic bradycardia remains, refer for permanent pacing.
  - Consider Holter monitoring in patients with possible episodic bradycardia. R–R intervals >2.5sec may require permanent pacing, especially if associated with symptoms.

Intraventricular conduction disturbances

Common causes of bundle branch block

- Ischaemic heart disease
- Hypertensive heart disease
- Valve disease (especially aortic stenosis)
- Conduction system fibrosis (Lev and Lenègre syndromes)
- Myocarditis or endocarditis
- Cardiomyopathies
- Cor pulmonale (RBBB) (acute or chronic)
- Trauma or post-cardiac surgery
- Neuromuscular disorders (myotonic dystrophy)
- Polymyositis.

Management

- General principles (see 📖 p.82) apply.
- Interventricular conduction disturbances on their own do not require temporary pacing. However, when associated with haemodynamic disturbance or progression to higher levels of block (even if intermittent), insertion of a transvenous pacing wire must be considered. The need for longer-term pacing is dependent on the persistence of symptoms and underlying cause. Consult a cardiologist. See 📖 p.758 for situations where temporary pacing is indicated.

Types of atrioventricular (AV) conduction block

First-degree heart block

Prolongation of the PR interval (>0.22sec, >5 small squares)

Second-degree heart block

- ***Mobitz type 1 (Wenckebach):*** progressive increase in PR interval with intermittent complete AV block (P wave not conducted).
- ***Mobitz type 2:*** the PR interval is constant but there is intermittent failure to conduct the P wave. Often occurs in the presence of broad QRS complex.
- ***2:1, 3:1 etc.:*** as in Mobitz type 2, PR interval is constant but every second (in 2:1) or third (in 3:1) P wave is not conducted on a regular basis.

Third-degree (complete) heart block

Complete AV dissociation. If the P and QRS rates are similar, a long rhythm strip or exercise (to speed up the atrial rate) will help demonstrate dissociation.

Causes

- Associated with acute infarction or ischaemia
- Drugs (β-blockers, digitalis, Ca^{2+}-blockers)
- Conduction system fibrosis (Lev and Lenègre syndromes)
- ↑vagal tone
- Trauma or following cardiac surgery
- Hypothyroidism (rarely thyrotoxicosis)
- Hypothermia
- Hyperkalaemia
- Hypoxia
- Valvular disease (aortic stenosis, incompetence, endocarditis)
- Myocarditis (diphtheria, rheumatic fever, viral, Chagas disease)
- Associated with neuromuscular disease, i.e. myotonic dystrophy
- Collagen vascular disease (SLE, RA, scleroderma)
- Cardiomyopathies (haemochromotosis, amyloidosis)
- Granulomatous disease (sarcoid)
- Congenital heart block
- Congenital heart disease (ASD, Ebstein's, PDA).

Management

- Principles are listed on 📖 p.82.
- In summary, all symptomatic patients must have temporary pacing. The higher the level of block (irrespective of symptoms) the greater the progression to complete heart block and/or chances of asystole.
- See 📖 p.758 for situations when temporary pacing is indicated.

Pulmonary oedema: assessment

Presentation

- Acute breathlessness, cough, frothy blood-stained (pink) sputum
- Collapse, cardiac arrest, or shock
- Associated features may reflect underlying cause:
  - Chest pain or palpitations: ?IHD/MI, arrhythmia
  - Preceding history of dyspnoea on exertion: ?IHD, poor LV
  - Oliguria, haematuria: ?acute renal failure (see 🕮 p.282)
  - Seizures, signs of intracranial bleed.

Causes

A diagnosis of pulmonary oedema or 'heart failure' is not adequate. An underlying cause must be sought in order to direct treatment appropriately. These may be divided into

- ↑pulmonary capillary pressure (hydrostatic)
- ↑pulmonary capillary permeability
- ↓intravascular oncotic pressure.

Often a combination of factors are involved (e.g. pneumonia, hypoxia, cardiac ischaemia) see 🕮 Box 1.19, p.89.

The main differential diagnosis is acute (infective) exacerbation of COPD (previous history, quiet breath sounds ± wheeze, fewer crackles). It may be difficult to differentiate the two clinically.

Principles of management

1. Stabilize the patient: relieve distress and begin definitive treatment.
2. Look for an underlying cause.
3. Address haemodynamic and respiratory issues.
4. Optimize and introduce long-term therapy.

Initial rapid assessment

- If the patient is very unwell (e. g. unable to speak, hypoxic, SBP <100mmHg), introduce stabilizing measures and begin treatment immediately before detailed examination and investigations (Box 1.18).
- If the patient is stable and/or if there is doubt as to the diagnosis, give O_2 and diuretic, but await the outcome of clinical examination and CXR before deciding on definitive treatment.

Urgent investigations for all patients

- ECG: sinus tachycardia most common. ?any cardiac arrhythmia (AF, SVT, VT). ?evidence of acute ST change (STEMI, NSTEMI, UA). ?evidence of underlying heart disease (LVH, p mitrale).
- CXR: to confirm the diagnosis, look for interstitial shadowing, enlarged hila, prominent upper lobe vessels, pleural effusion, and Kerley B lines. Cardiomegaly may or may not be present. Also exclude pneumothorax, pulmonary embolus (oligaemic lung fields), and consolidation.
- ABG: typically ↓P_aO_2. P_aCO_2 levels may be ↓(hyperventilation) or ↑ depending on severity of pulmonary oedema. Pulse oximetry may be inaccurate if peripherally shut down.

- U&Es: ?pre-existing renal impairment. Regular K^+ measurements (once on IV diuretics).
- FBC ?anaemia or leukocytosis indicating the precipitant.
- Echo: as soon as practical to assess LV function, valve abnormalities, VSD, or pericardial effusion.

Box 1.18 Investigations for patients with pulmonary oedema

All patients should have:
- FBC, U&Es, CRP
- Serial biochemical markers of myocardial injury (CK, CK-MB, troponins)
- LFTs, albumin, total protein
- ECG
- CXR
- Echo (± TOE)
- ABG.

Where appropriate consider:
- Septic screen (sputum, urine, blood cultures)
- Holter monitor (?arrhythmias)
- Coronary angiography (?IHD)
- Right and left heart catheter (if Echo unable to provide adequate information on pressures, shunts, valve disease)
- Endomyocardial biopsy (myocarditis, infiltration)
- MUGA scan
- Cardiopulmonary exercise test with an assessment of peak O_2 consumption.

Pulmonary oedema: causes

Look for an underlying cause for pulmonary oedema (Box 1.19).

Box 1.19 Causes of pulmonary oedema

Increased pulmonary capillary pressure (hydrostatic)

• ↑Left atrial pressure	• Mitral valve disease • Arrhythmia (e.g. AF) with pre-existing mitral valve disease • Left atrial myxoma
• ↑LVEDP	• Ischaemia • Arrhythmia • Aortic valve disease • Cardiomyopathy • Uncontrolled hypertension • Pericardial constriction • Fluid overload • High output states (anaemia, thyrotoxicosis, Paget's, AV fistula, beri-beri) • Reno-vascular disease
• ↑Pulmonary venous pressure	• L → R shunt (e.g. VSD) • Veno-occlusive disease
• Neurogenic	• Intracranial haemorrhage • Cerebral oedema • Post ictal

↑ pulmonary capillary permeability

• Acute lung injury	• ARDS, see 📖 p.22
• ↓intravascular oncotic pressure	

↓ intravascular oncotic pressure

• Hypoalbuminaemia	• ↑losses (e.g. nephrotic syndrome, liver failure) • ↓production (e.g. sepsis) • Dilution (e.g. crystalloid transfusion)

NB: the critical LA pressure for hydrostatic oedema = serum albumin (g/L) × 0.57.

Pulmonary oedema: management 1

Stabilize the patient

- Patients with acute pulmonary oedema should initially be continuously monitored and managed where full resuscitation facilities are available.
- Sit the patient up in bed.
- Give 60–100% O_2 by facemask (unless contraindicated, COPD).
- If the patient is severely distressed, summon the 'on-call' anaesthetist and inform ITU. If dyspnoea cannot be significantly improved by acute measures (see following text) the patient may require CPAP or mechanical ventilation.
- Treat any haemodynamically unstable arrhythmia—urgent synchronized DC shock may be required.
- Give:
  - Diamorphine 2.5–5mg IV (caution abnormal ABGs)
  - Metoclopramide 10mg IV
  - Furosemide 40–120mg slow IV injection.
- Secure venous access and send blood for urgent U&Es, FBC, and cardiac enzymes (including troponin).
- Unless thrombolysis is indicated take ABG.
- If the SBP is ≥90mmHg and the patient does not have aortic stenosis:
  - Give sublingual GTN spray (2 puffs)
  - Start IV GTN infusion 1–10mg/hour, increase the infusion rate every 15–20min, titrating against BP (aiming to keep SBP ~100mmHg).
- If the SBP is <90mmHg treat patient as cardiogenic shock (see 🕮 p.42).
- Insert a urinary catheter to monitor urine output.
- Repeat ABG and K^+ if the clinical condition deteriorates/fails to improve, or after 2h if there is improvement and the original sample was abnormal.
- Monitor pulse, BP, respiratory rate, O_2 saturation with a pulse oximeter (if an accurate reading can be obtained) and urine output.

Further management

The subsequent management of the patient is aimed at ensuring adequate ventilation/gas exchange, ensuring haemodynamic stability, and correcting any reversible precipitins of acute pulmonary oedema.

- ***Assess the patient's respiratory function:***
  - Does the patient require respiratory support? p.192
- ***Assess the patient's haemodynamic status:***
  - Is the patient in shock? p.9
- ***Look for an underlying cause*** p.89
- ***Conditions that require specific treatment:***
  - Acute aortic and mitral regurgitation p.114
  - Diastolic left ventricular dysfunction p.40
  - Fluid overload p.95
  - Renal failure p.284
  - Severe anaemia
  - Hypoproteinaemia p.95.

Pulmonary oedema: management 2

If the patient remains unstable and/or deteriorates take the following steps:

Assess the patient's respiratory function

- Wheeze may be caused by interstitial pulmonary oedema. If there is a history of asthma, give nebulized salbutamol (2.5–5mg), nebulized ipratropium bromide (500mcg), and hydrocortisone (200mg) IV. Consider commencing aminophylline infusion. This will relieve bronchospasm, as well as 'off-load' by systemic vasodilatation (see 📖 p.181). However, it may worsen tachycardia and it can be arrhythmogenic and lower K^+ (supplement to ensure K^+ 4–5mmol/L).
- Indications for further respiratory support include:
  - Patient exhaustion or continuing severe breathlessness
  - Persistent P_aO_2 <8kPa
  - Rising P_aCO_2
  - Persistent or worsening acidosis (pH <7.2).
- CPAP: this may be tried for cooperative patients, who can protect their airway, have adequate respiratory muscle strength, and are not hypotensive. The positive pressure reduces venous return to the heart and may compromise BP.
- Endotracheal intubation and mechanical ventilation may be required and some positive end expiratory pressure (PEEP) should be used (see 📖 p.781).
- Discuss the patient with the on-call anaesthetist or ITU team early.

Assess the patient's haemodynamic status

It is important to distinguish between cardiogenic and non-cardiogenic pulmonary oedema, as further treatment is different between the two groups. This may be difficult clinically. A PA (Swan–Ganz) catheter must be inserted if the patient's condition will allow.

- Non-cardiogenic pulmonary oedema occurs when the hydrostatic pressure within the capillary system overcomes the plasma oncotic pressure. In patients with hypoalbuminaemia this will occur at PCWP <15mmHg. The critical PCWP may be estimated by serum albumin (g/L) × 0.57. Thus a patient with a serum albumin of 15g/L will develop hydrostatic pulmonary oedema at a LA pressure of 8mmHg; a serum albumin of 30g/L will require an LA pressure of >17mmHg, etc.
- Cardiogenic pulmonary oedema is often associated with significant systemic hypotension or low output states. Contributing factors include conditions where there is 'mechanical' impairment to forward flow (e.g. valvular heart disease (especially if acute) VSD) or severe myocardial disease (large MI, myocarditis, cardiomyopathy).
- The gradient between PA diastolic pressure and PCWP (PAD–PCWP) is generally <5mmHg in cardiogenic and >5mmHg in non-cardiogenic pulmonary oedema (e.g. ARDS).
- The pulse and BP are most commonly elevated due to circulating catecholamines and over activity of the renin–angiotensin system. Examination reveals sweating, cool 'shut-down' peripheries, high pulse volume (assess carotid or femoral pulses).

Management (Box 1.20)

The general approach involves combination of diuretics, vasodilators ± inotropes. Patients may be divided into two groups:

- Patients in shock (with SBP <100mmHg) (see 📖 p.93)
- Haemodynamically stable patients with SBP >100mmHg (see 📖 p.93).

Box 1.20 Management key points: pulmonary oedema

- Sit the patient up in bed.
- O_2.
- IV diamorphine (+metoclopramide).
- IV furosemide.
- IV GTN infusion (titrate according to BP).
- Look for and treat underlying cause (e.g. ischaemia, arrhythmia).
- Consider CPAP or mechanical ventilation if dyspnoea is not improved by acute measures.

Pulmonary oedema: management 3

Patients with SBP <100mmHg

- The patient is in incipient (or overt) shock. The most common aetiology is cardiogenic shock but remember non-cardiogenic causes (e.g. ARDS, septic shock, see 🕮 p.310).
- Optimal monitoring and access: central line ± PA catheter (Swan–Ganz), urinary catheter, arterial line (monitoring BP and ABGs). Internal jugular lines are preferable as the risk of pneumothorax is lower.
- Ensure patient is not under filled using PCWP as a guide (<10mmHg) (mistaken diagnosis, e.g. septic shock from bilateral pneumonia).
- Is there a mechanical cause that may require emergency surgery?
  - Arrange an urgent Echo to rule out:
    —VSD and acute MR in all patients with recent MI with/without new murmur (see 🕮 p.32)
    —Prosthetic heart valve dysfunction (e.g. dehiscence, infection) or pre-existing native aortic or mitral disease that may require surgery.
  - Discuss patient early on with cardiologist/cardiac surgeon.

The choice of inotropic agent depends on the clinical condition of the patient and, to some extent, the underlying diagnosis.

- Treatment of septic shock is discussed elsewhere (see 🕮 p.316).
- SBP 80–100mmHg and cool peripheries: start dobutamine infusion at 5mcg/kg/min, increasing by 2.5mcg/kg/min every 10–15min to a maximum of 20mcg/kg/min until BP >100mmHg. This may be combined with dopamine (2.5–5mcg/kg/min). However, tachycardia and/or hypotension 2° to peripheral vasodilation may limit its effectiveness. Phosphodiesterase inhibitors (enoximone or milrinone) should be considered where dobutamine fails.
- SBP <80mmHg: give a slow IV bolus of adrenaline (2–5mL of 1 in 10 000 adrenaline solution Min-I-Jet®), equivalent to 0.2–0.5mg adrenaline, and repeat as necessary.
  - Dopamine at doses of >2.5mcg/kg/min has a pressor action in addition to direct and indirect inotropic effects and may be used at higher doses (10–20mcg/kg/min) if the BP remains low. However, it tends to raise the pulmonary capillary filling pressure further and should be combined with vasodilators (e.g. nitroprusside or hydralazine) once the BP is restored (see next section). Beware of arrhythmias at these doses.
  - Adrenaline infusion may be preferred to high-dose dopamine as an alternative inotrope. Once the BP is restored (>100mmHg), vasodilators such as nitroprusside/hydralazine or GTN infusion should be added to counteract the pressor effects. Adrenaline can be combined with dobutamine and/or a phosphodiesterase inhibitor, especially in the context of a poor ventricle.
- Intra-aortic balloon counter pulsation should also be used with/without inotropes in the context of a potentially reversible cause for the pulmonary oedema and shock (e.g. ongoing myocardial ischaemia, VSD, acute MR) (see 🕮 p.34).
- Further doses of diuretic may be given.

Patients with SBP ≥100mmHg

- Further doses of diuretic may be given—furosemide 40–80mg IV q3–4h or as a continuous infusion (20–80mg/hour).
- Continue the GTN infusion, increasing the infusion rate every 15–20min up to 10mg/hour, titrating against BP (aiming to keep SBP ~100mmHg).
- ACEIs can be used if BP is adequate and there are no other known contraindications (e.g. RAS, renal failure). Arteriolar vasodilators (nitroprusside or hydralazine) may also be added in or used instead of GTN (± ACEI) in patients with adequate BP. Arterial pressure should be monitored continuously via an arterial line to prevent inadvertent hypotension.

Long-term management

- Unless a contraindication exists, start an ACEI, increasing the dose to as near the recommended maximal dose as possible. In the context of LV impairment, ACEIs have significant prognostic benefit.
- If ACEIs are contraindicated or not tolerated, consider the use of hydralazine and long-acting oral nitrate in combination.
- If the patient is already on high doses of diuretics and ACEIs consider the addition of spironolactone (25–50mg) (NB: monitor renal function and serum potassium).
- In the context of stable patients (no clinical features of failure) and poor LV function β-blockers have significant mortality and some symptomatic benefit (NB: start at a very small dose and increase gradually every 2 weeks with regular monitoring). Bisoprolol, carvedilol, and metoprolol can all be used.
- Ensure all arrhythmias are treated (see 🕮 p.56).
- Digoxin can be used for symptomatic improvement.
- Consider multi-site pacing (biventricular) in the context of severe LV dysfunction, broad QRS complex ± MR on Echo.
- Patients with AF or poor LV function should be considered for long-term anticoagulation.
- Patients <60 years with severe irreversible LV dysfunction and debilitating symptoms must be considered for cardiac transplantation.

Pulmonary oedema: specific conditions

Diastolic LV dysfunction

- This typically occurs in elderly hypertensive patients with LV hypertrophy, where there is impaired relaxation of the ventricle in diastole. There is marked hypertension, pulmonary oedema, and normal or only mild systolic LV impairment.
- With tachycardia, diastolic filling time shortens. As the ventricle is 'stiff' in diastole, LA pressure is ↑ and pulmonary oedema occurs (exacerbated by AF as filling by atrial systole is lost).
- Treatment involves control of hypertension with IV nitrates (and/or nitroprusside), calcium blockers (verapamil or nifedipine), and even selective β-blockers (e.g. carvedilol).

Fluid overload

- Standard measures are usually effective.
- In extreme circumstances venesection may be necessary.
- Check the patient is not anaemic (Hb ≥10g/dL). Remove 500mL blood via a cannula in a large vein and repeat if necessary.
- If anaemic (e.g. renal failure) and acutely unwell, consider dialysis (see 🕮 p.282).

Known (or unknown) renal failure

- Unless the patient is permanently anuric, large doses of IV furosemide may be required (up to 1g given at 4mg/minute) in addition to standard treatment.
- If such treatment fails, or the patient is known to be anuric, dialysis will be required.
- In patients not known to have renal failure, an underlying cause should be sought (see 🕮 Box 4.2, p.287).

Anaemia

- Cardiac failure may be worsened or precipitated by the presence of significant anaemia. Symptoms may be improved in the long term by correcting this anaemia.
- Generally transfusion is unnecessary with Hb >9g/dL unless there is a risk of an acute bleed. Treatment of pulmonary oedema will result in haemoconcentration and a 'rise' in the Hb.
- If the anaemia is thought to be exacerbating pulmonary oedema, ensure that an adequate diuresis is obtained prior to transfusion. Give slow transfusion (3–4h per unit) of packed cells, with IV furosemide 20–40mg before each unit.

Hypoproteinaemia

- The critical LA pressure at which hydrostatic pulmonary oedema occurs is influenced by the serum albumin and approximates to [serum albumin concentration (g/L) × 0.57] (see 🕮 p.327).
- Treatment involves diuretics, cautious albumin replacement, spironolactone (if there is 2° hyperaldosteronism), and treatment of the underlying cause for hypoproteinaemia.

Infective endocarditis (IE)

Clinical presentation of IE is highly variable and dependent on a combination of intracardiac pathology, evolution of the infection, and possible extra cardiac involvement. Presentation can be insidious as in streptococcal infections with striking constitutional symptoms, such as *S. aureus*.

Presenting features can include the following:

- ***Symptoms and signs of the infection:*** these include malaise, anorexia, weight loss, fever, rigors, and night sweats. Long-standing infection produces anaemia, clubbing, and splenomegaly
- ***Cardiac manifestations of the infection:*** congestive cardiac failure, palpitations, tachycardia, new murmur, pericarditis, or AV block.
- ***Symptoms and signs due to immune complex deposition:***
  - Skin: petechiae (most common), splinter haemorrhages, Osler's nodes (small tender nodules (pulp infarcts) on hands and feet, which persist forh to days), Janeway lesions (non-tender erythematous and/or haemorrhagic areas on the palms and soles).
  - Eye: Roth spots (oval retinal haemorrhages with a pale centre located near the optic disc), conjunctival splinter haemorrhages, retinal flame haemorrhages.
  - Renal: microscopic haematuria, glomerulonephritis, and renal impairment
  - Cerebral: toxic encephalopathy.
  - Musculoskeletal: arthralgia or arthritis.

Complications of the infection

- *Local effects:*
  - Valve destruction results in a new or changing murmur. This may result in progressive heart failure and pulmonary oedema.
  - A new harsh pansystolic murmur and acute deterioration may be due to perforation of the interventricular septum or rupture of a sinus of Valsalva aneurysm into the right ventricle.
  - High degree AV block (2–4% of IE) occurs with intracardiac extension of infection into the interventricular septum (e.g. from aortic valve endocarditis).
  - Intracardiac abscess may be seen with any valve infection (25–50% of aortic endocarditis, 1–5% of mitral but rarely with tricuspid) and is most common in prosthetic valve endocarditis.
- *Embolic events:*
  - Septic emboli are seen in 20–45% of patients and may involve any circulation (brain, limbs, coronary, kidney, or spleen); pulmonary emboli with tricuspid endocarditis.
  - 40–45% of patients who have had an embolic event will have another.
  - The risk depends on the organism (most common with G–ve infections, *S. aureus or Candida)* and the presence and size of vegetations (emboli in 30% of patients with no vegetation on Echo, 40% with vegetations <5mm, and 65% with vegetations >5mm).

Ask specifically for a history of dental work, infections, surgery, IV drug use, or instrumentation, which may have led to a bacteraemia. Examine for any potential sources of infection, especially teeth or skin lesions. Risk factors for endocarditis are shown in Box 1.21.

Box 1.21 Risk factors for IE

- ***High risk:***
  - Prosthetic valves
  - Previous bacterial endocarditis
  - Aortic valve disease
  - Mitral regurgitation or mixed mitral disease
  - Cyanotic congenital heart disease
  - Patent ductus arteriosis
  - Uncorrected L → R shunt
  - Intracardiac and systemic–pulmonary shunts
- ***Moderate risk:***
  - MVP with regurgitation or valve thickening
  - Isolated mitral stenosis
  - Tricuspid valve disease
  - Pulmonary stenosis
  - Hypertrophic cardiomyopathy
  - Bicuspid aortic valve disease
  - Degenerative valve disease in the elderly
  - Mural thrombus (e.g. post infarction)
- ***Low risk:***
  - MVP without regurgitation
  - Tricuspid regurgitation without structural valve abnormality
  - Isolated ASD
  - Surgically corrected L → R shunt with no residual shunt
  - Calcification of MV annulus
  - Ischaemic heart disease and/or previous CABG
  - Permanent pacemaker
  - Atrial myxoma.

Other predisposing factors

- Arterial prostheses or arteriovenous fistulae
- Recurrent bacteraemia (e.g. IV drug users, severe periodontal disease, colon carcinoma)
- Conditions predisposing to infections (e.g. diabetes, renal failure, alcoholism, immunosuppression)
- Recent central line.

In many cases no obvious risk factor is identified.

IE: diagnosis

Clinical features can be non-specific and diagnosis difficult. A high index of suspicion must be maintained if patients present with unexplained fever, a predisposing cardiac lesion, bacteraemia, and embolic phenomenon.

The Duke classification has been devised to help diagnosis:

- *Definite endocarditis:* 2 major criteria, or 1 major and 3 minor criteria, or 5 minor criteria.
- *Possible endocarditis:* findings which fall short of definite endocarditis but are not rejected.
- *Rejected diagnosis:* firm alternative diagnosis, or sustained resolution of clinical features with <4 days of antibiotic therapy.

Major criteria

Positive blood culture

- Typical microorganism for IE from two separate blood cultures
- Persistently positive blood culture.

Evidence of endocardial involvement

- Positive echocardiogram:
  - Oscillating intracardiac mass (vegetation)
  - Abscess
  - New partial dehiscence of prosthetic valve
  - New valve regurgitation.

Minor criteria

- Predisposing condition or drug use.
- Fever >38°C.
- Vascular phenomena: arterial emboli, septic pulmonary infarcts, mycotic aneurysm, intracranial and conjunctival haemorrhage, Janeway lesions.
- Immunologic phenomena: glomerulonephritis, Osler's nodes, Roth spots, rheumatoid factor.
- Microbiological evidence: positive blood cultures but not meeting major criteria or serological evidence of organism consistent with IE.
- Echo: positive for IE but not meeting major criteria.

Box 1.22 Common organisms in IE

• 50–60%	Streptococci (especially *Strep. viridans* group)
• 10%	Enterococci
• 25%	Staphylococci: *S. aureus* = coagulase +ve *S. epidermidis* = coagulase –ve
• 5–10	Culture –ve
• <1%	Gram –ve bacilli
• <1%	Multiple organisms
• <1%	Diptheroids
• <1%	Fungi.

IE: investigations

- Blood cultures — Take 3–4 sets of cultures from different sites at least an hour apart and inoculate a minimum of 10mL/bottle for the optimal pick-up rate. Both aerobic and anaerobic bottles must be used. Lab should be advised that IE is a possibility especially if unusual organisms are suspected. In stable patients on antibiotic therapy, doses must be delayed to allow culture on successive days. Ask for prolonged (fungal) cultures in IV drug users.
- FBC — May show normochromic, normocytic anaemia (exclude haematinic deficiency), neutrophil leucocytosis, and perhaps thrombocytopenia.
- U&Es — May be deranged (this should be monitored throughout treatment).
- LFTs — May be deranged, especially with an increase in ALP and γ-GT.
- ESR/CRP: — Acute phase reaction.
- Urinalysis: — Microscopic haematuria ± proteinuria.
- Immunology — Polyclonal elevation in serum Igs, complement levels.
- ECG — May have changes associated with any underlying cause. There may be AV block or conduction defects (especially aortic root abscess) and rarely (embolic) acute MI.
- CXR — May be normal. Look for pulmonary oedema or multiple infected or infarcted areas from septic emboli (tricuspid endocarditis).
- Echo — TTE may confirm the presence of valve lesions and/or demonstrate vegetations if >2mm in size. TOE is more sensitive for aortic root and mitral leaflet involvement. A normal Echo does not exclude the diagnosis.
- MRI — Useful in investigation of paravalvular extension, aortic root aneurysm, and fistulas.
- Dentition — All patients should have an OPG (orthopentamograph—a panoramic dental XR) and a dental opinion.
- Swabs — Any potential sites of infection (skin lesions).
- V/Q scan — In cases where right-sided endocarditis is suspected this may show multiple mismatched defects.
- Save serum for — *Aspergillus* precipitins, *Candida* antibodies (rise in titre), Q fever (*Coxiella burnetti*), complement fixation test, *Chlamydia* complement fixation test, *Brucella* agglutinins, *Legionella* antibodies, *Bartonella* spp.

IE: antibiotics

'Blind' treatment for endocarditis

IE is usually a clinical diagnosis and must be considered in any patient with a typical history, fever, and a murmur with no other explanation. Often antibiotics need to be started before the culture results are available. Be guided by the clinical setting (Table 1.9); see Box 1.23 for suggested doses.

Table 1.9 Antibiotic treatment of IE*

Presentation	Choice of antibiotic
Gradual onset (weeks)	Benzylpenicillin + gentamicin
Acute onset (days) or history of skin trauma	Flucloxacillin + gentamicin
Recent valve prosthesis (possible MRSA, diptheroid, *Kelbsiella*, corynebacterium or nosocomial staphylococci)	Vancomycin (or teicoplanin) + gentamicin + rifampicin
IV drug user	Vancomycin

*Oakley CM (1995). *Eur Heart J* **16**(suppl.B): 90–3.

Box 1.23 Suggested antibiotic doses

Benzylpenicillin	4MU (2.4g) q4h IV
Flucloxacillin	2g qds IV
Vancomycin	15mg/kg q12h IV over 60min, guided by levels
Gentamicin	3mg/kg divided in 1–3 doses guided by levels
Rifampicin	300mg q12h PO
Ciprofloxacin	300mg q12h IV for 1 week, then 750mg q12h PO for 3 weeks

- Identification of an organism is invaluable for further management and blood cultures should be taken before antibiotics with meticulous attention to detail.
- Antibiotics should be administered IV, preferably via a tunnelled central (Hickman) line.
- If an organism is isolated, antibiotic therapy may be modified when sensitivities are known.
- Suggested antibiotic combinations are shown in Table 1.9; however, individual units may have specific policies. Patients should be discussed with your local microbiologist.

Duration of treatment

- This is controversial with a trend toward shorter courses. Microbiology and ID opinion is important especially in resistant and/or uncommon organisms. Box 1.24 shows one suggested protocol.
- The duration of treatment varies depending on the severity of infection and the infecting organism. IV therapy is usually for at least 2 weeks and total antibiotic therapy is for 4–6 weeks.
- If the patient is well following this period, antibiotic treatment may be stopped. Provided no surgery is indicated (see 📖 p.108), patient may be discharged and followed up in outpatient clinic.
- Patients should be advised of the need for endocarditis prophylaxis in the future (see 📖 Table 1.10, p.111).
- Patients with valvular damage following infection should be followed long term and patients with ventricular septal defects should be considered for closure.

Box 1.24 Suggested treatment protocol

- Viridans streptococci and *Strep bovis* (penicillin sensitive):
  - Benzylpenicillin only (4 weeks)
  - Vancomycin or teicoplanin (4 weeks)
  - Penicillin + aminoglycoside (2 weeks)
  - Ceftriaxone 2g (4 weeks)
- Group B, C, G streptococci, *Strep. pyogenes*, *Strep. Pneumoniae*:
  - Penicillin (4 weeks) + aminoglycoside (2 weeks)
  - Vancomycin (4 weeks) + aminoglycoside (2 weeks)
- Group A streptococci:
  - Penicillin (4 weeks)
  - Vancomycin (4 weeks)
- Enterococci:
  - Penicillin + aminoglycoside (4–6 weeks)
  - Vancomycin + aminoglycoside (4–6 weeks)
- Extra-cardiac infection from septic emboli:
  - Penicillin (4 weeks) + aminoglycoside (2 weeks)
  - Vancomycin (4 weeks) + aminoglycoside (2 weeks)
- *S. aureus* and coagulase-negative staphylococci:
  - Left-sided endocarditis:
    —Flucloxacillin (4–6 weeks) + aminoglycoside (2 weeks)
    —If MRSA: vancomycin+rifampicin (6 weeks) ± aminoglycoside (2 weeks)
  - Right-sided endocarditis:
    —Flucloxacillin (2 weeks) + aminoglycoside (2 weeks)
    —Ciprofloxacin (4 weeks) +rifampicin (3 weeks)
    —If MRSA: vancomycin (4 weeks)+rifampicin (4 weeks)
- Fungi:
  - Amphotericin B IV to a total dose of 2.5–3g.

IE: monitoring treatment

Patients need careful clinical monitoring both during and for several months after the infection. Reappearance of features suggestive of IE must be investigated thoroughly to rule out recurrent infection or resistance to treatment regimen.

Clinical features

- Signs of continued infection, persistent pyrexia, and the persistence of systemic symptoms.
- Persistent fever may be due to drug resistance, concomitant infection (central line, urine, chest, septic emboli to lungs or abdomen) or allergy (?eosinophilia, ?leucopoenia, ?proteinuria: common with penicillin but may be due to any antibiotic; consider changing or stopping antibiotics for 2–3 days).
- Changes in any cardiac murmurs or signs of cardiac failure.
- The development of any new embolic phenomena.
- Inspect venous access sites daily. Change peripheral cannulae every 3–4 days.

Echo

- Regular (weekly) TTEs may identify clinically silent, but progressive valve destruction and development of intracardiac abscesses or vegetations.
- The tips of long-standing central lines may develop sterile fibrinous 'fronds', which may be visible on TOE: change the line and send the tip for culture.
- 'Vegetations' need not be due to infection (see Box 1.25).

ECG

Looking specifically for AV block or conduction abnormalities suggesting intracardiac extension of the infection. A daily ECG must be performed.

Microbiology

- Repeated blood cultures (especially if there is continued fever).
- Regular aminoglycoside and vancomycin levels (ensuring the absence of toxic levels and the presence of therapeutic levels). Gentamicin ototoxicity may develop with prolonged use even in the absence of toxic levels.
- Back titration to ensure that minimum inhibitory and bactericidal concentrations are being achieved.

Laboratory indices

- Regular (daily) urinalysis.
- Regular U&Es and liver function tests.
- Regular CRP (ESR every 2 weeks).
- FBC: rising Hb and falling WCC suggests successful treatment; watch for β-lactam associated neutropoenia.
- Serum magnesium (if on gentamicin).

Box 1.25 Causes of 'vegetations' on Echo[1]

- IE
- Sterile thrombotic vegetations
- Libman–Sacks endocarditis (SLE)
- 1° antiphospholipid syndrome
- Marantic endocarditis (adenocarcinoma)
- Myxomatous degeneration of valve (commonly mitral)
- Ruptured mitral chordae
- Exuberant rheumatic vegetations (black Africans)
- Thrombus ('pannus') on a prosthetic valve
- A stitch or residual calcium after valve replacement.

Reference

1. Michel PL, Acar J (1995). Native cardiac disease predisposing to infective endocarditis. *Eur Heart J* **16**(suppl B): 2–6.

Culture-negative endocarditis

- The commonest reason for persistently negative blood cultures is prior antibiotic therapy and this affects up to 15% of patients with a diagnosis of IE (Box 1.26).
- If the clinical response to the antibiotics is good these should be continued.
- For a persisting fever:
  - Withhold antibiotics if not already started.
  - Consider other investigations for a 'PUO' (see 📖 p.440).
  - If clinical suspicion of IE is high, it warrants further investigation.
  - Repeated physical examination for any new signs.
  - Regular Echo and TOE. 'Vegetations' need not be due to infection (see 📖 Box 1.25, p.103).
  - Repeated blood cultures, especially when the temperature is raised. Discuss with microbiology about prolonged culturing times (4+ weeks) and special culturing and sub-culturing techniques. Most HACEK group organisms can be detected.
- Consider unusual causes of endocarditis.
- ***Q-fever*** (*Coxiella burnetii*): complement fixation tests identify antibodies to phase 1 and 2 antigens. Phase 2 antigens raised in the acute illness, phase 1 antigens raised in chronic illnesses such as endocarditis. PCR can be performed on operative specimens. Treat with indefinite (life-long) oral doxycycline ± co-trimoxazole, rifampicin, or quinolone.
- ***Chlamydia psittaci:*** commonly there is a history of exposure to birds and there may be an associated atypical pneumonia. Diagnosis is confirmed using complement fixation tests to detect raised antibody titres.
- ***Brucellosis:*** blood cultures may be positive though organisms may take up to 8 weeks to grow. Serology usually confirms the diagnosis.
- ***Fungi:*** Candida is the most common species *and* may be cultured. The detection of antibodies may be helpful though levels may be raised in normals. The detection of a rising titre is of more use. Other fungal infections (e.g. histoplasmosis, aspergillosis) are rare but may be diagnosed with culture or serology, though these are commonly negative. Antigen assays may be positive, or the organism *may* be isolated from biopsy material. Fungal IE is more common in patients with prosthetic valves and IV drug users. Bulky vegetations are common. Treatment is with amphotericin B ± flucytosine. Prosthetic valves must be removed. Mortality is >50%.

Box 1.26 Causes of culture-negative endocarditis

- Previous antibiotic therapy
- Fastidious organism
  - Nutritionally deficient variants of *Strep. viridans*
  - *Brucella, Neisseria, Legionella*
  - Nocardia
  - Mycobacteria
  - The HACEK* group of oropharyngeal flora
  - Cell-wall deficient bacteria and anaerobes
- Cell-dependent organisms
- Chlamydia, rickettsiae (Coxiella)
- Fungi

* HACEK = *Haemophilus, Acintobacillus, Cardiobacterium, Eikenella,* and *Kingella* spp.

Right-sided endocarditis

- May present as multiple infected pulmonary emboli (abscesses).
- Always consider this diagnosis in IV drug users (or patients with venous access).
- Endocarditis on endocardial permanent pacemaker leads is a rare but recognized cause.
- Patients most commonly have staphylococcal infection and are unwell, requiring immediate treatment and often early surgery.
- Lesions may be sterilized with IV antibiotics.
- Surgery may be required for:
  - Resistant organisms (*S. aureus*, *Pseudomonas*, *Candida*, and infection with multiple organisms)
  - Increasing vegetation size in spite of therapy
  - Infections on pacemaker leads (surgical removal of lead and repair or excision of tricuspid valve)
  - Recurrent mycotic emboli.

Prosthetic valve endocarditis (PVE)

Conventionally divided into early (<2 months postoperatively) and late (>2 months postoperatively).

Early prosthetic valve endocarditis

- Most commonly due to staphylococci, Gram –ve bacilli, diptheroids, or fungi.
- Generally infection has begun either perioperatively or in the immediate postoperative period.
- Often a highly destructive, fulminant infection with valve dehiscence, abscess formation, and rapid haemodynamic deterioration.
- Discuss with the surgeons early. They commonly require re-operation. Mortality is high (45–75%).

Late prosthetic valve endocarditis

- The pathogenesis is different. Abnormal flow around the prosthetic valve ring produces microthrombi and non-bacterial thrombotic vegetations (NBTVs), which may be infected during transient bacteraemia. The source is commonly dental or urological sepsis or indwelling venous lines.
- Common organisms are coagulase negative staphylococci, *S. aureus*, *Strep. viridans*, or enterococci.
- Frequently needs surgical intervention and this carries a high mortality, but less than for early PVE.
- It may be possible to sterilize infections on bioprostheses with IV antibiotics only. Surgery (see 📖 p.108) may then be deferred.

Surgery for IE

Discuss early with the regional cardiothoracic centre: immediate intervention may be appropriate.

- Surgical intervention may be necessary either during active infection or later because of degree of valve destruction. Optimal timing depends on a number of factors:
  - Haemodynamic tolerance of lesion
  - Outcome of the infection
  - Presence of complications.
- Choice of antimicrobial therapy should be modified depending on microbiological results from intraoperative specimens. Samples should be sent for culture, staining, immunological testing, and PCR depending on suspected organism.
- Duration of antimicrobial treatment is dependent on the clinical picture:
  - Culture-negative operative specimens: 2–3 weeks for valve infection and 3–4 weeks for abscess.
  - Culture-positive operative specimens: 3–4 weeks for valve infection and 4–6 weeks for abscess.
- Timing is dictated by clinical picture. Indications for urgent surgery are listed in Box 1.27. In patients with neurological injury, surgery should be delayed to avoid intracranial haemorrhage if cardiac function permits (embolic infarct: delay 10–14 days, haemorrhage: 21–28 days and when ruptured mycotic aneurysms have been repaired).
- Box 1.27 summarizes the absolute and relative indications for surgery.

Haemodynamic tolerance of lesion

- If the patient is haemodynamically stable, surgery may be delayed until after antibiotic course is completed. The final management depends on the valve affected, the degree of destruction, and its effect on ventricular function. Severe aortic and mitral regurgitation usually require surgery; tricuspid regurgitation, if well tolerated, is managed medically.
- Decompensation (severe congestive cardiac failure or low cardiac output syndrome with functional renal failure) may respond to surgery but the mortality is high.
- 'Metastable' patients who have been successfully treated after an episode of acute decompensation should be considered for early operation after 2–3 weeks of antibiotic therapy.

Outcome of the infection

- Persistence or relapse of infection (clinical and laboratory indices) despite appropriate antibiotics at an adequate dose may either be due to a resistant organism or an abscess (paravalvular, extra-cardiac). Consider valve replacement if no extra-cardiac focus found.
- The organism may influence the decision: consider early surgery for fungal endocarditis or prosthetic endocarditis with *E. coli* or *S. aureus*.

Presence of complications

Urgent surgery indications comprise:

- High degree AV block
- Perforation of interventricular septum

- Rupture of sinus of Valsalva aneurysm into RV
- Intracardiac abscess
- Recurrent septic emboli
- Prosthetic endocarditis especially associated with an unstable prosthesis.

Box 1.27 Indications for surgery in infective endocarditis

Absolute indications

- Moderate to severe heart failure 2° to valve regurgitation
- Unstable prosthesis
- Uncontrolled infection: persistent bacteraemia, ineffective antimicrobial therapy—IE 2° to fungi, *Brucella*, *Pseudomonas aeroginosa* (especially aortic and mitral valve)
- *S. aureus* prosthetic infection with an intracardiac complication.

Relative indications

- Perivalvular extension of infection
- Poor response to *S. aureus* native valve infection
- Relapse after adequate treatment
- Large (>10mm) hypermobile vegetations
- Persistent unexplained fever in culture-negative endocarditis
- Endocarditis 2° to antibiotic-resistant enterococci.

Endocarditis prophylaxis

NB: This is one regimen (after Leport *et al.*[1]). Refer to your local policy. See Boxes 1.28 and 1.29.

Box 1.28 Procedures that require antibiotic prophylaxis

• Dental:	• All procedures
• Upper respiratory tract:	• Tonsillectomy, adenoidectomy
• Gastrointestinal:	• Oesophageal dilatation or laser therapy
	• Oesophageal surgery
	• Sclerosis of oesophageal varicies
	• ERCP
	• Abdominal surgery
	• Barium enema
	• Sigmoidoscopy ± biopsy
• Urological:	• Instrumentation of ureter or kidney
	• Biopsy or surgery of prostate or bladder

Box 1.29 Procedures for which the risk of IE is controversial

• Upper respiratory tract:	• Bronchoscopy
	• Endotracheal intubation
• Gastrointestinal:	• Upper GI endoscopy ± biopsy
• Genital:	• Vaginal hysterectomy or delivery

- 📖 Box 1.21, p.97 shows cardiac conditions at risk of IE. High and moderate risk requires prophylaxis; 'low' risk does not.
- The regimen may be modified depending on the 'degree of risk' (both patient and procedure related) as shown in Table 1.10.

Table 1.10 Antibiotic prophylaxis

	1 hour before	6 hours after
Minimal regimen		
No penicillin allergy	Amoxicillin 3g PO	No 2nd dose
Allergy to penicillin	Clindamycin 300–600mg PO	No 2nd dose
Maximal regimen		
No penicillin allergy	Amoxicillin 2g IV	1–1.5g PO
	+	
	Gentamicin 1.5mg/kg IM/IV	No 2nd dose
	Vancomycin 1g IV over 1h	1g IV at 12h
Allergy to penicillin	+	
	Gentamicin 1.5mg/kg IM/IV	No 2nd dose

Flexible modifications depending on the 'degree of risk'

- Additional doses after procedure
- Additional aminoglycosides
- Parenteral administration

Reference

1. Leport C *et al.* (1995). Antibiotic prophylaxis from an international group of experts towards a European consensus. Group of Experts of the International Society for Chemotherapy. *Eur Heart J* **16**(suppl. B): 126–31.

Acute aortic regurgitation (AR)

Presentation

- Sudden, severe AR presents as cardiogenic shock and acute pulmonary oedema.
- The haemodynamic changes are markedly different from those seen in chronic AR. The previous normal-sized LV results in a smaller effective forward flow and higher LVEDP for the same degree of AR.
- Patients are often extremely unwell, tachycardic, peripherally shut down, and often have pulmonary oedema. Unlike chronic AR, pulse pressure may be near normal.
- If available, ask for a history of previous valvular heart disease, hypertension, features of Marfan syndrome, and risk factors for IE (see 🕮 Box 1.21, p.97).
- Physical signs of severe AR include a quiet aortic closure sound (S_2); an ejection systolic murmur over aortic valve (turbulent flow); high-pitched and short early diastolic murmur (AR); quiet S_1 (premature closure of the mitral valve).
- Examine specifically for signs of an underlying cause (see 🕮 Box 1.30, p.113).
- Where there is no obvious underlying cause (e.g. acute MI), assume IE until proven otherwise.

Diagnosis

Based on a combination of clinical features and TTE and/or TOE.

Management

Acute AR is a surgical emergency and all other management measures are only aimed at stabilizing patient until urgent AVR can take place. Patient's clinical condition will determine the urgency of surgery (and mortality). Liaise immediately with local cardiologists.

General measures

- Admit the patient to intensive care or medical HDU.
- Give O_2, begin treating any pulmonary oedema with diuretics.
- Monitor blood gases; mechanical ventilation may be necessary.
- Blood cultures × 3 are essential. See 🕮 IE: investigations, p.99.
- Serial ECG: watch for developing AV block or conduction defects.

Specific measures

- Every patient must be discussed with the regional cardiothoracic centre.
- In the context of good systemic BP, vasodilators such as sodium nitroprusside or hydralazine may temporarily improve forward flow and relieve pulmonary oedema.
- Inotropic support may be necessary if hypotensive. However, inotropes are best avoided as any increase in systemic pressures may worsen AR.
- All patients with haemodynamic compromise should have immediate or urgent aortic valve replacement.
- IE: indications for surgery are given in 🕮 Box 1.27, p.109.
- IABP must be avoided as it will worsen AR.

Box 1.30 Causes of acute AR

- IE
- Ascending aortic dissection
- Collagen vascular disorders (e.g. Marfan syndrome)
- Connective tissue diseases (large- and medium-vessel arteritis)
- Trauma
- Dehiscence of a prosthetic valve.

Acute mitral regurgitation (MR)

Presentation

- Patients most commonly present with acute breathlessness and severe pulmonary oedema. Symptoms may be less severe, or spontaneously improve, as left atrial compliance increases. There may be a history of previous murmur, angina, or MI.
- The signs are different to those seen in chronic MR because of the presence of a non-dilated and relatively non-compliant LA. Acute MR results in a large LA systolic pressure wave (*v*-wave) and hence pulmonary oedema.
- Patients may be acutely unwell with tachycardia, hypotension, peripheral vasoconstriction, and pulmonary oedema and a pan-systolic murmur of MR.
- Later in the illness, probably because of sustained high left atrial and pulmonary venous pressures, right heart failure develops.
- Examine for signs of any underlying conditions (see 📖 Box 1.31, p.115).
- The important differential diagnosis is a VSD. TTE and Doppler studies can readily differentiate between the two conditions. Alternatively, if Echo is not available, pulmonary artery catheterization in acute MR will exclude the presence of a left-to-right shunt and the PCWP trace will demonstrate a large *v*-wave.
- Where there is no obvious underlying cause (e.g. acute MI), assume the patient has IE until proven otherwise.

Diagnosis

Based on a combination of clinical features and Echo. TTE can readily diagnose and quantify MR. It also provides information on LV status (in particular, regional wall-motion abnormalities which can give rise to MR). TOE can provide specific information about aetiology of valve dysfunction including papillary muscle rupture and MV leaflet (anterior and posterior) structural abnormalities. This information will be vital for a decision regarding definitive management.

General measures

- Admit the patient to intensive care or medical HDU.
- Give O_2, begin treating any pulmonary oedema with diuretics.
- Monitor blood gases; mechanical ventilation may be necessary.
- Blood cultures × 3 are essential. See 📖 IE: investigations, p.99.
- If present, MI should be treated in the standard manner.

Specific measures

- Pulmonary oedema may be very resistant to treatment.
- In the presence of good BP, reduction in preload (GTN infusion) and afterload especially with ACEIs is important. Systemic vasodilators such as hydralazine (12.5–100mg tds) can also be added in.
- An IABP will help decrease LVEDP and also increase coronary blood flow.

- Patients may require inotropic support. There are multiple combinations and actiology of MR, haemodynamic status, and local policy/expertise should dictate choice of agent.
- CPAP and intubation and positive pressure ventilation are extremely useful and must be considered in all severe and/or resistant cases.
- Haemodynamic disturbance and severe pulmonary oedema in the context of acute MR is a surgical emergency.
- IE. Indications for surgery are given on p.108.
- Post-infarct MR. Management depends upon the patient's condition following resuscitation. Patients who are stabilized may have MVR deferred because of the risks of surgery in the post-infarct patient. Their preoperative management should consist of diuretics and vasodilators, including ACEIs if tolerated. Advise patients regarding endocarditis prophylaxis.

Box 1.31 Causes of acute MR

- IE
- Papillary muscle dysfunction or rupture (see post MI, p.114)
- Rupture of chordae tendinae (e.g. infection, myxomatous degeneration, SLE)
- Trauma (to leaflets, papillary muscle or chordae)
- Prosthetic valve malfunction (e.g. 2° to infection)
- Left atrial myxoma
- Acute rheumatic fever
- Collagen vascular disorders (e.g. Marfan syndrome)
- Connective tissue diseases (large- and medium-vessel arteritis).

Deep vein thrombosis (DVT): assessment

Presentation

- Most commonly asymptomatic. Minor leg discomfort or isolated swelling (>65%) in the effected limb are the most common clinical features. Breathlessness or chest pain may be 2° to PE.
- Signs include erythema and swelling of the leg, dilated superficial veins, and calf discomfort on dorsiflexion of the foot (Homan's sign). The thrombus may be palpable as a fibrous cord in the popliteal fossa. Confirm the presence of swelling (>2cm) by measuring the limb circumference 15cm above and 10cm below the tibial tuberosity.
- In all cases of leg swelling, abdominal and rectal (and pelvic in women) examination must be carried out to exclude an abdominal cause.

Risk factors for DVT

Pro-coagulant states

Congenital

- Factor V_{Leiden}
- Antithrombin III deficiency
- Protein C deficiency
- Protein S deficiency

Acquired

- Malignant disease (~5%)
- Antiphospholipid syndrome
- Myeloproliferative disorders
- Oral contraceptive pill (especially with Factor V_{Leiden} mutation)
- Nephrotic syndrome (via renal AT III losses)
- Homocystinuria
- Paroxysmal nocturnal haemoglobinuria

Venous stasis

- Immobility (e.g. long journeys)
- Recent surgery
- Pelvic mass
- Pregnancy or recent childbirth
- Severe obesity.

Miscellaneous

- Hyperviscosity syndromes (also see 📖 p.616)
- Previous DVT or PE
- Family history of DVT/PE.

Investigations

- Venous compression ultrasonography of leg veins is largely replacing venography as the initial investigation of choice. It is quick, and non-invasive, with sensitivity and specificity of >90% and does not carry the risk of contrast allergy or phlebitis. It can simultaneously assess extent of proximal progression of the thrombus in particular extension into pelvic vessels.
- D-dimers have a high negative predictive value for DVT. A low clinical probability of DVT and a negative D-dimer does not require

further investigation. A positive D-dimer result should be followed by ultrasonography.

- Venography: use if results uncertain and clinical suspicion is high.
- Consider baseline investigations—FBC, U&Es, ECG, CXR, urinalysis, and pulse oximetry (± ABG)—on all patients.
- If appropriate, look for an underlying cause.
    - Coagulation screen
    - Pro-coagulant screen: refer to local screening policy and get haematology advice (e.g. CRP, ESR, Protein C and S, antithrombin III levels, Factor V_{Leiden} mutation, auto-Ab screen, immunoglobulins and immunoelectrophoretic strip, anticardiolipin antibody, Ham test, etc.).
    - Screen for malignancy: ultrasound ± CT (abdomen and pelvis), CXR, LFTs, PSA, CEA, CA-125, CA-19.9, β-HCG, etc.

Table 1.11 Wells rule to estimate the probability of DVT

Clinical feature	Score
Active cancer (including treatment up to 6 months previously)	1
Paralysis, paresis, or recent plaster immobilization of the lower extremity	1
Recently bedridden for >3 days or major surgery within 4 weeks	1
Localized tenderness along the distribution of the deep venous system	1
Entire limb swollen	1
Calf swelling by >3cm when compared with the asymptomatic leg	1
Pitting oedema (greater in the symptomatic leg)	1
Dilated collateral superficial veins (nonvaricose)	1
Alternative diagnosis as likely or more possible than that of DVT	–2
Clinical probability of DVT with score	
Score > 3 High	
Score 1–2 Moderate	
Score < 1 Low	

Adapted from Oudega R, *et al* (2005). *Ann Intern Med* **143:** 101.

DVT: management

- If there is a high clinical suspicion of DVT (the presence of risk factors and absence of an alternative diagnosis), start empiric anticoagulation with LMWH. This may be stopped if subsequent investigations are negative.
- Below-knee DVT: thrombi limited to the calf have a lower risk of embolization and may be treated with compression stockings and SC prophylactic doses of LMWH until mobile to deter proximal propagation of thrombus. A brief period of systemic anticoagulation with LMWH may lessen the pain from below-knee DVT.
- Above-knee DVT: thrombi within the thigh veins warrant full anticoagulation with LMWH/UFH and subsequently warfarin.
- See management algorithm in Fig. 1.10.

Anticoagulation

Heparin

- LMWHs have now superseded UFH for management of both DVT and PE. They require no monitoring on a daily basis and also allow outpatient treatment.
- There must be period of overlap between LMWH/UFH therapies and anticoagulation with warfarin until INR is within therapeutic range and stable.
- LMWH are administered primarily as a once-daily SC injection and dosage is determined by patient weight.

Warfarin

- Always anticoagulate with LMWH/UFH before starting warfarin. Protein C (a vitamin K-dependent anticoagulant) has a shorter half-life than the other coagulation factors and levels fall sooner resulting in a transient pro-coagulant tendency.
- If DVT is confirmed commence warfarin and maintain on LMWH/UFH until INR >2.
- Anticoagulate (INR 2–2.5) for 3 months.
- If recurrent DVT, or patient at high-risk of recurrence, consider lifelong anticoagulation.

Thrombolysis

- This should be considered for recurrent, extensive, proximal venous thrombosis (e.g. femoral or iliac veins), as it is more effective than anticoagulation alone in promoting clot dissolution and produces a better clinical outcome.
- Catheter-directed thrombolytic therapy (rt-PA or SK) is superior to systemic thrombolysis.
- One approach is streptokinase 250,000U over 30min then 100,000U every hour for 24–72h (see data sheet). See 📖 p.22 for contraindications to thrombolysis.

Further management

- Women taking the combined OCP should be advised to stop this.
- If there are contraindications to anticoagulation, consider the insertion of a caval filter to prevent PE.
- All patients should be treated with thigh-high compression stockings to try to reduce symptomatic venous distension when mobilizing.

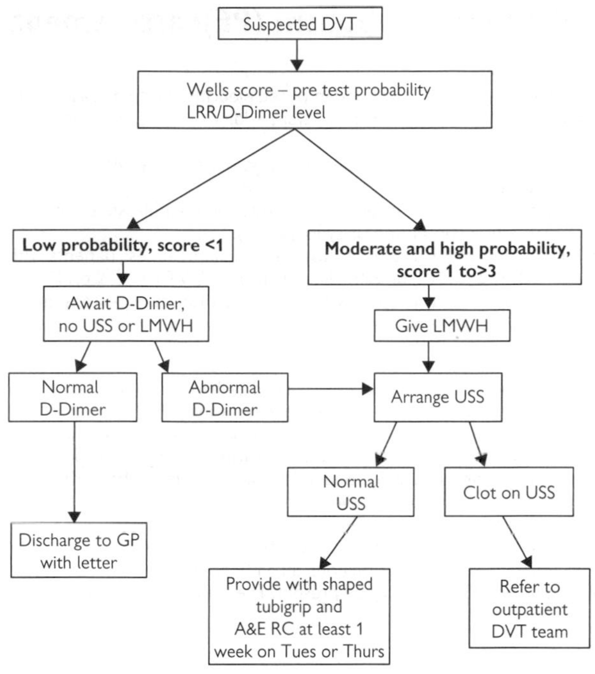

Fig. 1.10 DVT management algorithm.

Pulmonary embolism (PE): assessment

Symptoms

- Classically presents with sudden onset, pleuritic chest pain, associated with breathlessness and haemoptysis. Additional symptoms include postural dizziness or syncope.
- Massive PE may present as cardiac arrest (particularly with electromechanical dissociation) or shock.
- Presentation may be atypical, i.e. unexplained breathlessness or unexplained hypotension or syncope only.
- Pulmonary emboli should be suspected in all breathless patients with risk factors for DVT or with clinically proven DVT (see 📖 p.118).
- Recurrent PEs may present with chronic pulmonary hypertension and progressive right heart failure.

Signs

- Examination may reveal tachycardia and tachypnoea only. Look for postural hypotension (in the presence of raised JVP).
- Look for signs of raised right heart pressures and cor pulmonale (raised JVP with prominent 'a' wave, tricuspid regurgitation, parasternal heave, right ventricular S_3, loud pulmonary closure sound with wide splitting of S_2, pulmonary regurgitation).
- Cyanosis suggests a large PE.
- Examine for a pleural rub (may be transient) or effusion.
- Examine lower limbs for obvious thrombophlebitis.
- Mild fever (>37.5°C) may be present. There may be signs of coexisting COPD.

Causes

- Most frequently 2° to DVT (leg >> arm; see 📖 p.118).
- Other causes:
    - Rarely 2° to right ventricular thrombus (post MI)
    - Septic emboli (e.g. tricuspid endocarditis)
    - Fat embolism (post fracture)
    - Air embolism (venous lines, diving)
    - Amniotic fluid
    - Parasites
    - Neoplastic cells
    - Foreign materials (e.g. venous catheters).

Prognostic features

The prognosis in patients with pulmonary emboli varies greatly, associated in part with any underlying condition. Generally worse prognosis is associated with larger pulmonary emboli; poor prognostic indicators include:

- Hypotension
- Hypoxia
- ECG changes (other than non-specific T-wave changes).

Practice point

A normal D-dimer excludes pulmonary embolus with ~95% accuracy, but a positive D-dimer can be 2° to other disorders.

PE: investigations 1

General investigations

- ***ABG:*** normal ABG does not exclude a PE. ↓P_aO_2 is invariable with larger PEs. Other changes include mild respiratory alkalosis and ↓P_aCO_2 (due to tachypnoea) and metabolic acidosis (2° to shock).
- ***ECG:*** commonly shows sinus tachycardia ± non-specific ST- and T-wave changes in the anterior chest leads. The classical changes of acute cor pulmonale such as $S_1Q_3T_3$, right axis deviation, or RBBB are only seen with massive PE. Less common findings include AF.
- ***CXR:*** may be normal and a near-normal chest film in the context of severe respiratory compromise is highly suggestive of a PE. Less commonly may show focal pulmonary oligaemia (Westermark's sign), a raised hemidiaphragm, small pleural effusion, wedge-shaped shadows based on the pleura, sub-segmental atelectasis, or dilated proximal pulmonary arteries.
- ***Blood tests:*** there is no specific test. FBC may show neutrophil leukocytosis; mildly elevated CK, troponin, and bilirubin may be seen.
- ***Echo/TOE:*** insensitive for diagnosis but can exclude other causes of hypotension and raised right-sided pressures (e.g. tamponade, RV infarction, see 📖 p.28). In PE it will show RV dilatation and global hypokinesia, with sparing of apex (McConnell's sign), and pulmonary artery dilation. Doppler may show tricuspid/pulmonary regurgitation allowing estimation of RV systolic pressure. Rarely, the thrombus in the pulmonary artery may be visible.
- Underlying causes (see Box 1.32).

Specific investigations

D-dimer

- A highly sensitive, but non-specific test.
- Useful in ruling out PE in patients with low or intermediate probability.
- Results can be affected by advancing age, pregnancy, trauma, surgery, malignancy, and inflammatory states.

Ventilation/perfusion (V/Q) lung scanning

A perfusion lung scan (with IV technetium-99 labelled albumin) should be performed in all suspected cases of PE. A ventilation scan (inhaled xenon-133) in conjunction increases the specificity by assessing whether the defects in the ventilation and perfusion scans 'match' or 'mismatch'. Pre-existing lung disease makes interpretation difficult.

- A normal perfusion scan rules out significant-sized PE.
- Abnormal scans are reported as low, medium, or high probability:
  - A high probability scan is strongly associated with a PE, but there is a significant minority of false positives
  - A low probability scan with a low clinical suspicion of PE should prompt a search for another cause for the patient's symptoms
  - If the clinical suspicion of PE is high and the scan is of low or medium probability, alternative investigations are required.

Box 1.32 Investigations for an underlying cause for PEs

- USS deep veins of legs
- USS abdomen and pelvis (?occult malignancy/pelvic mass)
- CT abdomen/pelvis
- Screen for inherited pro-coagulant tendency (e.g. Protein C, S, antithrombin III, Factor V_{Leiden})
- Autoimmune screen (anticardiolipin antibody, ANA)
- Biopsy of suspicious lymph nodes/masses.

PE: investigations 2

CTPA

- This is the recommended initial lung imaging modality in patients with non-massive PE.
- Allows direct visualization of emboli as well as other potential parenchymal disease, which may explain alternative explanation for symptoms.
- Sensitivity and specificity are high (>90%) for lobar pulmonary arteries but not so high for segmental and sub-segmental pulmonary arteries.
- A patient with a positive CTPA does not require further investigation for PE.
- A patient with a negative CTPA in the context of a high/intermediate probability of a PE should undergo further investigation.

Evaluation of leg veins with US

- Not very reliable. Almost half of patients with PE do not have evidence of a DVT and therefore a negative result cannot rule out a PE.
- Useful second-line investigation as an adjunct to CTPA/V/Q scan.
- Outcome studies have demonstrated that it would be safe not to anticoagulate patients with a negative CTPA and lower limb US who have an intermediate/low probability of a PE.

Pulmonary angiography

- Is the 'gold standard' investigation.
- It is indicated in patients in whom diagnosis of embolism cannot be established by non-invasive means. Look for sharp cut-off of vessels or obvious filling defects.
- Invasive investigation and can be associated with 0.5% mortality.
- If there is an obvious filling defect, the catheter or a guide wire passed through the catheter may be used to disobliterate the thrombus.
- After angiography, the catheter may be used to give thrombolysis directly into the affected pulmonary artery (see 📖 p.126).
- The contrast can cause systemic vasodilatation and haemodynamic collapse in hypotensive patients.

MR pulmonary angiography

- Results are comparable to pulmonary angiography in preliminary studies.
- It can simultaneously assess ventricular function.

Fig. 1.11 summarizes one proposed pathway for investigation on potential PE patients.

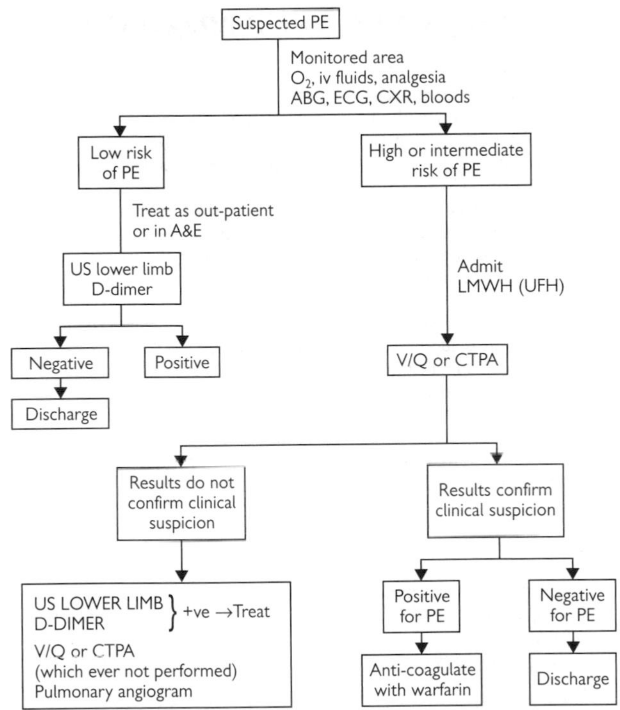

Fig. 1.11 Proposed pathway for investigation of patients with suspected PE.

Pulmonary embolism: management 1

1. Stabilize the patient

- Unless an alternative diagnosis is made the patient should be treated as for a pulmonary embolus until this can be excluded.
- Monitor cardiac rhythm, pulse, BP, respiration rate every 15min with continuous pulse oximetry and cardiac monitor. Ensure full resuscitation facilities are available.
- Obtain venous access and start IV fluids (crystalloid or colloid).
- Give maximal inspired O_2 via facemask to correct hypoxia. Mechanical ventilation may be necessary if the patient is tiring (beware of cardiovascular collapse when sedation is given for endotracheal intubation).
- *Give LMWH or UFH to all patients with high or intermediate risk of PE until diagnosis is confirmed.* Meta-analysis of multiple trials has shown LMWH to be superior to UFH with a reduction in mortality and bleeding complications. For doses consult local formulary.
- If there is evidence of haemodynamic instability (systemic hypotension, features of right heart failure) or cardiac arrest, patients may benefit from thrombolysis with rtPA or streptokinase—same doses used for treatment of STEMI (see Box 1.33).

2. Analgesia

- Patients may respond to oral NSAIDs.
- Opiate analgesia to be used with caution. The vasodilatation caused by these drugs may precipitate or worsen hypotension. Give small doses (1–2mg diamorphine IV) slowly. Hypotension should respond to IV colloid.
- Avoid IM injections (anticoagulation and possible thrombolysis).

3. Investigations with a view to a definite diagnosis

See 📖 pp.122–4.

4. Anticoagulate

- Patients with a positive diagnosis must undergo anticoagulation with warfarin. There should be period of overlap with LMWH/UFH until INR values are therapeutic. Target INR is 2–3 for most cases (see Box 1.34).
- Standard duration of anticoagulation is:
  - 4–6 weeks for temporary risk factor.
  - 3 months for first idiopathic cases.
  - At least 6 months for other cases.
  - With recurrent events and underlying predisposition to thromboembolic events (e.g. antiphospholipid antibody syndrome), lifelong anticoagulation may be needed (as well as higher target INR >3).

Box 1.33 Dosage of thrombolytic agents for pulmonary embolus

- Alteplase: 100mg over 2h or 0.6mg/kg over 15min (maximum of 50mg) followed by heparin
- Streptokinase: 250,000U over 30min followed by 100,000U/hour infusion for 24h

Box 1.34 Management key points: PE

- O_2
- Start LMWH when PE is suspected
- Start warfarin when PE is confirmed, continue LMWH until INR is therapeutic (2–3)
- Analgesia
- IV fluids if hypotensive
- If there is evidence of haemodynamic instability: consider thrombolysis.

Pulmonary embolism: management 2

Cardiac arrest

(Also see 📖 p.8.)

- Massive PE may present as cardiac arrest with EMD. Exclude the other causes of EMD (see 📖 p.8).
- Chest compressions may help break up the thrombus and allow it to progress more distally, thereby restoring some cardiac output.
- If clinical suspicion of PE is high and there is no absolute contraindication to thrombolysis, give rt-PA (similar in dose to STEMI with a maximum of 50mg (see 📖 Box 1.33, p.127) followed by heparin).
- If cardiac output returns, consider pulmonary angiography or inserting a PA catheter to try to mechanically disrupt the embolus.

Hypotension

The acute increase in PVR results in RV dilatation and pressure overload, which mechanically impairs LV filling and function. Patients require a higher than normal right-sided filling pressure, but may be worsened by fluid overload.

- Insert an internal jugular sheath prior to anticoagulation. This can be used for access, later if necessary.
- If hypotensive, give colloid (e.g. 500mL Haemaccel® stat).
- If hypotension, persists invasive monitoring and/or inotropic support is required. The JVP is a poor indicator of the left-sided filling pressures in such cases. Adrenaline is the inotrope of choice.
- Femoro-femoral cardiopulmonary bypass may be used to support the circulation until thrombolysis or surgical embolectomy can be performed.
- Pulmonary angiography in a hypotensive patient is hazardous as the contrast may cause systemic vasodilatation and cardiovascular collapse.

Pulmonary embolectomy

- In patients who have contraindications to thrombolysis and are in shock requiring inotropic support, there may be a role for embolectomy if appropriate skills are on site.
- This can be performed percutaneously in the catheterization laboratory using a number of devices or surgically on cardiopulmonary bypass.
- Percutaneous procedures may be combined with peripheral or central thrombolysis.
- Seek specialist advice early. Best results are obtained before onset of cardiogenic shock.
- Radiological confirmation of extent and site of embolism is preferable before thoracotomy.
- Mortality is ~25–30%.

IVC filter

- Infrequently used as little to suggest improved short- or long-term mortality.
- Filters are positioned percutaneously and if possible patients must remain anticoagulated to prevent further thrombus formation.

- Most are positioned infrarenally (bird's nest filter), but can also be suprarenal (Greenfield filter).
- Indications for IVC filter use include:
  - Anticoagulation contraindicated: e.g. active bleeding, heparin-induced thrombocytopenia, planned intensive chemotherapy
  - Anticoagulation failure despite adequate therapy
  - Prophylaxis in high-risk patients: e.g. progressive venous thrombosis, severe pulmonary hypertension.

Fat embolism

Commonly seen in patients with major trauma. There is embolization of fat and microaggregates of platelets, RBCs, and fibrin in systemic and pulmonary circulation. Pulmonary damage may result directly from the emboli (infarction) or by a chemical pneumonitis and ARDS (see 📖 p.198).

Clinical features

- There may be a history of fractures, followed (24–48h later) by breathlessness, cough, haemoptysis, confusion, and rash.
- Examination reveals fever (38–39°C), widespread petechial rash (25–50%), cyanosis, and tachypnoea. There may be scattered crepitations in the chest, though examination may be normal. Changes in mental state may be the first sign with confusion, drowsiness, seizures, and coma. Examine the eyes for conjunctival and retinal haemorrhages; occasionally fat globules may be seen in the retinal vessels. Severe fat embolism may present as shock.

Investigations

• ABG	Hypoxia and a respiratory alkalosis (with low P_aCO_2) as for thromboembolic PE.
• FBC	Thrombocytopenia, acute intravascular haemolysis.
• Coagulation	DIC.
• U&Es and glucose	Renal failure, hypoglycaemia.
• Ca^{2+}	May be low.
• Urine	Microscopy for fat and dipstick for haemoglobin.
• ECG	Usually non-specific (sinus tachycardia; occasionally signs of right heart strain.
• CXR	Usually lags behind the clinical course. There may be patchy, bilateral, air space opacification. Effusions are rare.
• CT head	Consider if there is a possibility of head injury with expanding subdural or epidural bleed.

Differential diagnosis

Pulmonary thromboembolism, other causes of ARDS ((see 📖 198), septic shock, hypovolaemia, cardiac or pulmonary contusion, head injury, aspiration pneumonia, transfusion reaction.

Management

- Treat respiratory failure (see 📖 p.196). Give O_2 (maximal via facemask; CPAP and mechanical ventilation if necessary).
- Ensure adequate circulating volume and cardiac output. CVP is not a good guide to left-sided filling pressures and a PA catheter (Swan–Ganz) should be used to guide fluid replacement. Try to keep PCWP 12–15mmHg and give diuretics if necessary. Use inotropes to support circulation as required (see 📖 p.202).
- Aspirin, heparin and dextran 40 (500mL over 4–6h) are of some benefit in the acute stages, but may exacerbate bleeding from sites of trauma.
- High-dose steroids (methylprednisolone 30mg/kg q8h for 3 doses) have been shown to improve hypoxaemia[1] but steroids are probably most effective if given prophylactically.

Reference

1. Lindeque BG *et al.* (1987). Fat embolism syndrome: A double blind therapeutic study. *Bone Joint Surg* **69:** 128–31.

Hypertensive emergencies

Hypertensive crisis

Hypertensive crisis is defined as a severe elevation in BP (SBP >200mmHg, DBP >120mmHg). Rate of change in BP is important. A rapid rise is poorly tolerated and leads to end-organ damage, whereas a gradual rise in a patient with existent poor BP control is tolerated better. Hypertensive crisis is classified as

- ***Hypertensive emergency***, where a high BP is complicated by acute target-organ dysfunction (see Box 1.35) and includes:
  - *Hypertensive emergency with retinopathy*, where there is marked elevation in BP (classically DBP >140mmHg) with retinal haemorrhages and exudates (previously called accelerated hypertension) and
  - *Hypertensive emergency with papilloedema*, with a similarly high BP and papilloedema (previously called malignant hypertension).
- ***Hypertensive urgency***, where there is a similar rise in BP, but without target organ damage.

Conditions which may present with hypertensive emergency

- Essential hypertension
- Renovascular hypertension: atheroma, fibromuscular dysplasia, acute renal occlusion
- Renal parenchymal disease: acute glomerulonephritis, vasculitis, scleroderma
- Endocrine disorders: pheochromocytoma, Cushing's syndrome, 1° hyperaldosteronism, thyrotoxicosis, hyperparathyroidism, acromegaly, adrenal carcinoma
- Eclampsia and pre-eclampsia
- Vasculitis
- Drugs: cocaine, amphetamines, MAOI interactions, ciclosporin, β-blocker and clonidine withdrawal
- Autonomic hyperactivity in presence of spinal cord injury
- Coarctation of the aorta.

Presentation

- Occasionally minimal non-specific symptoms such as mild headache and nose bleed.
- A small group of patients present with symptoms resulting from BP-induced microvascular damage:
  - Neurological symptoms: severe headache, nausea, vomiting, visual loss, focal neurological deficits, fits, confusion, intracerebral haemorrhage, coma.
  - Chest pain (hypertensive heart disease, MI, or aortic dissection) and congestive cardiac failure.
  - Symptoms of renal failure: renal impairment may be chronic (2° to long-standing hypertension) or acute (from the necrotizing vasculitis of malignant hypertension).

- Patients may present with hypertension as one manifestation of an underlying 'disease' (renovascular hypertension, chronic renal failure, CREST syndrome, pheochromocytoma, pregnancy).
- Examination should be directed at looking for evidence of end-organ damage even if the patient is asymptomatic (heart failure, retinopathy, papilloedema, focal neurology).

Box 1.35 Examples of hypertensive emergencies

- Hypertensive emergency with retinopathy/papilloedema
- Hypertensive encephalopathy
- Hypertension-induced intracranial haemorrhage/stroke
- Hypertension with cardiovascular complications
- Aortic dissection (see 📖 p.142)
- MI
- Pulmonary oedema (see 📖 p.87)
- Pheochromocytoma
- Pregnancy-associated hypertensive complications
- Eclampsia and pre-eclampsia
- Acute renal insufficiency
- Hypertensive emergency 2° to acute withdrawal syndromes (e.g. β-blockers, centrally acting antihypertensives)

Hypertensive emergencies: management

Priorities in management

- Confirm the diagnosis and assess the severity.
- Identify those patients needing specific emergency treatment.
- Plan long-term treatment.

Diagnosis and severity

- Ask about previous BP recordings, previous and current treatment, sympathomimetics, antidepressants, non-prescription drugs, recreational drugs.
- Check the BP yourself, in both arms, after a period of rest and if possible on standing. Monitor the patient's BP regularly while they are in A&E.
- Examine carefully for clinical evidence of cardiac enlargement or heart failure, peripheral pulses, renal masses or focal neurological deficit. Always examine the fundi: dilate if necessary.

Investigations

All patients should have:

- FBC: microangiopathic haemolytic anaemia with malignant HT
- U&E: renal impairment and/or ↓K^+ (diffuse intra-renal ischaemia and 2° hyperaldosteronism)
- Coag. screen: DIC with malignant HT
- CXR: cardiac enlargement:
  - Aortic contour (dissection?)
  - Pulmonary oedema
- Urinalysis: protein and red cells ± casts
- ECG: voltage criteria for LVH (Box 1.36).

Other investigations, depending on clinical picture and possible aetiology include:

- 24-hour urine collection:
  - Creatinine clearance
  - Free catecholamines, metanephrines, or VMA
- Echo: LVH, aortic dissection
- Renal USS and Doppler: size of kidneys and renal artery stenosis
- MR renal angiogram: renal artery stenosis
- CT/MR brain: intracranial bleed
- Drug screen: cocaine, amphetamine, others.

Indications for admission

- DBP persistently ≥120mmHg
- Retinal haemorrhages, exudates or papilloedema
- Renal impairment.

Box 1.36 Voltage criteria for LVH

- Tallest R (V4–V6)+deepest S (V1–V3) >40mm
- Tallest R (V4–V6) >27mm
- Deepest S (V1–V3) >30mm
- R in aVL >13mm
- R in aVF >20mm
- QRS complex >0.08s (2 small sq.)
- Abnormal ST depression or T inversion in V4–V6

Treatment principles

- Rapid reduction in BP is unnecessary, must be avoided, and can be very dangerous. This can result in cerebral and cardiac hypoperfusion (an abrupt change of >25% in BP will exceed cerebral BP autoregulation).
- Initial BP reduction of 25% to be achieved over 1–4h with a less rapid reduction over 24h to a DBP of 100mmHg.
- The only two situations where BP must be lowered rapidly are in the context of aortic dissection and MI.

Treatment

(Also see 🕮 p.136)

- The majority of patients who are alert and otherwise well may be treated with oral therapy to lower BP gradually.
- First-line treatment should be with a β-blocker (unless contraindicated) with a thiazide diuretic, or a low-dose calcium antagonist.
- Urgent invasive monitoring (arterial line) prior to drug therapy is indicated for patients with:
  - Evidence of hypertensive encephalopathy
  - Complications of hypertension (e.g. aortic dissection, acute pulmonary oedema, or renal failure)
  - Treatment of an underlying condition (e.g. glomerulonephritis, pheochromocytoma, CREST crisis)
  - Patients with persistent DBP ≥140mmHg
  - Eclampsia.
- Sublingual nifedipine must be avoided.

Conditions requiring specific treatment are listed in Box 1.37.

Long-term management

- Investigate as appropriate for an underlying cause.
- Select a treatment regimen that is tolerated and effective. Tell the patient why long-term therapy is important.
- Try to reduce all cardiovascular risk factors by advising the patient to stop smoking, appropriate dietary advice (cholesterol), and aim for optimal diabetic control.
- Monitor long-term control and look for end-organ damage (regular fundoscopy, ECG, U&Es). Even poor control is better than no control.

Box 1.37 Conditions requiring specific treatment

- Accelerated and malignant hypertension (see 🕮 p.138)
- Hypertensive encephalopathy (see 🕮 p.140)
- Eclampsia
- Pheochromocytoma
- Hypertensive patients undergoing anaesthesia.

Hypertensive emergencies: drug treatment

Table 1.12 Drugs for the treatment of hypertensive emergencies: IV therapy

Drug	Dosage	Onset of action	Comments
Labetalol	20–80mg IV bolus q10 min 20–200mg/min by IV infusion increasing every 15 min.	2–5 minutes	Drug of choice in suspected pheochromocytoma (p598) or aortic dissection (p170). Avoid if there is LVF May be continued orally (see below)
Nitroprusside	0.25–8mcg/kg/min IV infusion	Seconds	Drug of choice in LVF and/or encephalopathy.
GTN	1–10mg/hr IV infusion	2–5 minutes	Mainly venodilatation. Useful in patients with LVF of angina.
Hydralazine	5–10mg IV over 20 min 50–300mcg/min IV infusion	10–15 minutes	May provoke angina
Esmolol HCl	500mcg/kg/min IV loading dose 50–200mcg/kg/min IV infusion	Seconds	Short acting β-blocker also used for SVTs
Phentolamine	2–5mg IV over 2–5 minutes PRN	Seconds	Drug of choice in pheochromocytoma (p598) followed by labetalol (PO) when BP controlled

NB: It is dangerous to reduce the blood pressure quickly. Aim to reduce the diastolic BP to 100–110mmHg within 2–4 hours. Unless there are good reasons to commence IV therapy, always use oral medicines.

Table 1.13 Drugs for the treatment of hypertensive emergencies: Oral therapy

Drug	Dosage	Onset of action	Comment
Atendol	50–100mg PO od	30–60 minutes	There are numerous alternative β-blockers—see BNF
Nifedipine	10–20mg PO q8h (q12h if slow release)	15–20 minutes	Avoid sublingual as the fall in BP is very rapid
Labetalol	100–400mg PO q12h	30–60 minutes	Use if phaeochromocytoma suspected. Safe in pregnancy
Hydralazine	25–50mg PO q8h	20–40 minutes	Safe in pregnancy
Minoxidil	5–10mg PO od	30–60 minutes	May cause marked salt and water retention Combine with a loop diuretic (e.g. furosemide 40–240mg daily)
Clonidine	0.2mg PO followed by 0.1mg hourly max. 0.8mg total for urgent therapy, or 0.05–0.1mg PO q8h increasing every 2 days	30–60 minutes	Sedation common. Do not stop abruptly as here is a high incidence of rebound hypertensive crisis

NB: Aim to reduce diastolic BP to 100–110mmhg in 2–4 hours and normalize BP in 2–3 days.

Hypertensive emergency with retinopathy (accelerated and malignant hypertension)

This is part of a continuum of disorders characterized by hypertension (DBP often >120mmHg) and acute microvascular damage (seen best in the retina but present in all organs). It may be difficult to decide whether the damage in some vascular beds is the cause or effect of hypertension. An example is in the context of an acute glomerulonephritis.

- Accelerated hypertension (grade 3 retinopathy) may progress to malignant hypertension, with widespread necrotizing vasculitis of the arterioles (and papilloedema).
- Presentation is commonly with headache or visual loss and varying degrees of confusion. More severe cases present with renal failure, heart failure, microangiopathic haemolytic anaemia, and DIC.

Management

- Transfer the patient to medical HDU/ITU.
- Insert an arterial line and consider central venous line if there is evidence of necrotizing vasculitis and DIC. Catheterize the bladder.
- Monitor neurological state, ECG, fluid balance.
- Aim to lower the DBP to 100mmHg or by 15–20mmHg, whichever is higher, over the first 24h.
- Those with early features may be treated successfully with oral therapy (β-blockers, calcium channel blockers).
- Patients with late symptoms or who deteriorate should be given parenteral therapy aiming for more rapid lowering of BP.
- If there is evidence of pulmonary oedema or encephalopathy give furosemide 40–80mg IV.
- If there is no LVF, give a bolus of labetalol followed by an infusion. For patients with LVF, nitroprusside or hydralazine is preferable.
- Consult renal team for patients with acute renal failure or evidence of acute glomerulonephritis (>2+ proteinuria, red cell casts). ARF is managed as on 📖 p.288. Dopamine should be avoided as it may worsen hypertension.
- Consider giving an ACEI. High circulating renin levels may not allow control of hypertension, which in turn causes progressive renal failure. ACEIs will block this vicious circle. There may be marked first-dose hypotension so start cautiously.
- Haemolysis and DIC should recover with control of BP.

Hypertension in the context of acute stroke/intracranial bleed

- Stroke/bleed may be the result of hypertension or vice versa.
- In the acute setting there is impaired autoregulation of cerebral blood flow and autonomic function. Small changes in systemic BP may result in catastrophic falls in cerebral blood flow.
- Systemic BP should not be treated unless DBP >130mmHg and/or presence of severe cerebral oedema (with clinical manifestations).

- In most cases BP tends to settle over 24–36h. If treatment is indicated, BP reduction principles as listed earlier must be adhered to and a combination of nitroprusside, labetalol, and calcium channel blockers can be used.
- Centrally acting agents must be avoided as they cause sedation.
- In patients with SAH, a cerebroselective calcium channel blocker, such as nimodipine, is used to decrease cerebral vasospasm.
- Systemic BP must also be treated if it qualifies with the principles listed earlier and/or if it remains elevated after 24h. There is no evidence that this reduces further events in the acute phase.

Box 1.38 Hypertensive retinopathy

- Grade 1: tortuous retinal arteries, silver wiring
- Grade 2: AV nipping
- Grade 3: flame-shaped haemorrhages and cottonwool spots
- Grade 4: papilloedema.

Hypertensive encephalopathy

- Caused by cerebral oedema 2° to loss of cerebral autoregulatory function.
- Usually gradual onset and may occur in previously normotensive patients at BPs as low as 150/100mmHg. It is rare in patients with chronic hypertension and pressures are also much higher.

Symptoms

- Headache, nausea and vomiting, confusion, grade III and IV hypertensive retinopathy.
- Late features consist of focal neurological signs, fits, and coma.

Diagnosis

- A diagnosis of exclusion and other differential diagnosis must be ruled out (e.g. stroke, encephalitis, tumours, bleeding, vasculitis).
- History is helpful, particularly of previous seizures, SAH usually being sudden in onset and strokes being associated with focal neurological deficit.
- Always exclude hypoglycaemia.
- Starting hypotensive treatment for hypertension associated with a stroke can cause extension of the stroke.
- An urgent MRI or CT brain must be obtained to rule out some of the differential diagnosis.

Management

- The 1° principle of BP control is to reduce DBP by 25% or reduce DBP to 100mmHg, whichever is higher, over a period of 1–2h.
- Transfer the patient to ITU for invasive monitoring (see previous section).
- Monitor neurological state, ECG, fluid balance.
- Correct electrolyte abnormalities (K^+, Mg^{2+}, Ca^{2+}).
- Give furosemide 40–80mg IV.
- Nitroprusside is the first-line agent as it allows easy control of BP changes, despite its tendency to increase cerebral blood flow.
- Labetalol and calcium channel blockers are second-line agents and should be added in if necessary.
- It is vital to avoid agents with potential sedative action such as β-blockers, clonidine, and methyldopa.
- In selected patients who are stable and present at the very early stages, oral therapy with a combination of β-blockers and calcium blockers may be sufficient.

Aortic dissection: assessment

Aortic dissection is a surgical/medical emergency and untreated has a >90% 1-year mortality. Dissection begins with formation of a tear in the intima and the force of the blood cleaves the media longitudinally to various lengths. Predisposing factors are summarized in Box 1.39.

Classification

There are three classifications as illustrated in Fig. 1.12 (DeBakey, Stanford, and Descriptive). Dissections involving the ascending and/or aortic arch are surgical emergencies and those exclusive to the descending aorta are treated medically.

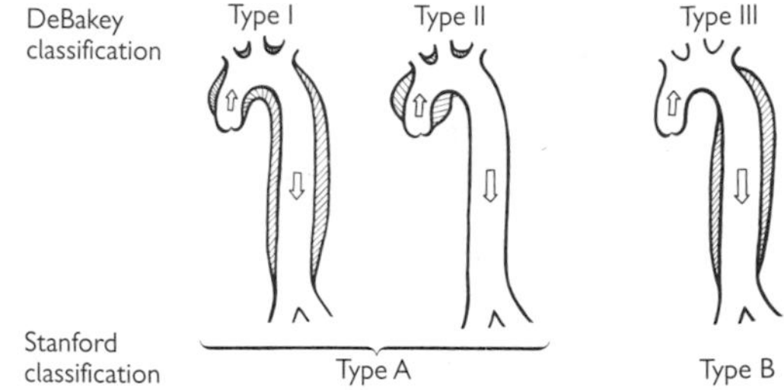

Fig. 1.12 Classification of aortic dissection.

Presentation

- ***Chest pain:*** classically abrupt onset of very severe, most commonly anterior chest pain radiating to the interscapular region. Usually tearing in nature and, unlike the pain of MI, most severe at its onset. Pain felt maximally in the anterior chest is associated with ascending aortic dissection, whereas interscapular pain suggests dissection of the descending aorta. Patients often use adjectives such as 'tearing', 'ripping', 'sharp', and 'stabbing' to describe the pain.
- ***Sudden death*** or ***shock:*** usually due to aortic rupture or cardiac tamponade.
- ***Congestive cardiac failure:*** due to acute aortic incompetence and/or MI.
- Patients may also present with symptoms and signs of occlusion of one of the branches of the aorta. Examples include:
  - Stroke or acute limb ischaemia: due to compression or dissection
  - Paraplegia with deficits: spinal artery occlusion
  - MI infarction: usually the right coronary artery
  - Renal failure and renovascular hypertension
  - Abdominal pain: coeliac axis or mesenteric artery occlusion.
- Aortic dissection may be painless.
- Ask specifically about history of hypertension, previous heart murmurs or aortic valve disease, and previous CXRs that may be useful for comparison.

Examination

- This may be normal.
- Most patients are hypertensive on presentation. Hypotension is more common in dissections of the ascending aorta (20–25%) and may be due to blood loss, acute aortic incompetence (which may be

accompanied by heart failure), or tamponade (distended neck veins, tachycardia, pulsus paradoxus).
- Pseudohypotension may be seen if flow to either or both subclavian arteries is compromised. Look for unequal BP in the arms and document the presence of peripheral pulses carefully. Absent or changing pulses suggest extension of the dissection.
- Auscultation may reveal aortic valve regurgitation and occasionally a pericardial friction rub. Descending aortic dissections may rupture or leak into the left pleural space and the effusion results in dullness in the left base.
- Neurologic deficits may be due to carotid artery dissection or compression (hemiplegia) or spinal artery occlusion (paraplegia with sensory loss).

Box 1.39 Conditions associated with aortic dissection

- Hypertension: smoking, dyslipidaemia, cocaine/crack
- Connective tissue disorders:
  - Marfan's syndrome*
  - Ehlers–Danlos syndrome
- Hereditary vascular disorders: bicuspid aortic valve
- Vascular inflammation:
  - Coarctation
  - Giant cell arteritis
  - Takayasu's arteritis
  - Behçet's disease
  - Syphilis
- Deceleration trauma:
  - Car accident
  - Falls
- Chest trauma
- Pregnancy
- Iatrogenic
  - Catheterization
  - Cardiac surgery.

*Marfan syndrome—arm span >height, pubis to sole >publis to vertex, depressed sternum, scoliosis, high-arched palate, upwards lens dislocation, thoracic aortic dilation/aortic regurgitation, ↑urinary hydroxyprolene (some).

Differential diagnosis

- The chest pain may be mistaken for acute MI and acute MI may complicate aortic dissection. Always look for other signs of dissection (see 🕮 Box 1.37, p.135), as thrombolysis will be fatal.
- Severe chest pain and collapse may also be due to PE, spontaneous pneumothorax, acute pancreatitis, and penetrating duodenal ulcer.
- Pulse deficits without backache should suggest other diagnoses: atherosclerotic pertipheral vascular disease, arterial embolism, Takayasu's arteritis, etc.
- Acute cardiac tamponade with chest pain is also seen in acute viral or idiopathic pericarditis and acute MI with external rupture.

Practice point

Unilateral tongue weakness after a car crash with whiplash injury suggests carotid artery dissection.

Aortic dissection: investigations

General

- ***ECG:*** may be normal or non-specific (LVH, ST/T abnormalities). Look specifically for evidence of acute MI (inferior MI is seen if the dissection compromises the right coronary artery ostium).
- ***CXR:*** may appear normal, but with hindsight is almost always abnormal. Look for widened upper mediastinum, haziness or enlargement of the aortic knuckle, irregular aortic contour, separation (>5mm) of intimal calcium from outer aortic contour, displacement of trachea to the right, enlarged cardiac silhouette (pericardial effusion), pleural effusion (usually on left). Compare with previous films if available.
- ***Bloods***: base FBC, U&E, cardiac enzymes as well as cross match. A novel monoclonal antibody assay to smooth muscle myosin heavy chains can accurately differentiate an acute dissection from a MI.

Diagnostic

- ***Echocardiography:*** TTE may be useful in diagnosing aortic root dilatation, AR, and pericardial effusion/tamponade. TOE is the investigation of choice as it allows better evaluation of both ascending aorta and descending aorta, may identify origin of intimal tear, allows evaluation of the origins of the coronary arteries in relation to the dissection flap, and provides information on aortic insufficiency. It is not good at imaging the distal ascending aorta and proximal arch.
- ***MRI angiography:*** is the gold standard for diagnosing aortic dissection. It has all the positive features of TOE and in particular also provides accurate information on all segments of ascending/arch/ descending aorta, entry/exit sites, and branch vessels. Images can be displayed in multiple views as well as reconstructed in three dimensions. However, there are a number of disadvantages including (1) availability of service out of hours and cost, (2) presence of metallic valves or pacemakers may preclude patient from having an MRI, (3) monitoring of unstable patients in the scanner can be difficult and unsafe.
- ***Spiral (helical) CT with contrast***: allows three-dimensional display of all segments of aorta and adjacent structures. True and false lumens are identified by differential contrast flow, enter and exit site of intimal flap, as well as pleural and pericardial fluid. However it cannot demonstrate disruption of the aortic valve, which may be associated with ascending aortic dissection.
- ***Angiography:*** using the femoral or axillary approach may demonstrate altered flow in the two lumens, aortic valve incompetence, involvement of the branches, and the site of the intimal tear. It is invasive and associated with a higher risk of complications in an already high-risk patient. It has largely been superseded by CT/MRI and TOE.

Selecting a diagnostic modality

- Confirm or refute a diagnosis of dissection.
- Is the dissection confined to the descending aorta or does it involve the ascending/arch?

- Identify extent, sites of enter and exit, and presence and absence of thrombus.
- To see whether there is AR, coronary involvement or pericardial effusions.

Box 1.40 Selecting a diagnostic modality

- Where available, TOE should be the first-line investigation. It is safe and can provide all the information necessary to take the patient to the operating theatre.
- If TOE is not available or if it fails to provide the necessary information a spiral contrast CT should be performed.
- MRI should generally be reserved for follow-up images.
- Angiography is rarely used, but is of value if other modalities have failed to provide a diagnosis and/or extensive information is needed on branch vessels.

Aortic dissection: management 1

Stabilize the patient

- If the diagnosis is suspected, transfer the patient to an area where full resuscitation facilities are readily available.
- Secure venous access with large-bore cannulas (e.g. grey venflon).
- Take blood for FBC, U&Es, and cross match (10 units).
- When the diagnosis is confirmed or in cases with cardiovascular complications, transfer to ITU, insert an arterial line (radial unless the subclavian artery is compromised when a femoral line is preferred), central venous line, and urinary catheter.
- Immediate measures should be taken to correct BP (see 📖 p.148).
- Adequate analgesia (diamorphine 2.5–10mg IV and metoclopramide 10mg IV).

Plan the definitive treatment (Box 1.41)

This depends on the type of dissection (see 📖 Fig. 1.12, p.142) and its effects on the patient. General principles are:

- Patients with involvement of the ascending aorta should have emergency surgical repair and BP control.
- Patients with dissection limited to the descending aorta are managed initially medically with aggressive BP control.

However, this may change in the near future with emerging encouraging data from deployment of endovascular stent-grafts.

Indications and principles for surgery

- Involvement of the ascending aorta
- External rupture (haemopericardium, haemothorax, effusions)
- Arterial compromise (limb ischaemia, renal failure, stroke)
- Contraindications to medical therapy (AR, LVF)
- Progression (continued pain, expansion of haematoma on further imaging, loss of pulses, pericardial rub, or aortic insufficiency).

The aim of surgical therapy is to replace the ascending aorta, thereby preventing retrograde dissection and cardiac tamponade (main cause of death). The aortic valve may need reconstruction and resuspension unless it is structurally abnormal (bicuspid or Marfan's), where it is replaced.

Indications and principles for medical management

Medical therapy is the treatment of choice for:

- Uncomplicated type B dissection
- Stable isolated arch dissection
- Chronic (>2 weeks' duration) stable Type B dissection.

In all but those patients who are hypotensive, initial management is aimed at reducing systemic BP and myocardial contractility. The goal is to stop the spread of the intramural haematoma and to prevent rupture. The best guide is control of pain. Strict bed rest in a quiet room is essential.

Box 1.41 Management key points: aortic dissection

- Monitor haemodynamically in ITU.
- Adequate analgesia: diamorphine (+ metoclopramide).
- Type A (involving the ascending aorta): emergency surgical repair and BP control.
- Type B (involving descending aorta): manage medically with BP control.
- Reduce BP (aim for systolic: 100–120mmHg): start on IV β-blocker (e.g. labetalol) if no contraindications.
- Resuscitate hypotensive patients with IV fluids.

Aortic dissection: management 2

Control blood pressure

Reduce SBP to 100–120mmHg.

- Start on IV β-blocker (if no contraindications) aiming to reduce the heart rate to 60–70/min (see Box 1.42).
- Once this is achieved, if BP remains high, add a vasodilator such as sodium nitroprusside (see Box 1.42). Vasodilators in the absence of β-blockade may increase myocardial contractility and the rate of rise of pressure (d*P*/d*t*). Theoretically this may promote extension of the dissection.
- Further antihypertensive therapy may be necessary and other conventional agents such as calcium channel blockers, β-blockers, and ACEIs can be used.
- In patients with AR and congestive cardiac failure, myocardial depressants should not be given. Aim to control BP with vasodilators only.

Hypotension

May be due to haemorrhage or cardiac tamponade.

- Resuscitate with rapid IV volume (ideally colloid or blood, but crystalloid may be used also). A pulmonary artery wedge catheter (Swan–Ganz) should be used to monitor the wedge pressure and guide fluid replacement.
- If there are signs of AR or tamponade, arrange for an urgent Echo and discuss with the surgeons.

Emerging indications and principles for interventional therapy

There are increasing reports and short case series demonstrating favourable outcome (prognostic as well as symptomatic) data on using endovascular stent-grafts in management of primarily type B and also to a lesser extent type A aortic dissections.

On the basis of the current evidence endovascular stent-grafts should be considered to seal entry to false lumen and to enlarge compressed true lumen in the following situations:

- Unstable type B dissection
- Malperfusion syndrome (proximal aortic stent-graft and/or distal fenestration/stenting of branch arteries)
- Routine management of type B dissection (under evaluation).

Cardiac tamponade

If the patient is relatively stable pericardiocentesis may precipitate haemodynamic collapse and should be avoided. The patient should be transferred to the operating theatre for direct repair as urgently as possible. In the context of tamponade and EMD or marked hypotension pericardiocentesis is warranted.

Long-term treatment

Must involve strict BP control.

Prognosis

- The mortality for untreated aortic dissection is roughly 20–30% at 24h and 65–75% at 2 weeks.
- For dissections confined to the descending aorta, short-term survival is better (up to 80%) but ~30–50% will have progression of dissection despite aggressive medical therapy and will require surgery.
- Operative mortality is of the order of 10–25% and depends on the condition of the patient preoperatively. Postoperative 5-year actuarial survival of up to 75% may be expected.

Box 1.42 Medical therapy of aortic dissection

β-blockade (aim for HR 60–70bpm)	
Labetalol	20–80mg slow IV injection over 10min then 20–200mg/hour IV, increasing every 15min 100–400mg PO q12h
Atenolol	5–10mg slow IV injection then 50mg PO after 15min and at 12h, then 100mg PO daily
Propranolol	0.5mg IV (test dose), then 1mg every 2–5min up to max. 10mg; repeat every 2–3h 10–40mg PO 3–4 times daily
When HR 60–70/min (or if β-blocker contraindicated) add:	
Nitroprusside	0.25–8mcg/kg/min IV infusion
Hydralazine	5–10mg IV over 20min 50–300mcg/min IV infusion 25–50mg PO q8h
GTN	1–10mg/hour IV infusion
Amlodipine	5–10mg PO od

Acute pericarditis: assessment

Presentation

- Typically presents as central chest pain, often pleuritic, relieved by sitting forward and can be associated with breathlessness.
- Other symptoms (e.g. fever, cough, arthralgia, rash, faintness/dizziness 2° to pain/↑HR) may reflect the underlying disease (see Box 1.43).
- A pericardial friction rub is pathognomonic. This may be positional and transient and may be confused with the murmur of TR or MR.
- Venous pressure rises if an effusion develops. Look for signs of cardiac tamponade (see 🕮 p.156).

Investigations

ECG

- May be normal in up to 10%.
- 'Saddle-shaped' ST-segment elevation (concave upwards), with variable T inversion (usually late stages) and PR-segment depression (opposite to P-wave polarity). Minimal lead involvement to be considered, typically including I, II, aVL, aVF, and V3–V6.
- ST segment is always depressed in aVR, frequently depressed or isoelectric in V1, and sometimes in depressed in V2.
- May be difficult to distinguish from acute MI. Features suggesting pericarditis are:
  - Concave ST elevation (versus convex)
  - All leads involved (versus a territory, e.g. inferior)
  - Failure of usual ST evolution and no Q-waves
  - No AV block, BBB, or QT prolongation.
- Early repolarization (a normal variant) may be mistaken for pericarditis. In the former, ST elevation occurs in pre-cordial and rarely in V6 or the limb leads and is unlikely to show ST depression in V1 or PR segment depression.
- Usually not helpful in diagnosing pericarditis post MI.
- The voltage drops as an effusion develops and in tamponade there is electrical alternans, best seen in QRS complexes.

Echo

- May demonstrate a pericardial collection.
- Useful to monitor LV function in case of deterioration due to associated myopericarditis.
- We recommend every patient has an Echo prior to discharge to assess LV function.

Other investigations depend on the suspected aetiology

All patients should have:

- FBC and biochemical profile
- ESR and CRP (levels rise proportionate to intensity of disease)
- Serial cardiac enzymes (CK, CK-MB, troponin). Elevations indicate sub-pericardial myocarditis
- CXR (heart size, pulmonary oedema, infection).

Where appropriate:
- Viral titres (acute +2 weeks later) and obtain virology opinion
- Blood cultures
- Autoantibody screen (RF, ANA, anti-DNA, complement levels)
- Thyroid function tests
- Fungal precipitins (if immunosuppressed), Mantoux test
- Sputum culture and cytology
- Diagnostic pericardial tap (culture, cytology).

Box 1.43 Causes of acute pericarditis

- Idiopathic
- Infection (viral, bacterial, TB, and fungal)
- AMI
- Dressler's syndrome, postcardiotomy syndrome
- Malignancy (e.g. breast, bronchus, lymphoma)
- Uraemia
- Autoimmune disease (e.g. SLE, RA, Wegner's, scleroderma, PAN)
- Granulomatous diseases (e.g. sarcoid)
- Hypothyroidism
- Drugs (hydralazine, procainamide, isonlazid)
- Trauma (chest trauma, iatrogenic)
- Radiotherapy.

Acute pericarditis: management

General measures

- ***Admit?*** Depends on clinical picture. We recommend admission of most patients for observation for complications especially effusions, tamponade, and myocarditis. Patients should be discharged when pain free.
- ***Bed rest.***
- ***Analgesia:*** NSAIDs are the mainstay. Ibuprofen is well tolerated and increases coronary flow (200–800mg qds). Aspirin is an alternative (600mg qds PO). Indometacin should be avoided in adults as it reduces coronary flow and has marked side effects. Use PPI (lansoprazole 30mg od) to minimize GI side-effects. Opioid analgesia may be required. Colchicine used as monotherapy or in addition to NSAIDs may help settle pain acutely and prevent recurrence.
- ***Steroids:*** these may be used if the pain does not settle within 48h (e.g. prednisolone EC 40–60mg PO od for up to 2 weeks, tapering down when pain settles). Use in conjunction with NSAID and taper steroids first before stopping NSAID. It is also of value if pericarditis 2° to autoimmune disorders.
- ***Colchicine:*** evidence suggests that either used as monotherapy or in conjunction with NSAIDs it may help to settle pain acutely and prevent relapses (1mg/day divided doses). Stop if patient develops diarrhoea, nausea. (1mg stat, 500mcg q6h for 48h).
- ***Pericardiocentesis:*** this should be considered for significant effusion or if there are signs of tamponade (see 🕮 p.156).
- ***Antibiotics:*** these should be given only if bacterial infection is suspected.
- ***Oral anticoagulants:*** should be discontinued (risk of haemo-pericardium). Patient should be given IV UFH, which is easier to reverse (IV protamine) if complications arise.

Bacterial pericarditis

- The commonest pathogens are pneumococcus, staphylococci, streptococci, Gram –ve rods, and *Neisseria* species.
- Risk factors include pre-existing pericardial effusion (e.g. uraemic pericarditis) and immunosuppression (iatrogenic, lymphoma, leukaemia, HIV).
- The infection may have spread from mediastinitis, IE, pneumonia, or sub-diaphragmatic abscess.
- Suspect in patients with high fever, night sweats, dyspnoea, and raised JVP (chest pain may be mild or absent); there may be other intrathoracic infection (e.g. pneumonia).
- If suspected, take blood cultures and start IV flucloxacillin (2g qds) and IV gentamicin or IV cefotaxime (2g tds). Adjust treatment when sensitivities known.
- Significant-sized pericardial collections should be drained to dryness if possible. Send fluid for Gram and ZN stain, fungal smear, and culture. Surgical drainage may be required for recurrent effusions.
- Patients with TB pericarditis are very prone to developing cardiac constriction. Steroids have not been shown to prevent this but they do prevent progression once constrictive symptoms develop. Surgical pericardectomy may be required. Take advice from cardiologists and infectious diseases team.

Viral pericarditis

- Pathogens include Coxsackie A + B, echovirus, adenovirus, mumps, EBV, VZV, CMV, hepatitis B, and HIV.
- Usually a self-limiting illness (1–3 weeks) and can be seasonal. Common in young individuals with no associated cardiac history.
- 20–30% develop recurrent pericarditis.
- Complications include recurrent pericarditis (20–30%), myocarditis, dilated cardiomyopathy, pericardial effusion and tamponade, and late pericardial constriction.
- Treatment is supportive (see previous section).

Uraemic pericarditis

This is an indication for urgent dialysis (see 📖 Box 4.3, p.289).

Dressler syndrome, postcardiotomy syndrome

- Complicates ~1% of acute MI and 10–15% patients following cardiac surgery presenting 2–4 weeks later (up to 3 months later).
- Consists of recurrent pericarditis, fever, anaemia, high ESR, neutrophil leucocytosis, pleural effusions, and transient pulmonary infiltrates on CXR.
- Treat with bed rest, NSAIDs (aspirin 600mg PO qds) and steroids for persisting symptoms (see above).
- Pericarditis following acute MI (see 📖 p.32).

Neoplastic pericarditis

- The 1-year survival of patients with malignant effusive pericarditis is ≤25%. The approach to treatment depends on the underlying malignancy and symptoms.
- Asymptomatic pericardial effusions do not require drainage. Treat the underlying malignancy (± mediastinal radiotherapy). Recurrent effusions may need formation of surgical pericardial window.
- Drainage is indicated for cardiac tamponade.

Myopericarditis

- Although it can occur with all cases of pericarditis it is more common in the context of AIDS, vasculitis/connective tissue disorders, rheumatic fever, and TB infection.
- Clinical suspicion should be higher in the context of pericarditis accompanied by significant arrhythmia (especially ventricular) and features of LV dysfunction and sinus tachycardia out of proportion to clinical picture (fever, pain, persistence >5–6 days).
- Biochemical markers of myocardial injury are often positive (especially TnT or TnI).
- In the absence of heart failure, treatment is as uncomplicated pericarditis. Steroids should be avoided unless indicated as part of treatment for underlying cause. Heart failure should be treated conventionally. Interferon can be used to treat enteroviral infections and globulins for CMV.
- Pericardial effusions must be drained with care as the effusion may be 'splinting' a dilated/myocarditic heart. Drainage can lead to rapid dilation and cardiovascular collapse.
- Prognosis is generally good and most recover unless there is severe LV impairment.

Cardiac tamponade: presentation

Cardiac tamponade occurs when a pericardial effusion causes haemodynamically significant cardiac compression. The presentation depends on the speed with which fluid accumulates within the pericardium. Acute tamponade may occur with 100–200mL in a relatively restricted pericardial sac. Chronic pericardial collections may contain up to 1000mL of fluid without clinical tamponade.

Causes

Acute tamponade

- Cardiac trauma
- Iatrogenic:
  - Post-cardiac surgery
  - Post-cardiac catheterization
  - Post-pacing/EP study
- Aortic dissection
- Spontaneous bleed
  - Anticoagulation
  - Uraemia
  - Thrombocytopenia
- Cardiac rupture post MI.

'Sub-acute' tamponade

- Malignant disease
- Idiopathic pericarditis: Uraemia
- Infections:
  - Bacterial
  - TB
- Radiation
- Hypothyroidism
- Post pericardotomy
- SLE.

Presentation

- Patients commonly present either with cardiac arrest (commonly electrical mechanical dissociation) or with hypotension, confusion, stupor, and shock.
- Patients who develop cardiac tamponade slowly are usually acutely unwell, but not in extremis. Their main symptoms include:
  - Breathlessness, leading to air hunger at rest.
  - There may be a preceding history of chest discomfort
  - Symptoms resulting from compression of adjacent structures by a large effusion (i.e. dysphagia, cough, hoarseness, or hiccough).
  - There may be symptoms due to the underlying cause (Box 1.44).
  - Insidious development may present with complications of tamponade including renal failure, liver and/or mesenteric ischaemia, and abdominal plethora.

Important physical signs

Most physical findings are non-specific. They include:

- Tachycardia (except in hypothyroidism and uraemia).
- Hypotension (± shock) with postural hypotension.
- Raised JVP (often >10cm) with a prominent systolic *x* descent and absent diastolic y descent (see Fig. 1.13). If the JVP is visible and either remains static or rises with inspiration it indicates concomitant pericardial constriction (Kussmaul's sign).
- Auscultation may reveal diminished heart sounds. Pericardial rub may be present and suggests a small pericardial collection.
- Look for pulsus paradoxus (a decrease in the palpable pulse and SBP of >10mmHg on inspiration). This may be so marked that the pulse and Korotkoff sounds may be completely lost during inspiration. This

can be measured using a BP cuff (Box 1.45) or arterial catheter if in situ already. Other conditions that can cause a pulsus paradoxus include: acute hypotension, obstructive airways disease, and pulmonary embolus.

- Other physical signs include cool extremities (ears, nose) tachypnoea, hepatomegaly, and signs of the underlying cause for the pericardial effusion.

Box 1.44 Causes of hypotension with a raised JVP

- Cardiac tamponade
- Constrictive pericarditis
- Restrictive pericarditis
- Severe biventricular failure
- RV infarction
- PE
- Tension pneumothorax
- Acute severe asthma
- Malignant SVC obstruction and sepsis (e.g. lymphoma).

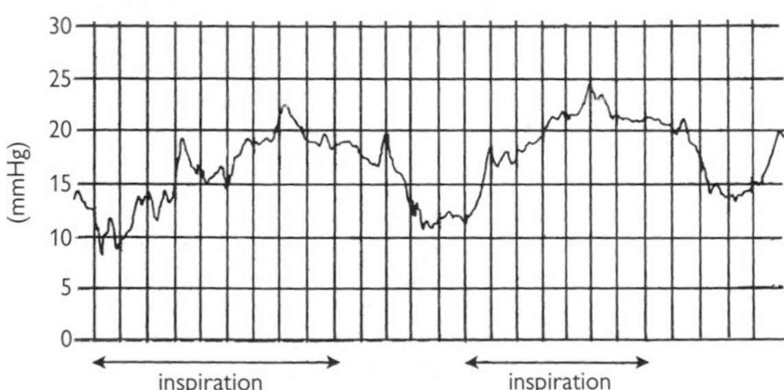

Fig. 1.13 Right atrial pressure (RAP) tracing in tamponade. There is a paradoxical rise in RAP during inspiration.

Box 1.45 Key point

To establish presence of pulsus paradoxus non-invasively, inflate BP cuff to 15mmHg above highest systolic pressure. Deflate cuff gradually until first beats are heard and hold pressure at that level concentrating on the disappearance and reappearance of sounds with respiration (bump–bump, silence–silence, bump–bump, where noise reflects expiration). Continue to deflate slowly, paying attention to same pattern until all beats are audible. The difference between the initial and final pressure should be >10mmHg.

Cardiac tamponade: management

Tamponade should be suspected in patients with hypotension, elevated venous pressure, falling BP, ↑HR and ↑RR (with clear chest), pulsus paradoxus especially if predisposing factors are present.

Investigations

- ***CXR:*** the heart size may be normal (e.g. in acute haemopericardium following cardiac trauma). With slower accumulation of pericardial fluid (>250mL) the cardiac silhouette will enlarge with a globular appearance. The size of the effusion is unrelated to its haemodynamic significance. Look for signs of pulmonary oedema.
- ***ECG:*** usually shows a sinus tachycardia, with low voltage complexes and variable ST-segment changes. With large effusions 'electrical alternans' may be present with beat-to-beat variation in the QRS morphology resulting from the movement of the heart within the pericardial effusion.
- ***Echocardiography:*** confirms the presence of a pericardial effusion. The diagnosis of tamponade is a clinical one. Echo signs highly suggestive of tamponade include:
  - Chamber collapse during diastole (RA, RV, RV outflow tract)
  - Marked variation in transvalvular flow
  - Dilated IVC with little or no diameter change on respiration.
- If available, examine the central venous pressure trace for the characteristic exaggerated x descent and absent y descent.

Management

Following confirmation of the diagnosis:

- While preparing for drainage of the pericardial fluid, the patient's circulation may temporarily be supported by loading with IV colloid (500–1000mL stat) and starting inotropes (i.e. adrenaline).
- In patients with an adequate BP, cautious systemic vasodilatation with hydralazine or nitroprusside in conjunction with volume loading may increase forward cardiac output. This is not to be recommended routinely as it may cause acute deterioration.
- The effusion should be urgently drained (see 🕮 p.766 for pericardiocentesis) guided by Echo or fluoroscopy. *In the event of circulatory collapse drainage must happen immediately without imaging.*
- Surgical drainage is indicated if the effusion is 2° to trauma.
- Avoid intubation and positive pressure ventilation as this reduces CO.
- In patients with cardiac arrest chest compression has little or no value, as there is no room for additional filling.
- Uraemic patients will also need dialysis.
- The cause of the effusion should be established (see 🕮 Box 1.43, p.151). Pericardial fluid should be sent for cytology, microbiology including TB, and if appropriate Hb, glucose, and amylase.

Further management is of the underlying cause.

Special cases

Recurrent pericardial effusion

In some cases pericardial effusion recurs. This requires either a change in the treatment of the underlying cause or a formal surgical drainage procedure such as a surgical pericardial window or pericardiectomy.

Low pressure tamponade

Seen in the setting of dehydration. The JVP is not raised, right atrial pressure is normal, and tamponade occurs even with small volumes of pericardial fluid.

- The patient may respond well to IV fluids.
- If there is a significant pericardial collection this should be drained.

Congenital heart disease in adults 1

Extra-cardiac complications

- ***Polycythaemia:*** chronic hypoxia stimulates erythropoietin production and erythrocytosis. The 'ideal' Hb level is ~17–18g/dL; some centres advocate venesection to control the haematocrit and prevent hyperviscosity syndrome (see 📖 p.616). Follow local guidelines. Generally consider phlebotomy only if moderate or severe symptoms of hyperviscosity are present and haematocrit >65%. Remove 500mL of blood over 30–45min and replace volume simultaneously with 500–1000mL saline, or salt-free dextran (if heart failure). Avoid abrupt changes in circulating volume. If hyperviscosity symptoms are the result of acute dehydration or iron deficiency, venesection is not required and patient must be rehydrated and/or treated with iron.
- ***Renal disease and gout:*** hypoxia affects glomerular and tubular function resulting in proteinuria, reduced urate excretion, ↑urate reabsorption and reduced creatinine clearance. Overt renal failure is uncommon. Try to avoid dehydration, diuretics, radiographic contrast. Asymptomatic hyperuricaemia does not need treatment. Colchicine and steroids are first-line agents for treatment of acute gout. NSAIDs should be avoided.
- ***Sepsis:*** patients are more prone to infection. Skin acne is common with poor healing of scars. Skin stitches for operative procedures should be left in for 7–10 days longer than normal. Dental hygiene is very important due to the risk of endocarditis. Any site of sepsis may result in cerebral abscesses from metastatic infection or septic emboli.
- ***Thrombosis and bleeding:*** multifactorial and caused by a combination of abnormal platelet function, coagulation abnormalities, and polycythaemia. PT and aPTT values may be elevated and 2° to a fall in Factors V, VII, VIII, and X. Both arterial ± venous thromboses and haemorrhagic complications (e.g. petechiae, epistaxes, haemoptyses) can occur. Dehydration or oral contraceptives are risk factors for thrombotic events. Spontaneous bleeding is generally self-limiting. In the context of severe bleeding general measures are effective including platelet transfusion, FFP, cryoprecipitate, and vitamin K. Aspirin and other NSAIDs should generally be avoided to decrease chances of spontaneous bruising/bleeding.
- ***1° pulmonary problems:*** include infection, infarction, and haemorrhage from ruptured arterioles or capillaries.
- ***Stroke:*** can be both thrombotic as well as haemorrhagic. Arterial thrombosis, embolic events (paradoxical emboli in R → L shunt) and injudicious phlebotomy lead to spontaneous thrombosis. Haemostasis problems (as indicated earlier) especially when combined with NSAIDs or formal anticoagulation can lead to haemorrhagic stroke. Any injured brain tissue is also a nidus for intracranial infection/abscess formation.
- ***Complications 2° to drugs, investigations, surgery:*** avoid abrupt changes in BP or systemic resistance. Contrast agents may provoke systemic vasodilatation and cause acute decompensation. They may also precipitate renal failure. Before non-cardiac surgery, try to optimize haematocrit and haemostasis by controlled phlebotomy and

replacement with dextran. High-flow O_2 is important before and after surgery. Extreme precaution with IV lines.

- ***Arthralgia:*** mainly due to hypertrophic osteoarthropathy. In patients with R → L shunt megakaryocytes bypass the pulmonary circulation and become trapped in systemic vascular beds, promoting new bone formation.

Cardiac complications

- ***Congestive cardiac failure:*** the aetiology can be complex and is often directly dependent on the underlying abnormality. Possibilities include valve dysfunction (calcification of an abnormal valve or 2° to supra- or subvalvular fibrosis and stenosis), ventricular dysfunction (hypertrophy, fibrosis, and failure), dysfunctioning surgical shunt, or pulmonary arteriolar disease and shunt reversal. Treat as usual taking special care not to dehydrate the patient or precipitate acute changes in BP (see 🕮 p.162).
- ***Endocarditis:*** the risk depends on the cardiac lesion and the pathogen. See 🕮 Box 1.21, p.97. The recommended antibiotic prophylaxis regimen is given on 🕮 p.110. Patients should be advised on careful skin care (e.g. acne) and antibiotic prophylaxis to prevent local infections that may 'metastasize' to heart or brain.
- ***Arrhythmias:*** treat in the standard way (see 🕮 pp.55–86).

Congenital heart disease in adults 2

Management

Patients can be very complex and must be discussed with their regular cardiologist and/or local congenital adult heart centre.

General measures

- Contact and take advice from the cardiologist normally involved in the patient's care.
- IV lines are potentially very hazardous due to the risk of sepsis and systemic embolization (air and particulate matter). Use an air filter if available. Remove IV cannulae if there are any local signs of thrombophlebitis.
- Avoid sudden changes in circulating volume (e.g. vomiting, diarrhoea, haemorrhage, venesection). Any acute fall in SVR may precipitate intense cyanosis and death and an acute rise in SVR may abruptly reduce systemic blood flow and cause collapse.
- Monitor for neurological signs and symptoms from cerebral thromboembolism or septic embolism.

Specific measures

- ***Haemoptysis:*** common. Most episodes are self-limiting and precipitated by infection. Differentiation from PE may be difficult. Try to keep the patient calm and ensure adequate BP control. Give high-flow O_2 by mask. If there is clinical suspicion of infection (fever, sputum production, leucocytosis, raised CRP, etc.) start broad-spectrum antibiotics. VQ scan may help in the diagnosis of pulmonary embolism (see 📖 p.120) but is often equivocal. Avoid aspirin and NSAIDs as these exacerbate the intrinsic platelet abnormalities. There is anecdotal evidence for the use of low-dose IV heparin, dextran 40 (500mL IV infusion q4–6h), acrid (Arvin®, reduces plasma fibrinogen by cleaving fibrin), or low-dose warfarin therapy for reducing thrombotic tendency in these patients. Severe pulmonary haemorrhage may respond to aprotinin or tranexamic acid.
- ***Breathlessness:*** may be due to pulmonary oedema or hypoxia (↑shunt) 2° to chest infection or pulmonary infarction. Do not give large doses of diuretics or nitrates as this will drop systemic pressures and may precipitate acute collapse. Compare CXR to previous films to try to assess if there is radiological evidence of pulmonary oedema. The JVP in patients with cyanotic CHD is typically high and should not be used as a sole marker of heart failure. Overall patients need a higher filling pressure to maintain pulmonary blood flow. Give high-flow O_2 by mask. Start antibiotics if there is a clinical suspicion of infection (see 📖 Table 2.1, p.171). Give oral diuretics if there is evidence of pulmonary oedema or severe right heart failure. Monitor haematocrit and renal function closely for signs of over-diuresis.
- ***Effort syncope:*** should prompt a search for arrhythmias, in particular VT (Holter monitor), severe valve disease, or signs of overt heart failure. Treat as appropriate.

- ***Chest pain:*** may be 2° to PE or infarction (spontaneous thrombosis), pneumonia, ischaemic heart disease, or musculoskeletal causes. It requires careful evaluation with the conventional diagnostic modalities already described.

Box 1.46 Congenital defects with survival to adulthood

Common

- Bicuspid aortic valve
- Coarctation of the aorta
- Pulmonary stenosis
- Ostium secundum ASD
- Patent ductus arteriosus
- Coronary or pulmonary AV fistulas
- Aneurysm of sinus of Valsalva.

Rarer

- Dextrocardia (situs solitus or invertus)
- Congenital complete heart block
- Congenitally corrected transposition
- Ebstein's anomaly.

Congenital defects with good prognosis after surgery

- Ventricular septal defect
- Fallot's tetralogy

Box 1.47 Causes of cyanosis in adults with congenital heart disease

- 'Eisenmenger reaction': R → L shunt through VSD, ASD or patent foramen ovale with pulmonary hypertension (pulmonary hypertension may be 2° to pulmonary vascular disease, pulmonary artery stenosis or banding, pulmonary valve stenosis, tricuspid atresia).
- Abnormal connection: transpositions, IVC or SVC to left atrium, total anomalous pulmonary venous drainage.
- Pulmonary AV fistulae.

Chapter 2

Respiratory emergencies

Acute pneumonia: assessment

Presentation

- Classically cough (productive or non-productive), fever, breathlessness, chest pain, abnormal CXR. There may be prodromal symptoms of coryza, headache, and muscle aches.
- The aetiological agent cannot be predicted from the clinical features (see Box 2.1).
- Immunocompromised patients may present with agitation, fever, tachypnoea, ↓ routine oximetry readings. CXR abnormalities may be subtle.
- Patients with right-sided endocarditis (e.g. IV drug users) may present with haemoptysis, fever, and patchy consolidation ± cavitation.

Severity assessment

- Severity assessment is the key to deciding the site of care (i.e. home, medical ward, or critical care ward) and guiding general management and antibiotic treatment.
- The 'CURB-65' score may be used[2] as a severity assessment tool (see Box 2.2):
  - *CURB-65 score ≥ 3*: high risk of mortality; should be admitted and managed as having severe pneumonia.
  - *CURB-65 score of 2*: ↑risk of mortality, need short stay in-patient treatment or hospital supervised outpatient treatment.
  - *CURB-65 score of 0–1*: low risk of mortality, may be suitable for home treatment.

Management[1]

General resuscitation and investigations

- Check 'ABC' (airway, breathing, and circulation). Arrange for urgent CXR.
- *Secure venous access:* if there are signs of dehydration, start IV crystalloids; examine regularly for signs of fluid overload.
- *Send bloods*: FBC, U&Es, LFT, CRP.
- *Check ABG*: correct hypoxia (P_aO_2 ≤10kPa) with O_2, at least 35%. If hypoxia fails to correct despite maximum inspired O_2 or there is hypercapnia (P_aCO_2 ≥6kPa) the patient is likely to require ventilation. Involve ITU early to plan the patient's care.
- Arrange for *urgent CXR*.
- Culture blood and sputum.
- *Pain relief*: paracetamol or a NSAID usually suffice. Morphine may be required; respiratory depression is unlikely to be a problem if the P_aCO_2 is low or normal and it may be reversed with naloxone.

Indications for intensive care

- Patients with >2 components of CURB (*C*onfusion, raised *U*rea, Raised *R*espiratory rate, low *B*P, see Box 2.2) who do not respond rapidly.
- Persisting hypoxia with P_aO_2 <8kPa despite maximal O_2 administration.
- Progressive hypercapnia (P_aCO_2 ≥6kPa), progressive exhaustion.
- Severe acidosis (pH<7.26).
- Shock, depressed consciousness.
- Involve ITU early—this may help avoid ventilation as an emergency.

Box 2.1 Causes of acute pneumonia in patients admitted to hospital

Community acquired
- Strep. pneumoniae (40%)
- H. influenzae (5%)
- *S. aureus* (2%)
- Moraxhella catarrhalis (2%)
- Gram –ve bacteria/anaerobes 1%
- Influenza A&B (11%)
- Other viruses (2%)
- Mixed pathogens (14%)
- No organism identified.

Atypicals
- Mycoplasma (11%)
- Legionella pneumophila (4%)
- Chlamydia pneumoniae (13%)
- Other *Chlamydia* species (4%).

Hospital acquired
- All of the above.

Immunocompromised
- All of the above.

Box 2.2 CURB-65 score*

CURB-65 score is a 6 point scale (0–5)—one point for each of the following on the initial assessment):
- *C*onfusion (defined as Mental Test Score ≤8, or new disorientation in time, person, or place)
- *U*rea >7mmol/L
- *R*espiratory rate (≥30/min)
- *B*lood pressure, low systolic (<90mmHg) or diastolic (≤ 60mmHg)
- Age ≥ ***65*** years.

Lim W.S., van der Eeden *et al.* (2003). Defining community acquired pneumonia severity on presenation to hospital: an international derivation and validation study. *Thorax* **58:** 377–82.

References

1. See British Thoracic Society guidelines. Guidelines for the Management of Community Acquired Pneumonia in Adults: http://www.brit-thoracic.org.uk/Portals/0/Clinical%20Information/Pneumonia/Guidelines/CAPGuideline-full.pdf

2. British Thoracic Society guidelines. Guidelines for the Management of Community Acquired Pneumonia in Adults: http://www.brit-thoracic.org.uk/Portals/0/Clinical%20Information/Pneumonia/Guidelines/CAPGuideline-full.pdf

Acute pneumonia: investigations

Investigations

All patients should have:

- ABGs (on air and O_2)
- FBC, U&Es, LFT, ESR, CRP
- ECG
- CXR (see Fig. 2.1)
- Blood cultures
- Sputum culture, Gram stain, ZN stain (if suspicious of TB), cytology
- Pleural fluid aspiration (if present) for MC&S, protein, and pH
- *Pneumococcal* antigen: urine, sputum, or blood
- Serology (acute and convalescent)
- Cold agglutinins (*Mycoplasma* day 7–14)
- Urine for *Legionella* antigen, sputum for *Legionella* culture, and direct immunofluorescence.

Where appropriate consider

- Bronchoscopy (±BAL) (if immunocompromised, or if fails to respond to first-line antibiotics and no organism identified)
- Echo (?right heart endocarditis, see 📖 p.96)
- CTPA (to exclude infected pulmonary infarct)
- Trans-bronchial or open lung biopsy
- Aspiration of pleural fluid for MC&S
- Viral titres.

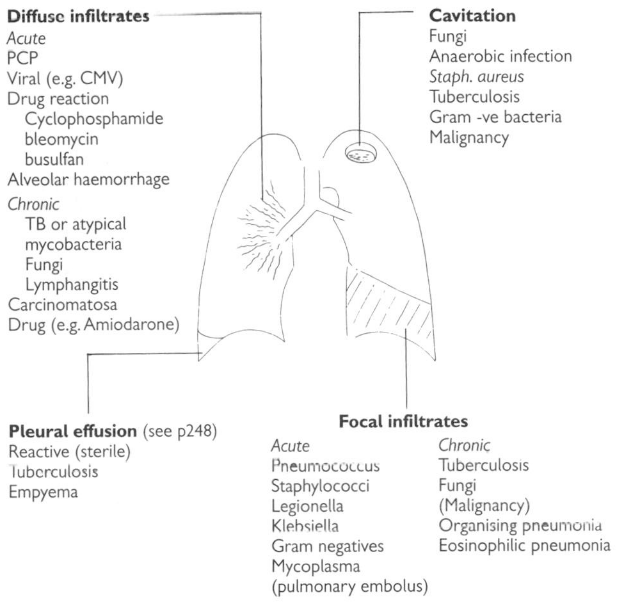
Diffuse infiltrates
Acute
PCP
Viral (e.g. CMV)
Drug reaction
Cyclophosphamide
bleomycin
busulfan
Alveolar haemorrhage
Chronic
TB or atypical
mycobacteria
Fungi
Lymphangitis
Carcinomatosa
Drug (e.g. Amiodarone)
Cavitation
Fungi
Anaerobic infection
Staph. aureus
Tuberculosis
Gram -ve bacteria
Malignancy
Pleural effusion (see p248)
Reactive (sterile)
Tuberculosis
Empyema
Focal infiltrates
Acute
Pneumococcus
Staphylococci
Legionella
Klebsiella
Gram negatives
Mycoplasma
(pulmonary embolus)
Chronic
Tuberculosis
Fungi
(Malignancy)
Organising pneumonia
Eosinophilic pneumonia

Fig. 2.1 Acute pneumonia: chest investigations.

Acute pneumonia: management

Treatment

- 'Blind' treatment should be started as soon as appropriate cultures have been sent (Table 2.1). Modify therapy in the light of subsequent investigations or positive cultures.
- Start on IV therapy (for at least 48h in patients with high CURB scores); adjust according to clinical condition and response (Table 2.1).
- In patients with COPD or asthma, consider treatment with salbutamol (2.5–5mg nebulized q4–6h) to relieve bronchospasm. This may also 'loosen secretions' and improve mucocilliary action.
- Continue IV fluids as necessary to keep the patient well hydrated.
- Monitor response to therapy with:
  - FBC, CRP
  - Pulse oximetry or blood gases
  - CXR at day 3–5 (sooner if deteriorating).
- Total duration of therapy usually 5–7 days (in low risk) up to 10 days (in high-risk patients).
- Follow-up CXR 4–6 weeks after discharge mandatory to exclude an underlying endobronchial lesion.
- Patients should not be discharged if they have more than one of the following features of instability: temperature > 37.8°C; pulse rate >100/min; respiratory rate >24/min; SBP <90mmHg; O_2 saturation <90%; abnormal mental status; inability to maintain oral intake.

Choice of antibiotics

In severely ill patients, the history may point to a likely pathogen:

- ***COPD:*** *S. pneumoniae, H. influenzae, M. catarrhalis*
- ***Alcoholism:*** *S. pneumoniae, S. aureus, H. influenzae, Klebsiella*, TB, anaerobes, Gram –ve bacteria
- ***Recent 'flu':*** S. aureus, S. pneumoniae, H. influenzae
- ***Risk of aspiration:*** anaerobes, Gram –ve bacteria
- ***Contact with birds:*** *C. psittaci*
- ***Haemoptysis:*** streptococci, *S. aureus*, lung abscess, necrotizing Gram –ve bacteria, invasive aspergillosis
- ***Diarrhoea, abdominal pain:*** *Legionella*
- ***Pharyngitis/otitsmedia:*** *Mycoplasma*, anaemia/cold agglutinins
- ***Risk factors for HIV:*** S. pneumoniae, H. influenzae, CMV, PCP, *Cryptococcus*
- ***Hospital acquired:*** Gram –ve bacteria, *S. aureus*
- ***Neutropenia:*** *P. aeruginosa*, Gram –ve bacteria, *Aspergillus*
- ***Drug addicts:*** *S. aureus, Candida*
- ***Nursing home patients:*** higher risk of aspiration: anaerobes, Gram –ve bacteria.

'Blind' treatment of pneumonia

- Most patients can be adequately treated with oral antibiotics.
- Consider IV antibiotics if adverse prognostic features (see 📖 p.166) present.

In patients with a good history of *penicillin allergy* (anaphylaxis, urticaria) alternatives include erythromycin, clarithromycin, levofloxacin, and moxifloxacin (NB: ciprofloxacin is not very active against *S. pneumoniae*). Alternatives for flucloxacillin include vancomycin, teicoplanin, or rifampicin: consult BNF for dosages.

Table 2.1 Empirical therapy for pneumonia

Community-Acquired Pneumonia (CAP)	
Mild or Moderate (CURB65 0–2)	Amoxicillin plus clarithromycin or doxycycline[1]
Severe (CURB65 3–5)	Co-amoxiclav 1.2g tds plus clarithromycin 500mg bd IV *or* cefuroxime/cefotaxime plus clarithromycin 500mg bd IV
Hospital-acquired pneumonia	Cefotaxime (or ceftazidime) ± metronidazole
Post-influenza pneumonia (*S. aureus* possible)	Cefuroxime (or amoxicillin + clarithromycin + flucloxacillin
If MRSA isolated or suspected	Switch flucloxacillin to vancomycin
Aspiration pneumonia	Cefuroxime + metronidazole or benzylpenicillin + gentamicin + metronidazole
Patient with risk factors for HIV and suspicion of PCP	As for CAP + high-dose IV co-trimoxazole

[1] If intolerant of B-lactam or macrolide, use fluoroquinolone with activity against *S. pneumoniae* (e.g. levofloxacin) or doxycycline (200mg then 100mg once daily).

Suggested antibiotic dosages

- Amoxicillin: 500mg –1g IV tds
- Benzylpenicillin: 1.2–2.4g IV qds
- Cefuroxime: 750mg –1.5g IV tds
- Cefotaxime: 1–2g IV tds
- Ceftazidime: 1–2g IV tds
- Co-amoxiclav: 1.2g IV tds
- Co-trimoxazole: 5mg/kg q6h of trimethoprim component.
- Clarithromycin: 500mg–1g PO bd
- Erythromycin: 500mg–1g IV (or PO) qds
- Flucloxacillin: 1–2g IV qds
- Gentamicin: loading dose (120mg IV) then 1–2.5mg/kg q8–12h guided by level
- Metronidazole: 500mg IV tds
- Vancomycin: 750mg–1g bd depending on size and renal function
- Teicoplanin: 200–400mg od IV for MRSA.

NB: IV erythromycin causes severe phlebitis. Use central line if available or change to oral preparation after 2–3 days. Clarithromycin is an alternative to erythromycin.

Acute pneumonia: specific situations

Community-acquired pneumonia

- Either *amoxicillin* 1g IV q8h or *cefuroxime* 750mg–1.5g IV q8h plus *erythromycin* 500mg–1g PO/IV q6h to cover atypicals plus flucloxacillin 1–2g IV q6h if *S. aureus* is suspected.
- *Penicillin allergy*: cephalosporins are usually safe where there is a history of rashes with penicillin. If there is history of anaphylaxis consider clarithromycin 500mg bd PO as sole therapy, or if unwell seek respiratory/microbiological advice.

Aspiration pneumonia

- Risk factors include: seizures, reduced conscious level, stroke, dysphagia, periodontal disease, 'down-and-out', general anaesthesia. Always admit.
- Clinical features include: wheeze and frothy non-purulent sputum (as soon as 2–4h after aspiration), tachypnoea, cyanosis, and respiratory distress.
- Gastric acid destroys alveoli resulting in ↑capillary permeability and pulmonary oedema. Haemorrhage is common. Severe necrotizing pneumonia may result.
- *Treatment: cefuroxime* (as for CAP) + *metronidazole* (500mg IV q8h). Amoxicillin + metronidazole + gentamicin.

Hospital-acquired pneumonia

- Most likely organisms are enteric Gram –ve ± anaerobes.
- *Treatment*: broad-spectrum cephalosporin (e.g. cefotaxime 2g tds IV) *metronidazole* (500mg IV tds). If intubated ≥48h use anti-pseudomonal antibiotic (e.g. ceftazidime 2g tds, modify dose in renal failure).

Pneumonia in the immunocompromised

- All 'routine' pathogens are possible; other infections depend on the nature of immunosuppression. TB and atypical mycobacteria are more common.
- Since the introduction of combination antiretroviral treatment opportunistic infections are less common and pulmonary Kaposi's sarcoma or lymphoma rarely seen. However, pulmonary opportunistic infection may be the first manifestation of HIV before it is diagnosed, the most common being *Pneumocystis carinii*. Fungal and viral (CMV) pneumonitis may also occur. Desaturation on exercise in the presence of a normal CXR or one with a diffuse interstitial shadowing is highly suggestive of PCP.
- Recipients of *organ transplants* have depressed cell-mediated immunity due to anti-rejection immunosuppressive therapy. Additional pathogens to which they are susceptible include PCP, viruses (e.g. CMV, RSV, influenza and parainfluenza, adenovirus), and fungi (*Aspergillus* spp., *Candida* spp.). The CXR abnormalities tend not to be specific for the pathogen and treatment should cover all possible pathogens.
- In general early bronchoscopy and BAL is indicated for diagnosis; management should be discussed early with a respiratory/infectious disease/microbiology team.

Acute pneumonia: complications

Community-acquired pneumonia that fails to respond

- Review the diagnosis (?PE, pulmonary oedema, pulmonary vasculitis, alveolar haemorrhage, cavitation, organizing pneumonia, eosinophilic pneumonia, bronchiectasis).
- Repeat CXR and arrange for CT chest to look for cavitation or empyema. Refer to Respiratory Team. Repeat culture of relevant specimens (e.g. sputum, blood). Consider possible resistant organism or underlying disease, e.g. bronchial carcinoma.
- Consider bronchoscopy to exclude TB, PCP, or an obstructing lesion.
- Review antibiotic dosages and intensify (e.g. inadequate oral erythromycin for *Mycoplasma* pneumonia).

Parapneumonic pleural effusion or empyema

- Parapneumonic pleural effusions develop in up to 50% of patients with bacterial pneumonia admitted to hospital.
- Diagnostic tap should be performed on all parapneumonic effusions to exclude an empyema. Sent pleural fluid for MC&S, urgent Gram stain, and pH analysis.
- Empyema (visibly cloudy fluid, pus, or organisms on Gram stain) or complicated parapneumonic effusion (visibly clear fluid with Ph <7.2) should be removed with pleural space drainage under ultrasound guidance. Discuss with respiratory physicians.
- Ultrasound may help look at the level of the effusion and demonstrate loculation with an empyema.
- If an empyema fails resolve with pleural space drainage, arrange chest CT and discuss with cardiothoracic surgeons (see 🕮 p.217).

Cavitation or abscess

Any severe pneumonia may cavitate, but particularly *S. aureus, Klebsiella* spp., TB, aspiration pneumonia, bronchial obstruction (foreign body, tumour) or pulmonary emboli (thrombus or septic emboli, e.g. from DVT with super-added infection or tricuspid endocarditis; see 🕮 p.106.)

Treatment

- Seek advice from respiratory team. Most respond to appropriate antibiotics but may require more prolonged course. Surgical drainage or CT-guided percutaneous aspiration may be necessary.
- 'Blind' treatment: cefuroxime 1.5g tds IV (or cefotaxime 2g tds IV) + flucloxacillin 1–2g qds IV + gentamicin loading dose (100–120mg IV) then 6–7mg/kg od (according to renal function and levels) ± metronidazole 500mg IV tds.
- Long-term antibiotics (4–6 weeks) likely to be required.

Other complications

- Respiratory failure: see 🕮 p.192
- Rhabdomyolysis: see 🕮 p.294
- DIC (especially *Legionella*): see 🕮 p.596.

Mycoplasma pneumonia

- Disease of young adults. Low-grade fever, dry cough, headache, and myalgia. Erythema multiforme may be seen in ~25%. ~5% have a meningoencephalitis.
- WCC is often normal, ESR is high, specific IgM is seen early then levels decline. ~50% develop cold agglutinins (also seen in measles, EBV) which may cause haemolysis. CXR may show reticulonodular shadowing (lower lobe > upper lobe) which may take over 6 weeks to resolve (unlike bacterial pneumonia).
- Treatment is with *erythromycin* 500mg qds PO/IV, *clarithromycin* 500mg bd PO/IV, or *tetracycline* 500mg qds PO/IV.

Legionella pneumonia

- Illness of middle-aged men; more severe in smokers. Incubation 2–10 days followed by high fever, rigors, headache, myalgia, dry cough, progressive respiratory distress, and confusion. Abdominal pain, diarrhoea, nausea and vomiting, and palpable hepatomegaly are seen in ~30%. Complications include pericarditis (± effusion), encephalopathy (CSF is usually normal) and rarely renal failure.
- Moderate leucocytosis ($\leq 20 \times 10^9$/L, neutrophilia, lymphopenia), hyponatraemia, deranged LFTs, proteinuria, haematuria, and myoglobinuria. Diagnosis: rise in specific IgM and IgG titres (urine, blood, sputum).
- CXR may show anything from diffuse patchy infiltrates to lobar or segmental changes and usually deteriorates in spite of treatment. Pleural effusions are seen in ~50%.
- Treatment is with *clarithromycin* 500mg bd PO/IV. Continue therapy for 14–21 days. Add *rifampicin* (600mg bd PO/IV) if symptoms do not settle within 72h.
- Pontiac fever is self-limiting (2–5 days) acute non-pneumonic *Legionella* infection with high fever, rigors, myalgia, headache, and tracheo-bronchitis.

Viral pneumonia

Clinical features resemble *Mycoplasma* pneumonia (see 📖 p.174). Diagnosis is by 4 × increase in specific antibody titres.

CMV

Commonest viral infection in AIDS and following solid organ or bone marrow transplantation, presenting as fever, dry cough, and progressive respiratory distress with hypoxia and bilateral crackles. CXR shows diffuse infiltrates; a miliary pattern is associated with rapid progression and poor outcome whereas an interstitial pattern has a better prognosis (see 📖 Fig. 2.1, p.169). Treat with *ganciclovir* 5mg/kg IV q12h for 2–3 weeks.

Coxsackie and echovirus

Titres often rise in 'epidemic pleurodynia' (Bornholm's disease), a self-limiting illness with chest pain exacerbated by coughing and deep breathing, myalgia, and muscle tenderness. Treatment: analgesia (paracetamol, NSAIDs).

Varicella pneumonia

More common in smokers and immunosuppressed patients. All patients with varicella pneumonitis should be treated with *aciclovir* 10mg/kg IV 8-hourly.

Chlamydia pneumonia

- *Chlamydia pneumoniae* presents in older adults with headaches and longer duration of symptoms before hospital admission. Extra-pulmonary manifestations may include meningoencephalitis, Guillian–Barré syndrome, arthritis, and myocarditis.
- Treatment: *erythromycin* 500mg qds PO/IV, *clarithromycin* 500mg bd PO/IV, or *tetracycline* 500mg qds PO/IV.

Psittacosis

- *Chlamydia psittaci* produces fever, cough, myalgia, and in severe cases, delirium (psittacosis). Complications include pericarditis, myocarditis, and hepatosplenomegaly. Diagnosis is by serology.
- Treat with *tetracycline* 500mg po qds for 2–3 weeks.

Miscellaneous conditions

Extrinsic allergic alveolitis may mimic viral pneumonia and present as breathlessness, dry cough, myalgia, and fever with neutrophilia (eosinophils usually normal acutely) and patchy radiographic changes. There is usually history of exposure to the allergen and serum precipitins are detectable. BAL shows predominance of mast cells and lymphocytes. Treatment is with steroids.

Pulmonary eosinophilia: this is a heterogenous group of disorders characterized by eosinophilic pulmonary infiltrates producing respiratory symptoms, CXR shadowing, and blood and sputum eosinophilia. The cause may be unknown as in cryptogenic eosinophilic pneumonia, or it may be due to drugs (e.g. nitrofurantoin, phenytoin, and ampicillin), helminth infections (e.g. *Ascaris lumbrocoides*, hookworms, *Strongyloides stercoralis*), tropical pulmonary eosinophilia (lymphatic filarial infection), or the small-vessel systemic vasculitis (Churg–Strauss).

Allergic bronchopulmonary aspergillosis is a hypersensitivity reaction of airways colonized by *Aspergillus* spp. producing pulmonary eosinophilia. It typically occurs in asthmatics with repeated episodes of bronchial obstruction, inflammation, and mucus impaction resulting in bronchiectasis and upper lobe fibrosis. Such patients are usually *Aspergillus* skin-prick test (IgE) and serum precipitins (IgG) positive. Treatment depends on the underlying condition.

COP may present with fever, malaise, cough, breathlessness, and pulmonary shadows on CXR. Characteristically infiltrates in different lobes over different time courses, or pneumonia unresponsive to antibiotics. Excessive proliferation of granulation tissue within small airways and alveoli, COP is the idiopathic form of bronchiolitis obliterans organizing pneumonia (BOOP). Organizing pneumonia can also be associated with collagen vascular diseases (rheumatoid arthritis, lupus, dermatomyositis), chronic infection (*Legionella*, CMV, *Mycoplasma*), and drugs (amiodarone, bleomycin). Treatment is with steroids.

Alveolar haemorrhage: intrapulmonary haemorrhage may present with cough, fever, and breathlessness. Haemoptysis may be absent in 30%. The CXR may show diffuse alveolar opacities. BAL shows predominantly RBCs. Causes include systemic vasculitis (e.g. Wegener's granulomatosis, microscopic polyangiitis), collagen vascular diseases (e.g. SLE), Goodpasture's syndrome, ARDS, and idiopathic pulmonary haemosiderosis. Treatment depends on the cause.

Bronchoalveolar cell carcinoma may mimic an acute pneumonia radiologically although typical symptoms of pneumonia are usually not present unless there is superadded infection. Diagnosis is made by lung biopsy.

Acute asthma: assessment

Presentation

- The classical triad is *wheeze, breathlessness*, and *cough*. Pleuritic pain may be due to diaphragmatic stretch, pneumothorax, or acute infection.
- Acute attacks may build up over minutes, hours, or days and the patients may deteriorate very rapidly and present as respiratory or cardiorespiratory arrest.
- Factors increasing the risk of severe life-threatening asthma include: previous ventilation, hospital admission for asthma in the last year, heavy rescue medication use, >3 classes of asthma medication, repeated attendances at A&E for asthma care, brittle asthma.

Precipitants

- No clear precipitating cause can be identified in over 30% of patients.
- Exposure to known allergen or irritant (e.g. pollens, animals, dusts, cigarette smoke).
- Upper respiratory tract infection (commonly viral).
- Chest infection: viral or bacterial.
- Neglect or poor compliance with regular inhaled or oral steroids.
- Emotional stress.
- Cold air or exercise-induced asthma.

Markers of severity

- For assessment of the severity of asthma, see Box 2.3.
- The severity of an attack may be easily underestimated. Assess:
  - the degree of airflow obstruction
  - the effect of ↑ work of breathing on the patient
  - the extent of ventilation–perfusion mismatch
  - any evidence of ventilatory failure.

(Patients with marked 'morning dips' in PEF are at risk of sudden severe attacks.)

Investigations

- ***ABG:*** hypoxaemia on room air is almost invariable. In attempting to maintain alveolar ventilation initially there is hypocapnia and respiratory alkalosis. ↑$PaCO2$ suggests incipient respiratory failure due to exhaustion; contact ITU immediately. Poorly controlled asthma over several days may be recognized by a mild 'non-anion gap' acidosis (serum bicarbonate 20–24mmol/L). A lactic acidosis seen with severe asthma.
- ***Pulse oximetry:*** continuous oximetry is essential; aim for ≥92%.
- ***CXR:*** exclude pneumothorax and to diagnose any parenchymal infection.
- ***ECG:*** usually normal; in severe asthmatics, signs of right heart strain may be present.
- ***FBC, U&E, CRP:*** assess for signs of infection; K^+ may be lowered by high doses of β-agonists.

Box 2.3 Assessment of severity of acute asthma*

A Near-fatal asthma

- Raised P_aCO_2 or immediate requirement for ventilation with raised inflation pressures.

B Life-threatening asthma

i Severe airways obstruction

- PEF <33% best or predicted
- Soft breath sounds or 'silent chest'
- Feeble respiratory effort.

ii Increased work of breathing and haemodynamic stress

- Exhaustion
- Hypotension (SBP <100mmHg)
- Bradycardia or arrhythmia.

iii Ventilation-perfusion mismatch

- Cyanosis
- Hypoxia (SpO_2 <92% and/or P_aO_2 <8kPa irrespective of inspired O_2 concentration).

iv Ventilatory failure

- Rising P_aCO_2 suggests 'near-fatal' asthma
- Confusion or coma.

C Acute severe asthma

- PEF 30–50% best or predicted
- Respiratory rate >25/min
- Tachycardia: heart rate >100/min
- Inability to complete sentences in one breath.

D Brittle asthma

- Type 1: wide PEF variation despite intensive and regular therapy
- Type 2: sudden severe asthma attacks on background of apparently well-controlled asthma

Admission is mandatory if *any* of the markers of severe, life-threatening, or near-fatal asthma are present.

*Adapted from BTS/SIGN (2003). British guidelines on management of asthma. *Thorax* **58** (suppl. 1) i1–94.

Acute severe asthma: immediate therapy

Priorities

1 Treat hypoxia.
2 Treat bronchospasm and inflammation.
3 Assess the need for intensive care.
4 Treat any underlying cause if present (e.g. infection, pneumothorax).

- Patients may deteriorate rapidly and should not be left unattended.
- *Remain calm:* reassurance is important in reducing the patient's anxiety which may further increase respiratory effort. (See Box 2.5)

Severe or life-threatening attack (Box 2.6)

1. Initial treatment

- Sit the patient up in bed.
- *O_2*: the highest percentage available, ideally at least 60% or 15L/min with a high-flow mask. CO_2 retention is not a problem in asthmatic patients. Maintain O_2 sats >92%.
- *Nebulized bronchodilators*: give nebulized salbutamol 5mg or terbutaline 10mg, administered via O_2 and repeat up to every 15–30min if required. Consider continuous nebulization of salbutamol 5–10mg/h if inadequate response to initial treatment.
- Add *ipratropium bromide* 0.5mg 4–6-hourly if initial response to β_2-agonists is poor.
- Obtain IV access.
- Start *steroids*: 200mg of hydrocortisone intravenously (steroids should still be used in pregnant women as the risk of fetal anoxia from the asthma is high). Continue either hydrocortisone 100mg qds IV or prednisolone 30–50mg od PO.
- *Antibiotics* should be given if there is evidence of chest infection (purulent sputum, abnormal CXR, raised WCC, fever). Yellow sputum may just be due to eosinophils and a raised WCC may be due to steroids. See 📖 p.170 for choice of antibiotics.
- *Adequate hydration* is essential and may help prevent mucus plugging. Ensure an intake (IV or PO) of 2–3L/day, taking care to avoid overload. Supplement potassium as required.

2. Monitoring progress

- Pre- and post-nebulizer peak flows.
- Repeated ABGs 1–2-hourly or according to response especially if SaO_2 <93%. Remember ABGs are painful—use topical anaesthetic cream and local anaesthetic or consider an arterial line if frequent sampling.

3. If response to treatment not brisk or if the patient's condition is deteriorating

- Continue O_2 and nebulized β_2-agonist every 15min.
- Give a single dose of IV magnesium sulphate (see Box 2.4).
- Consider starting an IV *aminophylline infusion* (see Box 2.4).
- Consider starting an IV *salbutamol infusion* (see Box 2.4).
- Summon anaesthetic help.

Box 2.4 Intravenous bronchodilators for asthma

Magnesium sulphate:
- 1.2–2g if infused over 20min.
- Give as a single dose only. Repeated doses may lead to hypermagnesaemia with muscle weakness and respiratory failure.

Salbutamol:
- *Loading dose:* 100–300mcg over 10min.
- *Maintenance infusion:* 5–20mcg/min (5mg in 500mL saline at 1–3mL/min).
- *Side effects:* tremor, tachycardia, hypokalaemia, hyperglycaemia common. Lactic acidosis may occur and responds within hours to reduction in salbutamol infusion rate.

Aminophylline:
- *Loading dose:* 250mg (4–5mg/kg) IV over 20min.
- *Maintenance infusion:* 0.5–0.7mg/kg/h (250mg in 1 litre N saline at 2–4 ml/kg/h).
- Do *not* give the loading dose if the patient is on oral theophyllines without checking a serum level.
- Halve the dose in patients with cirrhosis or CCF, or in those receiving erythromycin, cimetidine, or ciprofloxacin. Monitor levels every 24h (aim for levels of 10–20mg/L).

Box 2.5 Management of key points: acute asthma

- Oxygen
- Nebulized salbutamol and ipratropium bromide
- Steroids: iv hydrocortisone, followed by oral prednisolone
- Monitor PEFR and ABG
- If no improvement: iv magnesium sulphate. Consider iv aminophylline infusion or iv salbutamol.
- Summon anaesthetic help if patient is getting exhausted (PCO2 increasing)
- Monitor serum K^+ daily and supplement as necessary.
- Treat any underlying cause (e.g. infection, pneumothorax). Give antibiotics if there is evidence of chest infection (purulent sputum, abnormal CXR, raised WCC, fever).

Box 2.6 Indications for admission to intensive care unit

- Hypoxia (P_aO_2 <8kPa (60mmHg) despite FiO_2 of 60%
- Rising P_aCO_2 or P_aCO_2 >6kPa (45mmHg)
- Exhaustion, drowsiness, or coma
- Respiratory arrest
- Failure to improve despite adequate therapy.

Acute severe asthma: further management

- *Cautious CPAP* may help reduce the work of breathing in patients with respiratory muscle fatigue but may not increase the functional residual capacity further. Involve ITU early so as not to delay invasive ventilation.
- *Ketamine* (a dissociative anaesthetic agent) may be useful in ventilated patients (1–3mg/min) probably by increasing circulating catecholamines by blocking uptake into adrenergic nerve endings.
- *Inhalational anaesthetic agents* (e.g. halothane, enflurane, isoflurane) have been reported to improve bronchospasm and may be useful when initiating ventilation.
- *Mechanical ventilation* may be life saving but has a high risk of complications and an overall mortality of ~13%. Barotrauma is seen in ~14% (e.g. pneumothorax, pneumo-mediastinum, or subcutaneous emphysema) and hypotension in ~38% (usually a combination of ↑intrathoracic pressure, intravascular fluid depletion due to dehydration, and dilating effect of anaesthetic agents). Seek expert advice from your intensive care physician for the practical management of ventilation of the asthmatic patient.

General principles

- Adequate humidification and warming of inspired gases.
- Low frequency ventilation (6–10 breaths/min).
- Low tidal volumes (6–10mL/kg).
- Long expiratory phase of the cycle (I:E ratio 1:3 or longer).
- Minimize airway pressures (aim for <50cm H_2O, normal <25).
- Maintain P_aO_2 >8.0 kPa; allow P_aCO_2 to rise provided pH >7.2.
- Adequate sedation and paralysis to overcome respiratory drive.
- Avoid opiates and atracurium (may release histamine).
- Consider benzodiazepine, ketamine, vecuronium, isoflurane, etc.

Ongoing therapy

- Once improvement established continue nebulized β_2-agonist, reducing this to 4-hourly and PRN after 24–48h.
- Peak flow rate should be measured before and after each nebulizer.
- Maintain O_2 sats >92%.
- Continue nebulized ipratropium bromide 6-hourly until the condition is improving.
- Continue steroids, hydrocortisone 100mg q6h IV switching to 30–60mg od oral prednisolone when able to swallow, and continue for 10–14 days.
- Monitor IV aminophylline levels every 24h.
- Monitor serum K^+ daily whilst unwell and supplement as necessary.
- Discharge criteria (Box 2.7).

Box 2.7 Discharge after hospital admission

- The PEF should be ≥75% of best without significant morning dipping (diurnal variability ≤25%) and with no nocturnal symptoms.
- The patient should be established on inhalers with no requirement for nebulizers for 24–48h prior to discharge. Check inhaler technique
- Discharge drugs:
    - Prednisolone PO ≥30mg od for 1–3 weeks (plan gradual dose reduction if treatment >14 days)
    - Inhaled corticosteroids at high dose (usually 1000–1500mcg beclometasone via spacer) or equivalent.
    - Restart inhaled long-acting β_2-agonists if prescribed prior to admission.
    - Inhaled PRN β_2-agonist.
    - Oral theophyllines if required (confirm drug levels before discharge).
- Provide a written management plan.
- Provide PEFR meter and chart and arrange follow-up with GP or practice nurse (within 2 days) and chest clinic (within 1 month).
- Assess individual risk factors/precipitants.

Mild–moderate asthmatic attacks

Mild asthmatic attack

No severe features, PEF ≥75% of predicted (or of best when well).

- Administer the patient's usual bronchodilator (e.g. 2 puffs salbutamol by metered dose inhaler).
- Observe for 60min. If PEF remains ≥75% of predicted value, then discharge.
- Ensure patient is on at least 1000mcg inhaled beclometasone or equivalent per day.
- Advise the patient to get early GP follow-up, monitor PEF, and return to hospital early if the asthma deteriorates.

Moderate asthmatic attack

No acute severe features, PEF 51–75% of predicted (or of best when well).

- Administer nebulized β-agonist (salbutamol 5mg or terbutaline 10mg) and oral prednisolone 30–60mg.
- Re-assess after 30min. If worse or PEF ≤50% of predicted then admit and assess as follows for severe asthma.
- If PEF 51–75% predicted then repeat nebulizer and observe for a further 60min.
- The patient may be discharged from A&E if stable after 1–2 nebulizers and PEFR ≥75%.
- If after second nebulizer and a further 60min observation the patient is clearly improving and PEFR ≥50%, then discharge may be considered.
- Discharge on:
  - Oral prednisolone (usual dose 30–40mg od for 7 days)
  - Inhaled corticosteroid (≥1000mcg/day inhaled beclometasone)
  - Inhaled β-agonist.
- Advise the patient to seek GP follow-up within 48h and to return early to A&E if there is any deterioration.
- Consider referral to chest clinic.

Sending people home from A&E

- Mild–moderate exacerbations may be fit to be discharged from A&E.
- If there are any features of acute severe asthma (see 📖 Box 2.3, p.179) then admission is mandatory.
- A history of brittle asthma or previous attacks requiring mechanical ventilation is always a requirement for admission.

Acute exacerbation of chronic obstructive pulmonary disease (COPD): assessment

Presentation

- Deterioration of pre-existing symptoms of exertional breathlessness, cough (sometimes with daily sputum production) and wheeze.
- Respiratory failure (see 📖 p.192): may be Type 1 (normal P_aCO_2, low P_aO_2) or Type 2 (high P_aCO_2, low P_aO_2 reflecting severe bronchospasm and/or alveolar hypoventilation).
- Wheeze unrelieved or partially relieved by inhalers.
- ↑production of purulent sputum (i.e. infection as a precipitant).
- Positive smoking history (if not then late-onset asthma is likely).
- Confusion/impaired consciousness (exhaustion, CO_2 retention).

Causes

- Infective exacerbation (no new CXR changes): typically *H. influenzae*, *S. pneumoniae*, *Moraxella catarrhalis*. Commonly viral.
- Community acquired pneumonia (new CXR changes): see 📖 p.169.
- *Exposure to known allergen:* COPD may coexist with allergic asthma.
- *Pneumothorax* (see 📖 p.204), differentiate from large bullae).
- Expansion of large bullae.
- *Sputum retention* with lobar or segmental collapse (atelectasis): pneumonia, excessive sedation or opioid analgesia (trauma, post-surgery), impaired consciousness.
- *Confounding or contributing factors:* myocardial ischaemia, pulmonary oedema, cor pulmonale, PE.

Investigations

All patients should have:

- ***U&Es:*** look for dehydration, renal failure. Monitor K^+.
- ***FBC:*** look for leucocytosis or anaemia (chronic respiratory failure may produce a 2° polycythaemia).
- ***Pulse oximetry and ABGs:*** to assess degree of respiratory failure and pH, and guide appropriate O_2 treatment.
- ***Septic screen:*** sputum should be sent for culture. Blood cultures if febrile or CXR changes suggest pneumonia.
- ***Peak flows:*** ask what is normal for patient.
- ***CXR***: focal changes suggest pneumonia (see 📖 p.168).
- ***ECG:*** myocardial ischaemia or arrhythmia.

Assessment of severity

- ***History:*** assess the severity of COPD when stable and compare with current exacerbation. Ask about symptoms and functional capacity when well (distance walked on flat, stairs climbed, frequency of exacerbations, previous admissions, ever ventilated?). Assess level of usual treatment (regular nebulized bronchodilators or oral steroids, home O_2) and concurrent illnesses (IHD, renal impairment). Any previous documentation (PFTs, ABGs).
- ***Examination:*** assess for severity of respiratory distress (RR >25/min, use of accessory muscles or paradoxical chest wall movements), hypoxia (cyanosis), hypercapnia (CO_2 retention flap, confusion), cor pulmonale (peripheral oedema).

Box 2.8 Criteria for hospital admission

- Marked increase in symptoms
- Baseline of severe COPD
- New physical signs, e.g. cyanosis, peripheral oedema
- Failure to respond to initial management at home
- Significant comorbidities
- Diagnostic uncertainty
- Age >70 years
- Insufficient home support.

Acute exacerbation of COPD: management

Treat hypoxia and respiratory failure

- The distinction between 'pink puffers' (breathless to maintain P_aO_2 and so keep P_aCO_2 down) and 'blue bloaters' (lose breathless drive to maintain P_aO_2 and so P_aCO_2 rises) is unhelpful as most patients have features of both.
- ***Commence O_2 therapy*** Uncontrolled O_2 therapy may worsen CO_2 retention in some patients. While awaiting ABGs give controlled 24–28% O_2 via a Venturi mask. Nasal canulae give unreliable inspired O_2 concentration and may be dangerous. Once ABG results available, adjust FiO_2 accordingly.
- *ABGS:*
    - If patient is not retaining CO_2 (P_aCO_2 <6kPa) and is hypoxic (P_aO_2 <10kPa) then give O_2 28–40%. Repeat ABGs 30min later (sooner if conscious level deteriorates) to ensure correction of hypoxia and exclude rising P_aCO_2. Aim to maintain sats ≥92%.
    - If CO_2 retention is present then use 24–28% O_2 and repeat blood gases after 15–30min. Aim to keep P_aO_2 ≥7.3kPa and P_aCO_2 ≤7.5kPa, but these limits may not be achievable. Balance hypoxia (which may be fatal) against conscious level, arterial pH, and respiratory effort. Consider non-invasive ventilation, mechanical ventilation, or doxapram.
- ***NIV*** This is the first-line treatment of choice for COPD exacerbations with type 2 respiratory failure in patients who fail to respond to initial therapy. It is the first-line treatment of acidotic patients (on ABG). It allows the administration of higher O_2 concentrations without an uncontrolled rise in P_aCO_2. NIV reduces the need for intubation, decreases mortality and hospital stay, and should be considered in all patients with COPD exacerbations with P_aCO_2 ≥6.0kPa and pH ≤7.35 who have failed to respond to initial bronchodilator therapy.
- ***Mechanical ventilation*** This should be considered in patients unlikely or unable to tolerate NIV (see 📖 p.778).
- ***Respiratory stimulants*** These have generally been superseded by NIV. However where NIV is not available or has not been successful and mechanical ventilation is not considered appropriate, a trial of doxapram may be worthwhile. It is not beneficial in type 2 respiratory failure due to poor respiratory effort.

Treat bronchospasm and obstruction

- *Nebulized β-agonists* (salbutamol 5mg or terbutaline 10mg q4h and PRN) via O_2 or air if CO_2 retaining. (If patient is very hypoxic, give 2L/min O_2 via nasal cannulae whilst nebulizer in progress.)
- Patients with COPD may have relatively fixed bronchospasm, but where the patient is very unwell then consider IV aminophylline and/or IV β-agonists as for severe asthma (see 📖 Box 2.4, p.181).
- Include nebulized ipratropium bromide 500mcg 6-hourly.
- Give *steroids:* 200mg hydrocortisone IV or 30–40mg prednisolone PO.
- Urgent physiotherapy may help clearing bronchial secretions.

Box 2.9 Management key points: acute exacerbation of COPD

- O_2: initially 24–28% O_2 via a venturi mask (adjust FiO_2 when ABG results available).
- Nebulized salbutamol, ipratropium bromide.
- Steroids: IV hydrocortisone followed by oral prednisolone.
- Treat cause of exacerbation e.g. infective exacerbation or pneumothorax.
- Urgent physiotherapy may help clearing bronchial secretions.
- Consider NIV in type 2 respiratory failure patients who fail to respond to initial therapy. Mechanical ventilation should be considered in patients unable/unlikely to tolerate NIV.

Acute exacerbation of COPD

Mechanical ventilation

- COPD per se is not a contraindication to ventilation in appropriately selected patients. Ventilation should be considered where respiratory failure is present (P_aO_2 ≤7.3kPa) regardless of CO_2 levels and in those patients who have failed to respond to first-line treatment (including NIV), or who are very severely unwell and unlikely to respond to any other intervention.
- Discuss with a senior colleague or ITU staff prior to intubation.

In favour of a good outcome from ventilation

- Acute respiratory failure (normal bicarbonate, acute history)
- Relatively young patient
- Obvious remediable cause (e.g. pneumonia)
- Good recent exercise tolerance and quality of life
- Not previously known to retain CO_2 when well.

Against a good outcome from ventilation

- Relatively old
- Other comorbid conditions (e.g. IHD, renal failure)
- Previous difficulty weaning from ventilator
- On maximal therapy at home (home nebulizer, long-term O_2 therapy)
- Poor quality of life or poor exercise tolerance.

Management of gas exchange during ventilation

- Patients who are chronically hypoxic or CO_2 retainers will tolerate poor blood gases better than those patients with other causes of respiratory failure.
- When ventilating patients with COPD, achieving a 'normal' P_aCO_2 and P_aO_2 may not be appropriate. Those who are chronically hypoxic or who chronically retain CO_2 (as evidenced by previous abnormal gases or a raised bicarbonate with a normal or near-normal pH) are unlikely to breath spontaneously or wean from the ventilator unless their blood gases are allowed to mirror what is probably their chronic state. Thus a patient with chronic type 2 respiratory failure may need a P_aCO_2 of 6–7.5kPa ± mild hypoxia even on the ventilator to achieve successful weaning.

Treat cause of exacerbation

Infective exacerbation

- Suggested by purulent sputum or increase in sputum production.
- For lobar consolidation or bronchial pneumonia follow guidelines on 📖 pp.170–172. Otherwise treat with *amoxicillin* 500mg–1g tds PO/IV; if unwell or failure to respond treat *cefuroxime* 750mg tds IV for improved cover of resistant *Haemophilus* spp.
- Follow local protocols.

Pneumothorax Unless very small, consider aspiration ± drain, 📖 p.204

Pulmonary oedema 📖 p.87

Pulmonary embolism 📖 p.120.

Respiratory failure: assessment

Respiratory failure is present when gas exchange becomes significantly impaired. Clinically, it is not possible to predict the P_aO_2 or P_aCO_2 and so this diagnosis relies on ABG analysis. There are two types:

- ***Type 1*** Hypoxia P_aO_2 ≤8kPa on air or O_2 with normal or low P_aCO_2 (i.e. mainly ventilation–perfusion mismatch).
- ***Type 2*** Hypoxia P_aO_2 ≤8kPa on air or O_2 with raised P_aCO_2 (>6kPa) (i.e. predominantly alveolar hypoventilation).

In practice, both types may coexist.

Presentation

- *Shortness of breath* is the commonest presentation. Ask about the speed of onset (sudden onset may suggest pneumothorax, pulmonary embolus, or cardiac failure).
- Respiratory failure may present without dyspnoea, particularly exacerbations of COPD with hypoventilation ('blue bloaters'), and non-respiratory causes such as Guillain–Barré syndrome (📖 p.426) or drug overdose. Neuromuscular respiratory failure is discussed on 📖 p.416.
- *Confusion* may be the sole presentation in the elderly.

The history may point to the cause of respiratory failure:

- History of asthma/chronic bronchitis and smoking.
- History of other chronic lung disease (e.g. fibrosing alveolitis, sarcoidosis).
- Sputum production and fevers (pneumonia).
- Swollen legs due to the development of cor pulmonale or hypoxic/hypercapnic renal fluid retention in patients with chronic lung disease.
- Haemoptysis (pneumonia, PE).
- Cardiac history including palpitations and/or chest pain.
- Drug and/or overdose history.
- Neurological symptoms including painful legs and paraesthesiae (Guillain–Barré syndrome).
- Allergies.
- Try to assess the functional capacity when well, e.g. distance walked on flat, stairs climbed without stopping, frequency of attacks, previous admissions, ever ventilated?, concurrent illnesses (heart disease, renal impairment, liver impairment), etc.

Physical examination

- Listen to the breathing (stridor, wheeze, coarse crackles).
- Look for wheeze (airflow limitation, either localized (local obstruction) or generalized (e.g. asthma, COPD, pulmonary oedema), coarse crackles (infection, pulmonary oedema, or fibrosis), bronchial breathing (indicates consolidation or collapse, but may also occur with fibrosis or above a pleural effusion), signs of pneumothorax (hyper-resonance, ↓breath sounds), or pleural effusion (stony dull, ↓breath sounds).
- Palpate the upper chest and neck for crepitus (pneumothorax or pneumomediastinum).
- Look for signs of a DVT (swollen hot leg ± pain, see 📖 p.116).

Box 2.10 Causes of respiratory failure

Common

- Acute asthma (📖 p.178)
- Exacerbation of COPD (📖 p.188)
- Pneumonia (📖 p.166)
- Pulmonary oedema (📖 p.87)
- Pulmonary embolus (📖 p.120)
- Infection complicating kyphoscoliosis or other chronic lung disease
- Pleural effusion (📖 p.216)
- Pneumothorax (📖 p.204)
- ARDS/ALI (📖 p.198)
- Respiratory depression
- Drugs e.g. opiates.

Rarer

- Lung collapse/atelectasis (tumour, foreign body, sputum plug, infection)
- Acute respiratory muscle weakness Guillain–Barré syndrome (📖 p.426), myasthenia gravis (📖 p.420), poliomyelitis
- Upper airway obstruction (foreign body, tumour, epiglottitis) (📖 p.220)
- Chest trauma
- Anaphylaxis (📖 p.322).

Respiratory failure: investigations

Urgent investigations

- ***ABG:*** on air immediately, or if very unwell whilst on O_2 (note FiO_2).
- ***CXR:*** see 📖 Fig. 2.1, p.169.
- ***ECG:*** look for signs of PE (tachycardia, RBBB, anterior T-wave changes, RAD, rarely $S_1Q_3T_3$, see 📖 p.120), tachyarrhythmias, or myocardial ischaemia.
- ***Blood tests:*** FBC (anaemia, leucocytosis), U&Es, glucose.
- ***Inspect sputum:*** yellow, green, mucoid, streaky, or frank blood.
- ***FEV_1 and FVC:*** if suspected muscle weakness (e.g. Guillain–Barré).
- ***Septic screen:*** sputum culture, blood cultures if febrile or if CXR suggests infection.

Where indicated consider

- Aspirin and paracetamol levels.
- Plasma and urine for toxicology.
- Urinalysis for glucose and ketones.
- Examine the CXR systematically for any abnormality.

CXR assessment

- Consolidation/alveolar shadowing: may be lobar or patchy. Presence of an air bronchogram suggests pneumonia.
- Pulmonary oedema due to left ventricular failure (cardiogenic): typically perihilar ('bats-wing'), upper lobe venous congestion, Kerley B lines in peripheral lung fields, ± pleural effusions, ± cardiomegaly.
- Non-cardiogenic pulmonary oedema (ARDS/ALI): typically peripheral alveolar shadowing ± air bronchogram, *no* upper lobe venous congestion, Kerley B lines, pleural effusions, or cardiomegaly.
- Pleural effusions.
- Masses suggesting bronchogenic carcinoma.
- Pulmonary embolism: wedge-shaped peripheral opacities, small pleural effusions, localized areas of oligaemia, enlarged pulmonary artery.
- Pneumothorax (distinguish from large bullae).
- Trauma/rib fractures.
- Diffuse lung disease (e.g. fibrosing alveolitis): small lung fields, interstitial reticulo-nodular shadowing, peripherally and basally.

Respiratory failure: management

See 📖 p.416 for neuromuscular respiratory failure.

The severity of respiratory failure depends upon response to O_2. Failure of hypoxia to correct on 40–60% O_2 or progressive hypercapnia implies that non-invasive or mechanical ventilation may be necessary, depending on the clinical condition and underlying cause.

Poor prognostic signs on presentation include

- Inability to speak due to dyspnoea.
- Respiratory rate (>40/min).
- Peak flow ≤33% of predicted in acute asthma.
- Tachycardia HR ≥100bpm or bradycardia HR ≤60bpm.
- Exhaustion or coma (ventilatory support is required urgently).
- Stridor (this indicates upper airway obstruction, see 📖 p.220).
- Pulse oximetry saturation of <90%.
- Shock (tachycardia + hypotension). May indicate tension pneumothorax (📖 p.210), severe LVF (Pulmonary oedema: assessment)), severe pneumonia (📖 p.170), or large PE (📖 p.120).

Hypercapnia is the end result of many causes of respiratory failure (including asthma and pneumonia), not just COPD, and indicates a tiring patient. Even if relatively elderly the patient may respond well to ventilation with a satisfactory final outcome depending on the disease and premorbid condition.

General resuscitation (ABC)

- Ensure the airway is patent and the mouth is clear.
- If stridor is present request anaesthetic and/or ENT assistance urgently (📖 p.220).
- Sit the patient up (unless hypotensive) and administer O_2 at 60% unless there is a history of COPD (use 24–28% O_2).
- Ensure that respiratory effort is adequate and effective (measure respiratory rate and assess depth of respiration), use pulse oximetry to monitor the PaO_2.
- If the patient is exhausted with a failing respiratory drive, call for anaesthetic assistance and consider urgent transfer to ITU (Box 2.9).
- In comatose patients with poor respiratory effort consider drug overdose with opiates (pinpoint pupils) or benzodiazepines. Give naloxone 200–400mcg (2–4mcg/kg) IV bolus followed by infusion depending on response and/or IV flumazenil (200mcg over 15sec then 100mcg at 60-sec intervals if required—max. total dose 1mg (2mg if on ITU).
- Methods of respiratory support are discussed on 📖 p.776.
- Secure IV access.

- Measure the BP and HR, look for signs of cardiac failure (raised JVP, inspiratory crackles, oedema) or signs of PE (raised JVP, tachycardia, hypotension, normal breath sounds ± pleural rub).

Box 2.11 Indications for intensive care

- Progressive exhaustion or impaired conscious level
- Shock not responding rapidly to initial resuscitation
- Respiratory failure not responding rapidly to initial therapy.

Adult respiratory distress syndrome 1

ALI and its more severe subset, ARDS, is a common clinical disorder characterized by injury to the alveolar epithelial and endothelial barriers of the lung, acute inflammation, and protein-rich pulmonary oedema leading to acute respiratory failure. Often occurs in the setting of MOF.

Diagnostic criteria

- Acute onset of respiratory failure with one or more risk factors (see Box 2.10).
- Hypoxaemia:
  - ALI: ratio P_aO_2 (kPa):FiO_2 <40
  - ARDS: ratio P_aO_2 (kPa):FiO_2 <27.
- Bilateral infiltrates on CXR.
- Pulmonary capillary wedge pressure <19mmHg, with normal colloid oncotic pressure (in patients with hypoalbuminaemia, the critical PCWP is approx. serum albumin (g/L) × 0.57, see 🕮 p.327) or clinical exclusion of cardiac failure.

Investigations

- CXR.
- ABG (consider arterial line as regular samples may be required).
- Take blood for FBC, U&Es, LFTs and albumin, coagulation, X-match, and CRP.
- Septic screen (culture blood, urine, sputum).
- ECG.
- Consider drug screen, amylase if history suggestive.
- Pulmonary artery catheter to measure PCWP, cardiac output, mixed venous O_2 saturation and to allow calculation of haemodynamic parameters.
- Other investigations if appropriate:
  - CT chest
  - BAL for microbiology and cell count (?eosinophils)
  - Carboxyhaemoglobin estimation.

Management

- Almost all cases of ALI alone will require HDU/ICU care: liaise early.
- The main aim is to identify and treat the underlying cause whilst providing support for organ failure:
  - Respiratory support to improve gas exchange and correct hypoxia
  - Cardiovascular support to optimize O_2 delivery to tissues
  - Reverse or treat the underlying cause.

Box 2.12 Disorders associated with the development of ARDS

Direct lung injury

- Aspiration:
  - Gastric contents
  - Near drowning
- Inhalation injury:
  - Noxious gases
  - Smoke
- Pneumonia:
  - Any organism
  - PCP
- Pulmonary vasculitides
- Pulmonary contusion
- Drug toxicity or overdose:
  - O_2
  - Opiate overdose
  - Bleomycin
  - Salicylates

Indirect (non-pulmonary) injury

- Shock
- Septicaemia
- Amniotic or fat embolism
- Acute pancreatitis
- Massive haemorrhage
- Multiple transfusions
- DIC
- Massive burns
- Major trauma
- Head injury:
  - Raised ICP
  - Intracranial bleed
- Cardiopulmonary bypass
- Acute liver failure

Adult respiratory distress syndrome 2

Respiratory support

Spontaneously breathing patient

- In very mild ALI, hypoxia can be corrected with increased inspired O_2 concentrations (FiO_2 40–60%). However, such patients are rarely recognized as having ALI as a cause of their respiratory failure.
- Patients invariably require higher O_2 concentrations (non-rebreather masks with reservoir FiO_2 ~60–80%) or CPAP (see 🕮 p.777). Consider transfer to HDU/ICU.
- Indications for mechanical ventilation:
  - Inadequate oxygenation (P_aO_2 <8kPa on FiO_2 >0.6)
  - Rising or elevated P_aCO_2 (>6kPa)
  - Clinical signs of incipient respiratory/cardiovascular failure.

Mechanical ventilation

This is the realm of the ICU physician. Main aim is to improve oxygenation/ ventilation while minimizing the risk of further ventilator-induced lung injury; termed lung-protective ventilation.

General principles

- Controlled mechanical ventilation with sedation (± neuromuscular blockade).
- Aim for tidal volume ~6mL/kg. Recent evidence has confirmed that ventilation with smaller tidal volumes is associated with improved outcome compared to the traditional approach (~10–12mL/kg).
- Start with FiO_2 = 1.0. Subsequent adjustments are made to achieve O_2 saturation >90% with FiO_2 <0.6.
- Positive end-expiratory pressure (PEEP) improves oxygenation in most patients and allows reduction in FiO_2. Usual starting level, 5–10cm H_2O, with optimal levels in the range 10–15cm H_2O. Beware hypotension due to reduction in venous return.
- The use of smaller tidal volumes may impair CO_2 clearance with resulting acidosis despite high ventilatory rates (20–25 breaths/minute). Further increases in rate or tidal volume risk worsening ventilator-induced lung injury. Gradual increases in pCO_2 (up to ~13kPa) are well tolerated in most patients and acidosis (pH <7.25) can be treated with intravenous bicarbonate, so-called permissive hypercapnia.
- If oxygenation/ventilation cannot be improved despite these measures, the following can be considered:
  - Inverse ratio ventilation (🕮 p.778): may improve oxygenation, but pCO_2 may rise further.
  - Prone positioning: improves oxygenation in ~70% of patients with ARDS.
  - Inhaled vasodilators (nitric oxide, nebulized epoprostenol): may improve oxygenation.
- High-frequency ventilation: only available in specialist centres.

Adult respiratory distress syndrome 3

Cardiovascular support

- Arterial line essential for continuous BP measurements. Other invasive monitoring is invariably used (PA catheter, PiCCO, oesophageal Doppler), but their individual roles and effects on outcome are unclear.
- Most patients are haemodynamically compromised due to the underlying condition and/or ventilatory management, and benefit from fluid resuscitation. This may risk worsening capillary leak in the lung and compromise oxygenation/ventilation. Aim for a low-normal intravascular volume whilst maintaining cardiac index and mean arterial pressure.
- Inotrope and/or vasopressor support is commonly required and the choice of agent is usually decided on a combination of clinical evaluation and invasive haemodynamic monitoring (cardiac index, O_2 delivery, mixed venous/central venous saturation, lactate). Agents commonly employed include dobutamine, dopamine, adrenaline, noradrenaline.
- Repeated assessment is essential.

Ongoing management

- Look for and treat a precipitant (see 📖 Box 2.12, p.199).
- ***Sepsis:***
    - Fever, neutrophilia, and raised inflammatory markers are common in ALI/ARDS and do not always imply sepsis.
    - A trial of empiric antibiotics guided by possible pathogens, and following an appropriate septic screen (consider BAL once intubated and stable), should be considered. Antibiotics should be modified or discontinued in light of microbiological results.
    - Indwelling CVP catheters are a common source of sepsis.
    - Consider low-dose steroid infusion if (see below).
    - Consider activated protein C, which has been shown to improve survival in patients with septic shock with multi-organ failure.
- ***Renal failure:*** common and may require renal replacement therapy to control fluid balance and blood biochemistry.
- ***Enteral feeding:*** helps maintain integrity of the gut mucosa and is associated with a lower risk of systemic sepsis when compared to parenteral feeding (TPN). Delayed gastric emptying and reduced gut motility is common in ICU patients and may respond to pro-kinetic drugs (metoclopramide, erythromycin) or may require nasojejunal feeding. Stress ulcer prophylaxis (H_2-blockers) should be considered if mechanical ventilation >48h, or multi-organ failure.
- ***Coagulopathy:*** common and if mild does not require therapy. If severe/DIC, expert advice should be sought.
- ***Steroid therapy:***
    - ALI/ARDS: no benefit in the acute stage. Treatment (2mg/kg/day of methylprednisolone) later in the course of the disease (7–10 days) may improve prognosis but further studies are awaited.

- Sepsis: evidence suggests that some patients with refractory septic shock (ongoing/increasing vasopressor requirements) may have 'relative' or 'functional' adrenal insufficiency and may benefit from 'supraphysiological' steroid replacement (200–300mg/day hydrocortisone). Identification of patients likely to benefit unclear at present, but ACTH stimulation test may help discriminate.

Box 2.13 Causes of sudden deterioration in ARDS

Respiratory
- Pneumothorax
- Bronchial plugging
- Displaced ET tube
- Pleural effusion (haemothorax)
- Aspiration (e.g. NG feed).

Cardiovascular
- Arrhythmia
- Cardiac tamponade
- Myocardial infarction
- GI bleed ('stress' ulcer)
- Septicaemia.

Outcome

- The outcome for ALI/ARDS has improved in recent years, with overall mortality rates of ~40%.
- Patients with ALI/ARDS and sepsis, liver disease, non-pulmonary organ dysfunction, or advanced age have higher mortality rates.
- In survivors, although formal lung function tests are abnormal, respiratory compromise at 1–2 years is unusual.
- There is increasing evidence that survivors suffer considerable neuromuscular and psychological disability. This may reflect the period of prolonged critical illness rather than be specific for ALI/ARDS.

Further reading

1. Griffiths MJD, Evans TW (2002). Review series. The pulmonary physician in critical care: towards comprehensive critical care. *Thorax* **57**.

Pneumothorax: assessment

Presentation

Most individuals presenting to hospital with a spontaneous pneumothorax have no recognized underlying lung disease. The commonest presenting symptoms are:

- Breathlessness: usually abrupt in onset (young, fit patients may have very little, but patients with COPD or asthma may present with a sudden deterioration).
- Chest pain: dull, central, heavy; or there may be a pleuritic element.
- In an in-patient, consider the diagnosis in anyone who is:
  - Breathless after an invasive thoracic procedure (e.g. subclavian vein cannulation).
  - Increasingly hypoxic or has rising inflation pressures on mechanical ventilation.

Causes

- ***Primary/spontaneous:*** healthy subjects, no known underlying lung disease. More common in tall, young men who smoke, aged 20–40 years. Probably due to rupture of apical subpleural blebs/bullae.
- ***Secondary/spontaneous:*** pleural rupture due to underlying lung disease: emphysema, fibrosing alveolitis, cystic fibrosis, sarcoidosis
- ***Infection:*** cavitating pneumonia, e.g. staphylococcal, lung abscess, tuberculosis, PCP.
- ***Trauma:*** particularly chest trauma in RTA.
- ***Iatrogenic:*** after pleural biopsy or aspiration, transbronchial biopsy, percutaneous lung biopsy, subclavian vein cannulation, mechanical ventilation with high airway pressures.

Investigations: the chest radiograph

- The classical clinical signs may not always be present.
- In a supine patient a pneumothorax may not be easy to see. Look for hyperlucency of one lung field, and usually clear heart border, or a line parallel to the chest wall (caused by retraction of the R middle lobe).
- If a patient has COPD and marked bullous disease, take care that the suspected pneumothorax is not a large thin-walled bullus: with a pneumothorax the pleural line is usually convex to the lateral chest wall; with a bullus, the apparent pleural line is usually concave to the lateral chest wall. If there is any doubt, CT chest will be able to distinguish between the two.

Signs of a significant pneumothorax

- Tension pneumothorax: midline shift away from the pneumothorax, raised or obstructed JVP, hypotension, tachycardia, shock.
- Size of pneumothorax: percentages of pneumothorax are hard to estimate; classify according to the size of the visible rim between the lung margin and the chest wall on CXR:
  - Small pneumothorax: visible rim <2cm.
  - Large pneumothorax: visible rim >2cm.

  (NB: a large pneumothorax approximates to a 50% loss of lung volume).
- Hypoxia: $P_aO_2 \leq 10$kPa on air (may simply reflect underlying lung disease).
- Severe dyspnoea.

Pneumothorax: management

See 📖 Figs. 2.2 and 2.3, pp.208–209

Who to discharge from A&E

- Small spontaneous 1° pneumothorax, rim of air <2cm on CXR, no significant dyspnoea, and no underlying chronic lung disease.
- Large spontaneous 1° pneumothorax following successful aspiration (<2cm rim of air on repeat CXR), no significant dyspnoea or underlying lung disease.
- Follow up in chest clinic in 10–14 days with a repeat CXR.
- Advise the patient to return to A&E if breathless or increasing chest pain.

Who to admit for observation

- All patients with pneumothorax 2° to trauma or with underlying lung disease even if aspiration has been successful: discharge after 24h if follow-up CXR shows no recurrence.
- Patients in whom aspiration has failed to re-expand the lung fully.
- Give O_2 (>35% unless there is clinical evidence of COPD, in which case start with 24–28% and check ABGs). This accelerates the reabsorption of the pneumothorax up to 4-fold. Most of the pneumothorax is N_2 (air) and supplemental O_2 decreases the partial pressure of N_2 in the blood, increasing the gradient for its reabsorption.
- Once the air leak is sealed, the pneumothorax reabsorbs at a rate of ~1.25% of the volume of the hemithorax per day. A 15% pneumothorax will take approx. 3 weeks to reabsorb.

Attempt chest aspiration in patients with

- 1° pneumothorax: all large 1° pneumothoraces, whether symptomatic or not. Repeat aspiration is successful in up to 50%.
- 2° pneumothorax: all small 2° pneumothoraces, only if asymptomatic and <50 years. Admit for observation and if there is minimal or no pneumothorax on CXR after 24h, discharge with follow-up in chest clinic in 10–14 days with CXR.

Proceed to intercostal chest tube drainage in patients with

- 1° pneumothorax: failed aspiration after 1–2 attempts.
- 2° pneumothorax: small pneumothorax if symptomatic or >50 years; failed aspiration after 1 attempt.
- Miscellaneous: associated hydro- or haemopneumothorax, all mechanically ventilated patients with a pneumothorax, all patients with a pneumothorax requiring inter-hospital transfer.
- The technique for insertion of an intercostals drain is described on 📖 pp.788–790.
  - If the lung has re-expanded and the drain is not bubbling, wait 24h and repeat CXR to exclude recurrence, and remove the drain.
  - A collapsed lung and bubbling drain suggests persistent air leak and suction may be required. Use low-pressure suction (2–5kPa) via appropriate pump or modified wall suction on a specialist Respiratory Unit—discuss with chest team.

- A collapsed lung and no bubbling suggests the drain is blocked, displaced, or clamped. If a new drain is required it should be through a new incision.
- If there is a persistent air leak or failure of the lung to re-expand after 3–5 days consider surgical pleurodesis (consult the chest team and/or cardiothoracic team). Open thoracotomy and pleurectomy, or surgical talc pleurodesis, are more effective than medical pleurodesis (with talc, bleomycin, or tetracycline), which should only be considered for those unwilling or unable to undergo surgery.

Practice points

- There are ***NO*** indications in the standard management for a pneumothorax for clamping chest drains. If patients are to be moved, keep the drain bottle below chest height but ***DO NOT CLAMP.***
- ***NEVER*** clamp a chest drain unless you know what you are doing.

Acute pneumothorax: management

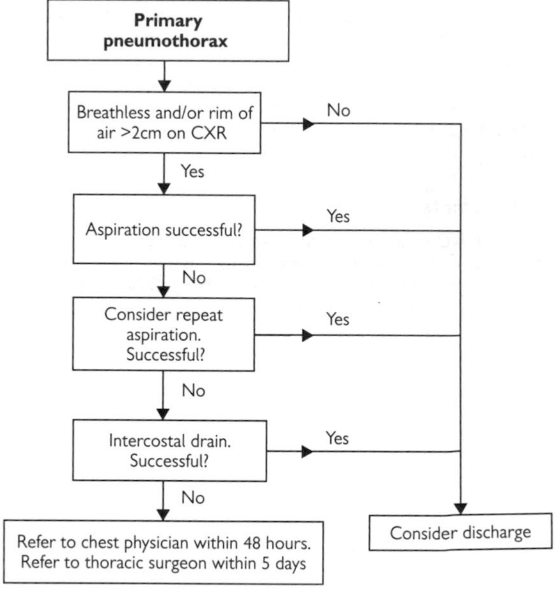

Fig. 2.2 Acute pneumothorax: management. Adapted from Henry M *et al.* (2003). BTS guidelines for the management of spontaneous pneumothorax. *Thorax* **58**(suppl.2): ii39–52.

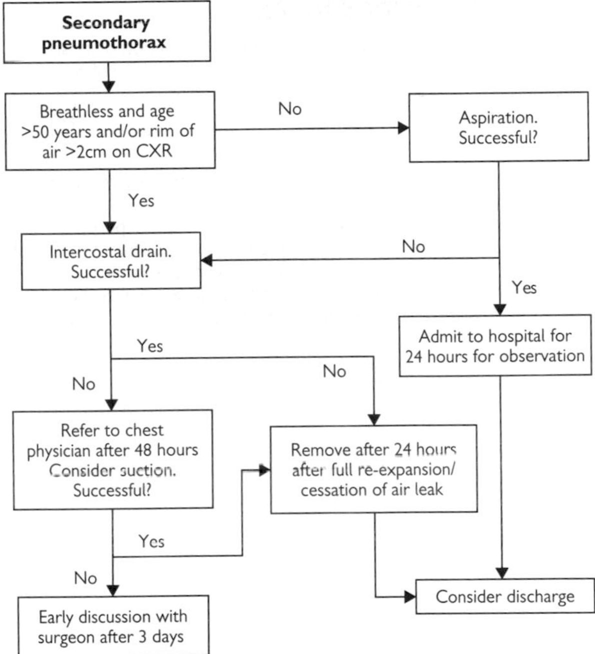

Fig. 2.3 Secondary pneumothorax: management. Adapted from Henry M *et al.* (2003). BTS guidelines for the management of spontaneous pneumothorax. *Thorax* **58**(suppl.2): ii39–52.

Tension pneumothorax

- Usually seen in patients receiving mechanical ventilation or post CPR.
- Patient is usually distressed, tachypnoeic with cyanosis, profuse sweating, and marked tachycardia and hypotension.
- This requires immediate attention.

Management

- Do not leave the patient unattended. Give maximal inspired O_2 to reverse hypoxia.
- Insert an 18G (green) cannula (or the largest available) perpendicular to the chest wall into the second intercostal space in the mid-clavicular line on the side with the pneumothorax on clinical examination (reduced breath sounds and trachea deviated away). Relief should be almost immediate. Leave the cannula in place until the air ceases to rush out.
- Insert a chest drain as soon as possible.
- If no air rushes out when the cannula is inserted, the patient does not have a tension pneumothorax and the cannula should be removed.

Haemoptysis: assessment

Presentation

- Haemoptysis is the coughing up of blood from the lungs or tracheobronchial tree (see Box 2.14).
- Massive haemoptysis is defined as ≥400mL over 3h or ≥600mL over 24h. The common causes of *massive* haemoptysis are bronchiectasis, bronchial carcinoma, infection (e.g. TB, lung abscess, or aspergilloma), or trauma.
- Often the cause is obvious from the history. Patients with large bleeds may be able to locate the site of bleeding by a 'gurgling' within the chest. Ask specifically for smoking and drug history.
- Examine for an underlying cause (see Box 2.14) and to assess the haemodynamic and respiratory effects of the bleed.
- Consider that the blood may be coming from somewhere other than the lungs: upper respiratory tract, GI tract, nasopharynx.

Poor prognostic factors

These include:

- Increasing age
- Pre-existing lung or cardiac disease
- Respiratory compromise (rate, cyanosis)
- Hypoxia (P_aO_2 ≤10kPa on air)
- Ongoing haemoptysis of large amounts of fresh blood
- Shock (postural or supine hypotension—rare).

Box 2.14 Common causes of haemoptysis

Lung disease

- Bronchiectasis (± infection)
- Bronchogenic carcinoma
- Infection:
  - TB
  - Pneumonia
  - Lung abscess
  - Aspergilloma
- Bronchitis
- Trauma
- AV malformation

Cardiovascular

- Pulmonary embolus
- Left ventricular failure
- Mitral stenosis
- Congenital heart disease with pulmonary hypertension
- Aortic aneurysm

Systemic vasculitis

- SLE
- Wegner's
- Goodpasture's
- Microscopic polyangiitis

Haemoptysis: management

Initial management

Stabilize the patient

- Massive haemoptysis should usually be managed at a hospital with cardiothoracic surgical back-up, and urgent transfer should be considered if this is not available.
- Give high inspired O_2.
- Place patient in the recovery position, with the bleeding lung down (if it is known which side the bleeding is from) to try to keep the unaffected lung free of blood.
- If aspiration of blood is threatened, get anaesthetic help urgently; anaesthetize, intubate, and ventilate. A double-lumen ET tube may be used to isolate the lungs but the narrow lumen may make subsequent flexible bronchoscopy difficult.
- Insert a large-bore peripheral cannula, followed by a central line if indicated; internal jugular route is preferred to minimize the risk of pneumothorax.
- Support the circulation: haemoptyses are rarely severe enough to warrant transfusion. If the patient has postural or supine hypotension use IV colloid until blood is available.
- Monitor the urine output, pulse, BP, and, if appropriate, CVP.

Investigations

All patients should have the following:

- Blood for FBC, U&Es, coagulation studies, X-match
- ABGs
- ECG
- CXR (± lateral)
- Sputum (microscopy and culture, cytology)
- Flexible bronchoscopy.

Diagnose the source of bleeding

- ***CXR*** This should be examined systematically for a mass lesion ± hilar nodes, bronchiectasis (tram-line shadows), old or new cavities which may suggest aspergillomas. Look for causes of minor haemoptysis, if this is the current problem.
- ***Fibreoptic or rigid bronchoscopy*** This should be performed urgently in all cases of massive haemoptysis. This is unlikely to localize the exact source, but may help localize the lung or lobe affected to guide surgeons or radiologists. Bleeding may be arrested by endoscopically administered adrenaline (1mL 1:10,000) or, in massive haemoptysis, a balloon catheter may be inflated for 24–48h within a segmental or sub-segmental bronchus.
- ***Selective pulmonary angiography*** Can identify the bleeding source in 90% of patients and, when combined with embolization, is effective in controlling bleeding in up to 90%. Multiple procedures may be necessary.
- ***High resolution CT chest*** May help identify parenchymal lesions and peripheral endobronchial lesions.

Specific therapeutic interventions

- Correct coagulopathy: if the haemoptysis is relatively minor it may be sufficient to correct an excessively elevated INR to a therapeutic range (INR 1.5–2.0) with FFP. In patients with a prosthetic valve and massive haemoptysis, the clotting must be normalized as best as possible. Discuss with your local haematologists or cardiologists. Support platelets if $<50 \times 10^9$/L.
- Consider nebulized β-agonist and/or IV aminophylline as a mucocilliary stimulant and to relieve bronchospasm in patients with asthma and COPD.
- Patients with minor haemoptysis should be fully investigated (see Box 2.15). No cause is found in ~10%.
- Patients with massive haemoptysis should undergo urgent fibreoptic bronchoscopy to locate the bleeding source.
- Angiography and embolization should be considered for all patients with massive haemoptysis prior to surgery.
- If angiography is not available, patients who continue to bleed >600mL/day or who have an identifiable lesion (e.g. lung abscess, aspergilloma, trauma) should have definitive surgery.
- Discuss all cases of haemoptysis with the chest team. Patients with massive haemoptysis should be managed in a specialist centre with appropriate cardiothoracic and radiological back-up. Transfer the patient (ventilated if unstable) if the patient is fit enough.
- Infection is a common precipitant (e.g. in bronchiectasis). Consider antibiotics (e.g. co-amoxiclav 1g IV q6–8h or cefotaxime 2g IV q8h) after appropriate cultures. TB or lung parasites will require specific antimicrobial therapy.

Box 2.15 Further investigation of haemoptysis

- Autoantibodies (ANA, ANCA, anti-GBM antibody)
- Serum for *Legionella* serology
- *Aspergillus* precipitins
- CT chest
- VQ scan
- Echo
- Pulmonary and bronchial artery angiogram
- Lung biopsy
- Pulmonary function tests with transfer factor.

Pleural effusions

Presentation

- Dyspnoea
- Chest discomfort or sensation of heaviness
- Symptoms of malignancy: loss of appetite, weight, energy
- Symptoms of infection: fever, cough, sputum, night sweats.

Severity depends on

- Speed of onset (e.g. traumatic or post-procedural)
- Haemodynamic compromise (hypotension, tachycardia)
- Hypoxia or respiratory failure
- Presence of underlying disease (e.g. heart failure, COPD).

Causes

Transudate (protein >30g/L)

- Raised venous pressure:
  - Cardiac failure
  - Constrictive pericarditis
  - Fluid overload
- Hypoproteinaemia:
  - Nephrotic syndrome
  - Cirrhosis with ascites
  - Protein-losing enteropathy
- Miscellaneous
  - Hypothyroidism
  - Meigs' syndrome
  - Yellow nail syndrome.

Exudate (protein >30g/L)

- Infection:
  - Pneumonia
  - Empyema (bacterial or TB)
  - Sub-phrenic abscess
- Malignancy:
  - 1° bronchial
  - Mesothelioma
  - 2° (and lymphoma)
  - Lymphangitis carcinomatosa
- Miscellaneous:
  - Haemothorax (trauma, iatrogenic)
  - Chylothorax (thoracic duct trauma)
  - Autoimmune (RA, SLE, Dressler's)
- Pancreatitis

Management

- If acute then stabilize the patient and insert a chest drain.
- If effusion is chronic then reach a diagnosis and treat accordingly.

Acute massive effusion

- Give O_2.
- IV access: via a wide-bore cannula or internal jugular central line. If central access is difficult then avoid attempting unless peripheral access is clearly inadequate. Attempt to cannulate (internal jugular veins only) on the normal side. A bilateral pulmonary problem will be a disaster.
- Take blood: for FBC, clotting, and urgent cross-match (6 units).
- Correct coagulopathies.
- Restore circulating volume: if BP low or tachycardic, then give a plasma expander 500mL stat, according to size of effusion drained and response.

- Insert a chest drain (see 📖 pp.788–791). The drain should be left unclamped and allowed to drain freely, the amount drained should be recorded.

Indications for specialist referral

- Traumatic haemothorax should be referred to the cardiothoracic surgeons.
- Haemothorax 2° to procedures should be referred if the patient is shocked and/or there is ongoing significant blood loss requiring transfusion at a rate ≥1 unit every 4h (approx.).
- When in doubt discuss the case with the surgical team.

Practice point

If there is ↓movement of one side of the chest, that is the side of pathology (e.g. fluid, infection, pneumothorax).

Chronic massive effusion

A unilateral chronic effusion will usually have accumulated over weeks or perhaps even months. The commonest causes are malignancy, empyema, TB, autoimmune diseases (e.g. rheumatoid), and cirrhotic ascites with transdiaphragmatic movement.

Investigation

- Diagnostic aspiration: ideally, the chest should be scanned and marked by ultrasound prior to tapping the effusion as underlying collapse may cause significant elevation of the hemidiaphragm.
- A sample should then be withdrawn (50mL) and split into three for:
  - ***Biochemistry:***
    —protein ≥30g/L implies an exudate
    —protein <30g/L implies a transudate
    —LDH to assess Light's criteria (see Box 2.16)
    —pH <7.2 suggests a possible empyema
    —glucose <3.3mmol suggests a possible empyema (also seen in TB and autoimmune-related effusions)
    —Amylase if acute pancreatitis suspected
    —Triglycerides if chylothorax suspected.
  - ***Microscopy/ microbiology:***
    —turbid fluid with neutrophils implies infection
    —blood-stained fluid implies malignancy but may be a haemothorax (check fluid haematocrit: if >1/2 blood haematocrit, suspect haemothorax)
    —ZN staining for AFB (+ve in only 20% of pleural TB)
    —culture for TB and routine culture.
  - ***Cytology:*** for 1° and 2° tumours. Positive in 60%, so negative does not exclude malignancy.
- Pleural biopsy should be performed if malignancy or TB is suspected.
- Chest CT with contrast may help differentiate benign from malignant disease, pleural thickening, mesothelioma, or intrapulmonary pathology.

Management

- The main priority is diagnosis.
- The fluid may be drained by repeated aspirations of 1L/day until dry, or by the insertion of a small-bore intercostal drain (see 📖 pp.788–791), which should be clamped and released to drain 1.5L/day (this is the only instance when a chest drain may be clamped).
- Drainage of >1.5L/day may result in reperfusion pulmonary oedema.
- If the malignant effusion reaccumulates rapidly, consider chemical or surgical pleurodesis.

Empyema

This is a serious complication of bacterial chest infection (📖 p.173). All effusions associated with a pneumonia (parapneumonic) should be tapped.

- To avoid long-term scarring and loculated infection the empyema requires urgent drainage by ultrasound guidance and usually the positioning of an intercostal drain.
- Frequently drainage fails as the empyema organizes with dense adhesions producing loculations. This can be assessed by ultrasound. Surgical drainage is the only option in this situation. The role of intrapleural thrombolytics remains unclear.
- Empyema should always be discussed with a respiratory physician or cardiothoracic surgeon.

Box 2.16 Light's criteria for pleural fluid analysis

The pleural fluid is an exudate if one or more of the following criteria are met:

- Pleural fluid protein divided by serum protein >0.5
- Pleural fluid LDH divided by serum LDH >0.6
- Pleural fluid LDH more than two-thirds the upper limit of normal serum LDH level

Acute upper airway obstruction

Presentation

- Stridor: inspiratory noise. Generated by the collapse of the extra-thoracic airway during inspiration
- Breathlessness
- Dysphagia
- Inability to swallow secretions (hunched forward, drooling)
- Cyanosis
- Collapse.
- Ask colleagues to call a senior anaesthetist and ENT assistance immediately while you continue your assessment.

Identify the cause (see Box 2.17)

- ***History*** Sudden onset, something in mouth or child playing with unsafe toy (foreign body), fever (epiglottitis, diphtheria, tonsillitis), hoarse voice (epiglottitis), sore throat (infective as listed), travel (Eastern Europe—diphtheria), smoker + longer history + systemic symptoms (?carcinoma), trauma.
- ***Examination*** Where infective cause is suspected then examination of oropharynx must be undertaken in area where patient may be immediately intubated, with an anaesthetist standing by.
- Fever, drooling, stridor. Bull neck, lymphadenopathy, pseudomembrane over oropharynx (diphtheria). Swollen throat + epiglottis on direct/indirect laryngoscopy (epiglottitis).
- ***Investigations*** Do not delay treatment if the patient is in distress. If the patient is relatively stable, perform a CXR (foreign body), lateral neck X-ray (swollen epiglottis). FBC, U&Es, blood gases.

Box 2.17 Causes of acute stridor

- Infective: acute epiglottitis, diphtheria, tonsillitis, or adenoiditis (children)
- Inhalation of foreign body
- Tumour of trachea or larynx
- Trauma
- Postoperatively (thyroid surgery).

Indications for ITU/surgical referral

- Prior to examination of oropharynx if infective cause suspected
- Failure to maintain adequate airway or oxygenation
- Inability to swallow secretions
- Ventilatory failure ($P_aO_2 \leq 10$kPa, $P_aCO_2 \geq 6$kPa)
- Collapse
- Severe dyspnoea.

Management

- If severe, liaise immediately with ITU and ENT or general surgeons (potential for urgent tracheostomy).
- Priorities are:
  - Stabilize the patient: ensure adequate airway
  - Identify cause of obstruction
  - Specific treatment measures.

Stabilize the patient

- Take ABGs and give high percentage O_2 (≥60%).
- If clear cause of obstruction (foreign body, postoperative thyroid surgery), then take appropriate measures to gain patient airway (see 📖 p.220).
- If patient is becoming increasingly exhausted or there is acute failure of ventilation then summon colleagues and be prepared to intubate or perform tracheostomy.

Foreign body

With total upper airway obstruction, perform Heimlich manoeuvre (stand behind patient, grip wrists across the patient's upper abdomen and tug sharply to raise intrathoracic pressure and expel foreign body). Otherwise perform CXR, liaise with respiratory/ENT/cardiothoracic teams for retrieval under direct vision.

Epiglottitis

Usually *Haemophilus influenzae* type b, also *Strep. pneumoniae*. Treat with 3rd-generation cephalosporin, e.g. cefotaxime 2g tds (adults). Children more likely to require intubation, but if any concerns over airway then patient (adult or child) should be monitored on ITU after anaesthetic assessment.

Diphtheria

Uncommon in UK, occasionally seen in patients returning from abroad. Toxin-mediated problems include myocarditis and neuritis. Treat with diphtheria antitoxin + antibiotic eradication of organism (consult microbiology).

Tumour obstruction

Unlikely to cause life-threatening obstruction without warning symptoms over ≥few days. If significant stridor present then administer 200mg hydrocortisone and thereafter prednisolone 40mg od PO. If laryngeal origin liaise with ENT regarding tracheostomy. Lung cancer in trachea, or extrinsic cancer eroding into the trachea, will require urgent radiotherapy (or occasionally laser or cryotherapy via bronchoscope).

Chapter 3

Gastroenterological emergencies

Acute upper gastrointestinal (GI) bleeding 1

Presentation

- Haematemesis (bright red, dark clots, coffee grounds).
- Melaena (black, sticky, smelly). This may arise from anywhere proximal to and including the caecum. Blood is cathartic and takes 4–6h to be passed. With massive bleeding (e.g. variceal) there may be dark clots in the stool. Other causes of dark stool include iron therapy, bismuth containing drugs, liquorice, or drinks (red wine).
- Weakness/sweating and palpitations.
- Postural dizziness and fainting.
- Collapse or shock.

Causes

	Approx %
• Peptic ulcer:	35–50%
• Gastroduodenal erosions:	8–15%
• Oesophagitis:	5–15%
• Varices:	5–10%
• Mallory–Weiss tear:	15%
• Upper GI malignancy:	1%
• Vascular malformations:	5%
• Rare miscellaneous:	5% (e.g. Meckel's, Crohn's disease)

Assessment of severity

It is essential to categorize patients at the time of admission into high or low risk of death (see Rockall's Score (Table 3.1)—BSG Guidelines[1]). Most deaths occur in the elderly with comorbid disease.

In general, high risk factors include the following:

- Age >60 years (30% risk of death if >90 years).
- Shock (BP <100mmHg systolic in patients <60 years or <120mmHg in patients >60 years. *Measure postural change* in BP in patients who are not shocked, and change in HR.
- Inappropriate bradycardia or HR >120bpm.
- Chronic liver disease.
- Other chronic disease (e.g. cardiac, respiratory, renal).
- Bleeding diathesis.
- ↓conscious level.

Management

Liaise with specialists early (on-call endoscopy team and surgeons). An experienced anaesthetist should be informed. Most patients will have stopped bleeding by the time they are seen: however, all upper GI bleeds should be taken seriously as they may re-bleed in hospital, and the mortality following a re-bleed is high.

Priorities are:

- Stabilize the patient: protect the airway, restore the circulating volume
- Identify the source of the bleeding
- Definitive treatment of the cause of bleeding.

Table 3.1 The Rockall score

Clinical variable	Points scored			
	0	**1**	**2**	**3**
Age (years)	<60 years	60–79 years	>80 years	
Shock	No shock	HR >100	HR >100	
		SBP >100	SBP <100	
Comorbidity	Nil		Cardiac	Liver
				Renal
				Malignancy
Diagnosis	Mallory–Weiss	All other	GI tract malignancy	
Stigmata of recent bleed	None or dark spot		Blood in upper GI tract	
			Adherent clot; spurter	
Score <3 = excellent prognosis				
Score >8 = high risk of death				

Reference

1. www.sign.ac.uk/PDF/sign105.pdf

Acute upper GI bleeding 2

Initial management (Box 3.1)

- ***Protect the airway:*** position the patient on side.
- ***IV access:*** insert 1–2 large bore (14G–16G) cannulae into peripheral vein for initial fluid resuscitation. If peripheral access is difficult, access via jugular, subclavian, or femoral vein may be necessary. CVP monitoring (see 🕮 p.742) allows early identification of bleeding, and is useful to prevent overfilling. It is essential in older patients or in those with massive haemorrhage. A fall of 5cm H_2O over 2h suggest re-bleed.
- Take blood for ***Hb*** and ***PCV***. These do not fall until the plasma volume has been restored, but if low at presentation suggests massive blood loss or acute-on-chronic bleeding. *WCC* may be elevated but usually <15000/mm^3. If WCC is elevated look for sepsis (sepsis predisposes to haemorrhage). ***Platelet count:*** if low suggests hypersplenism and chronic liver disease. ***U&Es:*** ↑urea out of proportion to the creatinine indicates significant GI bleed. Check ***PT and LFTs*** since liver disease is a common cause of GI bleeding, ***Group and X-match*** 4–8U. Monitor ***ABG*** in severely ill patients.
- ***Restore the circulating volume***
  - Tachycardia, hypotension, or a postural fall in BP or a postural increase in HR (by > 30bpm) suggests a low intravascular volume. Give 500mL–1L colloid over 1h or N\saline and continue until blood is available. Stable BP takes precedence over body sodium balance.
  - If there are no signs of haemodynamic compromise use a slow infusion of N saline (0.9%) to keep the IV line patent and for maintenance fluids.
  - Use compatible blood when it is ready (give 1U/h) until volume is restored or CVP 5–10cm. If the rate of bleeding is slow, packed cells are preferred. If there is massive haemorrhage, ask for 'O'-negative blood which may be given without X-matching. Save serum for retrospective cross-match.
- ***Monitor urine output*** and catheterize the patient if there are signs of haemodynamic compromise. Aim for >30mL/h. Prompt rescuscitation should restore urine output (see oliguria, 🕮 p.284).
- ***Watch for the usual signs of overload*** (raised JVP or CVP, pulmonary oedema, peripheral oedema). Too rapid transfusion may precipitate pulmonary oedema.
- ***Commence intravenous PPI***: re-bleeding occurs in ~20% of patients after endoscopic treatment of bleeding ulcers. IV omeprazole (80mg IV, followed by 8mg/h for 72h) decreases the risk of re-bleeding from >20% to ~7%. Many centres use IV pantoprazole. In patients admitted with upper GI bleeding, a single bolus of 80mg IV omeprazole followed by infusion (8mg/h) before endoscopy decreases endoscopic signs of bleeding and the need for endoscopic therapy.
- Keep the patient ***NBM*** for the endoscopy.

Box 3.1 Management key points: initial management of upper GI bleed*

- Protect the airway: position the patient on side.
- IV access: 2 large bore (14G–16G) cannulae. Insert a central line if peripheral access is difficult.
- G&S and X-match 4–8U.
- IV fluids: if haemodynamically compromised, initially give 500mL–1L colloid over 1h, then crystalloid and continue until compatible blood is available.
  - If there is massive haemorrhage, give 'O'-negative blood.
  - If there are no signs of haemodynamic compromise: give slow infusion of 0.9% saline to keep the IV line patent and for maintenance fluids.
- Consider central line insertion and CVP monitoring if initial Rockall score is ≥3.
- Commence IV PPI (80mg IV, followed by 8mg/h) pre-endoscopy and for 72h after endoscopy in patients who required ulcer haemostasis.
- Monitor pulse rate, BP, urine output and CVP (if appropriate).
- Keep the patient NBM for the endoscopy.

For variceal bleeding see 🕮 p.232.

Reference

1. Lau JY *et al.* (2007). Omeprazole before endoscopy in patients with gastrointestinal bleeding. *N Engl J Med* **356:** 1631–40.

Acute upper GI bleeding 3

Determine the source

- ***History:*** ask specifically about dyspepsia, alcohol, drug history (e.g. NSAIDs, anticoagulants), risk factors for liver disease, normal vomit prior to haematemesis (Mallory–Weiss tear, variceal bleed), previous GI bleeds, ulcers, or surgery.
- ***Physical examination:*** look for stigmata of chronic liver disease (including hepatomegaly and splenomegaly), scars of previous surgery, telangiectasia (Osler–Weber–Rendu syndrome), abdominal bruit, bruises. Rectal examination may reveal melaena or semi-fresh blood.
- ***Upper GI endoscopy*** should be done within 12h of the bleed. It may be difficult to precisely locate the site of bleeding due to clots in the stomach but it is easy to exclude possible areas of bleeding which may help decide further management. Remember upper GI bleeding in patients with cirrhosis has a non-variceal origin in ~30% of cases.
- ***Selective arteriography*** of the coeliac axis, superior mesenteric or inferior mesenteric artery is of value when the bleeding site cannot be identified, usually after 2 or more negative endoscopies and bleeding is brisk (0.5–1mL/min).
- ***Barium studies*** may be used to diagnose small bowel causes of melaena (e.g. Crohn's or tumour). Labelled RBC scans may also be useful. Meckel's scan may be useful in younger patients.
- ***Capsule endoscopy*** is used to diagnose causes of occult or recurrent but unidentified GI bleeding.

General measures to stop the bleeding

- ***Correct any coagulopathy***
  - Platelet count below 50,000/mm^3 should be treated with platelet support (6–12U of platelets).
  - If the patient is on anticoagulants, assess the need for anti-coagulation before reversal. The annual risk of embolization in non-anticoagulated patients with prosthetic heart valves is 4% for aortic and 8% for mitral valves overall with greater risk with caged ball valves. The annual risk of stroke in non-anticoagulated patients with AF is 3–5% (relative risk 2.5–3); but is much lower in those <75 years without comorbidity. Therefore, in patients with prosthetic valves correct with FFP (2–4U) and/or a very low dose of vitamin K (0.5–1 mg, IV). Otherwise give FFP and IV vitamin K (5–10 mg).
  - Cryoprecipitate may be required if the fibrinogen levels are low.
- ***Serum calcium*** may fall after several units of citrate-containing blood transfusion. Give 10mL (4.5mEq) of calcium gluconate for every 3–4U transfused. Supplement magnesium and phosphate as necessary.
- ***Ulcer healing agents:*** give an IV PPI such as pantoprazole (40mg IV daily) or omeprazole (80mg IV, followed by 8mg/h for 72h).
- ***Tranexamic acid*** (0.5–1g IV tds or 1–1.5g PO tds) increases the levels of fibrinogen and may be helpful. Likewise desmopressin may be useful in patients with renal failure.

Peptic ulcer disease

Bleeding peptic ulcers form the mainstay of upper GI bleeding, accounting for 60% of all cases and 1/3 of these have been taking a NSAID. Patients may give a history of epigastric distress relieved by food but often there is no prior history.

- ***Endoscopy*** allows the bleeding site to be visualized. Identification of the bleeding vessel or adherent clot has prognostic significance: >80% of these patients will re-bleed, cf. <5% without these stigmata.
  - The bleeding point may be treated endoscopically by electro-coagulation, injection of adrenaline, alcohol or endoclips around the bleeding point and into the base, heat probe, or laser photocoagulation, depending on the local facilities.
  - Keep the patient NBM for 6–8h post-endoscopy in case a repeat endoscopy or surgery is needed.
- ***Indications for surgery:*** see Box 3.2.
- ***Medical management:***
  - Treat with PPI for 4–8 weeks.
  - Repeat endoscopy at 6–8 weeks for all gastric ulcers to check the lesion has healed.
  - A biopsy should be taken at endoscopy for urease testing for *Helicobacter pylori*. Sensitivity affected by PPIs. Or use facial Ag testing. If positive add an *H. pylori* eradication regimen (see *BNF*).
- ***Prognosis:*** overall mortality is <10%. Mortality is reduced by early surgery in high-risk patients.

Practice point

In one major study, IV PPI infusion was almost as effective as therapeutic endoscopy in bleeding peptic ulcer disease.

Erosive gastritis/oesophagitis

These generally present as relatively minor bleeds but may be significant. Represent ~15% of upper GI bleeds, and are associated with prior use of aspirin or other NSAIDs in previously fit patients, or 'stress' in the critically ill patient.

- ***Management:*** at endoscopy there is commonly a generalized ooze of blood from the inflamed mucosa. Initial management is as before (Box 3.1).
- Give PPI or sucralfate 1–2g q6h PO or via NG-tube.
- PPIs are better than H_2-antagonists in healing oesophagitis and oesophageal ulcers.
- Correct any clotting disorder.
- If the lesions are too diffuse and the bleeding continues, partial gastric resection may be necessary.
- ***Prognosis:*** <5% of patients with haemorrhagic gastritis require surgery. Overall mortality is <10%.

Box 3.2 Relative indications for surgery

- Exanguinating haemorrhage (too fast to replace).
- Profuse bleeding:
  - >6U blood in initial resuscitation
  - Continued bleeding at >1 unit per 8h
  - Persistent hypotension.
- Re-bleed in hospital.
- Failed endoscopic therapy.
- Re-bleed after endoscopic therapy in patients >65 years.
- Lesions which are at high risk of re-bleeding, e.g. posterior DU with visible vessel or giant gastric ulcer.
- Special situations, e.g. patients with a rare blood group or patients refusing blood transfusion should be explored earlier.

Variceal haemorrhage: medical management

Oesophageal and gastric varices develop with portal hypertension of whatever cause. Bleeding from varices is typically vigorous and difficult to control and often occurs in the setting of abnormal clotting, thrombocytopenia, and sepsis.

Diagnosis

History and physical examination may raise the suspicion of a variceal source of bleeding but ~30% of cirrhotics have a non-variceal source of bleeding. The most reliable method is upper GI endoscopy which should be performed as soon as is feasible. Bleeding may occur from either gastric or oesophageal varices, or rarely portal hypertensive gastropathy.

Medical management

- Initial resuscitation is as described on 📖 p.226.
- Transfuse with blood, FFP, and platelets as necessary according to haematological parameters to try to stop the bleeding. Give vitamin K 10mg IV once only to exclude vitamin K deficiency. Avoid over-transfusion (may ↑the risk of rebleeding).
- ***Antibiotics:*** take blood, urine, and ascitic cultures ± microscopy. Start broad-spectrum antibiotics. Several studies have shown that variceal bleeding is associated with sepsis. Commence a third-generation cephalosporin or ciprofloxacin and amoxicillin. Treat for 5 days.
- ***Terlipressin***: (2mg initially, and then 1–2mg every 4–6h for up to 72h) is effective in controlling variceal bleeding by causing splanchnic vasoconstriction (relative reduction in mortality of ~34%). Avoid high doses (2mg) if possible. Serious side effects occur in 4% and include cardiac ischaemia, peripheral vasoconstriction, which may produce significant hypertension, skin, and splanchnic ischaemia. *Octreotide* is a synthetic analogue of somatostatin. A recent Cochrane review found that octreotide had no effect on mortality, and had a minimal effect on transfusion requirements.[1] It is not recommended.
- ***Band-ligation*** of the varices is most commonly used and is safer than injection sclerotherapy. It should be repeated at 2-weekly intervals until obliterated,
- ***Endoscopic injection*** of sclerosant into the varices or para-variceal can control the bleeding acutely. Side effects (serious in 7%) include retrosternal pain and fever immediately post injection, mucosal ulceration, late oesophageal strictures. Gastric varices should be injected with cyanoacrylate glue.
- ***Balloon tamponade***: a Sengstaken–Blakemore tube may be inserted (📖 p.794) with inflation of the gastric balloon **only**. This should not be left in place for >12h as ischaemic ulceration may occur.
- ***Liver failure regimen*** (📖 p.272): give lactulose 10–15ml q8h PO or per NG tube to prevent encephalopathy. In alcoholics give thiamine and multivitamins as necessary. Use phosphate enemas for patients with severe encephalopathy.

Box 3.3 Management key points: variceal haemorrhage

- Initial resuscitation: see Box 3.1 📖 p.227.Transfuse with blood, FFP, and platelets as necessary.
- Vitamin K (10mg IV once).
- Prophylactic antibiotics: a third-generation cephalosporin (e.g. ceftriaxone) or ciprofloxacin and amoxicillin (for 5 days).
- Terlipressin (2mg initially, and then 1–2mg every 4–6h for up to 72h).
- OGD: band ligation or sclerotherapy
- If bleeding is not controlled, balloon tamponade (e.g. a Sengstaken–Blakemore or Linton tube) may be used to temporarily stabilize the patient so that more definitive treatment (TIPS or surgery) can be instituted. These tubes should only be used in settings in which experienced staff are available
- Some centres are now using DANIS stents.

Reference

1. Cochrane Reviews ☞ www.cochrane.org/reviews/en/ab002147.html

Variceal haemorrhage: further management

Radiological management

TIPS is available in specialized units. Using a jugular or femoral approach, the hepatic veins are cannulated and an expandable stent is placed between the hepatic veins (low pressure) and the portal venous system (high pressure). The portal pressure should be decompressed to below 12mmHg.

Surgical management

This has been largely superseded by TIPS.

- *Emergency porto-caval shunting* is effective in controlling the bleed (>95%) but has a high operative mortality (>50%) and does not influence long-term survival. Few surgeons can do this now
- *Oesophageal transection* is never used now but remains an option.

Prognosis

- Overall mortality is 30%. This is highest in those with severe liver disease (Child's Grade C, see Table 3.2).
- Success rates for cessation of acute bleeding varices:
  - Injection sclerotherapy or banding: ~70–85%
  - Balloon tamponade: ~80%
  - Terlipressin:~70%

Long-term management

- *Band ligation* every 2 weeks until variceal obliteration more rapidly (39 days versus 72 days).
- *Injection sclerotherapy* is rarely used now.
- *Propranolol* (80mg tds: aim for a 30–40% reduction in resting heart rate, but confirm reduction of portal pressure by measurement of wedged hepatic venous pressure gradient) reduces the rate of re-bleeding from varices and portal hypertensive gastropathy. It has not been shown to decrease mortality.
- *TIPS* or shunt procedures provide a more definite cure and bleeding tends to recur only when the shunt blocks, but there is an ↑ incidence of chronic hepatic encephalopathy. It is very effective.

Mallory–Weiss tear

This is a tear in the mucosa at the gastro-oesophageal junction following severe retching and is particularly common following large bouts of alcohol. The vomit is normal initially and becomes bright red.

Management

- Most stop bleeding spontaneously.
- Tamponade with a Sengstaken–Blakemore tube may be used.
- Surgical over-sewing of bleeding point or selective arteriography and embolization of the feeding artery may be necessary.

Table 3.2 Child–Pugh score

Clinical or biochemical variable	Points scored		
	1	**2**	**3**
Encephalopathy grade	None	1–2	3–4
Ascites	Absent	Mild	Moderate–severe
Bilirubin (μmol/L)	<35	36–60	>60
Albumin (g/L)	>35	28–35	<28
PT (seconds prolonged)	1–4	4–6	>6
The Child–Pugh scoring system is a very effective way to get an index of the severity of liver disease in patients with cirrhosis. It is not directly applicable to patients with 1° biliary cirrhosis or sclerosing cholangitis.			
Child–Pugh A:	Score ≤6		
Child–Pugh B:	Score 7–9		
Child–Pugh C:	Score ≥10		

Acute gastroenteritis: assessment

Food poisoning is an acute attack of abdominal pain, diarrhoea ± vomiting 1–40h after ingesting contaminated foodstuffs and lasting 1–7 days. With the exception of an acute attack of inflammatory bowel disease and mesenteric ischaemia (see 📖 p. 248) the majority of acute-onset diarrhoea has an infective aetiology.

Differential diagnosis of acute diarrhoea

Common

- Gastroenteritis (bacterial, viral, protozoal)
- *Clostridium difficile* diarrhoea (pseudomembranous colitis)
- Inflammatory bowel disease.
- Food intolerance/allergy (e.g. lactase deficiency)
- Drugs (see 📖 Box 3.7, p.242)

Less common

- Coeliac disease
- Tumour (benign or malignant)
- Carcinoid syndrome
- Bacterial overgrowth
- Pancreatic insufficiency
- Bile salt enteropathy
- Hyperthyroidism
- Autonomic neuropathy.

Presenting features

Ask specifically about:

- Recent eating habits esp. restaurants and food prepared by caterers. Anyone else (family/friends) with similar symptoms?
- Time interval between eating any suspicious substance and onset of symptoms. Early onset of vomiting or diarrhoea (6–12h) suggests ingestion of preformed toxin (e.g. *Staph.* exotoxin). Enterotoxin-producing organisms may take 1–3 days to produce symptoms.
- Recent travel (enterotoxogenic *E. coli*, *Salmonella*, *Giardia*, or amoeba)? Recent medication? Any antibiotics (*C. difficile*)?
- PMH, e.g. gastric surgery or immunosuppression (drugs or HIV).
- Anal intercourse increases the risk of amoebiasis, giardiasis, shigellosis, rectal syphilis, rectal gonorrhoea, *Chlamydia trachomatis*, HSV of rectum and perianal area (diarrhoea in HIV-infected patients is discussed on 📖 p.500).
- The gross appearance of the diarrhoea may help: frankly bloody stool, *Campylobacter* or *Shigella*; watery, 'rice-water stool' classically secretory diarrhoea due to cholera, enterotoxogenic *E. coli*, or neuro-endocrine tumours. Typhoid produces greenish 'pea-soup' diarrhoea.
- Abdominal pain may be present: usually cramp-like or tenesmus.
- Fever: common with the severe bacterial diarrhoeas and acute exacerbations of Crohn's or UC.

Investigations

• *FBC*	↑WBC; ↑haematocrit (dehydration).
• *U&Es*	↑Urea (dehydration); ↓K^+.
• *Blood cultures*	Systemic infection may occur.
• *Stool cultures*	Fresh samples, mandatory for wet mount microscopy for ova, cysts, and parasites, culture, and antibiotic sensitivities. WBC in stool implies intestinal inflammation (mucosal invasion, toxin, inflammatory bowel disease, ischaemic colitis).
• *Clostridium difficile toxin*	Specifically request this for all patients who have recently taken antibiotics, or who develop diarrhoea in hospital.
• *Sigmoidoscopy and rectal biopsy*	Useful for persistent bloody diarrhoea (>4–5 days) without diagnosis or improvement.

Management

It is important to maintain hydration in patients with diarrhoea, and to avoid loperamide unless infective causes have been excluded. Box 3.4 contains general guidelines only.

Box 3.4 General approach to treat acute diarrhoea

Severity of symptoms	*Management*
• Mild (1–3 stools/day)	• Oral fluids only
• Moderate (3–5 stools/day)	• Oral fluids, loperamide
• Severe (>6 stools/day, fever).	• Fluids (± IVI), anti-microbial agent.

Note: avoid using loperamide unless you have excluded infectious causes of diarrhoea.

When to use antibiotics early

Unless shiga toxin-producing *E. coli* is suspected, it is reasonable to give antibiotics (e.g. ciprofloxacin) to all patients with an ↑risk of fatal or severe diarrhoea. These include frail elderly patients with achlorhydria (including patients on PPIs such as omeprazole), inflammatory bowel disease, poor haemodynamic reserve, or the immunocompromised.

Bacterial gastroenteritis

Salmonella spp.

May produce acute gastroenteritis (e.g. *S. enteritidis*, ~70–80% of cases), enteric fever (*S. typhi and S. typhimurium*, see 📖 p.466), or asymptomatic carriage. Acute gastroenteritis often occurs in epidemics, and is derived from poultry, eggs, or egg products, and occasionally pets (terrapins).

- ***Symptoms***: 8–48h after ingestion with headache, vomiting (worse than either *Shigella or Campylobacter*), fever, and diarrhoea lasting 2–4 days (rarely bloody with mucus). Reactive arthritis may occur (in HLA-B27 +ve). Enteric fever, see 📖 p.466.
- ***Management***: usually self-limiting after 2–5 days, and treatment is supportive for most cases. Some antibiotics can prolong carriage of the illness, and make clinical relapse more likely.

Clostridium perfringens (type A)

15–25% of cases of bacterial food poisoning. Spores are heat resistant and may germinate during reheating or slow cooking of meats. Enterotoxin is released when sporulation occurs in intestine. Incubation 8–22h.

- ***Symptoms***: diarrhoea, abdominal pain, nausea (rare to get vomiting). No fever. Lasts 12–24h.
- ***Management***: supportive.

Campylobacter

Campylobacter infections are common (5–10% of patients with acute diarrhoea). The incubation period is 3–7 days, symptoms last for 1–2 weeks. Presentation often follows eating contaminated poultry.

- ***Symptoms***: flu-like illness followed by headache, myalgia, abdominal pain (continuous then colicky), diarrhoea, rectal bleeding occasionally. Rarely complicated by reactive arthritis (1–2%), Guillain–Barré syndrome, or Reiter's syndrome.
- ***Management***: usually self-limiting <5 days. Treatment comprises either erythromycin or tetracycline. Antidiarrhoeals are contraindicated.

Staphlococcus aureus

(2–5% of cases) can multiply at room temperature in foods rich in carbohydrates and salt (dairy products, cold meats, mayonnaise). A heat-stable exotoxin produces nausea, vomiting, and diarrhoea 1–6h after ingestion. Fever is uncommon. Treatment is supportive.

Bacillus cereus

Associated with slow-cooking foods and reheated rice (fast-food takeaways). It produces a toxin that causes vomiting within 1–5h, and diarrhoea 8–16h later. Treatment is supportive.

Vibrio parahaemolyticus

Produces epigastric pain (cf. those above), diarrhoea, vomiting, and fever 12–18h after ingestion of raw seafood (shellfish). May last up to 5 days. ***Vibrio cholerae*** is uncommon in the Western nations. It produces profuse secretory diarrhoea. The disease is usually self-limiting (5–7 days) but tetracyclines may be used.

Yersinia enterocolitica

Incubation period 4–10 days after contact with infected animals, water, or ice cream.

- ***Symptoms:*** diarrhoea (80%), abdominal pain (80%), fever (40%), bloody stool in 10%, mesenteric adenitis, lymphadenopathy, reactive arthritis. Diagnosed by serology rather than culture.
- ***Management:*** supportive.

Shiga toxin-producing E. coli (e.g. O157:H7)

Infection is usually from contaminated meat/burgers. The incubation period is ~5 days. Stools become bloody over 24–48h, 2° to a diffuse colitis. Most patients resolve over 5–7 days without treatment. However, some, esp. children, may go to develop HUS with tiredness, microangiopathic anaemia, thrombocytopenia, renal failure, encephalopathy. Most recover with supportive care. Antibiotics are contraindicated, as some antibiotics increase shiga toxin production and exacerbate or cause the development of HUS.

Viral gastroenteritis

In addition to diarrhoea, URTI-like symptoms, abdominal cramps, headache, and fever may occur. The causative agent is usually not found but many viruses implicated (e.g. echovirus, Norwalk virus, and adenoviruses) Self-limiting illness (3–5 days).

Management

Oral fluids and restricting solid foods and dairy product intake usually suffice.

Clostridum difficile

Pseudomembranous colitis is caused by two necrolytic toxins (A and B) produced by *Clostridium difficile*. It is the commonest cause of hospital-acquired diarrhoea. Infection typically follows antibiotic therapy. Diarrhoea may occur during or up to 4 weeks following cessation of treatment.

Symptoms

Diarrhoea is usually profuse, watery, and without blood (may be bloody in ~5%). It is commonly associated with abdominal cramps and tenderness, fever, and an elevated white cell count.

Diagnosis

Diagnosis is based on detection of *C. difficile* toxin in stool. Culture of the organism itself is unhelpful; ~5% of healthy adults carry the organism. Sigmoidoscopy is not diagnostic, but may show mucosal inflammation together with multiple yellow plaques.

Management

Patients should be isolated and barrier nursed. Rehydrate and correct electrolyte abnormalities. Mild disease responds to oral metronidazole (500mg tds). Oral vancomycin 250mg qds for 7–14 days is an alternative. Severe disease requires IV therapy. Complications include toxic megacolon and colonic perforation.

Giardiasis

Giardia lamblia is transmitted by the faeco-oral route. Risk factors include recent travel, immunosuppression, homosexuality, and achlorhydria.

Symptoms

More chronic diarrhoeal illness with epigastric discomfort due to duodenal infestation. Malaise, bloating, flatulance, and occasionally malabsorption occur. Diagnosis is by stool microscopy for cysts or trophozoites or duodenal aspiration. If negative, consider blind therapeutic trial.

Management

Metronidazole is the treatment of choice, 2g daily for 3 days or 400mg tds for 5 days orally. Alternatives include tinidazole (2g single dose) or mepacrine hydrochloride 100mg tds for 5–7 days. Lactose intolerance post infection may persist for up to 6 weeks.

Travellers' diarrhoea

Travel through developing countries is commonly associated with self-limiting acute diarrhoeal illness transmitted through food and water. The most frequent pathogen is enterotoxigenic *E. coli* (40% of cases). The illness lasts 3–5 days with nausea, watery diarrhoea, and abdominal cramps. Oral rehydration is usually sufficient. Antimotility agents (e.g. loperamide) may be used with caution. Antibiotic treatment (ciprofloxacin 500mg bd) may help patients with more protracted illness. Alternatives include doxycycline or co-trimoxazole. Diarrhoea that persists for >7 days requires further investigation including stool microscopy and culture, serology, sigmoidoscopy, and biopsy (see table opposite). A 3–5-day course of a broad-spectrum antibiotic such as ciprofloxacin may terminate the illness.

Box 3.5 Causes of travellers' diarrhoea

Bacterial
- Enterotoxigenic *E. coli* (40%)
- Shigellas and enteroinvasive
- *E. coli* (10%)
- *Salmonella* (5%)
- *Campylobacter* (3%)
- Aeromas/plesiomonas (5%)
- Vibrioparahaemolyticus (1%).

Not-identified (22%)

Viruses (10%)
- Norwalk
- Rotavirus.

Protozoa (4%)
- *Giardia*
- *Entamoeba*
- *Cryptosporidium*
- *Microsporidium.*

Box 3.6 Causes of persistent diarrhoea in travellers

Protozoa
- *Giardia lamblia*
- *Entamoeba histolytica*
- *Cyclospora cayetanensis.*

Bacteria
- *Salmonella*
- *Campylobacter.*

Helminths
- Strongyloides
- Colonic schistosomiasis (rare).

Box 3.7 Common drugs that may cause acute diarrhoea

- Laxatives
- Antacid (Mg^{2+}, Ca^{2+})
- Lactulose
- Diuretics therapy
- Antibiotics
- Colchicine
- Quinidine
- Digitalis
- Theophyllines
- Cholinergic agents
- Propranolol
- Aspirin
- NSAIDs
- Cytotoxic
- Captopril

There are many drugs other than those listed here that can cause diarrhoea

Bloody diarrhoea

Causes

- Acute infectious colitis:
  - Bacillary dysentery (*Shigella* spp.)
  - Salmonellosis (📖 p.466)
  - *Campylobacter* (📖 p.238)
  - Haemorrhagic colitis (shiga-like toxin-producing *E. coli*)
  - Pseudomembranous colitis (📖 p.240)
- Inflammatory bowel disease (IBD, UC, or Crohn's).

Presenting features

- Ask about duration of symptoms and recent eating habits. Others affected? Recent travel (enterotoxogenic *E. coli, Salmonella, Giardia*, or amoeba)? Recent medication? Any antibiotics (*C. difficile*)?
- The gross appearance of the stool may help. Inflammatory bowel disease may result in rectal bleeding (fresh red blood) in patients with disease largely confined to the rectum and sigmoid colon. Diffuse disease tends to be associated with diarrhoea. Infectious colitis results in frankly bloody stool (*Campylobacter or Shigella*).
- Abdominal pain may be present: usually cramp-like, or tenesmus.
- Vomiting is uncommon in acute IBD.
- Systemic features such as general malaise and lethargy, dehydration electrolyte imbalance, or fever are seen with the severe bacterial diarrhoeas and acute exacerbations of Crohn's or UC. Skin, joints, and eyes may be involved in either IBD or follow acute infection.
- Previous altered bowel habit, weight loss, smoking history, vascular disease (mesenteric infarction), mesenteric angina may be relevant.

Examination

Look for:

- Fever, signs of dehydration (tachycardia, postural hypotension), abdominal distension. Abdominal tenderness or rebound over affected colon (IBD) may indicate colonic dilatation or perforation. An abdominal mass may indicate tumour or inflammatory mass.
- Mouth ulcers and perianal disease are common in active IBD.
- Erythema nodosum and pyoderma gangrenosum occur in inflammatory bowel disease; *Yersinia* may produce erythema nodosum. Rose spots indicate typhoid fever.
- Joint involvement (often an asymmetrical, non-deforming synovitis, involving large joints of the lower limbs) may occur in active IBD, but also in infectious colitis (e.g. *Campylobacter, Yersinia*).
- Uveitis is associated with both IBD and acute infectious colitis.

Investigations

The priority is to exclude any infectious cause for the bloody diarrhoea and to monitor for complications.

- ***Blood tests*** FBC, U&Es, LFTs, CRP, ESR, coagulation studies.
- ***Microbiology*** Stool MC&S, blood cultures, *C. difficile* toxin.

- ***Sigmoidoscopy biopsy*** May help to distinguish between acute infectious colitis and IBD (↑risk of perforation during colonoscopy).
- ***Imaging*** Plain AXR may help monitor colonic dilatation. Contrast studies are contraindicated acutely. Nuclear imaging studies (e.g. WBC scans) are used in IBD to demarcate extent of disease.

Practice points

- Always test for *C. difficile* in patients with new onset bloody diarrhoea.
- Unexplained extreme leucocytosis (e.g. WBC >35,000), consider *C. difficile*.

Bacterial dysentery

This is due to infection with *Shigella (S. dysenteriae, S. flexneri, S. boydii, S. sonnei)* or some shigella-like *E. coli* (0157:H7). Transmitted by the faeco-oral route, and clusters of cases are often found.

Symptoms

- It causes mild diarrhoea to a severe systemic illness between 1–7 days following exposure.
- Fever (usually resolves in 3–4 days).
- Abdominal cramps with tenesmus.
- Watery diarrhoea ± nausea and vomiting (resolves by day 7). Bloody diarrhoea occurs later (after 24–72h) due to invasion of the mucosa.
- Diagnosed by stool culture. *E. coli* infections may be complicated by haemolytic uraemic syndrome.

Management

- Patients may require IV fluid replacement
- Antibiotics should be reserved for the most severe cases. Ampicillin (250mg PO qds × 5–10 days) is usually effective, but in resistant cases co-trimoxazole or ciprofloxacin may be used.
- Anti-motility agents such as loperamide and codeine are contraindicated as they prolong carriage and worsen symptoms.

Amoebic dysentery

Entamoeba histolytica can produce intermittent diarrhoea or a more severe illness that resembles IBD. There is an ↑risk in homosexuals, and in those with recent travel to third world countries. It is transmitted by the faeco-oral route.

Symptoms

- Diarrhoea or loose stool (± blood), abdominal discomfort, mild fever. In severe cases, liver abscess.
- Fulminant attacks present abruptly with high fever, cramping abdominal pain, and profuse bloody diarrhoea.
- Marked abdominal tenderness is present.
- Diagnosis is made by identifying amoebic cysts on stool microscopy.
- May be complicated by late development of amoebic liver abscess.

Treatment

- Aimed at replacement of fluid, electrolyte, and blood loss, and eradication of the organism.
- In acute-invasive intestinal amoebiasis oral metronidazole 800mg tds, for 5–10 days is the treatment of choice. Tinidazole (2g daily for 2–3 days) is also effective. This should be followed with oral diloxanide furoate 500mg tds for 10 days to destroy gut cysts.
- Metronidazole (or tinidazole) and diloxanide furoate are also effective for liver abscesses, and USS-guided aspiration may help improve penetration of the drugs and shorten illness.
- Diloxanide furoate is the treatment of choice for asymptomatic patients with *E. histolytica* cysts in the stool as metronidazole and tinidazole are relatively ineffective.

Inflammatory bowel disease (IBD) 1

IBD includes Crohn's disease and UC. Crohn's disease is a chronic inflammatory disease of any part of the GIT, characterized by granulomatous inflammation. UC is a chronic inflammatory disease of the colon of unknown aetiology. It always affects the rectum, and extends proximally to a variable extent of the colon.

Ulcerative colitis

Presentation

- Gradual onset of progressively more severe symptoms.
- Diarrhoea is dependent on disease activity and extent. Nocturnal diarrhoea and urgency are common symptoms of severe UC.
- Mucus and frank pus, or blood, is often mixed in with the stool.
- Occasionally abdominal pain (not a prominent feature, though lower abdominal cramping pains relieved by defecation is common; severe abdominal pain suggests a severe attack with acute dilatation or perforation, or ischaemic colitis).
- Urgency and tenesmus.
- In severe disease there is severe (>6 motions/day) and nocturnal diarrhoea, anorexia, and weight loss. Blood may be altered in colour.
- Aphthous ulcers (also present in Crohn's).
- Ask about recent cessation of smoking (precipitant).

Examination

Look for *fever*, signs of dehydration (tachycardia, postural hypotension), and abdominal distension. *Abdominal tenderness* ± rebound may indicate colonic dilatation or perforation. This may be masked if the patient is on steroids. An abdominal mass may indicate tumour or inflammatory mass. *Systemic features*: examine for extra-intestinal manifestations (Box 3.8).

Crohn's disease

Presentation

- Diarrhoea 80%.
- Abdominal pain 50% (colic and vomiting suggest ileal disease).
- Weight loss 70% and fever 40%.
- Obstructive symptoms (colic, vomiting).
- Rectal bleeding 50% (commoner in colonic disease, but is present in 50% with ileal disease; colonic disease is associated with perianal disease in 30%).
- Extra-intestinal manifestations such as erythema nodosum (5–10%), arthropathy (10%), or eye complications (5%) (Box 3.9)
- Symptoms of anaemia (iron, B12, or folate deficiency) or nutritional deficiencies.

Examination

Examine nutritional status and for evidence of malabsorption. Examine for evidence of intestinal obstruction (strictures). Fistulae may occur between the bowel and other organs (bladder, vagina). Toxic megacolon (>6cm on AXR) occurs but is much rarer than in UC. Bloody diarrhoea is occasionally massive.

Box 3.8 Extra-intestinal manifestations of UC

Related to disease activity
- Aphthous ulcers
- Fatty liver
- Erythema nodosum
- Peripheral arthropathy
- Episcleritis
- ± Pyoderma gangrenosum
- ± Anterior uveitis.

Unrelated to disease activity
- Sacroiliitis
- Ank. spondylitis
- 1° sclerosing cholangitis
- Cholangiocarcinoma (usually with PSC).

Box 3.9 Extra-intestinal manifestations of Crohn's disease

Related to disease activity
- Aphthous ulceration (20%)
- Erythema nodosum (5%)
- Pyoderma gangrenosum (0.5%)
- Acute arthropathy (8%)
- Eye complications (5%)
  - Conjunctivitis
  - Episcleritis
  - Uveitis.

Unrelated to disease activity
- Sacroiliitis (15%)
- Ank. spondylitis (4%)
- Liver disease (5%)
  - Gall stones common
  - Chronic active hepatitis (2%)
  - Cirrhosis (2%)
  - Fatty change (5%).

Inflammatory bowel disease 2

Markers of a severe attack of IBD

- >6 bloody stools/day
- Systemically unwell: pyrexia and tachycardia
- Hb <10g/dL
- Albumin <30g/L
- Toxic dilatation (colon >6cm).

Although the presence of these symptoms, signs, or findings indicate severe IBD (UC or Crohn's), it should be noted that severe Crohn's disease may be present in the absence of any of the listed markers.

Investigations

- ***Blood tests*** Anaemia may be present if the colitis is acute and florid severe and iron-deficiency picture may be observed. ↑WCC (neutrophilia) and ↑ platelets. ↓K+ may follow severe diarrhoea. There may also be an element of pre-renal dehydration. In severe colitis albumin often falls to 20–30g/L. ESR and CRP reflect disease activity, though are often not elevated in distal (rectal) disease. They are useful to monitor therapy.
- ***Stool culture and microscopy***
- ***Supine AXR ± erect CXR*** To look for wall thickening (moderate–severe) and mucosal oedema, with loss of haustration and colonic dilatation (more severe cases). Colonic diameter >6cm indicates toxic dilatation, with risk of perforation. The extent of the disease can be indirectly assessed; distal colitis is often associated with proximal faecal loading. In the acute stages of a severe attack abdominal films should be performed daily, or twice daily if there is borderline toxic dilatation. Free air under the diaphragm on an erect CXR indicates perforation.
- ***White cell scan*** ^{111}Indium-labelled WBC accumulate in areas of active inflammation, and are a useful adjunct to plain AXR to assess the extent of active disease. Crohn's typically shows patchy uptake and involvement of the small bowel while UC is commonly limited to colon.
- ***Sigmoidoscopy ± colonoscopy*** Bowel preparation is unnecessary and may cause reddening of the mucosa. Flexible sigmoidoscopy has a lower risk of bacteraemia and is easier than rigid sigmoidoscopy. Non-specific findings such as hyperaemia and contact or spontaneous bleeding are common. Ulceration suggests acute disease; pseudopolyps and atrophy of the bowel mucosa indicate chronic UC. Rectal biopsy from the posterior wall below 10cm should be taken from all patients (less risk of perforation).

Inflammatory bowel disease 3

Management

- Rehydrate patient with IV fluids and correct any electrolyte imbalance (hypokalaemia in particular). Inform and discuss the patient with surgical colleagues, especially if moderate–severe (Box 3.11).
- The differential diagnosis is wide (Box 3.10). Exclude infectious colitis (normal stool microscopy and culture) and systemic infections as far as possible.
- Avoid anti-motility and opiate drugs (such as loperamide and codeine) and anti-spasmodics as they cause proximal constipation and may precipitate paralytic ileus and megacolon.
- ***Corticosteroids*** Acute attacks of UC may respond to rectal steroids (e.g. Predfoam® or Predsol® enema, 20mg 1–2 times daily) especially if disease is confined to the rectum. However severe attacks require IV steroids (hydrocortisone 100mg qds IV) until remission is achieved. Crohn's disease is only treated if it is causing symptoms. Severe Crohn's disease should be treated with IV steroids (hydrocortisone 100mg qds IV).
- ***Aminosalicylates*** In patients with UC, mesalazine should be started (800mg bd or tds orally) ± mesalazine foam enema (1g od PR) in addition to steroids: they help induce, and maintain, remission after steroids are tailed off. Use mesalazine for small bowel Crohn's.
- ***Elemental diets*** Elemental diets are as effective as steroids for the treatment of Crohn's disease. However, it is difficult to get patients to comply.
- ***Other agents*** UC: there are few data to support the use of azathioprine, ciclosporin, or methotrexate in acute attacks. Two trials have reported that nicotine patches significantly improve symptoms and help to induce remission of UC. Crohn's disease: each of these agents has been tried with variable success (they take up to 16 weeks to become effective). Azathioprine (2mg/kg daily) may be useful for maintenance of remission.
- ***Antibiotics*** There is no evidence that broad-spectrum antibiotics are useful in UC. Metronidazole is useful in the treatment of perianal Crohn's fistulae. Ciprofloxacin may also be useful in Crohn's disease. Other antibiotics should only be used if specifically indicated and should be considered for patients developing toxic megacolon.
- ***Infliximab*** is being increasingly used (with success) for perianal and fistulating Crohn's disease as well as severe Crohn's disease in general.
- ***Nutrition*** There is no evidence for keeping the patient 'nil by mouth'. However a low residue and early institution of TPN may be of benefit, especially if the patient is likely to come to surgery. When the patient is recovering, stool-bulking agents (e.g. methylcellulose) may be used to adjust stool consistency.
- ***Smoking*** Encourage patients who smoke to stop, as this enhances remission rates.

Box 3.10 Differential diagnosis of inflammatory bowel disease

Bacteria
- *Shigella*
- *Salmonella*
- *E. coli*
- *Camplyobacter*
- *C. difficile*
- TB
- *Gonococcus*
- *Chlamydia*
- *Yersinia.*

Parasites
- Amoebiasis
- Schistosomiasis.

- ***Miscellaneous***
- Ischaemic colitis
- Lymphoma
- Trauma
- Radiation colitis.

Indications for surgery

- Failure of symptoms to resolve after 5 days is an indication for proctocolectomy (7–10 days in some centres).
- Colonic perforation, uncontrollable bleeding, toxic megacolon, and fulminating disease require urgent proctocolectomy; ~30% of all patients with UC will require a colectomy at some stage.
- Toxic dilatation prior to treatment is not an indication for surgery (failure of the colonic diameter to decrease after 24h). The development of dilatation during treatment is an indication for surgery.
- Surgery in Crohn's disease is not 'curative' and is only indicated for perforation, obstruction, abscess formation, and fistulae (enterocutaneous or enterovesical). High recurrence rate after surgery.

Box 3.11 Management key points: acute management of inflammatory colitis

- IV fluids: rehydrate patient and correct any electrolyte imbalance (e.g. hypokalaemia). Correct anaemia.
- Corticosteroids: IV hydrocortisone 100mg qds (+ rectal steroids in acute UC or Crohn's with distal colonic disease).
- Prophylactic heparin (5000U SC bd).
- Metronidazole for colonic Crohn's disease.
- Avoid anti-motility drugs, opiates, and anti-spasmodics (cause proximal constipation and may precipitate paralytic ileus and megacolon).
- Inform and discuss the patient with surgical colleagues.
- Nutrition: a low residue and early institution of TPN may be of benefit, especially if the patient is likely to come to surgery.

Jaundice: assessment

Jaundice requires urgent investigation and diagnosis. It may herald the onset of a severe hepatitis and acute liver (±renal) failure (see 📖 p.268). It may indicate an obstructive jaundice which can be complicated by cholangitis and septicaemia (📖 p.264).

History

- Non-specific symptoms include anorexia, pruritus, malaise, lethargy, drowsiness, confusion, or coma. Dark urine and pale stools may be features of either obstructive jaundice or hepatitis.
- Colicky RUQ pain, previous biliary colic, or known gallstones suggests biliary colic (see 📖 p.264). Fever, rigors, abdominal pain, and fluctuating jaundice should raise the suspicion of cholangitis. Painless jaundice and weight loss suggest pancreatic malignancy.
- Take a detailed drug history including homeopathic or proprietary preparations. Ask specifically about use of paracetamol and alcohol.
- Risk factors for infectious hepatitis: blood transfusion, IV drugs, homosexual, travel, ethnic origin, ingestion of shellfish.

Examination

- Note the degree of jaundice and look for stigmata of chronic liver disease (spider naevi or telangiectasia, palmar erythema, Dupuytren's contractures, etc.). Lymphadenopathy may reflect malignancy. Hepatic encephalopathy results in falling conscious level, and liver flap.
- Note the BP and the diastolic carefully: it falls with liver failure. Oliguria or shock may occur with acute liver failure (see 📖 p.268). Examine for pleural effusions (may occur with ascites).
- Examine the abdomen for ascites, hepatomegaly, splenomegaly (portal hypertension or intravascular haemolysis), or masses.

Urgent investigations for jaundice (on day of admission)

- *U&Es, LFTs* — Exclude renal failure (hepatorenal syndrome 📖 p.296).
- *Glucose* — DM is common in haemochromatosis or pancreatic
- *PT* — ↑ in severe liver injury or DIC.
- *FBC* — ↓ platelets (chronic liver disease with hypersplenism,
- *Urinalysis* — Absence of bilirubin in the urine in a jaundiced patient
- *Septic screen* — e.g. Blood cultures, ascitic tap if relevant
- *CXR* — Tumour or metastases, effusion assoc. with ascites.
- *USS* — If patient is unwell or septic, exclude biliary obstruction
- *Paracetamol* — If overdose is suspected or possible.

Non-urgent investigations for jaundice

- ***Viral serology*** Anti-HAIgM, HBsAg and anti-HBc, anti-HCV, ± EBV or CMV serology.
- ***Immunology*** ANA, anti-SM, AMA and Igs (CAH, PBC).
- ***Ferritin, iron, transferrin*** ↑ferritin is seen in any acute illness, but may indicate haemochromatosis (↑in alcoholic liver hepatitis).

Causes of jaundice

- Viral hepatitis
- Alcoholic hepatitis ± cirrhosis
- Drug-induced hepatitis (including paracetamol)
- End-stage cirrhosis (alcoholic, chronic viral hepatitis, haemochromatosis, Wilson's, cryptogenic cirrhosis, etc.)
- Haemolytic anaemia
- Gilbert's syndrome (mild jaundice)
- Biliary obstruction (stones or turnover)
- Intrahepatic cholestasis, post hepatitic (1° biliary cirrhosis, 1° sclerosing cholangitis, sepsis, drugs).
- Autoimmune hepatitis
- Ischaemic hepatitis
- Sepsis.

Viral hepatitis

Hepatitis A, hepatitis B or delta co-infection of HBV carriers can lead to an acute hepatitis with jaundice. Acute hepatitis C can present with jaundice but this is less usual. EBV infection frequently causes abnormal liver function tests including mild or moderate jaundice, and is often associated with splenomegaly during the acute phase. Patients should be asked about IV drug use, recent tattoos, sexual contacts and any familay or contact history of jaundice or hepatitis.

- Prodromal 'flu-like' illness and very high transaminase (up to ~4000U/L) with a small increase in alkaline phosphatase activity.
- If there is no coagulopathy, encephalopathy, or renal failure, send the patient home, and await virology results. Arrange repeat LFTs and clotting at 2–3 day intervals, and see the results (but not necessarily the patient). See the patient again within a week. Instruct the patient and carers to return if increasingly unwell, or drowsy.

Hepatitis A

Patients with acute hepatitis A (anti-HAV IgM positive) require no specific treatment but all household and school contacts should be immunized with HAV vaccine. This replaces previous guidelines that state that contacts should receive normal human immunoglobulins. Patients with acute hepatitis A may rarely develop acute liver failure, although the prognosis is relatively good (>80% survival) with conservative management. Acute hepatitis A may be associated with a high fever (40°C).

Hepatitis B

HBsAg appears in serum 1 to 10 weeks after an acute exposure to hepatitis B, and prior to the onset of symptoms or increased ALT. As HBsAg disappears from serum, HBsAb appears, and there may be a window period when both are negative. The detection of anti-HBc IgM is usually regarded as an indication of acute HBV infection, however, anti-HBc IgM may remain detectable up to two years after the acute infection, and anti-HBc may increase to detectable levels during exacerbations of chronic hepatitis B.

In the majority of patients who recover, HBsAg becomes undetectable after 4 to 6 months. Persistence of HBsAg for more than 6 months suggests chronic infection. The rate of progression from acute to chronic hepatitis B is less than 1-5% for adult-acquired infection. Patients with acute HBV do not require acute antiviral treatment. However, many clinicians treat patients with a severe hepatitis (e.g. INR >1.5) or protracted symptoms or marked jaundice for > four weeks after presentation, as well as those who are immunocompromised, or have preexisting liver disease, since this may reduce the likelihood of re-infection post-liver transplant.

For HBsAg positive patients, family and close contacts should be tested for HBsAg, HBsAb and antiHB core IgM. Prophylactic-specific hepatitis B immunoglobulin ('HBIG' 500 units im) is protective if given within 10 days of exposure to HBV: however only use for persons with clear exposure to HBsAg-contaminated material (needle-stick or sexual contacts who are HBsAb negative). Follow-up for at least 6 months.

Hepatitis C

HCV RNA is usually detectable in serum by PCR within 8 weeks following exposure, but may be earlier. Transmission is predominantly through blood exposure. Sexual or peri-natal transmission are rare (<5% risk). Acute hepatitis C accounts for less than 5% of cases of acute viral hepatitis in the UK. Most cases are asymptomatic, less than 25% develop an increase in serum bilirubin, and serum ALT is usually <1000U/L. The presence of HCV RNA in serum is the first evidence of HCV infection, and is detectable within 2 months following exposure. Anti-HCV ELISA tests become positive between 2–6 months after exposure.

About 80% of patients develop chronic HCV but a significant number clear the virus. All patients with diagnosed HCV should be followed-up and treated once it is established that they have chronic disease.

Treatment of acute hepatitis C with pegylated interferon: There are some data which suggest that treatment of acute hepatitis with pegylated interferon improves the eradication of hepatitis C virus.

For anti-HCV positive patients, try and determine the source. Check LFTs and HCV RNA, and follow up since the majority of untreated patients will need treatment with pegylated interferon and ribavirin.

Alcoholic hepatitis

- Acute hepatitis may be asymptomatic or present with nausea, vomiting, and anorexia, rarely RUQ pain. Fever may reflect severe liver damage but infection needs to be excluded. Most patients who present with alcoholic hepatitis have cirrhosis at presentation.
- The term alcoholic hepatitis is misnomer, as the transaminases rarely exceed 200U/L and are always <400U/L. The AST is always higher than the ALT (this is in contrast to most other liver diseases).
- Investigations: ↑bilirubin may be up to 800μM; albumin is often reduced; a prolonged PT usually signifies underlying cirrhosis; ↑WBC with left shift may occur (even without proven infection), anaemia and thrombocytopenia suggests cirrhosis; renal failure (HRS) may occur in severe alcoholic hepatitis.
- Screen for bacterial or fungal infections (blood, urine ascitic microscopy, and culture. If clinically suspected start broad-spectrum antibiotics (e.g. cefotaxime ± fluconazole (50–100mg IV daily) as prophylaxis against fungal infections.
- Admit most patients to hospital, unless mild (bilirubin <50μM, normal PT) or patient in abstinent environment. Give thiamine (100–200mg/day), folic acid, and multivitamins. Monitor and correct K^+, Mg^{2+}, PO_4^{3-} and glucose. Start a high-calorie, high-protein diet. Low-protein diets are contraindicated.
- Delirium tremens or severe agitation may be managed with low dose diazepam or oral chlomethiazole PO (📖 pp.414, 674). Treat seizures in the standard way (📖 pp.390, 414). Avoid chlordiazepoxide in patients with cirrhosis since the half life may be as long as 7 days in patients with liver disease.
- Calculate the Glasgow Alcoholic Hepatitis Score (see Table 3.3)
- Calculate the discriminant index for alcoholic hepatitis (see Box 3.12).

Practice points

- The AST level is normally > the ALT and both are usually <200U/L in alcoholic hepatitis. Never diagnose alcoholic hepatitis if the AST or ALT exceed 400U/L.
- Muscle injury or excessive exercise can increase both AST and ALT.
- A very high AST or ALT (i.e. >10,000 U/L) should suggest paracetamol (acetaminophen) overdose or ischemia.

Table 3.3 Calculation of Glasgow Alcoholic Hepatitis score (GAHs)

Score given	1	2	3
Age	<50	≥50	–
WCC (× 109/L)	<15	≥15	–
Urea (mM)	<5	≥5	–
INR	<1.5	1.5–2.0	≥2.0
Bilirubin (μM)	<125	125–250	>250

A score >9 = 50% mortality at 28 days

Box 3.12 Calculation of Discriminant Index (DF)

$$DF = \frac{\text{Bilirubin} + (\text{Prolongation of PT} \times 4.6)}{17}$$

e.g. serum bilirubin = 340μmoles/L, PT = 17s (control 12s) would score (340 ÷ 17) + [(17 − 12) × 4.6], i.e. 20 + 23 = 43

- There is a 32% mortality if DF>32
- A value >32 should be treated with prednisolone 40mg/day for 4 weeks. The only practical contraindication is untreated sepsis. If there is doubt, then give broad-spectrum antibiotics for 24–48h prior to steroids.

Management

Patients with severe alcoholic hepatitis (Glasgow alcoholic hepatitis score > 9) should be treated with prednisolone at 40mg/day for 4 weeks. The only practical contraindication is untreated sepsis. If there is doubt, then give broad-spectrum antibiotics for 24–48 hours prior to steroids. For patients with a GAHS greater than or equal to 9 the 28-day mortality for corticosteroid-treated patients is 22% with untreated patients having a mortality of 48%. An alternative to treatment with steroids is pentoxyfylline (400mg tds orally), and has been suggested to have an improved outcome in patients compared with steroids, however, further studies are needed.

Drug-induced hepatitis

Patients with drug-induced jaundice should be monitored 3 times per week or admitted for observation, as many are serious and may not resolve. Stop suspected drug immediately and observe. Look for rash and eosinophilia and exclude other causes (see Box 3.13). (For paracetamol overdose, see 🕮 p.268). Drugs causing jaundice are listed in Box 3.13. Drugs causing a rise in transaminases, but rarely causing jaundice, are not listed. All drug-induced causes of jaundice should be reported to the CSM (yellow pages at the back of the *BNF*).

Box 3.13 Common drugs that cause jaundice

Hepatitic	*Cholestatic*	*Mixed*
• Paracetamol	• Chlorpromazine	• Sulphonamides
• Rifampicin	• Flucloxacillin	• Sulfasalazine
• Allopurinol	• Azathioprine	• Carbamazepine
• NSAIDs	• Captopril	• Dapsone
• Halothane	• Co-amoxiclav	• Ranitidine
• Methyldopa	• Penicillamine	• Amitriptyline
• Hydralazine	• Erythromycin	• Nitrofurantoin
• Isoniazid	• Anabolic steroids	• Co-amoxiclav.
• Phenytoin.	• Oral contraceptive.	

Autoimmune hepatitis

This is characterized by elevated transaminases, up to a few thousand, usually <2000U/L, anti-smooth muscle antibody positive, ANA positive, and raised IgG (polyclonal). The total globulins (total protein-albumin) should be <35g/L in normals. ↑globulin (>45g/L) should always raise suspicion of autoimmune hepatitis. Confirm with liver biopsy. Treatment: steroids (prednisolone 30–40mg od) ± azathioprine (1mg/kg) as a steroid-sparing agent once viral hepatitis has been excluded (i.e. HBsAg negative). If there is failure to respond in a young patient (<30 years), consider Wilson's disease.

Acholuric jaundice

This is characterized by the absence of bilirubin in the urine. This may be caused by haemolytic anaemia (previous history, excess urinary urobilinogen, splenomegaly, reticulocytosis, etc.) or a congenital disorder of conjugation (Gilbert's syndrome, 2% of population). Fasting (<400 calories) for 48–72h (or IV nicotinic acid 50mg) will increase serum unconjugated bilirubin in patients with Gilbert's (bilirubin rarely >80μM).

Sepsis

Any severe infections may cause jaundice (incl. pneumonia). Most severe with intra-abdominal sepsis. LFTs may be cholestatic, or characterized by a predominant rise of the bilirubin only. Exclude other causes and treat infection with antibiotics ± surgical drainage.

Ischaemic hepatitis

Presentation

Occurs with significant hypotension or hepatic arterial occlusion. Predisposing factors include congestive cardiac failure±hypoxia. In its mildest form it manifests as mildly deranged LFTs (hepatitic picture, ↑PT) in a patient with CCF and in its most severe form may present as acute liver failure. Look for hypoxia, hypotension (may have normalized by the time of assessment), signs of arteriopathy (abdominal bruits from hepatic arterial occlusion), and signs of right ventricular failure. May cause confusion ± encephalopathy. Exclude other causes of hepatitis (📖 p.254).

Management

Most will respond to correction of the underlying aetiology. Correct hypotension (see 📖 p.312) and give O_2 to correct hypoxia. If hepatic artery or coeliac axis are occluded prognosis is poor, and depends on the extent of hepatic necrosis. Usually age and extent of disease preclude salvage surgery. Discuss with specialist centre. If signs of severe (acute) liver failure present, see 📖 p.270 for guidance. Most patients are not fit enough for liver transplantation.

Obstructive jaundice

See 📖 p.264.

Gallstone disease

Gallstone disease affects 10–20% of the population. The stones may be predominantly cholesterol (>80%), pigment stones (<25% cholesterol; multiple, irregular, friable), or mixed (faceted, calcium containing). The majority are asymptomatic and diagnosed incidentally.

Complications of gallstones

- Biliary colic
- Obstructive jaundice
- Cholecystitis ± empyema and gangrene of gallbladder
- Cholangitis septicaemia or liver abscesses
- Acute pancreatitis (📖 p.276)
- Perforation and peritonitis
- GB fistula, gallstone ileus.

Biliary colic

Presentation

Abdominal pain (RUQ) radiating to epigastrium, back, or shoulders associated with nausea and vomiting. Attacks commonly follow a heavy meal and pass spontaneously. Differential diagnosis includes acute MI, leaking aortic aneurysm, peptic ulcer, intestinal obstruction or ischaemia, pancreatitis, renal colic, and pneumonia.

Investigations

USS to detect the stone and gallbladder distention. Urine microscopy, CXR, ECG will help exclude other conditions.

Management

- Pain relief (pethidine 50–100mg IM q4h + prochlorperazine 12.5mg IM q8h); avoid morphine.
- Laparascopic cholecystectomy in the longer term.

Acute cholecystitis

Presentation

Sudden onset severe RUQ pain and symptoms similar to biliary colic with fever and persisting symptoms. Persistent vomiting suggests a bile duct stone. Physical signs include fever, tachycardia, sweating, RUQ tenderness, and peritonism, especially in inspiration (Murphy's sign) ± palpable gall-bladder. Jaundice (~33%) suggests obstruction of CBD. Acalculous chole-cystitis is seen in elderly or patients with coexisting disease or trauma, in the ITU, and patients on TPN. Mortality may be high.

Investigations

- ***Blood tests*** ↑WCC is usual. LFTs may show ↑bilirubin, and cholestatic liver function tests; ± ↑amylase.
- ***USS*** Should demonstrate gallstones or biliary sludge ± thickening of gallbladder wall.
- ***AXR*** Gallstones visible in ~10% of patients. Local peritonitis may produce a 'sentinal loop'.
- ***HIDA Scan*** Using ^{99}Tc-label is usually diagnostic.

Management

- NBM and IV fluids; insert an NG-tube if there is severe vomiting.
- Antibiotics should cover enteric organisms and *Enterococcus* (e.g. cefuroxime 750mg IV q8h + metronidazole 500mg IV q8h).
- Early laparoscopic cholecystectomy is the treatment of choice.
- Complications include perforation, gallstone ileus, or fistula.

Biliary obstruction

Biliary obstruction or apparent biliary obstruction will be associated with either a dilated or non-dilated biliary system and the patient may be either septic or aseptic. Biliary dilatation in patients with mechanical biliary obstruction may not always be apparent on USS.

Presentation

- Jaundice (painful or painless) ± fluctuation
- RUQ pain ± tenderness
- Fever (indicates infection or cholecystitis)
- Itching
- Dark urine ± pale stools (not very useful in practice)
- Septic shock.

Investigations

- ***Blood tests*** ↑WCC indicates sepsis. U&Es may indicate renal failure or pre-renal uraemia. LFTs show ↑bilirubin, ↑↑ALP, and ↑↑γ-GT; ↑amylase with concomitant pancreatitis; transient i ALT, AST with passage of a stone and persistent in cholangitis (usually "≤400U/L; higher suggests hepatitis). Blood cultures and CRP mandatory.
- ***USS*** This is mandatory, and should be performed within 12h if possible, to demonstrate the presence of dilated ducts ± gall stones. Post cholecystectomy slight dilatation (~0.8cm) of CBD is normal.
- ***AXR*** Aerobilia may indicate a gas-forming organism or recent instrumentation. There may be localized ileus.
- ***ERCP*** Shows stones in CBD and allows examination of GIT and ampulla to exclude other pathology. Give broad-spectrum antibiotics if intervention is planned.
- ***MRCP*** Magnetic resonance cholangio panereatography is a very accurate non-invasive investigation.

Poor prognostic features (depend on the cause)

- Elderly (>65 years)
- Shock
- Renal failure
- Cholangitis with cirrhosis, liver abscess, or high malignant stricture
- Cholangitis following transhepatic percutaneous cholangiography
- Acute pancreatitis.

Management

See algorithm opposite.

- Analgesia (pethidine 50–100mg IM q4h), NBM, IV fluids.
- Antibiotics (e.g. cefotaxime or ciprofloxacin + amoxicillin) if septic.
- Emergency decompression of the biliary system by:
  - ERCP
  - Percutaneous drainage
  - Surgical decompression.

- Follow up with LFTs, CRP, and temperature.
- Repeat ERCP when well to exclude missed stones or further anatomic abnormality.
- Repeat USS or CT liver scan to look for hepatic abscesses.

Box 3.14 Causes of biliary obstruction

Mechanical obstruction
- Gallstones
- Malignancy (pancreatic carcinoma, nodes, 2° deposits, cholangiocarcinoma)
- Postoperative stricture
- Cavernous transformation of portal vein
- Parasitic infection (e.g. onchocerciasis)

Intra-hepatic cholestasis
- 1° sclerosing cholangitis
- 1° biliary cirrhosis
- Cholestatic drug reaction

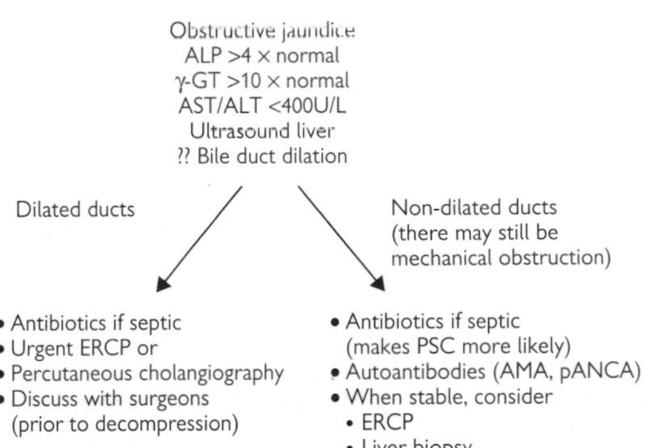

Fig. 3.1 Management algorithm for biliary obstruction. NB In cirrhosis there may be no duct dilatation with biliary obstruction.

Ascites

Presentation

The patient may present with symptoms due to the fluid (abdominal distension, weight gain, abdominal pain), the underlying cause (jaundice, haematemesis, fever, or night sweats, frothy urine due to proteinuria), or complication of the ascites (dyspnoea, anorexia, reflux oesophagitis, herniae, pleural effusions, scrotal or leg oedema, peritonitis). Ask specifically about alcohol, risk factors for chronic liver disease, GI bleeding (portal hypertension), previous pancreatitis, risk factors for TB, cardiac history, exercise tolerance, and menstrual history (?ovarian malignancy) (Box 3.15).

Differential diagnosis

- Ovarian cyst
- Obesity (simple or metabolic)
- Pregnancy
- Abdominal mass.

Investigations

• ***Blood tests***	U&Es, glc, FBC, PT, LFTs, blood cultures. Amylase.
• ***Ascitic tap (see* 🕮 *p.792)***	An ascitic tap should be carried out in all patients unless a diagnosis of malignant ascites is certain. Inoculate blood culture bottles and send fluid in sterile pot for microscopy and WBC
• ***Imaging***	Plain AXR shows a glass ground pattern with loss of psoas shadow. USS can detect as little as 30mL. Note the size and texture of the liver and spleen, check patency of hepatic veins. CT scan may be required.
• ***Urine***	Urine sodium (cirrhotic ascites), 24-h protein.

Management

Admit all patients with symptomatic ascites. Treat the underlying cause.

- *Cirrhotic ascites*: do not start diuretics if there is renal impairment.
- *Salt restrict* to 90mmol/day.
- *Paracentese* if tense or moderate ascites: drain *all* ascites as quickly as possible (maximum 25L in 5h), and then give 8g albumin per litre of ascites removed as 20% albumin. Start *spironolactone* at 100mg/day increasing to 400mg/day. Add furosemide 40mg/day if response is poor.
- If there is renal impairment (creatinine >140μM) give an extra *colloid and crystalloid volume challenge* (e.g. 500mL gelofusine, over 1h followed by 1L N saline over 4h). Do not commence diuretics; more harm is done by diuresing patients who are hypovolaemic.
- *Malignant ascites*: treatment is palliative, and may include total paracentesis to make the patient more comfortable. Specialist advice should be sought for future management of the malignancy.
- *Pancreatic ascites*: usually associated with a pancreatic pseudocyst and should be managed in consultation with surgical colleagues.
- *Spontaneous bacterial peritonitis* occurs in up to ~15% of patients admitted with cirrhotic ascites, and is frequently asymptomatic.

It rarely, if ever, occurs in non-cirrhotic ascites. The risk is ↑ with low ascitic protein. It is important to inoculate ascitic fluid into blood culture bottles at the bedside since this increases the positive culture yield to >90%. Diagnosis: ascitic WCC >250PMN/mm^3. If culture +ve but acsitic WBC low, repeat tap for microscopy and treat if WBC 250PMN/mm^3. Treat with broad-spectrum antibiotic for enteric organisms and G +ve cocci (e.g. cefotaxime). Suspect TB ascites if there is a predominant lymphocytosis. In patients with spontaneous bacterial peritonitis, the administration of IV albumin (1.5g/kg) at the time of diagnosis of infection and a second dose of 1.0g/kg on day 3 of antibiotic therapy may reduce the incidence of renal impairment and mortality.

Box 3.15 Causes of ascites

- Cirrhosis and portal hypertension
- Malignant ascites
- Congestive cardiac failure
- Pancreatic ascites
- Hepatic venous obstruction
- Nephrotic syndrome
- Hypothyroidism
- Infection (e.g. TB).

Ascites does not occur with portal vein thrombosis, congenital hepatic fibrosis, or other causes of non-cirrhotic portal hypertension except during a major insult such as GI bleeding.

Acute liver failure: assessment and investigations

Acute liver failure (fulminant hepatic failure) is defined as a potentially reversible severe liver injury, with an onset of hepatic encephalopathy within 8 weeks of the appearance of the first symptoms and in the absence of pre-existing liver disease. A more recent classification is: hyperacute liver failure: encephalopathy within 7 days of jaundice; acute liver failure: encephalopathy within 8–28 days of jaundice; sub-acute liver failure: encephalopathy within 29–84 days of jaundice.

Presentation

- The history may point to a cause (see Box 3.16). Ask specifically about recent viral illnesses, paracetamol, alcohol, and drug history. Signs of chronic liver disease are typically not present (unless 'acute-on-chronic'). Splenomegaly does not occur. If present consider an acute presentation of Wilson's disease, autoimmune chronic active hepatitis, or lymphoma. Frequently the presenting feature is a complication of liver failure. Patients with paracetamol overdose may present with severe abdominal pain and retching.
- **Encephalopathy**. Present in all cases (by definition) and conventionally divided into 4 grades (see Box 3.17). Cerebral oedema is heralded by spikes of hypertension, dysconjugate eye-movements, papilloedema is rare. Unless treated this progresses to decerebrate posturing (back, arms and legs rigid, hands in flexion, opisthonus), and brainstem coning.
- Metabolic disturbances. Hypoglycaemia and hyponatraemia are common. Other abnormalities include ↓K^+, respiratory alkalosis, and severe hypophosphataemia. Lactic acidosis carries a poor prognosis.
- **Cardiovascular abnormalities**. Spikes of systolic hypertension may reflect cerebral oedema. The diastolic BP falls as disease progresses with a vasodilated hyperdynamic circulation (↓SVR, ↑cardiac output).
- **Respiratory failure**. Hypoxia is relatively common and may be worsened by localized infection, aspiration, or atelectasis. Non-cardiogenic pulmonary oedema is seen in ~10%.
- **Renal failure**. Indicates a worse prognosis with conservative treatment, and may be due to hepatorenal syndrome (see 📖 p.296) or ATN (paracetamol).
- **Bleeding problems**. The PT is prolonged and reflects the progression of the disease. Low-grade DIC may occur with bleeding from the GI tract from gastritis or elsewhere. Sub-conjunctival haematoma is common in paracetamol-induced liver failure.
- **Infections**. Bacterial and fungal infections (septicaemia, pneumonia, peritonitis, UTIs) are more frequent due to impaired neutrophil function.

Box 3.16 Causes of acute liver failure in the UK

- ***Drug-induced hepatitis*** (58%) (see 📖 p.260) Paracetamol OD (📖 p.722). Less commonly halothane, isoniazid, sulphonamides, NSAIDs, phenytoin, valproate, penicillins, MAOIs, ecstasy, sulfasalazine, disulfiram, ketoconazole.
- ***Viral hepatitis*** (36%) (see 📖 p.256) Hepatitis A, B, delta co-infection in HBsAg +ve carrier, NANB (not HCV in UK), E, less commonly CMV, EBV, and HSV.
- ***Toxins*** *Amanita phalloides* (these mushrooms are available in the UK), herbal remedies, CCl_4.
- ***Malignancy*** Lymphoma, malignant infiltration.
- ***Vascular*** Budd–Chiari syndrome, veno-occulive disease, ischaemic injury (shock and hypotension).
- ***Miscellaneous*** Wilson's (not strictly acute, as many are cirrhotic, but in all clinical respects similar), autoimmune hepatitis, malignant hyperthermia (incl. ecstasy), fatty liver of pregnancy, PET/HELLP syndrome, Reye syndrome.

Box 3.17 Grades of hepatic encephalopathy

- ***Grade 1*** Drowsy but coherent; mood change.
- ***Grade 2*** Drowsy, confused at times, inappropriate behaviour.
- ***Grade 3*** Very drowsy and stuparose but rousable; alternatively restless, screaming.
- ***Grade 4*** Comatose, barely rousable.

Investigations

- ***Blood tests (daily)*** U&Es, glucose (and 2-hourly BM stix), FBC, PT, LFTs (albumin is usually normal on admission unless 'acute-on chronic'), phosphate, arterial blood gases. Blood group and X-match on admission.
- ***Blood tests (for diagnosis)*** Viral serology (A IgM, HBsAg, HBcore Ab IgM, delta in HBsAg +ve, EBV, CMV, HSV), drug screen (esp. paracetamol), plasma caeruloplasmin (if <50 years ± 24-h urine copper).
- ***Bacteriology*** Blood cultures, urine, and sputum MC&S daily (incl. fungal cultures). Throat and vaginal swabs.
- ***USS (liver)*** To assess hepatic veins, portal vein patency, size (if possible), spleen size, nodes lymphoma).
- ***ECG/CXR*** Repeat CXR daily (infection/ARDS).
- ***EEG*** May be helpful in the assessment of hepatic encephalopathy though not widely used.
- ***Liver biopsy*** Rarely necessary but will exclude underlying malignant infiltration or cirrhosis where the diagnosis is in doubt. The transjugular approach is preferred as it carries lower risk of haemorrhage (📖 p.795).

Acute liver failure: management

The mainstay of treatment is support until the acute insult resolves. If a patient fulfils criteria for liver transplantation (see Box 3.19) on or during their admission they should be referred to a centre where liver transplantation is available.

*It is **vital** to discuss all cases of severe liver injury with one of the regional liver transplant centres* even though patients may not fulfil the criteria (Box 3.18), as it generally takes up to 48h to obtain an emergency graft, and delay in referral can result in failure to procure an adequate graft. All of these centres are also experienced in managing this serious illness. None of the known causes of acute liver failure respond well to medical therapy. Steroids may be of benefit in patients with lymphoma or autoimmune hepatitis, but by the time most patients present it is usually too late. All patients should be admitted to a high dependency or intensive therapy unit.

- ***Paracetamol overdose*** Give N-acetylcysteine (see 🕮 p.722). The benefit of N-acetylcysteine may be evident up to 48h and possibly longer.
- ***General measures*** Nurse supine (not 45° as often stated). Keep in a peaceful environment. Insert an arterial line and CVP line for monitoring and if possible a pulmonary artery catheter (Swan–Ganz) to optimize the haemodynamic status.
- ***Coagulopathy*** The PT is the best indicator of liver function. Avoid giving FFP unless there is bleeding or unless undergoing surgical procedures or line insertion. Factor concentrates may precipitate DIC. The PT may rise and fall precipitously and should be measured twice daily if deteriorating. Give vitamin K 10mg once only IV. Give platelet support if thrombocytopenic and bleeding.
- ***Encephalopathy*** see 🕮 p.273.
- ***Cerebral oedema*** Cerebral oedema develops in 75–80% of patients with grade IV encephalopathy. ICP monitoring is used in some centres. If signs of cerebral oedema are present then give mannitol (100mL of 20% mannitol); if in renal failure, watch for fluid overload. Hyperventilation decreases ICP at the expense of cerebral blood flow and should be avoided. Epoprostenol and N-acetylcysteine may decrease ICP. Hypertension is almost always 2° to raised ICP and should be treated with mannitol as alrady described; antihypertensive drugs may precipitate brainstem coning. There is no evidence that giving lactulose or neomycin affects prognosis or prevents grade 3–4 encephalopathy. Flumazenil is reported to improve encephalopathy but does affect outcome. Seizures should be treated in the usual way (🕮 p.390).
- ***Haemodynamic support*** Correct hypovolaemia with colloid or blood but avoid fluid overload. Persistent hypotension may respond to noradrenaline infusion or glypressin.
- ***Metabolic changes*** Monitor glucose 2-hourly, and give 10% or 50% glucose to keep glc >3.5mM. Monitor serum phosphate (often very low), replace with IV (9–18mmol/24h) if <0.4mM. Nutrition: ileus is often present, but drip enteral feeding (10–20mL/h) is enterop-protective.

- ***Renal failure*** See 📖 p.296. Monitor renal function (renal failure occurs in ~70% cases). Treat by haemodiafiltration rather than haemodialysis.
- ***Respiratory support*** Monitor O_2 saturations continuously and give oxygen by mask if SaO_2 <90%. Ventilate when grade 3 or 4 coma (avoid ETT ties which compress the IJ veins).
- ***Infection*** Start prophylactic antibiotics and anti-fungals (e.g. cefotaxime and fluconazole).
- ***Wilson's disease*** Consider penicillamine and IV vitamin E.

Box 3.18 Management key points: acute liver failure

- Discuss all cases with the regional liver transplant centre.
- Nurse supine and keep patient in a peaceful environment.
- ***Correct hypovolaemia*** (colloid or blood) ***and electrolyte disturbances*** (e.g. hypokalaemia, hypophosphataemia). Avoid fluid overload. Persistent hypotension may respond to noradrenaline or vasopressin infusion.
- ***Encephalopathy:*** lactulose 10–15mL tds. Phosphate enemas.
- ***Cerebral oedema:*** If signs of cerebral oedema (e.g. hypertension) are present give mannitol (100mL of 20% mannitol).
- ***Coagulopathy:*** monitor PT, Give vitamin K (10mg IV once only). Avoid FFP unless if bleeding or undergoing surgical procedures. Platelet support if thrombocytopenic and bleeding.
- ***Hypoglycaemia:*** monitor BM 2-hourly, and treat with10% or 50% glucose to keep glucose >3.5mM.
- ***Hepatorenal syndrome:*** terlipressin and IV albumin (see 📖 p.296).
- ***Sepsis:*** prophylactic antibiotics/antifungals (e.g. cefotaxime and fluconazole)
- ***Treat the underlying cause:*** e.g. in paracetamol overdose: N-acetylcysteine; stop the suspected drug.
- ***Monitor:*** pulse rate, BP, O_2 saturations, CVP, urine output/fluid balance, grade of encephalopathy, and renal function closely in the high dependency or intensive therapy unit.

Box 3.19 Indications for liver transplantation

Paracetamol OD with arterial pH <7.3 (admission)
Grade 3 or 4 encephalopathy and PT >100s
or in the absence of above

ALL 3 of the following or	*Any 3 of the following*
• PT >100s	• PT >50s
• Creatinine >300μM	• Jaundice to encephalopathy >7 days
• Grade 3–4 encephalopathy	• Age <10 years or >40 years
	• Bilirubin >300μM
	• Unfavourable aetiology (i.e. non-paracetamol, not Hep A, not Hep B).

'Acute-on-chronic' liver failure

Patients with chronic liver disease from cirrhosis may present with acute decompensation due to a variety of causes (see Box 3.20).

Clinical features

- Ask specifically for a history of previous hepatitis, jaundice, alcohol intake, previous drug history. Weight loss may point to a malignancy. Pruritus, pigmentation, and xanthelasma in a young woman may be due to 1° biliary cirrhosis.
- Examine for evidence of long-standing liver dysfunction: leuconychia, palmar erythema, clubbing, spider naevi, gynaecomastia, and small testes. Splenomegaly and distended abdominal veins signify portal hypertension.
- Examine specifically for features of decompensation: encephalopathy (confusion, 'liver flap'), ascites, oedema, jaundice, or fever.

Investigations

Unless the cause for the decompensation and the diagnosis for the pre-existing liver disease are known the patient warrants full investigation (see 📖 p.254).

Management

As for patients with acute liver failure, the mainstay of treatment is supportive. The decision on how aggressively you manage the patient (i.e. admission to ICU, invasive monitoring, etc.) depends on the previous diagnosis, on a reversible element to the acute insult, and whether the patient is a candidate for liver transplantation. They have less capacity to regenerate their hepatocytes and prognosis of patients requiring mechanical ventilation and haemodynamic support is very poor without a transplant.

Sepsis

Start 'blind' treatment if there is a fever or ↑WCC (e.g. cefotaxime) and be guided by culture results (e.g. a third-generation cephalosporin, bacterial peritonitis, see 📖 p.266. Add IV fluconazole as an anti-fungal agent.

Box 3.20 Causes of acute decompensation of chronic liver disease

- Intercurrent infection:
  - Spontaneous bacterial peritonitis
  - Pneumonia
  - Skin infections
- Acute GI haemorrhage
- Additional hepatotoxic insult:
  - Alcoholic binge
  - Acute viral hepatitis
  - Hepatotoxic drugs
- Drugs:
  - Sedatives/narcotics
  - Diuretics
- Metabolic derangement:
  - Hypoglycaemia
  - Electrolyte disturbance
- Major surgery
- Constipation
- Progression of disease.

Hepatic encephalopathy

Hepatic encephalopathy is a neuropsychiatric disturbance of cognitive function in a patient with acute-on-chronic liver disease (see 📖 p.272). It is said that patients with cirrhosis do *not* develop cerebral oedema, although we have seen extensor posturing in alcoholic cirrhotics following variceal haemorrhage.

Clinically there is usually altered conscious level, asterixis (liver flap), abnormal EEG, impaired psychometric tests, and an elevated arterial ammonia concentration. Patients may present with parkinsonian features. However, in patients with chronic liver disease, it may be sub-clinical with subtle changes in awareness or attention span. It is graded as in 📖 Box 3.17, p.269.

Treatment

The aim of treatment is to improve morbidity.

- Exclude other causes of confusion (see 📖 p.410).
- Identify and correct the precipitating causes e.g. infection (including spontaneous bacterial peritonitis), hypovolaemia, hypokalaemia, hypoxias, hypoglycaemia, GI bleeding, constipation, drugs (sedatives or tranquilizers) or rarely hepatoma or hepatic or portal vein thrombosis.
- Give lactulose: this semi-synthetic disaccharide is poorly absorbed. It is digested in the large bowel and undergoes fermentation. This alters faecal pH and nitrogen utilization by bowel flora. Lactulose enemas can be given if the patient cannot take lactulose orally.
- Lactitol has a similar action to lactulose but has fewer side effects.
- Phosphate enemas help to purge the large bowel. Most useful in the context of an acute food load (e.g. GI bleeding).
- Dietary restriction is controversial, and may be harmful in malnourished patients. Ensure adequate calorie intake.

Liver abscesses

Presentation

- Commonly present with fever and night sweats, weight loss, or RUQ or intercostal pain.
- The underlying cause (e.g. appendicitis) may be silent or barely noticed. Ask about recent abdominal pain, altered bowel habit, diarrhoea, biliary colic, blood PR, or IBD.
- The travel history, occupation (farming is a risk factor for amoebiasis), or contact with infected persons (TB) may help.
- Examine for jaundice, hepatomegaly, pleural effusions (commonly right-sided), intercostal tenderness (characteristic of amoebic abscesses), abdominal masses (tumour or inflammatory mass), and lymphadenopathy. Perform a rectal examination for pelvic tumour.
- Severe infection may be associated with septic shock (see 🕮 p.316).

Causes

- Pyogenic organisms (appendicitis, diverticulitis, carcinoma, biliary)
- Amoebic abscess (*Entamoeba histolytica*)
- Hydatid cyst (*Echinococcus granulosus*)
- TB (very rare).

Investigations

- U&Es (renal impairment with sepsis). LFTs (non-specific, tend to be cholestatic; may be normal with amoebic abscess).
- Prothrombin time may be prolonged with multiple abscesses.
- FBC (leucocytosis, eosinophilia, non-specific anaemia).
- Blood cultures, CRP, ESR.
- Amoebic and hydatid serology.
- Stool may contain amoebic cysts or vegetative forms.
- CXR (looking for effusion, or pulmonary TB).
- USS of liver, biliary tree, and abdomen (iliac fossae in particular) ± CT scan with contrast, looking for masses. Both pyogenic and amoebic abscesses tend to be thick walled; hydatid cysts are thin walled and there may be daughter cysts. Solid tumours are echodense but may have necrotic hypodense centres.
- Gallium scan (or indium-111 labelled WBC scan) will show up pyogenic foci in the liver and elsewhere (e.g. terminal ileitis); amoebic abscesses do not take up the label.
- Aspirate any large abscesses and send for Gram stain, and culture. If there is a suspicion of hydatid disease aspiration is contraindicated.

Management

- Aspirate any large abscesses under USS. It is pointless to try and drain multiple abscesses. If there is a continuing intra-abdominal source it is virtually impossible to eradicate liver abscesses without removing or dealing with that source (e.g. appendix).
- Pyogenic abscess: percutaneous aspiration of any large abscesses. Broad-spectrum antibiotics (e.g. cefotaxime and metronidazole).

- Amoebic abscess: see 📖 p.247. Treat with metronidazole (or tinidazole) followed by diloxanide furoate. USS-guided aspiration may help improve penetration of the drugs and shorten illness. 2° bacterial infection occurs in up to 20%.
- Hydatid disease: open surgical drainage is the treatment of choice. Albendazole may help reduce the risk of recurrence post surgery or be used in inoperable cases.
- Anti-tuberculous therapy for tuberculous abscesses.

Acute pancreatitis: assessment

Acute pancreatitis is occasionally managed by physicians, particularly if it presents in an unusual way (e.g. chest pain).

Presentation

- Abdominal pain: epigastric or generalized, of rapid onset, but may occur anywhere (including chest); dull, constant, and boring. Radiation to the back or between the scapulae, often relieved by leaning forward (differential diagnosis is leaking aortic aneurysm).
- Nausea, vomiting, and dehydration ± jaundice.
- Peritonitis with epigastric tenderness, localized rebound tenderness, or generalized abdominal rigidity. An abdominal mass may indicate a pancreatic pseudocyst or abscess. Bowel sounds usually absent.
- Tachycardia and hypotension; shock/collapse and respiratory failure in severe cases (especially in the elderly).
- Very rarely signs of bleeding in the pancreatic bed, Grey–Turner's sign (ecchymosis in the flanks) or Cullen's sign (peri-umbilical bruising), tender red skin nodules (due to subcutaneous fat necrosis).
- Hypocalcaemic tetany.

Investigations

- ***Amylase*** Elevated, but not specific (see 📖 Box 3.21), especially if only up to 4 × upper limit of normal. A persistently raised amylase (several days to weeks) may indicate the development of a pseudocyst.
- ***FBC*** Raised haematocrit and leucocytosis.
- ***U&Es*** Urea may be raised with hypovolaemia.
- ***Glucose*** May be raised.
- ***LFTs*** AST and bilirubin often elevated especially in gallstone pancreatitis. Disproportionately elevated γ-GT may indicate an alcohol aetiology.
- ***Calcium*** Hypocalcaemia (unless precipitant was ↑Ca^{2+}).
- ***CRP*** Elevated: used to monitor progression of the attack.
- ***ABGs*** Mandatory. Hypoxia ± metabolic acidosis.
- ***AXR*** Generalized ileus or sentinel loops (dilated gas-filled loops in the region of the pancreas). Look for evidence of pancreatic calcification or biliary stone.
- ***CXR*** May show a pleural effusion, elevated diaphragm, or pulmonary infiltrates.
- ***USS*** May confirm diagnosis and detect gallstones ± biliary obstruction, pseudocysts, and abscesses
- ***CT abdomen*** Dynamic contrast-enhanced is reliable at detection of pancreatic necrosis and grading severity.

Assessment of severity

- The severity of disease has no correlation with the elevation of serum amylase. Several prognostic indices have been published, but it takes 48h to fully appreciate disease severity. See Box 3.22.

- The mortality from acute pancreatitis is ~10%, and rises to 40% in those developing a pancreatic abscess. The mortality is highest in those with a first episode of pancreatitis. Around 15% of patients presenting with acute pancreatitis have recurrent disease.

Box 3.21 Causes of abdominal pain and elevated serum amylase

- Acute pancreatitis
- Stomach or small bowel perforation
- Perforated peptic ulcer
- Mesenteric infarction
- Acute liver failure
- Acute cholecystitis or cholangitis
- Renal failure (modest elevation)
- Diabetic ketoacidosis.

Box 3.22 Markers of severity in acute pancreatitis

At presentation

- Age >55 years
- WBC >16 × 10^9/L
- Glucose >10mM (non-diabetic)
- LDH >350IU
- AST >250IU/L.

During the first 48h

- Haematocrit fall >10%
- Urea rise >10mM
- Serum Ca^{2+} <2.0mmol/L
- Base excess >4mmol/L
- PaO_2 <8kPa
- Serum albumin <32g/L
- Estimated fluid sequestration >6L.

Mortality: 0–2 criteria = 2%; 3–4 = 15%; 5–6 = 40%; >7 = 100%.

Practice point

Severe acute abdominal pain is nearly always due to a surgical cause.

Acute pancreatitis: management

The principles of management are

- Liaise with surgeons
- Supportive measures: the majority will subside in 3–10 days
- Careful observation for the development of complications
- Identify the cause (see Box 3.23)
- Key points in management (see 📖 Box 3.24, p.280).

Supportive treatment

- Establish IV access. If there is shock, markers of moderate–severe pancreatitis, elderly patient, hypoxia not readily correcting with O_2 or other co-existent disease, insert a CVP line to help control fluid balance.
- Patients are usually severely volume depleted: give prompt fluid replacement with colloid (e.g. Haemaccel®) or 0.9% saline. Monitor urine output and insert a urinary catheter if required.
- Oxygen should be given if there is hypoxia on air (use continuous pulse oximetry in severe cases and 6-hourly for the first 48h for rest, to monitor for respiratory failure).
- Keep NBM.
- The use of NG suction is unproven. Enteral nutrition (nasojejunal) should be commenced early in acute pancreatitis.
- Monitor blood glucose regularly and treat with insulin if high.
- Pethidine causes the least spasm of the sphincter of Oddi.
- Antibiotic prophylaxis with cefuroxime decreases 2° infections.
- Octreotide (somatostatin analogue): this suppresses pancreatic enzyme secretion but is of unproven benefit.
- Peritoneal lavage: there is no proven benefit.
- H2-antagonists have not been shown to affect mortality.

Complications (seen in ~20%)

Local

- Abscess
- Pseudocyst infection
- Biliary obstruction
- Ascites, pleural effusion
- Fistula
- Splenic, portal, or mesenteric.

Systemic

- Electrolyte imbalance
- ↓Ca^{2+}, ↓Mg^{2+}
- Acute renal failure
- Shock
- Respiratory failure
- Sepsis vein obstruction.

Septic complications

Sepsis is the most common cause of death. This should be suspected when there is a persistent fever, leucocytosis, pain/tenderness, or an overall clinical deterioration. These signs are an indication for multiple blood cultures and an abdominal CT. Pancreatic pseudocysts are more common in alcoholic pancreatitis (15% versus 3% in gallstone AP), but infection is more common in gallstone pancreatitis.

Biliary pancreatitis

Urgent ERCP within 72h of presentation reduces complications and mortality in patients with severe gallstone pancreatitis. The benefit has not been demonstrated in mild cases. There is a growing vogue for the use of MRCP (magnetic resonance cholangiopancreatogaphy) to diagnose biliary disease prior to ERCP.

Indications for surgery

Infected pancreatic necrosis or pancreatic abscess. Radiologically guided percutaneous drainage is now preferred to surgery for pancreatic pseudocysts.

Box 3.23 Causes of acute pancreatitis

Common (80%)
- Gallstones (including biliary microlithiasis or sludge) (60%)
- Alcohol (20%)

Rare (10%)
- Iatrogenic (ERCP or any form of abdominal surgery)
- Trauma (even seemingly minimal trauma, as pancreas is in a very vulnerable position, e.g. 'seat-belt sign' or bicycle handle-bar injury)
- Infections
    - Viral: mumps, rubella, coxsackie B, EBV, CMV, Hep A and B)
    - Bacterial: mycoplasma
    - Others: ascaris, flukes (*Clonorchis sinensis*)
- Systemic vasculitis (SLE, polyarteritis nodosa, etc.)
- Drugs (e.g. thiazides, furosemide, NSAIDs, sulphonamides, azathioprine, tetracyclines, and valproate; possibly steroids)
- Hypertriglyceridaemia (serum amylase falsely low)
- Hypercalcaemia or iv calcium infusions
- Hypothermia
- Pancreatic carcinoma (3% present with acute pancreatitis)
- Misc.: anatomical abnormalities (pancreas divisum, duodenal or peri-ampullary diverticulae), scorpion bites, cystic fibrosis

Unknown (10%)

Box 3.24 Management key points: acute pancreatitis

- Liaise with surgeons.
- Keep NBM.
- IV fluids.
- Analgesia (pethidine causes the least spasm of the sphincter of Oddi).
- Antibiotic prophylaxis (e.g. cefuroxime) decreases 2° infections.
- O_2 should be given if there is hypoxia on air.
- Gallstone pancreatitis: ERCP within 72h of presentation in severe cases.
- Monitor urine output, O_2 sats, blood glucose, and CVP (if there is shock or markers of moderate–severe pancreatitis).
- Enteral nutrition (nasojejunal).
- Careful observation for the development of complications.

Chapter 4

Renal emergencies

Acute kidney injury (AKI) 1

AKI or acute renal failure (ARF) is a common clinical presentation, representing 5% of acute hospital admissions, and 30% of admissions to ITU. It has 50% mortality. The term AKI replaces the term ARF. It is a clinical syndrome characterized by a rapid reduction in renal excretory function and GFR over hours to weeks leading to impaired control of extracellular volume, electrolytes, and acid–base balance. AKI is classically divided into pre-renal, renal (intrinsic), and post-renal. AKI has to be *distinguished from acute on chronic renal failure*. The latter is normally associated with anemia, abnormal calcium, and small kidneys on USS ± history of pre-existing renal disease.

Definition

Acute kidney injury (AKI) is defined as an abrupt (within 48 hours) reduction in kidney function currently defined as an absolute increase in serum creatinine of ≥ 26 µmol/l, or a > 50% increase in serum creatinine from baseline, or a reduction in urine output (documented oliguria of less than 0.5 ml/kg per hour for more than 6h).

Presentation

- May be asymptomatic
- Elevated creatinine (or urea) during biochemical screening
- Detection of oliguria by nursing staff
- Malaise, confusion, seizures, or coma
- Nausea, anorexia, or vomiting
- Oliguria or abnormal urine colour
- Haematuria (pink rather than frank blood)
- Drug overdose (e.g. paracetamol)
- Constitutional symptoms (arthralgia, rhinitis, respiratory)
- Vasculitic rash
- Multi-organ failure.

Diagnosing the cause of AKI

In 80% of cases, renal impairment can be resolved by adequate volume replacement, treatment of sepsis, and stopping nephrotoxic drugs. There are many causes of acute renal impairment, some of which, such as multi-system vasculitis or rhabdomyolysis, are important as their early diagnosis and treatment may have a profound effect on outcome (see Box 4.1).

The priorities are:

- ***Volume assessment*** and fluid challenge (unless fluid overloaded) to ensure adequate intravascular volume. Give 1L of N/saline or Hartmann's solution over 2h, assess urine output.
- ***Stop all nephrotoxic drugs*** and review drug history.
- ***Is the patient septic?*** (pyrexia, high CRP, leucocytosis).
- ***History:*** is there a history of hypertension, diabetes, prostatism, haematuria or vascular disease?
- ***Urgent ultrasound scan*** to look for obstruction, blood flow, size, cysts, and symmetry.
- ***Urinalysis and microscopy*** to look for red or white cell casts, myoglobinuria, and haematuria.

Points to note in the history

- History of fluid loss (D&V, diuretics, bleeding, fever). Diarrhoea may suggest hypovolaemia or haemolytic–uraemic syndrome (HUS).
- History of sepsis (e.g. UTI, fever, or hypothermia, bacterial endocarditis. Symptoms may be non-specific in elderly).
- Drug history: NSAIDs, ACEI, antibiotics (in particular aminoglycosides and amphotericin), drugs for HIV disease.
- Non-specific symptoms (e.g. myalgia, arthralgia), neurological signs, ophthalmic complications, sinusitis, haemoptysis, and skin rashes may suggest vasculitis.
- Past history of BP, DM, renovascular disease, prostatism, or haematuria.
- Patients with diabetes or myeloma have an ↑risk of contrast-induced renal impairment (avoid volume depletion).
- Are there symptoms or signs of liver disease?
- Backache may suggest pelvi-ureteric obstruction. Consider aortic aneurysm or retroperitoneal fibrosis.
- Cholesterol emboli (aneurysms, absent pulses, rash, history of recent vascular intervention e.g. angiography).
- Post-partum (HELLP syndrome, HUS, fatty liver, pre-eclampsia).

Box 4.1 Causes of AKI

Pre-renal

- Hypovolaemia
- Hypotension, shock (📖 p.310)
- Renal artery emboli
- Renal artery stenosis + ACEI
- Hepatorenal syndrome.

Post-renal (obstructive)

- Renal vein thrombosis
- ↑intra-abdominal pressure
- HIV drugs (indinavir)
- Intratubular (uric acid crystals)
- Ureteric
    - Stones
    - Retroperitoneal fibrosis/ tumour
- Urethral
    - Prostatic hypertrophy.

Renal (parenchymal)

- Vasculitis (SLE, PAN)
- Glomerulonephritis
- Acute tubular necrosis
    - Ischaemia (e.g. hypotension)
    - Septicaemia
    - Toxins (myoglobin, BJ proteins)
    - Drugs (e.g. gentamicin) or radio contrast media
    - Prolonged pre-renal oliguria
    - Malaria
- Thrombotic microangiopathy
    - Accelerated hypertension
    - HUS/TTP/DIC (📖 p.598)
- Scleroderma crisis
- Sepsis
    - Interstitial nephritis
    - Drugs (NSAIDs, antibiotics)
    - Infections (*Strep.*, *Staph.*, *Leptospirosis*, *Brucella*, G –ve sepsis, *Legionella*)
- Calcium, urate, oxalate overload
    - Tumour lysis syndrome (📖 p.617).

The urine appearance my help, see Box 4.10 (📖 p.307).

AKI 2

Assessment of severity

- ***Fluid overload*** (dyspnoeic with signs of pulmonary oedema, high JVP or CVP, peripheral oedema, gallop rhythm) or dehydration (postural hypotension, tissue turgor).
- ***Hypotension*** is a common cause of AKI and should be corrected.
- ***Urine output:*** anuria occurs in complete obstruction (usually low, e.g. prostate), rapidly progressive glomerulonephritis, or dissection of the aorta.
- ***Hyperkalaemia*** can be life threatening. Look at ECG for signs, and measure serum potassium.
- ***Acidosis*** causes hyperventilation and cardiac instability.

Poor prognostic features include

- Age >50 years
- Infection (esp. septicaemia)
- Burns (>70% surface area)
- Rising urea (>16mmol/24h)
- Oliguria for >2 weeks
- Multi-organ failure (>3)
- Jaundice.

The main priorities are to:

- Resuscitate and correct volume if depleted
- Remove nephrotoxic drugs or agents
- Identify if the patient is septic and treat with antibiotics
- Exclude obstruction or major vascular injury
- Identify the minority (~5%) that have intrinsic renal disease since these are best managed by a specialist centre. These include:
  - Myeloma
  - Glomerulonephritis
  - Rhabdomyolysis (high CPK)
  - Vasculitis
  - Interstitial nephritis.

Assessment of patients with AKI

- Is there life-threatening hyperkalaemia or pulmonary oedema?
- What is the likely cause?
- Is the patient still passing urine?
- Does it look normal?
- ECG
- Urgent U&Es + ABGs
- CXR.

Pre-renal (75%)

- Check postural BP, HR
- Assess volume status, measure CVP
- Sepsis screen.

Renal (20%)

- Urinalysis and microscopy for blood/casts
- Vasculitis screen
- Drug history
- CPK/myoglobin in urine.

Post renal (5%)

- May or may not have complete anuria

Patients should be stabilized on a general intensive care unit with haemofiltration and support until safe to transfer care to a renal unit. It is particularly important to transfer care for patients with intrinsic renal disease.

AKI: investigations

Blood tests

• *U&Es*	Urea is disproportionately raised in pre-renal failure, GI bleeds, catabolic states. Creatinine may be disproportionately elevated in acute liver failure with renal failure.
• *Calcium, phosphate*	Acidaemia increases ionized calcium. Rhabdomyolysis may be associated with high or low calcium.
• *FBC*	Anaemia suggests chronic or acute on chronic renal failure. ↓platelets suggest liver disease, HELLP (haemolytic uraemic syndrome, elevated liver enzyme, low platelet count), sepsis. Blood film (HUS (haemolytic uraemic syndrome), myeloma, left shift). ↑platelets: vasculitis (e.g. Wegener's) eosinophilia, Churg–Strauss syndrome, interstitial nephritis
• *Coagulation*	Abnormal in DIC, liver disease, SLE, HELLP syndrome. The PT and PTT are usually normal in HUS.
• *LFTs*	Acute hepatitis, paracetamol overdose, cirrhosis. Alkaline phosphatase often ↑ in vasculitis
• *LDH/HBD*	↑ in HUS/ITP/DIC
• *CPK*	Very high in rhabdomyolysis
• *Blood cultures*	Take BC in all patients with AKI (ARF)
• *Immunology*	ANCA, anti-GBM, Igs, C3/C4, Rh factor, ANA, ENA, dsDNA, cryoglobulins, anti-cardiolipin and anti-β2-glycoprotein-1 antibodies (anti-phospholipid syndrome)
• *ESR/CRP*	CRP and ESR are elevated in vasculitis. CRP may be normal in SLE.
• *Protein strip*	For paraproteins (myeloma, light chain disease)
• *HIV, HBsAg, HCVAb*	Serology may be required for dialysis.

Urine

- Inspect the urine yourself. Contact the renal registrar or microbiology technician on call to arrange urgent microscopy. Save urine for cytology if haematuria is the dominant symptom, and do urine dipstick for nitrites, protein, and blood.
- Send a specimen to microbiology for microscopy and culture.
- *RBC casts* suggest glomerulonephritis (refer to renal physician urgently); *pigment casts* suggest myoglobinuria; *WBC casts* suggest acute pyelonephritis. *Excess eosinophils* in the urine are associated with interstitial nephritis.
- Urine Bence–Jones protein, present in 75% of myeloma.
- *Urine electrolytes and osmolality:* these may help but do not replace careful clinical examination and are unreliable when diuretics have been given or established AKI. They may be less reliable in the elderly when sub-clinical renal impairment may be present. See Box 4.2.

Other investigations

- ***USS*** All patients with AKI (ARF) should have an *urgent* renal ultrasound to exclude obstruction and to assess kidney size (small or asymmetric in acute-on-chronic failure), and blood flow on Doppler imaging.
- ***CXR*** Look at the heart size (dilated, pericardial effusion), pulmonary vasculature (pulmonary oedema, Kerley lines), lung fields ('fluffy' shadows: oedema, haemorrhage of ANCA associated vasculitis).
- ***ECG*** Look for changes of hyperkalaemia (tented T-waves, QRS broadening) and signs of myocardial ischaemia or pericarditis.

Box 4.2 Urinary electrolytes and osmolality in renal failure

Urine electrolytes are generally not very useful in clinical practice. A high urine osmolality (>550) with a low urine sodium (<10mM) indicates hypovolaemia.

AKI: management

Hyperkalaemia

In general terms the absolute K^+ concentration is less important than the effect on the cardiac-conducting tissue (tented T waves, broad QRS, flattened P wave; Fig. 4.1), but if the K^+ is >7mmol/L then treat urgently. If hyperkalaemia is unexpected with no ECG signs of hyperkalaemia, then repeat K^+ urgently.

If there are ECG changes or K^+ >7mmol/L, contact renal team.

- Record 12-lead ECG, attach to cardiac monitor.
- If ECG shows signs of hyperkalaemia give *10mL of 10% calcium gluconate IV*, repeated every 10–20min until ECG normalizes (patients may require up to 50mL). IV calcium does not lower the potassium level but reduces cardiac excitability.
- Give *nebulized salbutamol* (5mg) to drive K^+ intracellularly (use lower doses in patients with ischaemic heart disease).
- *50mL 50% glucose with 5U soluble insulin* over 15–30min and monitor blood glucose; this should lower K^+ for several hours.
- *50–100mL 8.4% bicarbonate IV via central line over 30min* (or 500mL 1.26% peripherally).
- 250mg *furosemide* or 5mg *bumetanide* IV over 1h.
- Polystyrene sulphonate resin enema (*Calcium Resonium®*) 30g increases gut losses of potassium. Follow with 15g PO tds with regular lactulose. This takes 24h to work.
- Lactulose 20mL tds.
- Monitor serum K^+ frequently to assess response to treatment.

Fluid balance

- Manage on HDU or ITU (Box 4.3 for indications for dialysis).
- Measure weight, BP (supine and sitting or upright), and HR.
- Assess hydration (dry axillae, central skin turgor, mucous membranes, and JVP).
- Insert central venous line and measure CVP. Monitor PCWP in patients who are hypoxic or severely compromised.
- Examine fluid and weight charts, and operation notes if applicable.

If volume depleted

- If patient has a low or normal CVP ± postural hypotension give a trial of volume expansion (500mL of colloid or N saline) over 30min. Monitor urine output response and CVP. Continue fluids until CVP is at least >5cm at midaxillary line.
- When adequately filled (e.g. CVP >10 and/or PCWP >15) reassess urine output. Do not give furosemide or a loop diuretic until the patient is adequately filled. Some clinicians use high doses of furosemide (120mg–250mg IVI max. followed by a furosemide infusion of 5–10mg/h) to maintain urine output and help with fluid and electrolyte management. However a recent meta-analysis of randomized controlled trials showed that furosemide is not associated with any significant clinical benefits in the treatment of AKI in adults and high doses may be associated with an ↑risk of ototoxicity.

- If hypotension persists (MAP <60mmHg) in spite of adequate volume replacement (i.e. CVP of >10cm), commence inotropic support (see 📖 p.315).

If fluid overloaded

- Give O_2 to maintain SaO_2 >95%. Consider CPAP (📖 p.777).
- Start IV nitrates (e.g. GTN 2–10mg/h IV).
- Give IV furosemide: 120mg–500mg, then infuse 5–10mg/h.
- Paracentesis if tense ascites is present (📖 p.793).
- Avoid opiates, although a single dose (e.g. 2.5mg diamorphine IV) may help relieve anxiety and breathlessness.
- If no response, consider urgent haemofiltration, dialysis, or venesection (remove 250–500mL) (Box 4.3.).

Box 4.3 Indications for dialysis or haemofiltration

- Persistent hyperkalaemia (K^+ >7mmol/L)
- Fluid overload (e.g. refractory pulmonary oedema)
- Pericarditis (heralds the risk of tamponade, 📖 p.150)
- Acidosis (arterial pH <7.1, bicarbonate <12mmol/L)
- Symptomatic uraemia (tremor, cognitive impairment, coma, fits, urea typically >45mmol/L).

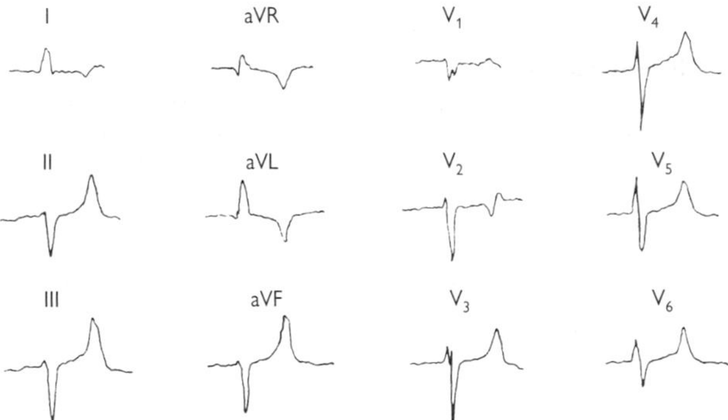

Fig. 4.1 Patients with hyperkalaemia develop tall tented T waves and a shortened QT interval. Later there is widening of the QRS complex and VT or VF.

AKI: further management

Treatment of life-threatening hyperkalaemia, severe fluid overload, or dehydration take priority (see 📖 p.288).

Correct other abnormalities

- ***Acidaemia*** Classically produces sighing respirations (Kussmaul's breathing) and may worsen hypotension (impaired cardiac function):
    - If pH is <7.2 give 100mL of 8.4% bicarbonate via central line over 30min (or 500mL 1.26% bicarbonate peripherally)
    - Arrange urgent dialysis
    - Correction can cause symptomatic hypocalcaemia.
- ***Hyponatraemia*** Usually dilutional (relative water excess). Management is discussed on 📖 p.538.
- ***Hyperphosphataemia*** is more a problem of chronic renal failure. If the product of [Ca^{2+}] × [phosphate] is >4.6 the risk of 'metastatic' precipitation is high. Give oral phosphate binders (e.g. calcium carbonate 300–1200mg q8h PO) to lower phosphate to <1.8mmol/L. Phosphate levels decrease with dialysis or haemofiltration.
- ***Nutrition*** There is no role for protein restriction. Institute enteral or parenteral feeding early. In patients with diabetes, insulin requirements fall with renal impairment.
- ***Sepsis*** Common precipitant/complication of AKI. Culture blood, urine, and specimens from other potential sites of infection. Treat with appropriate antibiotics remembering to adjust the daily dose in view of the renal impairment (septic shock is discussed on 📖 p.316).

Further measures

The causes of AKI are listed in 📖 Box 4.1, p.283. Most cases are multi-factorial with volume depletion or hypotension, sepsis, and drugs (e.g. injudicious use of ACEI and NSAIDs), urinary tract obstruction, and/or pre-existing chronic renal disease. It is essential to identify treatable conditions.

Patients should be divided into those with pre-renal, renal, and post-renal AKI using *clinical assessment*, *filling pressures* (CVP, PCWP), and *USS*. Whilst sepsis is included as a renal cause, much of the early deleterious effects (i.e. hypotension) are potentially reversible with appropriate management. The principles of further management are:

- *Optimize fluid balance*: there is no substitute for painstaking physical examination. Careful fluid balance charts and daily weights guide replacement. Limit fluid intake to total fluid output plus 500mL/day. The best sign of intravascular volume depletion is postural drop in BP.
- *Intrinsic renal disease*: oliguria is reversed by restoration of circulating volume or BP, but takes up to 8h to respond fully. It is important that fluid balance is optimized (CVP of 5–10cm, MAP of >75mmHg). If diuretics fail to improve urine output, ATN is likely to be established, and the patient will require renal support.

- Patients with severe portal hypertension and ascites may be oliguric (~250mL urine per day) with a concentrated urine virtually devoid of sodium. These patients may maintain a normal plasma creatinine. They are often resistant to diuretics, but may respond transiently to volume expansion. Beware of precipitating electrolyte or renal dysfunction by over-diuresis.

Box 4.4 Management key points: AKI

- Treat ***hyperkalaemia*** (if ECG changes or K^+ >7mmol/L):
  - 10mL of 10% calcium gluconate IV
  - 50mL 50% glucose with 5U soluble insulin over 15min
  - Nebulized salbutamol
  - Contact renal team and arrange for dialysis if appropriate.
- Treat ***metabolic acidosis*** (if pH <7.2):
  - 50–100mL of 8.4% bicarbonate via central line over 15–30min.
- Treat ***pulmonary oedema***:
  - O_2, consider CPAP
  - IV GTN 2–10mg/h
  - IV furosemide: 250mg over 1h, followed by infusion (5–10mg/h)
  - IV diamorphine (*single* dose of 2.5mg) relieves anxiety and breathlessness
  - Haemofiltration or dialysis (venesect ~250–500mL if delay for dialysis).
- ***Assess hydration and fluid balance***. PR, lying and standing BP, JVP, skin turgor, chest auscultation, ?peripheral oedema, CVP, fluid and weight charts.
- ***IV fluids*** if volume depleted: 500mL colloid or 0.9% saline over 30min, assess response, i.e. urine output/CVP), continue fluids until CVP ~5–10cm. ***Inotropes*** if hypotension persists in spite of CVP of >10cm.
- ***Treatment of infection***—remember to adjust the dose of antibiotics in view of the renal impairment.
- ***Stop the nephrotoxic drugs*** (e.g. ACEI and NSAIDs) and non-essential drugs.
- ***Identify intrinsic renal disease*** and treat.
- ***Relieve the obstruction*** e.g. urinary catheter, nephrostomies.
- ***Optimize nutritional support.***
- ***Identify and treat bleeding tendency***—prophylaxis with PPIs or H_2 antagonist, transfuse if required, avoid aspirin.

Anuria

Anuria implies that there is no urine output.

Causes

- Obstructed urinary tract—bilateral ureteric or bladder outflow.
- Renal infarction, e.g. prolonged hypotension in patients with dissection involving renal arteries.
- Rapidly progressive glomerulonephritis.
- Other causes of AKI may rarely cause anuria.

Assessment

Assess as for AKI (ARF). However, also:

- Ask specifically about symptoms of prostatism, or haematuria (tumour) and backache (stones, aneurysm).
- Drug history (ACEIs) as a possible cause of renal infarction, recent antibiotics, NSAIDs rarely.
- Recent renal angiography or angioplasty (renal infarction, contrast nephropathy).
- Constitutional symptoms suggestive of glomerulonephritis.
- Has the patient previously lost a kidney?

Management

(See 📖 p.288.)

If patient is anuric:

- Examine for palpable bladder, enlarged prostate, or other pelvic masses. Insert urinary catheter to exclude retention.
- If the bladder is empty, an urgent ultrasound is needed to confirm renal perfusion, and exclude urinary tract obstruction (or obstruction of solitary functioning system). Antegrade imaging can determine the level of obstruction, but consult with urologists and radiologists.
- The absence of hydronephrosis does not exclude obstruction.
- USS with Doppler of renal vessels. Arrange a CT scan ± contrast if USS normal and dissection is suspected.
- If no evidence of obstruction (one cannot exclude acute obstruction on USS) an isotope renogram will provide further information on renal perfusion.
- If there is renal perfusion, then a retrograde ureterogram will determine whether there is obstruction. Absent renal perfusion suggests renal infarction.

Interstitial nephritis

This is caused by inflammatory cell infiltration of the renal parenchyma, usually induced by drugs (NSAIDs, penicillin, cephalosporins, sulphonamides, allopurinol, rifampicin, mesalazine, interferon), some infections (e.g. *Legionella*, *Leptospirosis*, viral), granulomatous interstitial nephritis (e.g. sarcoidosis). Other causes include DM, sickle cell disease, reflux nephropathy, renal transplant rejection.

Presentation

Non-oliguric AKI, fever, rash common), eosinophilia, and urinary eosinophils. Precipitating cause usually precedes renal impairment by a few days to 2 weeks (very variable).

Diagnosis

Renal biopsy.

Treatment

Stop offending drug. The use of steroids in this setting remains controversial, and no controlled clinical trials have ever shown benefit. However, may continue to give steroids in hope.

Rhabdomyolysis

This is the development of AKI (ARF) 2° to extensive muscle damage and release of myoglobin. Approx. 7% of all cases of AKI. For causes, see Box 4.5.

Presentation

- Most cases occur following muscle trauma (e.g. crush syndrome) or severe physical exertion (e.g. marathon running or military training].
- Prolonged immobility (e.g. after drug overdose and coma) may result in pressure necrosis of the muscles.
- Malignant hyperthermia or malignant neuroleptic syndrome.
- Symptoms include swollen tender muscles, dirty red-brown urine (like Coca-Cola® mixed with urine) and/or oliguria.
- Myoglobin is present in muscle as ferrous myoglobin (Fe^{2+}), and myoglobin is deposited in the kidney as ferric myoglobin (Fe^{3+}). Further oxidation of myoglobin by hydroperoxides generates a potent oxidizing species ferryl-myoglobin (Fe^{4+}) that causes renal injury. Alkalinization works by stabilizing the ferryl-myoglobin and making it less reactive.

Investigations

- ***U&Es*** Typically marked increase in serum K^+, ↑creatinine:urea ratio.
- ***Ca^{2+}*** (may be high or low); ***phosphate*** (may be high).
- ***Urate*** Usually ↑ with tissue necrosis, also ↓excretion.
- ***LFTs*** AST very high: from skeletal muscle.
- ***CPK*** Very high (up to 1 million U/L).
- ***ABG*** Metabolic acidosis, hypoxic if there is associated acute lung injury (trauma) or infection.
- ***Urine*** The urine looks red-brown. Urinalysis is positive for blood (myoglobin tests positive), but no RBC seen on microscopy. Urinary myoglobin is diagnostic.
- ***Miscellaneous*** FBC, glucose, blood cultures, ESR, CRP, serum for toxicology ± virology, plasma myoglobin, ECG. Serum looks clear (cf. haemolysis) as myoglobin does not bind haptoglobins and is cleared by kidneys.

Management

Patients are often febrile, volume depleted, and unwell. The priorities are:

- Hyperkalaemia needs urgent treatment (see 📖 p.288).
- Volume replacement: in elderly patients or if oliguric, insert a central line and be guided by CVP. Avoid fluid overload.
- Alkaline diuresis with 1.26% sodium bicarbonate or 8.4% centrally (see 📖 p.728): alkalinization stabilizes the oxidizing form of myoglobin. It is usually effective within the first 8h. Test urine regularly with pH strips to maintain urine pH >7.
- Paracetamol may also prevent oxidative cycling of haem proteins (use ig qds for 24h).
- Analgesia: avoid NSAIDs: use opiate analgesia if required.
- Refer for a surgical opinion. Fasciotomies or debridement of necrotic tissue may be needed for compartment syndrome.

- Avoid Ca^{2+} infusion to treat hypocalcaemia: it may cause metastatic calcification in damaged muscle and cause further tissue necrosis. However, IV Ca^{2+} is indicated for patients with severe hyperkalaemia
- Treat the underlying cause (see Box 4.5).
- Dialysis or haemofiltration may be necessary for the short term but full recovery of renal function is likely.

Box 4.5 Causes of rhabdomyolysis

- Crush injury
- Severe exertion, heat stroke
- Prolonged convulsions
- Prolonged immobility
- Polymyositis or viral myositis
- Malignant hyperpyrexia
- Acute alcoholic binge
- McArdle's syndrome
- Hypokalaemia
- CO poisoning (📖 p.702)
- Burns
- Diabetics ketoacidosis (📖 p.516)
- Ecstasy abuse (📖 p.710)
- Snakebite
- Electric shock
- Neuroleptic malignant syndrome (📖 p.570).

Hepatorenal syndrome

This is defined as the onset of renal failure or AKI in patients with severe liver disease in the absence of renal pathology. It may occur in either cirrhosis or acute liver failure. It may be characterized by a low urine sodium (<10mM), but this is not a criterion in the diagnosis. It may be acute (type 1) or insidious in development in patients with refractory ascites (type 2).

Presentation

- An increase in serum creatinine is most commonly found as incidental finding during biochemical screening of patients with ascites (cirrhosis), or jaundice (esp. common in alcoholic hepatitis).
- Causes of renal failure in cirrhosis that should be excluded before the diagnosis of HRS is made include hypovolaemia, shock, parenchymal renal disease, and concomitant use of nephrotoxic drugs.
- The most common precipitant of HRS in patients with advanced liver disease is sepsis. 30% of patients with spontaneous bacterial peritonitis develop HRS.

There are many causes of renal failure and liver disease which are ***not*** synonymous with hepatorenal syndrome. These include

- Hypovolaemia: caused by bleeding, over-diuresis, or post paracentesis circulatory dysfunction.
- Nephrotoxic drugs given to patients with liver disease (e.g. gentamicin).
- Chronic viral hepatitis (HBV or HCV) with glomerulonephritis.
- Leptospirosis (marked hyperbilirubinaemia, liver enzymes near normal).
- Paracetamol overdose.
- Rhabdomyolysis may mimic liver disease and HRS by causing DIC (high PT) and high AST (muscle injury).

Investigations

- See 🕮 p.286.

Management (Box 4.6)

- Exclude other causes of renal failure in liver disease (see 'Presentation').
- ± Insert a urinary catheter and monitor urine output.
- Volume challenge (1L Hartmann's over 2h) and continue. Stop diuretics). ± IV albumin (e.g. 200mL 20%).
- Ideally central venous pressure should be monitored to help in the management of fluid balance, and particularly to prevent volume overload.
- Broad-spectrum antibiotics (e.g. cefotaxime + metronidazole).
- Based on current evidence, terlipressin should be considered to be the first-line therapeutic agent for patients presenting with type 1 HRS. Most studies have used terlipressin together with albumin therapy (1g/kg day 1 then 40g daily). Terlipressin and albumin therapy leads to reversal of type 1 HRS in approximately 40% of patients, but has no clear benefit on 3-month survival.

- If terlipressin is unavailable use noradrenaline (1–10mcg/min).
- N-acetylcysteine 100mg/kg bd by IV infusion may improve renal function if all else fails. Controlled trials are needed.
- If there is tense ascites, a total paracentesis will decrease the renal venous pressure and enhance renal blood flow (see 📖 p.793), but there are no data of efficacy on outcome.
- Haemofiltration or dialysis: patients tolerate haemofiltration better than haemodialysis.
- Patient with HRS and a reversible cause of liver failure (i.e. acute liver failure or acute alcoholic hepatitis should be considered for full renal support.
- There is no value in dialysing patients with end-stage cirrhosis and HRS unless the patient is going to have a liver transplant.
- Patients with HRS should be discussed with a liver transplant centre. HRS can be reversed by liver transplantation, but the prognosis from liver transplantation is worse in this group.
- Hyperkalaemia and acidosis are rarely a problem.
- For management, see Box 4.6.

Box 4.6 Management key points: hepatorenal syndrome

- IV fluids (1L Hartmann's over 2h ± albumin).
- Stop all diuretics.
- Antibiotics (e.g. cefotaxime + metronidazole) after cultures.
- Terlipressin (0.5–1mg IV every 4–6h) with albumin (1g/kg and 40g daily thereafter, or noradrenaline (1–10mcg/min) if MAP <75mmHg. Assess response by urine output.
- N-acetylcysteine 100mg/kg bd by IV infusion may improve renal function if the above fail.
- Haemofiltration or dialysis if appropriate.
- Paracentesis for tense ascites (no data available on efficacy).
- Monitor urine output/fluid balance.
- Hyperkalaemia and acidosis are rarely a problem.
- Discuss with a liver transplant centre.

Acute upper urinary tract infections

Infection of the upper urinary tract may result in acute pyelonephritis, renal abscess, pyonephrosis, or perinephric abscess (see Fig. 4.2). Infection with obstruction causes rapid tissue destruction unless the obstruction is relieved. This is a urological emergency.

Predisposing factors

- Either an ascending infection or haematogenous spread.
- Organisms: *E. coli* 60%, *Proteus* 20%, *S. faecalis* 10%, *Klebsiella* 5%.
- Female (short urethra)
- Renal stones
- Bladder catheter
- Chronic liver disease
- Structural abnormality of renal tract
- Pregnancy
- Diabetes mellitus
- IV drug abuse
- IE.

Presentation

- Classical symptoms are loin pain, fever, and rigors.
- Non-specific symptoms may predominate: e.g. nausea, vomiting, anorexia, malaise, confusion, or weakness.
- Up to 75% have preceding lower urinary tract symptoms (frequency, dysuria). There may be associated haematuria.
- Severe, bilateral pyelonephritis or acute-on-chronic pyelonephritis may result in AKI.
- A preceding history of intermittent loin pain may imply intermittent obstruction with pyonephrosis. Renal abscesses occur with IV drug use, endocarditis, or skin infections.
- Ask specifically about any predisposing factors.
- Signs include fever, abdominal or loin tenderness, a palpable mass in the loin, and with severe infection, scoliosis, hypotension, and shock (septicaemia).
- Symptoms and signs may be difficult to distinguish from pneumonia or other causes of an acute abdomen (e.g. cholecystitis, diverticulitis).

Investigations

- Urinalysis commonly shows blood and protein. Urine nitrite is often positive. White cells, bacteria, WBC casts may be seen on microscopy. Culture may be negative in infections confined to the renal cortex.
- All patients should have U&Es (for renal dysfunction–dehydration, acute-on-chronic failure), glc, FBC (anaemia, leucocytosis) and blood cultures.
- AXR: stones, soft tissue mass, or loss of psoas line on affected side.
- USS to exclude obstruction and delineate renal and peri-renal collections. Arrange CT without contrast if surgery is planned.

Management (Box 4.7)

- Stabilize the patient: resuscitate severely ill patients with IV fluids ± inotropes, guided by CVP and BP (see Box 4.7).
- Give IV antibiotics, e.g. a bolus of gentamicin (dose dependent on serum creatinine) and cefuroxime 750mg tds and modify treatment in light of results of cultures. Continue antibiotics for 7–14 days.
- Organize drainage of infected and obstructed urinary system.
- Fluid balance: maintain high fluid intake (e.g. 3L/24h). Monitor fluid balance and urine output carefully for the first 48–72h.
- Analgesia: try opiates.
- Pyonephrosis, renal or perinephric abscess: requires urgent advice: contact the urologists. Save a sample for MC&S.
- When patient recovered, investigate for any underlying cause: IVU, DMSA, and DTPA scans will determine anatomy, extent of renal damage, and remaining function.

Box 4.7 Management key points: acute pyelonephritis

- Analgesia.
- IV fluids (if dehydrated); maintain high fluid intake.
- IV antibiotics: cefuroxime or ciprofloxacin may also be used; give a bolus of gentamicin as you initiate treatment. Modify antibiotics when culture/sensitivity results are known.
- Monitor BP, fluid balance, and urine output.
- Contact urologists if pyonephrosis, renal/perinephric abscesses are suspected.
- Investigate for an underlying cause (IVU, DMSA, and DTPA scans).

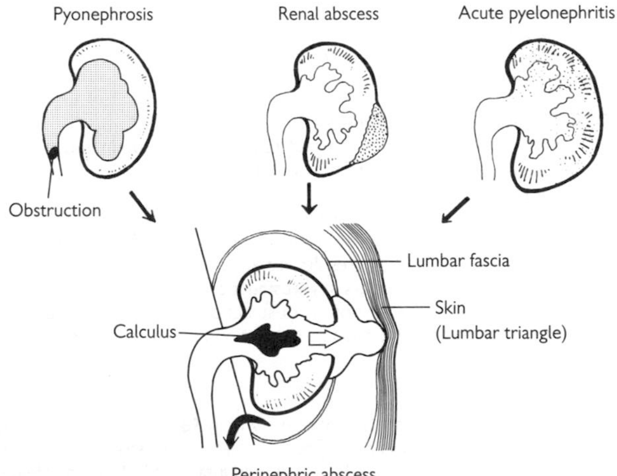

Fig. 4.2 Patterns of renal infections.

Renal colic and renal stones

Spasmodic pain radiating from loin to groin is usually due to stones or blood clots (see Box 4.8). ~2–3% of population have a stone in the upper urinary tract. Pain can also be caused by a sloughed papilla, 2° to diabetes, sickle cell disease, or analgesics.

Presentation

- May be painless.
- Pain: the site of the pain may vary; stones in the renal pelvis cause dull loin ache; ureteric stones produce severe colicky pain often of sudden onset radiating from loin to groin; bladder stones cause suprapubic and perineal or testicular ache.
- Haematuria (often frank) may be the only feature.
- With severe pain the patient will be restless, sweaty, pale, nauseated, and very distressed.
- Is there a history of previous episodes? Ask re: UTIs, fluid intake, occupation, residence in hot climates, symptoms of hypercalcaemia, or family history of stone disease.
- On examination note any fever, abdominal tenderness (especially loin or subcostal), palpable kidneys. Do not miss a leaking abdominal aortic aneurysm that may be producing similar symptoms.

Investigations

- Bloods: U&Es (for renal dysfunction) and glucose, FBC (for Hb, WCC).
- Urine: dipstick urinalysis for blood and formal microscopy for crystals, pyuria, and bacteria. Culture for infection.
- AXR: >90% of renal stones are radio-opaque. Most but not all stones can be detected on a plain AXR.
- USS or CT KUB will show obstruction.
- Tests to consider include serum Ca^{2+} and urate and 24-h urine for Ca^{2+}, phosphate, oxalate, urate to detect a stone-forming metabolic defect, or citrate levels.

Management of acute renal colic

- Analgesia: diclofenac sodium 75mg IM repeated after 30min. If needed pethidine 50–100mg IM q4h PRN with an antiemetic.
- High fluid intake.
- Beware of infection above the stone and pyonephrosis (see 📖 Fig. 4.2, p.299). If there is fever, bacteriuria, or obstruction treat empirically until culture results are known (e.g. cefuroxime 750mg IV tds) and decompress any obstruction.
- Large-sized stones with infection or obstruction require urological management such as ureteroscopic extraction or extracorporeal shock wave lithotripsy, or surgery.

Prognosis

~60% of all stones will pass (half of these within 48h). ~30% will require surgical removal, and 10% will recur. The risk of idiopathic stone recurrence is altered slightly by diet, but is ↓ by a high fluid intake (>1.5L per day leads to 6-fold decrease). It is important to control hypercalciuria if present (low-calcium diet, thiazide diuretics), treating hypercalcaemia if present (📖 p.544), urinary alkalinization (hyperuricaemia, renal tubular acidosis, cystinuria), urinary acidification to pH <5.5 ± urease inhibitors (struvite stones), allopurinol (urate stones), or D-penicillamine (cystine stones).

Box 4.8 Causes of renal colic

Renal stones

Usually divided into:

- *Radio-opaque (90%):* contain Ca^{2+} or Mg^{2+}, e.g. calcium oxalate (hypercalciuria, hypercalcaemia, dehydration, renal tubular acidosis, medullary sponge kidney, hyperoxaluria), calcium phosphate (as before and UTIs), magnesium ammonium phosphate (UTIs with urease-positive organisms, e.g. *Proteus*). Cystine stones are 'semi-opaque' due to their sulphur content.
- *Radiolucent:* urate or xanthine or rarely 2,8 dihydroxyadenine.

Indinavir crystal deposition (HIV drug)

Renal papillary necrosis

DM, sickle cell disease, analgesic nephropathy. Pain occurs when a papilla 'sloughs' into the ureter.

Blood clots

Due to trauma, tumour (parenchymal or urothelial), bleeding diathesis, or polycystic kidney disease.

Haematuria

History

Haematuria is either visible and symptomatic or microscopic and asymptomatic.

- Severity of haematuria: pink urine, frank blood, or clots?
- The timing of haematuria: bleeding occurs at start or end of micturition suggests bladder neck, prostate, or urethral source. Blood mixed with the stream suggests a source higher in the urinary tract.
- History of trauma: even seemingly minor trauma can cause bleeding from congenital lesions of the urinary tract.
- Unilateral loin pain: consider calculi, tumour, cystic disease, or hydronephrosis. Painless haematuria suggests neoplasm.
- Disturbance of micturition: frequency, urgency, dysuria, hesitancy, poor stream, and dribbling suggest cystitis. Bleeding and pain at the end of the stream is typical of a bladder stone.
- Constitutional symptoms: sore throats, arthralgia, malaise, and rash may indicate glomerulonephritis. AF is associated with renal emboli. Fever, dysuria, or abdominal pain may indicate infection. Bruising or other bleeding may indicate a bleeding diathesis.

Physical examination

- **General examination** Hypertension (chronic or acute renal disease incl. polycystic disease), irregular pulse or heart murmurs (source of emboli), anaemia, bruising or purpura, oedema or pleural effusions.
- **Urinary tract examination** Loin or abdominal tenderness, renal mass, pelvic mass, prostate enlargement, testes. Inspect the urine.

Investigations

• Urinalysis	Positive result seen with myoglobinuria (📖 p.294) and haemoglobinuria. Proteinuria suggests renal pathology
• Microscopy	RBC casts or dysmorphic red cells suggest glomerular origin. WBC casts suggest pyelonephritis. Other findings include crystals (stone disease), ova (schistosomiasis), and malignant cells
• FBC	Thrombocytopenia anaemia (haemolysis, leukaemia), leucocytosis may indicate infection
• U&Es	For renal function
• Clotting	For coagulopathy
• G&S	If post traumatic or severe
• ASOT	If glomerulonephritis is suspected. Consider measuring autoantibodies. Refer to renal team
• Ultrasound	May diagnose polycystic disease, ureteric obstruction by stone or tumour, or gross renal abnormalities
• CT scan	May demonstrate stones, hydronephrosis, renal injury or tumour, cystic disease, or urothelial tumour
• Cystoscopy	To exclude other causes of bleeding from the lower urinary tract.

Management

- Admit patients with:
  - Post-traumatic haematuria (refer to urology).
  - Severe unexplained haematuria (incl. bleeding diathesis) esp. if there is clot retention. Insert a large (22G) triple lumen urinary catheter for continuous bladder irrigation with monosol (not glucose) to wash out clots.
  - Haematuria and renal impairment (?glomerulonephritis). Arrange for urgent renal referral and biopsy.
  - Severe infection, e.g. pyelonephritis. Commence antibiotics (e.g. cefuroxime or gentamicin) after taking cultures.
- Pain relief (pethidine 25–50mg IV with an antiemetic). Propantheline bromide 15mg tds PO relieves painful bladder spasm of haemorrhagic cystitis and clot retention (may cause urinary retention).
- Correct any bleeding diathesis (FFP or Vit K for warfarin).

Box 4.9 Causes of haematuria

• ***Trauma***	Blunt and penetrating injuries, iatrogenic (e.g. recent TURP or renal biopsy), severe exercise, foreign body
• ***Stones***	Renal, ureteric, or bladder
• ***Infections***	Pyelonephritis, haemorrhagic cystitis, acuteprostatitis: bacterial, TB, or parasitic (e.g. schistosomiasis)
• ***Tumours***	Urothelial, renal parenchymal, prostatic
• ***Bleeding diatheses***	Haemophilia, thrombocytopenia
• ***Renal pathology***	Glomerulonephritis, renal arterial emboli, renal vein thrombosis
• ***Drugs***	Anti-coagulants, cyclophosphamide, D-penicillamine
• ***Congenital***	Polycystic disease, sickle cell disease (papillary necrosis), Alport's syndrome, hydronephrosis.

NB: Discoloured urine may also be due to beetroot, porphyria, rifampicin, co-danthramer, and vegetable dyes.

Renovascular disease

Renal artery stenosis may be atherosclerotic (common in the elderly and diabetics) or fibromuscular dysplasia (young patients). Fibromuscular dysplasia occurs in young patients, usually female, and may involve other vascular beds such as peripheral, coronary, or cerebral. Renal artery stenosis should be considered in all patients with:

- Flash pulmonary oedema (sudden unexpected onset)
- Peripheral vascular disease, aortic dissection, type 2 diabetes
- Unequal kidneys on USS
- Impaired renal function in context of ACEI use
- Hypertension/coronary or carotid artery disease
- Complete anuria in a patient who has previously lost a kidney.
- Patients with hypokalaemia.

Investigations

- USS: to look at renal size and asymmetry and Doppler flow through the renal arteries.
- Isotope renogram (rarely done now).
- MRA is taking over from angiography as the gold standard investigation in some hospitals: Avoid a gadolinium scan in patients with a GFR of <30mL/min as this is associated with nephrogenic sclerosing dermopathy.
- Be guided by your local radiologists.
- Digital subtraction angiography is sometimes used.

Management

- Optimize fluid status with sodium bicarbonate (1.26%)
- There is often a fine balance between pulmonary oedema and pre-renal uraemia.
- Avoid ACEIs and NSAIDs.
- Refer to a dedicated team of interventional radiologists and vascular surgeons if there is >70% stenosis, intractable hypertension (>5 drugs), or flash pulmonary oedema. However, the recent ASTRAL trial suggests that patients do ***not*** benefit from stents, and this is changing clinical practice.
- Most patients with atheromatous renovascular disease die from their associated ischaemic heart disease.

Cholesterol embolism

Most commonly seen in arteriopaths after manipulation of vasculature (e.g. angiography) and is followed by AKI. Usually silent. There is partial occlusion of small- and medium-sized arteries resulting in ischaemic atrophy. More florid presentation includes: widespread purpura, dusky and cyanotic peripheries with intact pedal pulses, GI bleeding, myalgia, and AKI. It can be spontaneous or follow therapy with heparin or warfarin.

Diagnosis

Eosinophilia, renal impairment, hypocomplementaemia, ESR, ANCA negative. Urinary sediment is usually benign; mild proteinuria may be seen. Renal biopsy shows cholesterol clefts.

Management

The renal impairment is usually irreversible or only partially reversible (in contrast to ATN). Anticoagulation is contraindicated. Treatment is supportive.

Contrast nephropathy

This is acute impairment of renal function, which follows exposure to radiocontrast materials. Incidence in an unselected population is 2–7% but increases to 25% if renal function is already impaired. Pre-expand plasma volume with normal saline or Hartmann's solution.

Risk factors

- Pre-existing renal disease (incidence up to 60% if Cr >400μM)
- Renovascular disease
- Proteinuria (increases risk 3-fold)
- DM (risk depends on renal function; incidence of AKI (ARF) ~100% if Cr >400μM)
- Congestive cardiac failure (incidence 7–8%)
- Multiple myeloma
- Pancreatitis
- Dehydration
- Jaundice
- Congestive cardiac failure
- Concomitant nephrotoxins (e.g. gentamicin).

Management

There is no specific treatment. Prevention is the best policy.

- Monitor U&Es, creatinine.
- Ensure good hydration pre-procedure (give patients who are at risk IV fluids if they are to be kept NBM for the procedure).
- Maintain high urine output. Stop nephrotoxic drugs (esp. NSAIDs) peri-procedure.
- Outcome in one study: 68% regain normal renal function, 14% had partial recovery, 18% death, dialysis, or transplantation.
- N-acetylcysteine is no longer thought to be effective.

Box 4.10 Causes of contrast nephropathy

Pre-renal

- Hypovolaemia:
  - Vomiting and diarrhoea
  - Haemorrhage
- Decrease in effective circulating volume:
  - Cardiac failure
  - Septic shock
  - Cirrhosis
- Drugs: ACEIs.

Intrinsic

- Glomerular: glomerulonephritis
- Tubular
  - Acute tubular necrosis
  - Rhabdomyolysis
  - Myeloma
- Interstitial: interstitial nephritis.

Post-renal

- Renal calculi
- Retroperitoneal fibrosis
- Prostatic hypertrophy
- Cervical carcinoma
- Urethral stricture
- Obstructed urinary catheter
- Intra-abdominal hypertension.

Urine appearance

Typical urine is pale yellow to amber in colour. Other colours do not necessarily imply pathology:

- ***Red:*** haematuria, haemoglobinuria, beetroot, rifampicin, senna, porphyrinuria
- ***Brown:*** haematuria, haemoglobinuria, myoglobinuria, jaundice, chloroquine, carotene
- ***Black:*** haematuria, haemoglobinuria, myoglobinuria, alkaptonuria (black on standing)
- ***Green:*** triamterene, propofol
- ***Darkening on standing:*** porphyrinuria (fluorescence in UV light), metronidazole, imipenem or cilastatin.

Chapter 5

Shock

Shock

Shock is defined as inadequate perfusion of vital organs. Concurrent hypotension need not necessarily be present. The drop in BP is a late finding, particularly in young, fit people, so resuscitation should ideally commence before this point is reached.

Priorities

- *If the BP is unrecordable, call the cardiac arrest team.* Begin basic life support and establish venous access.
- Seek specialist help early.
- The cause of hypotension is often apparent. If it is not, then one can usually make a rapid clinical assessment of likely causes:
  - Cardiac pump failure
  - Hypovolaemia
  - Systemic vasodilatation, including neurogenic shock
  - Anaphylaxis
  - Obstruction (e.g. PE, tension pneumothorax, tamponade).

Differential diagnosis of shock

Cardiac pump failure

- Myocardial infarction (📖 p.12)
- Dissection of thoracic aorta (📖 p.142)
- Cardiac arrhythmias (📖 p.55)
- Acute valvular failure or acute VSD (📖 p.34)
- Drug overdose (cardiac depressants, see 📖 p.692)
- Myocarditis.

Hypovolaemia

- Haemorrhage (GI tract (📖 p.224), aortic dissection or leaking AAA, trauma (fractures, liver or spleen injury, haemothorax, occult)
- Fluid losses (diarrhoea, vomiting, polyuria, or burns)
- '3rd space' fluid losses (acute pancreatitis (📖 p.276)
- Adrenal failure (📖 p.548).

Systemic vasodilatation

- Sepsis
- Liver failure (📖 p.268)
- Drug overdose (calcium antagonists or other vasodilators, drugs causing multi-organ failure, e.g. paracetamol, paraquat)
- Adrenal failure (may be both hypovolaemic and vasodilated)
- Neurogenic shock (bradycardia and hypotension, autonomic failure).

Anaphylaxis

- Recent drug therapy
- Food allergy (e.g. peanut)
- Insect stings.

Obstruction

- Cardiac tamponade (📖 p.156)
- Pulmonary embolus (📖 p.120)
- Tension pneumothorax (📖 p.210).

Shock: assessment

If the BP is unrecordable then call the cardiac arrest team. Begin basic life support (Airway, Breathing, and Circulation) and establish venous access. If the cause of hypotension is not obvious, perform a rapid clinical examination looking specifically for the following:

- Check the airway is unobstructed. Give high-flow (60–100%) O_2 by mask or ETT if airway unprotected or breathing inadequate. Check both lungs are ventilated (?tension pneumothorax).
- Note the respiratory rate (↑ in acidosis, pneumothorax, embolus, and cardiac failure, but often ↑ regardless of cause).
- Check cardiac rhythm and treat if abnormal (see 📖 pp.56–87).
- Is the JVP elevated (see Box 5.1)?
- Is the BP the same in both arms (thoracic aortic dissection)?
- Are there any unusual cardiac murmurs? (Acute valvular lesion, flow murmurs are often heard in vasodilated patients.)
- Is the patient cold and clammy? This suggests cardiac pump failure or hypovolaemia; NB patients with septic shock may also be peripherally shut down. Check for fever (temperature may be sub-normal, especially in the elderly and children).
- Is the patient warm and systemically vasodilated (feel finger pulp and feet). Palpate for bounding pulses.
- Examine the abdomen. Is there a fullness or pulsatile mass in the abdomen (ruptured aneurysm)? Is there evidence of an acute abdomen (aneurysm, pancreatitis, perforated viscus)?
- Is there evidence of trauma or fractures?
- Is the patient clinically dehydrated or hypovolaemic (skin turgor, mucous membranes, postural fall in BP)?
- Any evidence of haematemesis (blood around mouth) or melaena (PR examination)?
- Is there any evidence of anaphylaxis such as urticaria, wheezing, or soft tissue swelling (e.g. eyelids or lips)?
- Is conscious level impaired?

Investigations

- ***ECG*** Acute MI, arrhythmias, PE (right heart strain with S1, Q3, T3).
- ***CXR*** Pneumothorax, PE, dissection, tamponade, pleural effusion.
- ***Blood tests*** *U&Es* (renal impairment, adrenal failure), *FBC* (haemorrhage, ↓platelets in liver disease and sepsis), *glucose, clotting studies* (liver disease, DIC), *LFTs*, *X-match.*
- ***ABGs*** Acidaemia (renal, lactate, ketoacidosis).
- ***Septic screen*** Culture blood, urine, sputum.
- ***Miscellaneous*** Echo (suspected tamponade, dissection, valve dysfunction), LP, USS, or CT abdomen and head.

Box 5.1 Causes of hypotension with a raised CVP

- Pulmonary embolus
- Cardiac tamponade (📖 p.156)
- Cardiogenic shock (📖 p.42)
- Fluid overload in shocked vasodilated patients
- Right ventricular infarction (📖 p.28)
- Tension pneumothorax (📖 p.210).

Shock: management

General measures

- Check the airway, give O_2 (60–100%) by face mask to optimize O_2 saturation. If conscious level is impaired (GCS <8), airway is unprotected, and/or breathing is inadequate, consider intubation.
- Lie the patient flat.
- Insert 2 large-bore IV cannulae and commence infusion of a crystalloid (ideally Hartmann's solution, or N saline. In most cases of shock, including cardiac causes, it is usually beneficial and safe to give a crystalloid such as N saline (200mL over 5–10min) while a more detailed assessment is being carried out. If the fluid challenge brings improvement, give a further fluid challenge while assessing the situation. If large volumes of crystalloid are needed it is better to give Hartmann's solution to avoid causing hyperchloraemia and metabolic acidosis with N saline.
- Send blood for U&Es, glucose, FBC, X-match, and blood cultures.
- Once resuscitation is underway and it is safe, insert a central venous line to monitor CVP, and for inotrope infusions as necessary. Insert arterial line for more accurate assessment of BP. Catheterize the bladder to monitor urine output.
- Titrate fluid replacement according to BP, CVP, and urine output. Over-enthusiastic fluid administration in patients with cardiac pump failure will precipitate pulmonary oedema (see 🕮 p.327).
- Persistent hypotension despite adequate filling is an indication for inotropic support, assuming that tension pneumothorax, and pulmonary embolus have been excluded. The choice of first-line agent varies to some extent depending upon the underlying diagnosis.
- Treat the underlying condition and *enlist specialist help early*.
- Ensure someone takes time to talk to the relatives to explain the patient is seriously ill and may die. Discuss resuscitation status.

Cardiogenic shock (cardiac pump failure)

- Manage cardiac ischaemia, arrhythmias, and electrolyte disturbances.
- Possible concurrent hypovolaemia? Consider cautious IV fluids. Optimize filling, guided by physical signs and response in filling pressures and stroke volume to fluid challenges (100–200mL colloid)
- If BP allows, start a nitrate infusion (e.g. GTN 5mg/h).
- If very hypotensive, start an IV inotrope infusion. Dopamine is the preferred agent for patients with cardiogenic shock.
- A small amount of diamorphine (e.g. 2.5mg) is beneficial as it vasodilates, reduces anxiety, and lowers metabolic rate.
- Consider non-invasive or invasive ventilation in patients with severe heart failure as this decreases the work of breathing and benefits both left ventricular afterload and preload.
- If there is a potentially reversible cause for cardiogenic shock, consider intra-aortic balloon counterpulsation (🕮 p.774).

Hypovolaemic shock

- Fluid replacement with crystalloids are as good as colloids.[1]
- Give blood to maintain Hb ≥8g/dL.
- Na^+ and K^+ abnormalities should be treated. Metabolic acidosis often responds to fluid replacement alone.
- If the patient remains hypotensive in spite of fluids, consider other causes (sepsis, tamponade, tension pneumothorax, etc.). Reperfusion injury may occasionally manifest itself as a hypotensive, vasodilated circulation. If fluid replete, commence inotropes: dopamine if a low cardiac output state is suspected, or noradrenaline if there is a vasodilated circulation.
- If oliguria persists despite adequate resuscitation, furosemide (40–80mg IV) may be given to try and maintain a urine output, as this may make fluid management easier. There is no evidence that furosemide improves outcome.

Practice point

In one major study involving ~7000 patients, saline was equally effective as albumin for fluid resuscitation.[1]

Box 5.2 Management key points: shock

- ABC, O_2 (60–100%), consider intubation if GCS <8.
- IV access and fluids: titrate according to BP, CVP, and urine output. (In most cases it is safe to give 200mL colloid over 5–10min and assess response.)
- Inotropes: if there is persistent hypotension in spite of adequate filling.
- After initiating inotropes assess patients frequently for tachyphylaxis (may require dose titration) and additional haemodynamic insults.
- Treat the underlying condition e.g. infections, cardiac ischaemia or arrhythmia.
- Talk to the relatives. Discuss resuscitation status.

Reference

1. Finfer S *et al.* (2004). *N Engl J Med* **350**: 2247–56.

Sepsis syndrome and septic shock

Definitions

- ***Bacteraemia*** Positive blood cultures.
- ***Sepsis*** Evidence of infection plus systemic inflammatory response such as pyrexia or tachycardia.
- ***Sepsis Syndrome*** Systemic response to infection plus evidence of organ dysfunction: confusion, hypoxia, oliguria, metabolic acidosis.
- ***Septic shock*** Sepsis syndrome plus hypotension refractory to volume replacement.

Presentation

Sepsis is now defined as infection with evidence of systemic inflammation, consisting of 2 or more of the following: ↑ or ↓ temperature or leucocyte count, tachycardia, and rapid breathing. Septic shock is sepsis with hypotension that persists after resuscitation with IV fluid.

General symptoms

Sweats, chills, or rigors. Breathlessness. Headache. Confusion in 10–30% of patients, especially the elderly. Nausea, vomiting, or diarrhoea may occur.

Examination

Hypotension (SBP <90mmHg or a 40mmHg fall from baseline), tachycardia, with peripheral vasodilatation (warm peripheries, bounding peripheral pulse, bounding pulses in forearm muscles) are the hallmarks of early sepsis, but patients do become shut down eventually. SVR is reduced and cardiac output is ↑ initially but severe myocardial depression may occur. Other features include fever >38°C or hypothermia <35.6°C (immunocompromised or elderly patients may not be able to mount a febrile response), tachypnoea and hypoxia, metabolic acidosis, oliguria. Focal physical signs may help to localize the site of infection.

Investigations

- ***Blood tests*** Blood cultures, U&Es, blood sugar, FBC, coagulation studies, LFTs, CRP, group and save serum, lactate, ABGs. Amylase, CK and serology.
- ***Culture*** Blood, sputum, urine, line-tips, wound swabs, throat swab, drain fluid, stool, CSF (as indicated).
- ***Imaging*** CXR, USS or CT brain, chest, abdomen, and pelvis for collections. Echo if endocarditis suspected.

Continuous assessments in ICU/HDU

Patients should be monitored in either an ICU or HDU. An arterial line should be inserted for continuous BP monitoring and intermittent blood sampling. It is important in the management of such critically ill patients *not* to lose sight of the needs of the patient. It is easy in an ICU setting not to examine patients but to look at charts. Always examine the patient at least twice a day and determine whether the clinical parameters match those on the ICU chart.

Ask yourself twice a day

- Fluid requirements (what is the fluid balance, is the patient clinically dry, euvolemic or oedematous?)
- Is the circulation adequate? Note the BP (and MAP), filling pressures, and cardiac output. Examine the peripheries (are they cool and shut down, or warm?). Is the urine output satisfactory? Is there a swing on the arterial trace, suggestive of hypovolaemia? Is there a developing metabolic acidosis, which may indicate tissue hypoperfusion?
- Is gas exchange satisfactory? Watch for developing ARDS (📖 p.198). Examine the chest daily for deterioration that may be masked on ABG by adjustments of mechanical ventilation and do a CXR if needed.
- Are there signs of sepsis? Is there a new focus of infection?
- What do the tests show (U&Es, LFTs, Ca^{2+}, PO_4^{3-}, Mg^{2+}, CRP, cultures (blood, urine, sputum, line tips, etc.)?
- Is the patient receiving adequate nutrition (TPN or enteral)? Always give enteral nutrition if possible. Even enteral nutrition at 10ml/h will benefit the gut mucosa. Give with TPN if the gut function is not adequate but ensure regular aspiration of any unabsorbed feed.

Prognosis

The incidence of bacteraemia is 7/1000 admissions to hospital. Of these 20% develop septic shock and approximately 50% of these die (Table 5.1). Also see Box 5.3.

Table 5.1 Mortality in sepsis

	Mortality
Bacteraemia	15–20%
Bacteraemia plus shock	30–40%
Shock plus ARDS	40–60%

Box 5.3 Poor prognostic features in sepsis syndrome

- Age >60
- Multi-organ failure (>3 organs)
- Renal failure
- Respiratory failure (ARDS)
- Hepatic failure
- Hypothermia or leucopenia
- Hospital-acquired infection
- DIC
- Underlying disease (e.g. immunocompromised, poor nutritional status, malignancy).

Septic shock: management

Patients with established shock require adequate haemodynamic monitoring and high-dependency facilities.

Check the airway is clear. Give high-flow O_2: if there is refractory hypoxia, intubate and ventilate. Insert a large-bore peripheral venous cannula to begin fluid resuscitation. Insert central line and arterial line.

Key recommendations from the updated Surviving Sepsis Campaign guidelines (2008)[1] for management of severe sepsis and septic shock are summarized here:

- *Early goal-directed resuscitation:* during the first 6h after recognition (in patients with hypotension or serum lactate >4 mmol/L).
- *Resuscitation goals include:*
  - Mean arterial pressure ≥65 mmHg.
  - Target CVP of 8–12mmHg (12–15mmHg if ventilated).
  - Central venous O_2 saturation ≥70%.
  - Urine output ≥0.5mL/kg/h.
- *Source identification:*
  - Within first 6h of presentation.
  - Blood cultures before antibiotic therapy.
  - Culture all sites as clinically indicated.
  - Imaging studies performed promptly to confirm potential source of infection.
- *Broad-spectrum antibiotics:*
  - Within 1h of diagnosis of septic shock/ severe sepsis (give first dose of antibiotics yourself).
  - Daily reassessment of antimicrobial therapy with microbiology and clinical data.
  - Antibiotic therapy guided by clinical response; normally 7–10 days but longer if response is slow, there are undrainable foci of infection or immunologic deficiencies.
- *Source control:* abscess drainage, tissue debridement or removal IV access devices if potentially infected as soon as possible following successful initial resuscitation (exception: infected pancreatic necrosis, where surgical intervention is best delayed).
- *IV fluids:*
  - Crystalloid or colloid; fluid challenge (e.g. 1L of crystalloids or 300–500mL of colloids over 30min) to restore circulating volume.
  - Rate of fluid administration should be reduced if cardiac filling pressures increase without concurrent haemodynamic improvement.
- *Vasopressors:*
  - Noradrenaline or dopamine (administered centrally) are first line.
  - Terlipressin may be subsequently added to, or used to replace noradrenaline.
- *Inotropic therapy:* consider dobutamine when cardiac output remains low despite fluid resuscitation and vasopressor therapy.
- *Steroids:* in the Corticus study[2] it was shown that hydrocortisone (50mg 6-hourly) reversed septic shock more rapidly in some patients, but had no effect on outcome.

- *Recombinant activated protein C:* this has anti-inflammatory, anti-coagulant and profibrinolytic properties. Consider in patients with severe sepsis and clinical assessment of high risk for death (typically APACHE (APACHE, Acute Physiology and Chronic Health Evaluation) II ≥ 25 or multiple organ failure) if there are no contraindications.
- *Blood products:*
  - Target haemoglobin of 7–9g/dL, Aim for a higher target in the presence of tissue hypoperfusion, coronary artery disease, or acute haemorrhage.
  - Do not use FFP to correct laboratory clotting abnormalities unless there is bleeding or planned invasive procedures.
  - Administer platelets when platelet counts are <40 $\times 10^9$/L and there is significant bleeding risk.
- *Ventilation:*
  - A low tidal volume and limitation of inspiratory plateau pressure strategy for ALI/ARDS.
  - Application of at least a minimal amount of positive end-expiratory pressure in ALI.
  - Head of bed elevation in mechanically ventilated patients unless contraindicated.
  - Avoid routine use of pulmonary artery catheters in ALI/ARDS.
- *Glucose control:* use IV insulin to control hyperglycaemia; targeting a blood glucose <8.3 mmol/L after initial stabilization.
- *Renal replacement:* continuous haemofiltration is the preferred method.
- *DVT prophylaxis:* low-dose UFH or LMWH, unless contraindicated; compression stockings when heparin is contraindicated.
- *Stress ulcer prophylaxis:* H_2 blockers or proton pump inhibitors.
- *Consideration of limitation of support* (where appropriate): discuss advance care planning with patients and families. Describe likely outcomes and set realistic expectations.

References

1. Dellinger RP *et al.* (2008). Surviving Sepsis Campaign: International guidelines for management of severe sepsis and septic shock: 2008 [published correction appears in *Crit Care Med* 2008; **36:** 1394–6]. *Crit Care Med* **36:** 296–327.

2. Sprung C *et al.* (2008). Hydrocortisone therapy for patients with septic shock. *N Engl J Med* **358:** 111–24.

Sepsis syndrome/septic shock: antibiotics

Antibiotic choice is dictated by the suspected site of infection and probable microbe, host factors such as age, immunosuppression, and hospitalization, and local antibiotic-resistance patterns. A suggested empiric regimen in patients with sepsis syndrome and the following source of infection is as follows:

• ***Pneumonia: community-acquired***	Co-amoxiclav or Cefotaxime + clarithromycin
• ***Pneumonia: hospital-acquired***	Ceftazidime alone or Piperacillin + gentamicin NB: if *S. aureus* suspected, use teicoplanin or vancomycin (if MRSA), flucloxacillin (if MSSA)
• ***Intra-abdominal sepsis***	Cefotaxime + metronidazole or Piptazobactam or gentamicin
• ***Biliary tract***	Piptazobactam or gentamicin
• ***Urinary tract: community-acquired***	Co-amoxiclav or cefotaxime
• ***Urinary tract: hospital-acquired***	Ceftazidime or Piptazobactam or gentamicin
• ***Skin and soft tissue***	Co-amoxiclav or Amoxicillin + flucloxacillin
• ***Sore throat***	Benzylpenicillin
• ***Multiple organisms (anaerobes, E. coli, Strep.)***	Vancomycin+ gentamicin + metronidazole or Clindamycin or gentamicin
• ***Meningitis***	Cefotaxime or (if pen. and cef. allergic) Vancomycin or rifampicin Many now suggest chloramphenicol

NB: consult your microbiologists for local antibiotic policy.

Remove infective foci

It is essential to identify and drain focal sites, e.g. obstructed urinary tract or biliary tree, drain abscesses, and resect dead tissue.

Causes of treatment failure

- Resistant or unusual infecting organism
- Undrained abscess
- Inflammatory response (raised CRP, raised WCC) may persist despite adequate anti-microbial therapy
- Advanced disease.

Toxic shock syndrome

- Distinct clinical illness caused by toxin-producing Gram-positive bacteria, usually staphylococci or streptococci.
- Infection is often localized and illness is manifest by the toxins.
- 85% of cases are female.
- Association with the use of tampons and postpartum in females or following nasal packing (either sex).
- May occur with any focal infections due to a toxin-producing strain, including postoperative wound infections.

Clinical features

- Fever: >38.9°C.
- Rash: diffuse macular (seen in ≥95%), mucous membrane involvement common. Desquamation 1–2 weeks later, palms and soles (consider drug reaction in differential diagnosis).
- Hypotension: SBP <90mmHg, or postural hypotension.
- Diarrhoea and vomiting are common.
- NSAIDs may mask symptoms.
- DIC and petechial rash.
- Multi-organ failure may follow.

Laboratory findings

- Normochromic normocytic anaemia (50%) and leucocytosis (>80%).
- Renal/hepatic failure (20–30%).
- Myalgia and elevated CPK are common.
- DIC.
- Pyuria.
- CSF pleiocytosis (sterile).
- Blood cultures rarely positive.
- Vaginal swabs, throat swab, and wound swabs.
- Toxin-producing *S. aureus* in 98% of menses-associated cases.

Therapy

- Limit toxin production/release.
- Drain any focal collections and remove foreign bodies.
- Anti-*Staph.* antibiotics (high-dose flucloxacillin, teicoplanin or clindamycin intravenously).
- Supportive care as for any patient with shock.

Anaphylaxis

Anaphylaxis is a severe, life-threatening, generalized or systemic hypersensitivity reaction, characterized by rapidly developing life-threatening airway and, or breathing and, or circulation problems usually associated with skin and mucosal changes. The UK incidence of anaphylactic reactions is increasing.

Atopic individuals are particularly at risk, but it may occur in some in the absence of past history. Precipitants include

- Insect bites (especially wasp and bee stings)
- Foods and food additives (e.g. peanuts, fish, eggs)
- Drugs and IV infusions (blood products and IV immunoglobulin, vaccines, antibiotics, aspirin and other NSAIDs, iron injections, heparin).

Presentation

Cutaneous features include skin redness, urticaria, conjunctival injection, angioedema, and rhinitis. More severe manifestations include laryngeal obstruction (choking sensation, cough, stridor), bronchospasm, tachycardia, hypotension, and shock.

Management (Fig. 5.1)

- *Maintain the airway:* if respiratory obstruction is imminent, intubate, and ventilate or consider emergency cricothyroidotomy (see 📖 p.782). A 14G needle and insufflation with 100% O_2 can temporize until the anaesthetist arrives.
- *Give 100% O_2:* if there is refractory hypoxaemia, intubate, and ventilate.
- Lie the patient flat with head-down tilt if hypotensive.
- *Give intramuscular adrenaline 0.5–1mg* (0.5–1mL of 1 in 1000 adrenaline injection) and repeat every 10min according to BP and pulse.
- *If IV access is present, use small IV doses of adrenaline (0.1–0.2mg) then review response.* SC adrenaline should not be given in anaphylactic shock due to variable absorption.
- Establish venous access and start IV crystalloid fluids (e.g. 500mL Hartmann's or N saline over 30min). Persistent hypotension requires a continuous adrenaline infusion titrated to a BP response.
- Give IV hydrocortisone 200mg and chlorphenamine 10mg.
- Continue H_1-antagonist (e.g. chlorphenamine 4mg q4–6h) for at least 24–48h longer if urticaria and pruritus persist.
- If the bronchospasm does not subside, treat as severe asthma (including salbutamol, nebulized or intratracheal adrenaline, aminophylline).

Angioneurotic oedema (C_1-esterase inhibitor deficiency)

See 📖 p.652.

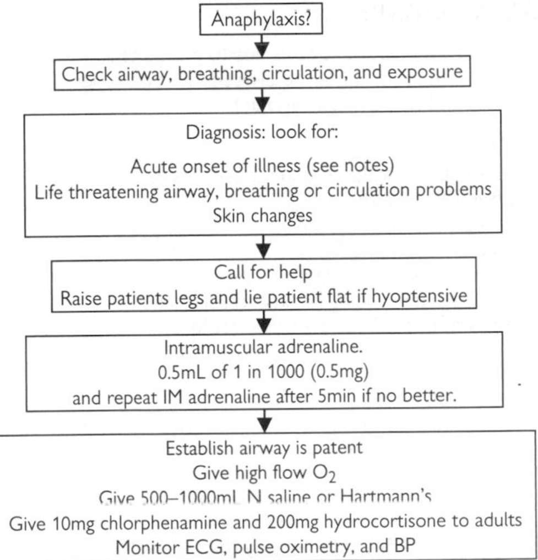

Acute onset of illness:

- *Airway:* swelling, hoarse voice, stridor
- *Breathing:* wheeze, shortness of breath, respiratory arrest
- *Circulation:* pale, clammy, tachycardia, shock, cardiac arrest.

Skin changes may be subtle or dramatic, involving both skin or mucosae. There may be erythema, or there may be urticaria which can appear anywhere on the body. The weals are usually itchy and may be pale, pink or red, or look like nettle stings. They can be different shapes and sizes, and are often surrounded by a red flare.

Fig. 5.1 Treatment algorithm for anaphylaxis.

Lactic acidosis

Lactic acidosis is a metabolic acidosis due to excess production or reduced metabolism of lactic acid. It may be divided into two types, *type A* (due to tissue hypoxia) and *type B* (non-hypoxic).

Presentation

Patients are usually critically ill. Clinical features include

- Shock (often BP <80/40)
- Kussmaul respiration
- Tachypnoea
- Deteriorating conscious level
- Multi-organ failure including hepatic, cardiac, and renal failure
- Clinical signs of poor tissue perfusion (cold, cyanotic peripheries).

Investigations

- ABGs (pH <7.34, severe if pH <7.2)
- Serum electrolytes including bicarbonate and chloride to calculate anion gap, if lactate unavailable. Raised anion gap >16mmol/L [anion gap = $(Na^+ + K^+)$ – (bicarbonate + chloride)]
- FBC (anaemia, neutrophilia)
- Blood glucose
- Blood lactate level >5mmol/L (mainly done on ABG analysers)
- Screen for sepsis (blood cultures, CRP, MSU, etc.)
- Spot urine (50mL) for drug screen if cause unknown
- CXR looking for consolidation or signs of ARDS.

Assessment of severity

Severity is assessed by the blood lactate concentration and the degree of acidaemia. This may be confounded by the presence of acute renal failure. In the early stages, the arterial pH may be normal or even raised as elevated lactate levels in the CNS cause hyperventilation with a compensatory respiratory alkalosis. The best predictor of survival is the arterial pH. Patients presenting with a lactate of >5mmol/L and a pH <7.35 have a mortality >50%.

Management

The principle of management is diagnosis and treatment of the cause (Box 5.4). All patients should be managed in a higher dependency area.

- ***Sepsis*** Start broad-spectrum antibiotics (e.g. cefotaxime plus metronidazole).
- ***Diabetic lactic acidosis*** Insulin and fluids as needed (see 🕮 p.516).
- ***Shock*** Consider invasive haemodynamic monitoring (see 🕮 p.314).
- ***Renal failure*** Treat by continuous haemofiltration. These patients are usually too unstable to tolerate haemodialysis.
- ***Methanol*** Infuse ethanol or fomepizole (competitive metabolism, see 🕮 p.718).
- ***Acidaemia*** The role of bicarbonate is controversial as it may lower CSF pH. There is no benefit of bicarbonate over equimolar saline in controlled trials.

Box 5.4 Causes of lactic acidosis

Type A

- Tissue hypoperfusion (shock)†
- Severe anaemia
- Severe hypoxia (same as†)
- Catecholamine excess (e.g. phaeochromocytoma or exogenous)
- Severe exercise.

Type B

- Sepsis
- Renal/hepatic failure
- Diabetes mellitus (uncontrolled)
- Malignancy (leukaemia, lymphoma)
- Acute pancreatitis
- Paracetamol (acetaminophen) overdose

Drug-induced

Metformin, methanol, ethanol, salicylates, ethylene glycol and cyanide.

Rare causes

Heriditary enzyme defects such as glucose-6-phosphatase and fructose 1,6 diphosphatase deficiency.

Appendix 1: haemodynamic calculations

In general most systems these days calculate all the parameters that you require, and the formulae below should not be necessary. It is important to distinguish between indexed (modified for body surface area) and non-indexed values. Indexed values are signified by the letter I. Thus cardiac output (CO) becomes CI and systemic vascular resistance (SVR) becomes SVRI.

Mean arterial pressure (MAP)

MAP = Diastolic pressure +1/3 (systolic − diastolic pressure)
e.g. BP 120/60 = MAP of 60 +1/3 (120 − 60) = 80mmHg

R. atrial pressure	NR	1–7mmHg
R. ventricular systolic pressure	NR	15–25mmHg
R. ventricular diastolic pressure	NR	1–7mmHg
PA systolic pressure	NR	20–25mmHg
PA diastolic pressure	NR	3–12mmHg
Mean PA pressure	NR	9–16mmHg
Pulmonary artery wedge pressure	NR	3–12mmHg

The PAWP is ↑ in mitral regurgitation, and it may be difficult or impossible to obtain a typical 'wedged' tracing.

Cardiac output (CO) NR 4.0–6.2L/min

Cardiac index (CI)

$$CI = \frac{\text{Cardiac Output}}{\text{Body surface area}} \quad NR \quad 2.8-3.6\text{L/min/m}^2$$

Systemic vascular resistance (SVR) and SVRI

$$SVR = \frac{(MAP - RAP) \times 80}{CO} \quad NR \quad 800-1500\text{dyne/S/cm}^5$$

$$SVRI = \frac{(MAP - RAP) \times 80}{CI} \quad NR \quad 1760-2600\text{dyne/S/cm}^5/\text{m}^2$$

Pulmonary vascular resistance (PVR)

$$PVR = \frac{(\text{Mean PA} - PAWP)}{CO} \quad NR \quad 20-120\text{dyne/S/cm}^5$$

O2 delivery

$DO_2 = CO \times CaO_2$ NR 900–1000mL/min

O_2 consumption

$VO_2 = (CaO_2 - CvO_2) \times CO$ NR 230–250L/min

CaO_2 = oxygen content of arterial blood (measured by haemoglobinometer or derived from arterial gases)

CvO_2 = oxygen content of mixed venous blood (obtained from PA distal line)

Oxygen content = Hb (g/L) × 1.34 × oxygen sat.

Oxygen extraction ratio (OER)

OER= VO_2/DO_2 NR 0.22–0.3 (22–30%)

Appendix 2: understanding circulatory failure

Intelligent manipulation of the filling pressures and inotropic support of a patient with shock or heart failure requires a basic understanding of the way in which the left and right ventricles respond to changes in filling pressure and what effect different clinical conditions have on their function. The following is a somewhat simplified approach.

The stroke volumes of the right and left ventricles are identical but since the resistance of the pulmonary bed is much lower than the systemic bed, the right ventricle is able to function well at a lower filling pressure (than the left ventricle). Raising the right atrial pressure with iv fluids will increase the stroke volume of the right ventricle. The left atrial pressure (and thus the LVEDP) will rise, keeping the stroke volume of both sides of the heart matched.

Sepsis, acidosis, ↑K^+, ↓Ca^{2+}, MI, or ischaemia, and certain drugs (e.g. β-blockers) are known to impair myocardial function. Inotropes will improve cardiac function.

Expanding the circulation with IV fluids becomes progressively less effective in increasing the stroke volume (and so cardiac output) as the function become more depressed, i.e. the increase in stroke volume per unit transfused becomes progressively less. Furthermore it increases the risks of precipitating pulmonary oedema (see next section).

Pulmonary oedema occurs when the hydrostatic pressure within the capillary overcomes the plasma oncotic pressure (the major determinant of which is the serum proteins and albumin). The critical PCWP for hydrostatic pulmonary oedema is approx. = serum albumin (g/L) × 0.57 (i.e. with an albumin of 40g/L, critical PCWP = 22mmHg. The lungs will of course get 'stiffer' as the PCWP rises and the patient may get breathless before this pressure is reached.

Thus, even in normal patients, continued IV transfusion will eventually raise the right- and left-sided filling pressures sufficiently to precipitate pulmonary oedema.

The circulation in sepsis

Sepsis produces a systemic inflammatory response that results in 'leaky' capillaries, in the lungs and elsewhere, as well as hypoalbuminaemia from a combination of impaired production and loss into extravascular spaces. Thus patients are at risk of pulmonary oedema at lower values of PCWP. Furthermore, the cardiac function is depressed so that IV fluids will produce less increase in stroke volume and cardiac output. There are 2 debates, fluids or vasopressor support. Generally, most clinicians advocate fluids and more fluids until there is a downturn.

Appendix 3: inotrope support

Inotropes

General points

- Ensure all patients given inotropes have an adequate intravascular volume (CVP or Swan–Ganz catheter).
- The aim of inotropic support is to maximize tissue oxygenation (e.g. as assessed by plasma lactate and mixed venous oxygenation) and not cardiac output.
- The inotropes in widespread clinical use are catecholamines or their derivatives. Their haemodynamic effects are complex and reflect the relative importance of a and b adrenergic effects for each agent. They are summarized in Table 5.2.

Table 5.2 Haemodynamic effects of inotropes

	HR	SVR	MAP	CO	CP
Isoprenaline	+++	–	+/–	+	±
Adrenaline	+	+	+	++	++
Dopamine (low dose)	+	–	±	+	+
(high dose)	++	++	++	++	±
Dobutamine	++		–/+	++	++
Noradrenaline	–	++	++	–/+	–/+

Abbreviations: HR, heart rate; SVR, systemic vascular resistance; MAP, mean arterial pressure; CO, cardiac output; CP, coronary perfusion; +, increase; –, decrease; ±, no change.

Box 5.5 Key points: mechanism of action of inotropes

- Activation of α-1 adrenergic receptor →vasoconstriction (↑SVR*).
- Activation of β-1 adrenergic receptor →↑heart rate/contractility (↑CO).
- Activation of β-2 adrenergic receptor →vasodilation (↓SVR).
- Dopamine: at <2mcg/kg/min causes vasodilation/↑renal blood flow (unclear clinical significance).
- Dopamine at 2–10mcg/kg/min causes ↑CO (β-1 receptor effect).
- Dopamine at >10mcg/kg/min causes ↑SVR (α-receptor effect).

Box 5.6 Key points: choice of inotrope

- Anaphylaxis: adrenaline (β-1 receptor effect).
- Hyperdynamic septic shock (high cardiac index, warm extremities): noradrenaline (acts on α1 and β-1 receptors). (Dobutamine is relatively contraindicated).
- Hypodynamic septic shock (low cardiac index, cold extremities): dopamine (↑MAP with minimal ↑ of the SVR). Monitor for lack of response and the need for a 2nd agent e.g. noradrenaline. Cardiogenic shock: Dopamine (2–10mcg/kg/min): ↑MAP with minimal ↑SVR.
- Dobutamine is suggested in patients with hypotension (SBP 70–100mmHg) who do not have clinical evidence (symptoms/signs) of shock: ↑cardiac output: β-1 receptor effect and causes vasodilation/↓SVR: β-2 receptor effect.

Table 5.3 Preparation of inotrope infusions for a typical 70kg patient

Inotrope	Formulation	Volume to add to 500ml 5% glucose	Starting infusion rate	Maintenance dose
Adrenaline	1:1000 soln	2mL (2mg)	15mL/h (1µg/min)	15–180mL/h (1–12mcg/min)
Dopamine	40mg/mL	20ml (800mg)	6Ml/h (2.25mcg/kg/min)	'Renal' dose 25–13ml/h (1–5mcg/kg/min)
				'Cardiac' dose 13–26mL/h (5–10 mcg/kg/min)
Dobutamine	12.5mg/mL	40ml (500mg)	10 mL/h (2.5mcg/kg/min)	10–60mL/h (2.5–15mcg/kg/min)
Noradrenaline	2mg/mL	2ml (4mg)	15mL/h (2mcg/min)	7.5–90mL/h (1–12mcg/min)
Isoprenaline	1mg/mL	5ml (5mg)	3ml/h (0.5mcg/min)	3–60mL/h (0.5–10mcg/min)

Appendix 4: sodium bicarbonate

Pharmacology

Sodium bicarbonate is an important buffering mechanism *in vivo*. Its effects are short lived. The administration of sodium bicarbonate results in the generation of carbon dioxide, which may cause an intracellular acidosis, and is negatively inotropic, and for these reasons should be used cautiously. It may also produce a left shift in the oxygen dissociation curve, and decrease effective oxygen delivery. Mild acidosis also causes cerebral vasodilatation, and thus correction could compromise cerebral blood flow in those with cerebral oedema.

Uses

- Severe metabolic acidaemia (use in DKA is controversial)
- Severe hyperkalaemia
- Its use is best avoided in cardiac resuscitation, since adequate ventilataion and chest compression usually suffice.

Dosing

It is available as either an 8.4% solution (hypertonic, contains 1mmole HCO_3-/mL) or a 1.26 % solution (isotonic). It is usually administered as intermittent boluses of 50–100mL 8.4% sodium bicarbonate to increase arterial pH to a safe level (>7.1), and the effect on arterial pH and haemodynamics monitored.

Side effects

- Tissue extravasation causes severe necrosis. Give via a central line where possible.
- It precipitates in the line when given with calcium chloride, and can cause microemboli.

Drug interactions

Precipitates with calcium salts.

Contraindications

Arterial pH>7.2.

Chapter 6

Neurological emergencies

Coma: assessment

Presentation

Coma is a 'state of *unarousable unresponsiveness*'.

- *No evidence of arousal:* there is no spontaneous eye opening, comprehensible speech, or voluntary limb movement.
- *Unresponsive* to external stimuli and surrounding environment, although abnormal postures may be adopted, eyes may open, or grunts may be elicited in response to pain.
- *Involuntary movements*, e.g. seizures or myoclonic jerks, may occur.
- GCS (📖 p.432) is a useful way of assessing and monitoring level of consciousness.
- *Signs of brain shift* (📖 p.438) may accompany decreasing level of consciousness.

Causes

For practical purposes, it is best to divide these into

• Metabolic • Toxic • Infective • Structural lesions	with or without	• Focal brainstem signs • Lateralizing cerebral signs • Meningeal irritation.

In general, toxic and metabolic causes usually do not produce focal signs (except rarely with hypoglycaemia, liver, or renal failure), whereas infections and structural lesions do. Meningism offers a very useful clue about the cause of coma (see 'Coma with meningism').

Coma without focal/lateralizing neurological signs

- Anoxia/hypoperfusion
- Metabolic: e.g. hypo-/hyperglycaemia, acidosis/alkalosis, hypo- or hypernatraemia, hypercalcaemia, hepatic or renal failure
- Intoxications: e.g. alcohol, opiates, benzodiazepines, tricyclics, neuroleptics, lithium, barbiturates, carbon monoxide
- Endocrine: hypothyroidism
- Hypo- or hyperthermia
- Epilepsy
- Hypertensive encephalopathy.

Coma with focal/lateralizing neurological signs (due to brainstem or cerebral dysfunction)

- Vascular: cerebral haemorrhage or infarction
- Supra- or infratentorial space-occupying lesion: tumour, haematoma, abscess. In order to produce coma these either have to be within the brainstem or compress it by producing brain shift (📖 p.438).

Coma with meningism

- Meningitis, encephalitis
- Subarachnoid haemorrhage.

Assessment of severity

- GCS (📖 p.432)
- Signs of brain shift (📖 p.438) and/or brainstem compromise.

Coma: immediate management

Priorities

1. Stabilize the patient (airway, breathing, circulation). Give O_2.
2. Consider giving thiamine, glucose, naloxone, or flumazenil.
3. Examine patient. Is there meningism? Establish Glasgow Coma Scale score. Is there evidence of brainstem failure? Are there focal or lateralizing signs?
4. Plan for further investigations.
5. Observe for signs of deterioration and attempt to reverse them.

Stabilize the patient

- *Open the airway* by laying the patient on their side. Note the pattern of *breathing* (see 📖 pp.436–437). If there is apnoea or laboured or disturbed breathing, intubation and ventilation should be considered. Measure ABGs.
- *Support the circulation*. Correct hypotension with colloid and/or inotropes. If prolonged therapy is required, both require careful and frequent monitoring of CVP and/or PAWP. Search for any occult source of bleeding, e.g. intra-abdominal.
- *Treat seizures* with usual drugs (📖 p.390) but beware of over-sedation and hypotension.
- Take blood for *glucose, U&Es, calcium, liver enzymes, albumin, clotting screen, FBC, toxicology* (including urgent paracetamol and salicylate levels). Urine should be saved for *toxicology screen*.

Give thiamine, glucose, naloxone, or flumazenil

- Check blood glucose. There is a good argument for giving 50mL of 50% glucose immediately for presumed hypoglycaemia because this will usually not cause any harm.
- The only concern is that glucose may precipitate Wernicke's encephalopathy in malnourished individuals. Some clinicians therefore favour giving a bolus of *thiamine* 100–200mg IV beforehand.
- *Naloxone* should only be given if opiate intoxication is likely (small pupils) and the patient is in coma or has a markedly reduced respiratory rate. In adults naloxone 0.8–2.0mg IV should be given at intervals of 2–3min to a maximum of 10mg.
- *Flumazenil* should only be administered if benzodiazepine intoxication is likely; it is contraindicated in epileptics who have received prolonged benzodiazepine therapy. In adults flumazenil 200mcg should be given over 15sec; further 100mcg boluses may be given at 1-min intervals (usual dose is 300–600mcg maximum total dose outside intensive care setting is 1mg).
- Both naloxone and flumazenil may be given as IV infusions if drowsiness recurs but intensive care monitoring is advisable.

Box 6.1 Key points: treatments to be considered in coma

- Resuscitate (ABC, O_2).
- IV fluids to correct hypotension (and inotropes if necessary).
- Glucose (50mL of 50%) for hypoglycaemia.
- Thiamine 100–200mg IV in malnourished/alcoholic individuals before glucose (to avoid precipitating Wernicke's encephalopathy).
- Naloxone: if opiate intoxication is likely (small pupils or reduced respiratory rate). In adults 0.4–2.0mg IV may be given at intervals of 2–3min to a maximum of 10mg.
- Flumazenil: if benzodiazepine intoxication is likely. In adults: 200mcg over 15sec; further 100-mcg boluses may be given at 1-min intervals (maximum total dose outside ITU is 1mg).

Coma: clues from examination

History

If available, the assessment may be made easier. Even if the history is not extensive, a witness may help to establish whether coma commenced suddenly (suggestive of a vascular event) or whether there was a gradual decline in level of consciousness over hours or even days. Individuals known to suffer from specific diseases may be wearing a Medicalert bracelet or carrying their regular medication. An enormous amount may be learned from a rapid but thorough examination.

General examination[1,2]

This should establish the following.

- ***Core temperature*** A fever usually indicates infection but sometimes results from diencephalic lesions. Hypothermia is often forgotten as a cause for coma; the possibility of myxoedema should be considered.
- ***Heart rate and rhythm*** May indicate a dysrhythmia as the reason for poor cerebral perfusion.
- ***Blood pressure*** Prolonged hypotension of any cause will lead to anoxia and ischaemia. Apart from a cardiac cause, occult bleeding, a cause of sepsis, and drug intoxication need to be considered.
- ***Respiratory pattern*** Shallow, slow breathing should alert the examiner to the possibility of drug intoxication, e.g. opiates. Deep, rapid Kussmaul breathing suggests acidosis. Brainstem compromise can cause distinctive patterns of breathing (see 📖 Fig. 6.2, p.437).
- ***Breath*** Alcohol, ketones, hepatic, or uraemic fetor?
- ***Skin*** There may be signs of trauma to the head. Bruising over the scalp or mastoids, blood in the nostrils, or external auditory meatus raises the possibility of a basal skull fracture. A rash suggests the possibility of meningitis. Look for signs of chronic liver disease or sallow discoloration of uraemia. IV drug abuse may be suggested by needle tracks.
- ***Heart*** Occasionally bacterial endocarditis or vasculitides associated with heart murmurs present with coma.
- ***Abdomen*** Look for enlargement of organs which may give clues to the cause of coma. It is important not to miss an acute intra-abdominal event such as perforation of a viscus or a leaking aortic aneurysm.
- ***Fundi*** Papilloedema indicates raised ICP but its absence does *not* exclude that possibility. Subhyaloid haemorrhages are pathognomonic of subarachnoid haemorrhage but are rare. Changes of diabetic or hypertensive retinopathy suggest the possibility of encephalopathy 2° to these conditions.

Is there meningism?

Neck stiffness should be assessed only if it is certain that there has been no trauma to the cervical spine. ↑stiffness suggests meningeal irritation, either because of inflammation or infiltrative processes affecting the meninges, or because of the presence of blood. Meningism raises the possibility of meningitis, encephalitis, or subarachnoid haemorrhage. Start antibiotics immediately if meningitis is suspected.

Assess the GCS

This may reveal brainstem dysfunction or lateralizing signs. When testing the motor response decorticate or decerebrate posturing may become evident (see 📖 p.434). If there is a change in these signs, it may indicate brain shift (see 📖 p.438).

Look for evidence of brainstem dysfunction?

See 📖 p.434 for details.

- Test and observe:
  - Pupillary response
  - Corneal reflex
  - Resting position of eyes
  - Spontaneous eye movements
  - Oculocephalic response/doll's head manoeuvre (if no C-spine injury)
  - Oculovestibular response/caloric stimulation
  - Swallowing
  - Respiratory pattern.
- There will be evidence of brainstem failure either because there is structural damage (intrinsic lesion or extrinsic compression due to brain shift, see 📖 p.438) or because of metabolic coma such as drug intoxication with diffuse, usually reversible, dysfunction.
- If there is focal brainstem dysfunction the cause is most likely structural or intrinsic brainstem disease.
- If there is rostro-caudal progression of brainstem signs consider a herniation syndrome (📖 p.438).
- If there appears to be diffuse brainstem dysfunction, it may not be easy to distinguish between structural and metabolic aetiologies. The most important clue is that in metabolic coma, irrespective of their size, the pupils continue to react except in very few exceptional cases (atropine, hyoscine, or glutethimide intoxication will depress brainstem function and produce pupillary abnormalities).

Are there lateralizing signs?

Testing of brainstem reflexes, assessing the GCS, and general examination may reveal facial asymmetry, and differences in muscle tone, reflexes, and plantar responses between the two sides. All these features point toward the possibility of a structural lesion, although occasionally metabolic coma is associated with focal neurological signs.

References

1. Posner JB *et al.* (2007). *Plum and Posner's Diagnosis of Stupor and Coma* (Contemporary Neurology 71), 4th edn. Oxford University Press, New York.

2. Bates D (1993). The management of medical coma. *J Neurol Neurosurg Psychiat* **56:** 589–98.

Coma: management

Plan for further investigations

The history, physical examination, and/or laboratory studies may help make the diagnosis. Often, however, a diagnosis cannot be reached so rapidly. The practical approach is to divide patients according to the following scheme.

Brainstem function intact

Urgent CT head scan. This will reveal one of the following:

- Operable lesions (e.g. subdural haematoma, subarachnoid or intracerebral haemorrhage); refer as appropriate.
- Inoperable lesions; treatment is supportive.
- Normal CT: a lumbar puncture should be performed. Measure opening pressure. CSF analysis may suggest an infective process (e.g. meningitis, encephalitis) (p.355). If the CSF is normal, the most likely diagnosis is a metabolic coma.

Brainstem function not intact

- Consider whether there are signs of brain shift (p.438).
- If a herniation syndrome appears to be progressing rapidly, mannitol should be given, hyperventilation commenced, and a surgeon contacted urgently (see p.372).
- If the tempo of events is not so rapid, mannitol may be given and an urgent CT scan arranged.
- Even if the brainstem signs appear to be non-progressive, a CT scan should be arranged to exclude the possibility of an operable posterior fossa mass or haemorrhage (e.g. cerebellar haemorrhage).
- If the CT is normal, a lumbar puncture should be performed to exclude infection. If this too is normal the diagnostic possibilities are intrinsic brainstem disease not detected by CT, metabolic coma, or possibly infection, e.g. encephalitis, without leucocytic response.
- MRI is more sensitive in detecting intrinsic brainstem pathology.
- Lumbar puncture should be repeated the next day if there is no improvement in the patient's condition. Treatment is supportive.

Monitoring progress

- Regular observations of vital signs and neurological state (and GCS).
- An important cause of deterioration in structural brain lesions is brain shift leading to herniation syndromes (p.438). The emergency treatment of raised ICP is discussed on p.374.
- Other reasons for deterioration are electrolyte or metabolic changes, hypovolaemia, or fluid overload. Monitor regularly.

Prognosis

In coma due to head injury, prognosis is clearly related to GCS. Patients scoring 8 or less have a poor prognosis. In non-traumatic coma, GCS alone is not a very good predictor. Patients with drug intoxications may have low scores on admission but, in general, have good outcomes.

Prognosis in non-traumatic coma is gauged by simple features of the examination. (e.g. if after 24h pupillary responses, corneal reflexes, and oculovestibular response remain absent, survival is extremely unlikely).[1]

Reference

1. Levy DE *et al.* (1981). Prognosis in nontraumatic coma. *Arch Int Med* **94**: 293–301.

Limb weakness: assessment

History

The history should establish if there has been:

- Sudden onset or gradual progression
- Weakness or incoordination
- Upper limb or facial weakness
- Asymmetrical or symmetrical weakness
- Associated sensory symptoms, e.g. paraesthesiae or numbness
- Difficulty with swallowing, speech, micturition, or defecation
- Back or neck pain
- Systemic symptoms, e.g. malaise, fever, diarrhoea and vomiting, arthralgia
- Recent trauma
- Previous medical history, e.g. hypertension, ischaemic heart disease, stroke, diabetes, connective tissue diseases, immunosuppression
- Drug history, e.g. phenytoin, isoniazid, vincristine, metronidazole.

Examination

- ***What is the pattern of weakness?*** Some common patterns, together with associated features, are illustrated on 📖 p.342. This should help to localize the level of the lesion in the nervous system.
- ***Is the weakness upper or lower motor neuron/combination?***
- ***If upper motor neuron, is it pyramidal?*** I.e. extensor more than flexor weakness in upper limbs; flexor greater than extensor weakness in lower limbs.
- ***Is there fatiguable weakness with repetitive effort?*** As in myasthenia.
- ***Are there any involuntary movements?*** Tremor, myoclonic jerks, or fits may be noted.
- ***What is the gait like?*** This is important to test if at all possible. It may demonstrate, for example, a hemiplegic gait, ataxia (cerebellar or sensory), a waddling (myopathic) gait, steppage (lower motor neuron) gait, festinating movements of the parkinsonian patient.
- ***Is there any sensory loss? Where? Is there a 'sensory level'?*** Sensory changes are often the most difficult to elicit. Do not forget to test all modalities or to test the back of the legs up to the anal sphincter.
- ***What modalities of sensation are lost?*** Dorsal column loss produces a 'discriminatory' loss with impaired two-point discrimination, joint-position and vibration loss, and sensory ataxia. Spinothalamic loss usually produces a lack of awareness of pain and temperature.

The history and examination should help to localize the lesion and, together with the patient's age, give an indication of the likely pathological process involved.[1]

Investigations

The initial investigation of choice depends upon the likely diagnosis. Investigations to consider are given in Box 6.2.

Diagnoses not to miss

- Spinal cord compression 📖 p.422
- Guillian–Barré syndrome 📖 p.426
- Subdural haematoma 📖 p.382
- Stroke 📖 p.394.

Diagnoses to consider

- Demyelination (multiple sclerosis, post infectious, etc.)
- Malignancy (carcinomatous meningitis, intracranial mass)
- Syringomyelia
- Motor neuron disease
- Vitamin deficiency (sub-acute combined degeneration-B_{12})
- Peripheral neuropathy (toxic, DM, autoimmune, amyloid, etc.)
- TB, syphilis.

Box 6.2 Investigations to consider

- Blood tests: FBC, U&Es, LFTs, ESR, CRP, prostate specific antigen, B_{12}/folate, protein strip, syphilis serology
- CT scan
- MRI brain ± spine
- CSF analysis: protein, cells, oligoclonal bands
- Visual evoked potentials
- EMG
- NCS
- Tensilon® test
- Muscle biopsy.

Practice point

A patient who can cycle easily, but only walk yards, usually has lumbar stenosis.

Reference

1. Adapted from Lindsay KW *et al.* (1991). *Neurology and Neurosurgery Illustrated*, 2nd edn, pp.191–4. Churchill Livingstone, London.

Limb weakness: localizing the lesion

Table 6.1 Patterns of limb weakness

Monoplegia	Lesion site	Other features
Arm ± face	Contralateral cortex	• Visual field defect • Dysphasia (dominant hemisphere lesion) • Cortical sensory loss (↓ JPS and 2-point discrimination)
Leg only	Contralateral cortex	• With ipsilateral sensory deficit
	Ipsilateral spinal lesion	• Contralateral pain and temperature loss • JPS lost on same side
Hemiplegia	**Lesion site**	**Other features**
Face + arm + leg	Contralateral hemisphere	• UMN VII involvement • Impaired conciousness • Visual field defect • Dysphasia (if dominant hemisphere lesion)
	Contralateral internal capsule	• UMN VII involvement • Alert • No dysphasia (even with a dominant hemisphere lesion)
	Contralateral mid-brain lesion	• Contralateral IIIrd palsy • Impaired upgaze
Arm (± face) or leg alone	Contralateral cortex	• VII unaffected • Visual field defect • Dysphasia (if dominant hemisphere lesion) • Cortical sensory loss (↓ JPS and 2-point discrimination)
	Contralateral medullary	• Ipsilateral pain and temperature loss • Contralateral Horner's syndrome • Contralateral palatal and tongue weakness
	Ipsilateral spinal lesion	• Pain and temperature loss in contralateral leg • Ipsilateral loss of JPS • Ipsilateral Horners's
Arm, leg, and opposite face	Contralateral pons	• LMN face involvement on opposite side to weak limbs • Conjugate gaze deviation towards weak side

UMN = upper motor neurons; JPS = joint position sense

Hemiplegia	Lesion site	Other features
Arm and opposite leg 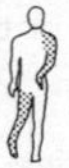	Medullary lesion	• Palatal and tongue weakness on the side of arm weakness

Paraplegia	Lesion site	Other features
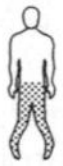	Mid-line cortical lesion	• Cortical sensory loss (JPS and 2-point discrimination) • 'Frontal' incontinence • Normal pain and temperature
	Thoracic spine	• 'Sensory level' • Acute urinary retention or hesitancy of micturition

Tetraplegia	Lesion site	Other features
Face and all four limbs involved 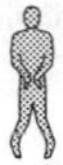	Pontine lesion	• 'Locked-in' syndrome: only vertical eye movements possible
Face spared 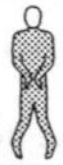	Cervical spine lesion	• No cranial nerve lesion • High lesions (C1–3) require ventilation • Lesions at C4 have intact diaphragmatic breathing
	Medullary lesion	• No palatal or tongue movement or speech but intact facial movements

Combined UMN and LMN signs
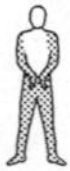 • The LMN signs point to the level of the lesion • Two lesions (e.g. cervical and lumbar spondylosis) may produce mixed signs in limbs

LMN limb weakness (unilateral or bilateral)
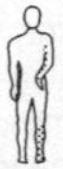 • Nerve root distribution? • Plexopathy? • Peripheral nerve distribution (mono- versus polyneuropathy) • Presence of reflexes suggests a myopathy (cf. neuropathy) • Specific distribution seen in e.g. fascioscapulohumoral dystrophy • Fatiguability suggests neuromuscular junction disease

LMN = Lower motor neurone

Acute dizziness: assessment

History

Determine whether:

- ***There is true vertigo:*** i.e. a hallucination that either the patient or their environment is rotating.
- ***Symptoms started acutely*** are progressively worsening, or are transient (see 'vertebrobasilar TIAs', 📖 p.408). Vestibular neuritis typically begins over a period of a few hours, peaks in the first day, and then improves within days. Infarction causes a vestibular syndrome that typically has an abrupt onset. TIAs often last for <30min. Abrupt onset of vertigo for seconds after a change in head position is characteristic of benign positional vertigo.[1]
- ***Symptoms worse with certain postures:*** vertigo is worse with certain head positions in benign position vertigo and some cases of central nystagmus (see Box 6.3). Postural hypotension is frequently caused by drugs and can be caused by acute blood loss; uncommonly it is due to autonomic failure. Neck movements in cervical spondylosis or carotid sinus hypersensitivity may also lead to dizziness.
- ***There is associated tinnitus*** (as in Ménière's disease).
- ***Hearing loss*** is present in Ménière's disease, cerebellopontine angle lesions, e.g. acoustic neuromas.
- ***Ear discharge*** may occur with middle ear disease.
- ***Associated focal neurological symptoms:*** e.g. unilateral weakness, clumsiness, paraesthesiae, or numbness.
- ***Headache:*** sudden onset in intracerebral haemorrhage; progressive with features of ↑ICP in mass lesions (e.g. acoustic neuroma).
- ***Any recent head injury?***
- ***Systemic symptoms:*** e.g. weakness and lethargy in anaemia.
- ***Previous medical/psychiatric history,*** e.g. hypertension, ischaemic heart disease, diabetes, risk factors for stroke or TIAs (📖 p.408), episodes of neurological disturbance, panic attacks, and anxiety.
- ***Drug history*** is pertinent to both true vertigo (e.g. phenytoin, gentamicin, furosemide) and dizziness (e.g. antihypertensives, antidepressants, drugs for Parkinson's disease, hypoglycaemics).

Examination

- ***Ear*** Is there a discharge? Is the tympanic membrane normal?
- ***Neurological examination*** should discover whether there are any focal signs due to brainstem or cerebellar disease (📖 p.434). Non-contiguous brainstem pathology may be due to patchy demyelination. Do not forget to assess the *corneal reflex*, the absence of which is one of the earliest signs of an ipsilateral acoustic neuroma. Observe the *gait* if possible; it may be ataxic. Examine *extraocular eye movements*. Is there an intranuclear ophthalmoplegia (vascular/demyelinating brainstem disease)? Examine carefully for *nystagmus* (see Box 6.3). *Hallpike manoeuvre* involves positioning the patient's head over one side of the bed and watching for nystagmus. *Benign positional vertigo:* nystagmus develops after a brief delay, but it fatigues and, with

repetition, adapts. *Central nystagmus:* no initial delay, fatigueability, or adaptation. *Fundoscopy* may reveal papilloedema (suggestive of intracranial space-occupying lesion) or optic atrophy (which occurs with previous demyelination in multiple sclerosis).
- ***General examination:*** *measure BP* (lying and standing). Postural hypotension is a common cause of dizziness.

Box 6.3 Classification of nystagmus

- ***First-degree nystagmus*** occurs only when the eyes are deviated to one side. If it occurs in the midline position as well, it is ***second degree***. Nystagmus in all directions of gaze is termed ***third degree***
- ***Vestibular nystagmus*** is due to dysfunction of the labyrinth or vestibular nerve. The slow phase is towards the lesion; the quick phase is away from the lesion. There may be rotatory nystagmus
- ***Central nystagmus*** is due to brainstem dysfunction (vestibular nuclei or their connections); there may be no vertigo associated with this form of nystagmus. The nystagmus may be horizontal, vertical, or rotatory; sometimes it is present in one eye only. The quick phase is determined by direction of gaze: it is multi-directional
- ***Positional nystagmus*** may occur in benign positional vertigo but with repeated testing it adapts. It may also occur with posterior fossa, e.g. cerebellar lesions (quick phase tends to be toward the lesion) in which there is no adaptation.

Reference

1. Hotson JR and Baloh RW (1998). Acute vestibular syndrome. *N Engl J Med* **339:** 680–5.

Acute dizziness: management

Investigations

These depend upon the likely diagnosis.

- Cerebellopontine angle lesions such as acoustic neuroma may be imaged by *CT with contrast* but, in general, posterior fossa and brainstem disease is better appraised by *MRI scanning*.
- *Pure tone audiometry* is a sensitive way of detecting sensorineural loss.
- *Cervical spine films* may reveal degenerative disease compromising vertebral artery circulation.
- Measure ***blood sugar*** and ***FBC*** if indicated.
- For management see Boxes 6.4 and 6.5.

Box 6.4 Approach to true vertigo

	Management
• ***Acute labyrinthitis***	• Bed rest • Consider cyclizine or prochlorperazine
• ***Benign positional vertigo***	• Avoid precipitating position • Epley manoeuvre
• ***Ménière's disease*** (sensorineural deafness and tinnitus)	• Bed rest • Consider cyclizine or prochlorperazine • Pure tone audiometry • ENT referral
• ***Middle ear disease***	• ENT referral
• ***Brainstem/cerebellar*** disease (stroke, see 📖 p.394; demyelination; vertebrobasilar insufficiency; migraine; vasculitis)	• Consider CT/MRI
• ***Cerebellopontine angle*** lesions (e.g. acoustic neuroma)	• Pure tone audiometry • CT, MRI scan

Box 6.5 Dizziness but no true vertigo

	Management
• *Hypotension*	Postural, cardiac, volume loss, or autonomic failure
• *Anaemia*	FBC, blood film, other investigations as necessary
• *Hypoglycaemia*	Diabetic on hypoglycaemics or insulin, insulinoma
• *Hyperventilation*	Attempt to reproduce symptoms. Explain
• *Cervical spondylosis*	A collar may be useful, if only to act as reminder
• *Carotid sinus hypersensitivity*	See 📖 p.84.

Acute loss of vision

History

Determine whether:

- Visual loss is or was monocular or binocular, complete or incomplete, e.g. hemianopia, central or peripheral loss, haziness or complete obscuration of vision.
- Loss of acuity occurred instantly ('like a curtain') as in amaurosis fugax.
- Period for which it lasted.
- There were any other associated visual symptoms, e.g. scintillations ('flashing lights and shapes') occur in retinal migraine.
- The eye is painful ± red.
- Headache or facial pain: unilateral or bilateral.
- Associated focal neurological symptoms, e.g. unilateral weakness, clumsiness, paraesthesiae, or numbness.
- Any recent trauma?
- Systemic symptoms, e.g. malaise, aches, and pains.
- Previous medical history, e.g. hypertension, ischaemic heart disease, diabetes, other risk factors for stroke or TIAs (📖 p.408), migraine, connective tissue diseases.

Examination

- ***External appearance of the eye*** Is it red (📖 p.352) Is there corneal clouding?
- ***Visual acuity*** should be measured for each eye with a Snellen chart. Near vision should be tested (with newsprint if necessary). If none of these are possible, the patient's acuity for counting number of fingers, or perceiving hand movement or light should be noted. Ideally, colour vision should also be examined with Ishihara plates.
- ***Plot the visual fields*** Often careful bedside examination is sufficient; perimetry available in ophthalmological departments is more sensitive and should be done to document the defect and recovery. The loss of vision may be incomplete.
- ***Is there an afferent pupillary defect?*** (Swinging torch test.)
- ***Fundoscopy*** may reveal a retinal embolus, changes of central/ branch retinal artery occlusion, swollen or pale optic nerve head, papilloedema, or hypertensive changes.
- ***Is the temporal artery tender?*** It need not be in temporal arteritis.
- ***Complete neurological examination*** is necessary to discover if there are any other associated signs.
- ***Listen for carotid bruits*** although they may not be present in patients with symptomatic carotid stenosis.
- ***Assess heart rhythm (including ECG) and cardiovascular*** *system* for possible cardiogenic source of embolus.
- ***Measure BP (lying and standing) and blood sugar*** Hypotension in the presence of arteriosclerosis can lead to occipital lobe ischaemia. Hypertension and diabetes are risk factors for TIAs.

Investigations

See 📖 p.398.

NB: An *ESR* should be performed in any patient aged >50 years who presents with monocular blindness and unilateral headache. It is rarely normal in temporal arteritis. If the ESR is elevated and the presentation is compatible with temporal arteritis, high-dose corticosteroid therapy should be considered (initially 60mg/day orally) because the other eye is also at risk of anterior ischaemic optic neuropathy.

Approach to acute/sub-acute visual loss

Monocular transient loss without prominent unilateral headache

- Amaurosis fugax (see 'TIAs', 📖 p.408. In the elderly this may be due to embolism. In some younger patients it is probably due to vasospasm (a diagnosis of exclusion).
- Hyperviscosity syndrome (e.g. polycythaemia, myeloma, sickle cell anaemia), hypercoagulable state, vasculitis: blood film, protein electrophoresis, autoimmune screen, other haematological investigations as required (📖 p.616).
- Postural hypotension (may exacerbate vertebrobasilar ischaemia): stop any exacerbating drugs. Exclude autonomic neuropathy.

Monocular transient loss with prominent headache

Migraine (usually there are positive phenomena, e.g. scintillations): observe, give analgesics/ergot derivative. Arrange neurological consultation.

Monocular sustained loss with red eye

- Acute glaucoma (dilated pupil and corneal clouding): urgent ophthalmology referral.
- Acute uveitis (inflammation of iris and ciliary body with small pupil), keratitis (corneal inflammation), endophthalmitis (involvent of vitreous, uvea, and retina with cellular debris/pus in anterior chamber), or ocular trauma. Urgent ophthalmic referral.

Monocular sustained loss without red eye

Central scotoma with relative afferent pupillary defect

- Optic neuritis ± orbital pain exacerbated by eye movement. The commonest cause is demyelination but consider the possibility of mass lesions compressing the optic nerve (consider evoked potentials, CT orbit).
- Anterior ischaemic optic neuropathy due to presumed atherosclerosis of posterior ciliary arteries or to temporal arteritis (consider steroids, perform ESR, temporal artery biopsy).

Central scotoma without relative afferent pupillary defect

- Vitreous haemorrhage
- Macular disorder: macular degeneration, haemorrhage, or exudate
- Branch or central retinal vein/artery occlusion.

Peripheral visual field loss

- Retinal detachment
- Chorioretinitis
- Intraocular tumour
- Retinal vascular occlusion.

Binocular sustained loss

- Field loss (e.g. quadrantonopia, hemianopia, bitemporal) → CT scan.
- Hypotension (e.g. cardiac failure) → posterior circulation insufficiency. Dysrhythmias or vertebrobasilar insufficiency may produce transient episodes of binocular visual loss. CT scan.
- Toxic optic neuropathies (e.g. tobacco, alcohol, methanol).
- Genetic (e.g. Leber's heriditary optic neuropathy).

Painful red eye: assessment

History

This should establish if there has been:

- ***Ocular trauma or foreign body (including contact lens) in the eye.***
- ***Sudden or gradual onset of symptoms, nature, and location of pain:*** irritation, soreness, or gritty sensations may occur with conjunctivitis but the pain is severe in acute glaucoma.
- ***Diminution of visual acuity*** occurs with conditions affecting the cornea (variable reduction), iris (mild reduction), and glaucoma (severe reduction of acuity).
- ***Discharge*** (not simply lacrimation) *from eyes* may be mucopurulent with bacterial or chlamydial conjunctivitis. It may be mucid and stringy with allergic conditions or dry eyes.
- ***Headache or facial pain*** is common with orbital cellulitis. It may precede cavernous sinus thrombosis or herpes zoster ophthalmicus.
- ***Photophobia*** suggests corneal involvement or iritis.
- ***Systemic symptoms***: e.g. malaise/fever, occurs with orbital cellulitis and cavernous sinus thrombosis, vomiting is a feature of acute glaucoma, arthralgias + urethral discharge suggests Reiter's or chlamydial infection.
- ***Previous history:*** recurrent red eyes may occur with episcleritis, iritis, herpes simplex corneal ulcer. Ask specifically about ↑BP, heart disease, diabetes, connective tissue diseases, and atopy.

Examination

- ***What is red?*** The conjunctiva, iris, sclera, or episclera (which lies just beneath the conjunctiva and next to the sclera), eye lid, skin around orbit? Is there a visible haemorrhage, either sub-conjuctival or in the anterior chamber (hyphaema)? In conjunctivitis there is 'injection' or ↑filling of existing light red vessels, with individual branches distinctly visible; the vessels can be moved with the conjunctiva over the sclera. Ciliary or circumcorneal injection refers to a blue–red discolouration, most conspicuous at the limbus (cornea–scleral border) and occurs in anterior uveitis or iritis and keratitis (corneal inflammation). Mixed injection (conjunctival + ciliary) also occurs in uveitis.
- ***Is there proptosis?*** Suggests a retro-orbital/intraoribtal mass or cavernous sinus thrombosis in which it may become bilateral.
- ***Is it pulsatile?*** As in a carotico-cavernous fistula, with an audible bruit.
- ***Is there ophthalmoplegia?*** (Mass lesion or cavenous sinus thrombosis.)
- ***Is visual acuity diminished?*** A Snellen chart should be used and near vision tested (with newsprint if necessary). In acute glaucoma, there is marked reduction in acuity; in acute iritis or keratitis, acuity is only modestly diminished; in conjunctivitis it is normal.
- ***What is the size of the pupil?*** Fixed and dilated in acute glaucoma; small with reduced reaction to light in iritis; normal in conjunctivitis.
- ***Is the red reflex normal?*** *If it is, does the cornea appear normal?* The red reflex may be impaired in keratitis, central corneal ulcer or oedema, anterior chamber hyphaema (blood in anterior chamber after blunt trauma), anterior uveitis, glaucoma, or endophthalmitis (involvent of vitreous, uvea, and retina with cellular debris/pus in anterior chamber). *Fundoscopy* may not be possible as with the corneal clouding of acute glaucoma.

- ***Are there any anterior chamber abnormalities?*** In acute anterior uveitis there are exudates in the anterior chamber.
- ***Is there a rash or vesicles on the face, nose, or eyelid?*** Herpes zoster can lead to conjunctivitis, iritis, corneal ulceration, and 2° glaucoma.

Table 6.2 Differential diagnosis of 'red-eye'*

	Conjunctiva	Iris	Pupil	Cornea	Anterior chamber	Intraocular pressure	Appearance
Acute glaucoma	Both ciliary and conjunctival vessels injected. Entire eye is red	Injected	Dilated, fixed, oval	Steamy, hazy	Very slow	Very high	
Iritis	Redness most marked around cornea Colour does not blanch on pressure	Injected	Small, fixed	Normal	Turgid	Normal	
Conjunctivitis	Conjunctival vessels injected, greatest toward fornices Blanch on pressure. Mobile over sclera	Normal	Normal	Normal	Normal	Normal	
Subconjunctival haemorrhage	Bright red sclera with white rim around limbus	Normal	Normal	Normal	Normal	Normal	

*After Judge RD *et al.* (1989). *Clinical Diagnosis*, 5th edn. Little Brown, Boston, MA http://iww.com

Painful red eye: management

With a careful history and examination, the diagnosis may become clear. *Unless you are absolutely sure of the diagnosis, discuss the patient with an ophthalmologist.*

Diagnosis of painful red eye in non-traumatic cases

With prominent ocular discharge

- Viral/bacterial conjunctivitis (watery/mucopurolent discharge, normal red reflex, normal pupil)
- Bacterial/fungal keratitis (mucopurolent discharge, opaque cornea with impaired red reflex, normal or slightly reduced pupil)
- Keratoconjunctivitis sicca or atopic response (dry eye, mucoid strands).

Without prominent discharge and normal red reflex

Normal cornea

- Episcleritis, scleritis, or sub-conjunctival haemorrhage
- Orbital cellulitis (skin around orbit erythematous and tender)
- Carotico-cavernous fistula (dilated conjunctival vessels, forehead veins, and choroidal vessels because of 'arterialization', reduced acuity because of optic nerve ischaemia, pulsatile proptosis, and bruit)
- Cavernous sinus thrombosis (fever, acute onset painful ophthalmoplegia, conjunctival oedema and congestion, proptosis, oedema over mastoid (emissary vein) → may progress to meningitis).

Abnormal cornea

Corneal abrasion or ulcer (NB: herpes simplex and herpes zoster).

Without prominent discharge and impaired red reflex

- Acute glaucoma (severe pain, markedly reduced acuity, cloudy cornea, purple congestion at limbus, fixed dilated pupil, rock–hard globe)
- Acute anterior uveitis (malaise, clear cornea, blue–red congestion at limbus, anterior chamber exudate, iris muddy and injected, small pupil with reduced response to light)
- Endophthalmitis (reduced acuity, eyelid swelling, conjunctival injection, anterior chamber cellular debris, vitreous clouding, retinal haemorrhages)
- Keratitis (red congestion at limbus, pupil normal or reduced in size, cornea opaque)
- Central corneal ulcer.

Acute bacterial meningitis: assessment

Presentation

- ***Headache, fever, neck stiffness (absent in 18% of patients),***[1] ***photophobia*** (often over hours to days).
- ***Rash:*** meningococcal meningitis is most commonly associated with a macular rash progressing to petechiae or purpura (see 📖 p.462) but other organisms may also cause a rash.
- ***Confusion, psychiatric disturbance*** (e.g. mania) or ***altered level of consciousness.*** In the elderly (especially those with diabetes mellitus or cardiopulmonary disease) and the immunocompromised or neutropenic, there may be little other than confusion.
- ***Focal neurological signs*** complicate meningitis in at least 15% of cases. These can suggest cerebral damage (e.g. hemiparesis following venous infarction or arteritis) or indicate cranial nerve and brainstem involvement by basal exudation and inflammation (e.g. in *Listeria monocytogenes* meningitis). They can also indicate brain shift 2° to raised ICP (see 📖 p.438). Consider the possibility of brain abscess or encephalitis if focal signs or seizures are prominent.[2] Papilloedema is uncommon (<1%) and should suggest an alternative diagnosis.
- ***Seizures*** are the presenting feature in up to 30%.

Predisposing factors

Usually none, but acute otitis media, mastoiditis, pneumonia, head injury, sickle cell disease, alcoholism, previous influenza infection, and immunocompromised states are all associated.

Causes in adults

Common
- Neisseria meningitidis
- *Strep. pneumoniae*

Rarer
- Gram-negative bacilli (in elderly)
- *Listeria* (in elderly)

Assessment of severity

Mortality ↑ as consciousness ↓ (~55% for adults in coma). *However*, meningitis can proceed with alarming rapidity even in the most alert patients.

Management

1. Stabilize the patient (Airway, Breathing, Circulation); give O_2.
2. Commence antibiotics. It is *not* necessary to await CSF analysis.
3. CT scan prior to lumbar puncture (this is the safest option).
4. Make a definitive diagnosis with lumbar puncture.
5. Reconsider antibiotic regimen after CSF analysis. Consider adjunctive corticosteroid therapy.
6. Arrange for contacts (including medical/nursing staff) to have prophylaxis. Notify the public health service.
7. Observe for and, if necessary, treat complications.

References

1. Consensus Statement on Diagnosis, Investigation, Treatment and Prevention of Acute Bacterial Meningitis in Immunocompetent Adults (1999). *J Infect* **39:** 1–15.

2. Anderson M (1993). Management of cerebral infection. *J Neurol Neurosurg Psychiat* **56:** 1243–58.

Acute bacterial meningitis: immediate management

Antibiotic therapy: follow your hospital guidelines if available

- Adult patients with a typical meningococcal rash should be given IV *benzylpenicillin* 2.4g (4MU) every 4h. Adults between 18–50 without a rash should receive *cefotaxime* 2g q8h or *ceftriaxone* 2g every 12h. For adults over 50 without a rash, consider addition of 2g ampicillin every 4h to cefotaxime or ceftriaxone as above (to cover *Listeria*). If the patient comes from an area of the world where penicillin and cephalosporin-resistant pneumococci are common (e.g. mediterranean countries) then add IV *vancomycin* 500mg every 6h. If the individual is allergic to penicillin, consider IV *chloramphenicol* 25mg/kg every 6h with *vancomycin* 500mg every 6h. Additional co-trimoxazole should be given in those over 50. Discuss the case with your microbiologist.
- *Blood cultures* should be taken but it is dangerous to withhold IV antibiotics until these are taken or lumbar puncture is performed. Most organisms will be diagnosed from blood cultures.
- Meningococcal infections are discussed on 📖 p.462.

CT scan

Our policy is that all patients should have a CT scan prior to lumbar puncture. Others suggest this need be performed only if there is ↓level of consciousness, focal signs, papilloedema (very unusual in meningitis), or signs suggesting impending cerebral herniation (📖 p.438). You should discuss the patient with a senior member of your team.

Lumbar puncture

- ***Measure opening pressure*** CSF pressure is often raised (>14cm CSF) in meningitis and there are only a few reports of cerebral herniation (coning) following the procedure. If the pressure is raised the patient must be observed closely at no less than 15-min intervals. A CT scan is required to exclude a complication of meningitis or a space-occupying lesion, e.g. cerebral abscess.
- ***Analysis of CSF*** (see Table 6.3)
  - *CSF WCC:* bacterial meningitis characteristically demonstrates a high (usually >1000/mm^3) WCC with predominance of neutrophils. A low CSF WCC (0–20/mm^3) with high bacterial count on Gram stain is associated with a poor prognosis
  - *CSF glucose:* usually reduced (CSF:blood glucose ratio <0.31 in ~70%) but may be normal
  - *CSF protein*: usually elevated (>1.0 g/L)
  - *Gram stain:* is positive in 60–90% but may not be if there has been a delay between starting antibiotics and lumbar puncture. Also the yield of CSF culture falls to <50% from 70–85%.

This CSF profile may also occur with viral and TB meningitis in the early phase, but repeat CSF analysis shows transformation to a lymphocytic predominance. Patients with a CSF profile characteristic of bacterial meningitis should be treated as if they have this condition until proven otherwise.

Table 6.3 CSF composition in meningitis

	Bacterial	Viral	TB meningitis
Appearance	Turbid	Clear	Clear
Cells (per mm^3)	5–2000	5–500	5–1000
Main cell type	Neutrophil	Lymphocyte	Lymphocyte
Glucose (mM)	Very low	Normal	Low
Protein (g/L)	Often >1.0	0.5–0.9	Often >1.0
Other tests	Gram stain	PCR	Ziehl–Neelsen
	Bacterial antigen		Fluorescent test
			PCR

See 📖 p.808 for reference intervals for CSF analysis

Box 6.6 Management key points: bacterial meningitis

- GPs should give benzylpenicillin or a third-generation cephalosporin (cefotaxime or ceftriaxone) before urgent transfer to hospital. Give chloramphenicol if there is a history of anaphylaxis to penicillin or cephalosporins.
- Initial blind therapy: third-generation cephalosporin (cefotaxime 2g qds or ceftriaxone 2g bd)
- Meningococci: benzylpenicillin or third-generation cephalosporin for at least 5 days. (Chloramphenicol if there is history of anaphylaxis to these). Give rifampicin for 2 days to patients treated with benzylpenicillin or chloramphenicol (to eliminate nasopharyngeal carriage).
- Pneumococci: third-generation cephalosporin or benzylpenicillin (if penicillin-sensitive) for 10–14 days. If penicillin- and cephalosporin-resistant pneumococci: add vancomycin (+ if necessary rifampicin)
- *Haemophilus influenzae*: third-generation cephalosporin for at least 10 days (chloramphenicol if there is history of anaphylaxis to penicillin or cephalosporins or if the organism is resistant to these)
- *Listeria*: amoxicillin + gentamicin.
- Adjunctive dexamethasone in suspected pneumococcal or *H. influenzae* meningitis. Avoid in septic shock, meningococcal disease, immunocompromised patients or in meningitis following surgery.
- Notify public health services and consult a consultant in communicable disease control for advice regarding chemoprophylaxis and vaccination for close contacts:
  - *Neisseria meningitides* (to eradicate pharyngeal carriage) in adults: rifampicin (600 mg PO, every 12h, total of 4 dose) or ciprofloxacin (500 mg PO once) or ceftriaxone (250 mg IM once).
  - *H. influenzae:* rifampicin (600mg od for 4 days in adults).

Acute bacterial meningitis: continuing therapy

Reconsider antibiotics? Adjunctive steroids?

- ***CSF lymphocytosis:*** if the CSF pleocytosis is predominantly lymphocytic the diagnosis is unlikely to be bacterial meningitis. This is discussed further on 📖 p.360
- ***CSF polymorphs >50,000/mm³*** suggests possibility of cerebral abscess. A CT brain scan should be performed.
- ***CSF Gram stain:*** if Gram –ve diplococci are visible, continue with 2.4g *benzylpenicillin* IV every 4h or 2g *ampicillin* IV 4-hourly. Discuss the case with your microbiologist. If Gram +ve diplococci are visible give 2g *cefotaxime* IV 6-hourly and consider adding *vancomycin* 500mg IV 6-hourly. If Gram +ve cocco-bacilli suggestive of *Listeria monocytogenes* are visible give *ampicillin* 2g 4-hourly IV and *gentamicin* 5mg/kg/24h IV as a single daily dose or divided into 8-hourly doses.
- ***Adjunctive corticosteroid therapy*** has been shown to reduce the incidence of neurological sequelae in adults and children, especially in pneumococcal meningitis[1,2] and many neurologists now favour its use to reduce inflammation. In patients with raised ICP, stupor, or impaired mental status, give 10mg dexamethasone IV loading dose, followed by 4–6mg PO q6h.

Prophylaxis for contacts should be given immediately

- ***Public health services*** should be notified of any case of bacterial meningitis. They will be able to give advice on current prophylactic treatment and vaccination (possible with some strains of meningococcus); they will also assist in contact tracing. Patients with meningococcus are infectious and can spread organisms to others. Liaise with your local microbiologists.
- ***Prophylaxis*** should be given as soon as the diagnosis of bacterial meningitis is suspected. In the UK, for adult contacts, rifampicin 600mg bd for 2 days is recommended. The alternative for adults is ciprofloxacin 750mg as a single dose (for children older than 1 year: 10mg/kg bd for 2 days; for children 3 months–1 year: 5mg/kg bd for 2 days).

References

1. De Gans J *et al.* (2002). Dexamethasone in adults with bacterial meningitis. *N Engl J Med* **347:** 1549–56.

2. Van de Beek D *et al.* (2003). Corticosteroids in acute bacterial meningitis. *Cochrane Database Syst Rev* **3:** CD004405.

Acute bacterial meningitis: complications and their treatment

- ***Raised ICP*** may respond to steroids and, as discussed earlier, some neurologists give this routinely to reduce inflammatory reaction. In the acute situation, if there is evidence of brain shift or impending transtentorial herniation (📖 p.438) mannitol should be given 1g/kg over 10–15min (~250mL of 20% solution for an average adult) and the head of the bed elevated to 30° (see 📖 p.373). Oral glycerol has also been shown to be effective in some small trials.
- ***Hydrocephalus*** (diagnosed by CT) may require an intraventricular shunt and should be discussed urgently with neurosurgeons. It can occur because of thickened meninges obstructing CSF flow or because of the adherence of the inflamed lining of the aqueduct of Sylvius or fourth ventricular outflow. Papilloedema may not be present.
- ***Seizures*** should be treated as seizures of any other aetiology (see 📖 p.390).
- ***Persistent pyrexia*** suggests that there may be an occult source of infection. The patient should be carefully re-examined (including oral cavity and ears).
- ***Focal neurological deficit*** may occur because of arteritis or venous infarction or space-occupying lesion, e.g. subdural empyema. Inflammatory reaction at the base of the skull may lead to cranial nerve palsies. A CT scan should be requested if it has not already been performed. Anticoagulation is not of benefit for treatment of thromboses.
- ***Subdural empyema*** is a rare complication. Focal signs, seizures, and papilloedema suggest the diagnosis. It requires urgent surgical drainage.
- ***Disseminated intravascular coagulation*** is an ominous sign. Platelet and FFP may be required. The use of heparin should be discussed with a haematologist and neurologist.
- ***Syndrome of inappropriate ADH*** may occur. Fluid balance and electrolytes need to be checked regularly.

Meningitis with lymphocytic CSF

Presentation

- Viral meningitis may be indistinguishable on clinical grounds from acute early bacterial meningitis but it is usually self-limiting.
- TB meningitis is usually preceded by a history of malaise and systemic illness for days to weeks before meningeal features develop. However, it may present very acutely. TB meningitis may be associated with basal archnoditis, vasculitis, and infarction leading to focal neurological signs, e.g. cranial nerve palsies, obstructive hydrocephalus with papilloedema.
- Cryptococcal or syphilitic meningitis in the immunocompromised present with features indistinguishable from TB meningitis.

Causes

Viral

- Coxsackie
- Echo
- Mumps
- Herpes simplex type 1
- Varicella zoster
- HIV
- Lymphocytic choriomeningitis virus

Non-viral

- TB
- Cryptococcus
- Leptospirosis
- Lyme disease
- Syphilis
- Brucellosis
- Paramenigeal infection with a CSF reaction

CSF findings

The CSF usually demonstrates a lymphocytosis but the CSF in viral meningitis may initially demonstrate predominantly neutrophils. It is important not to dismiss the possibility of TB meningitis if CSF glucose is normal; it may be in ~20% of cases and the tuberculin test may also be negative initially in a similar percentage. *M. tuberculosis* is seen in the initial CSF of approximately 40% of patients with TB meningitis. Send CSF for viral and TB PCR.

Treatment regimens

- *Viral meningitis:* usually supportive treatment only.
- *TB meningitis:* pyrazinamide 30mg/kg/day and isoniazid 10mg/kg/day (up to a max of 600mg/day) achieve best CSF penetration. Give pyridoxine 10mg daily as prophylaxis against isoniazid neuropathy. For the first 3 months, add rifampicin (450mg/day if wt <50kg or 600mg/day if wt >50kg) and ethambutol (25mg/kg/day) if the patient is not unconscious. Thereafter, for the next 7–10 months, give isoniazid (at a lower dose of 300mg/day) and rifampicin. Consult your local respiratory/ID specialists for advice. Consider HIV status.
- There are several other regimens in use for *M. tuberculosis* meningitis; *M. avium intracellulare* requires a different combination of drugs.[1] *Corticosteroids* are often prescribed if there are focal signs, raised ICP, or very high levels of CSF protein (see 📖 p.358).

- *Cryptococcal meningitis:* several regimens are used. Amphotericin 0.6–1.0mg/kg/day alone or at a lower dose of 0.5mg/kg/day in conjunction with flucytosine 150mg/kg/day for 6 weeks appears effective. Fluconazole (400mg/day initially, then 200–400mg/day for 6–8 weeks) is an alternative which appears to be as effective in AIDs.

Reference

1. Berger JR (1994). Tuberculous meningitis. *Curr Opin Neurol* **7:** 191–200.

Acute viral encephalitis

Presentation

- *Change in personality.*
- *Confusion, psychiatric disturbance or altered level of consciousness.*
- *Headache, fever and some neck stiffness.* Meningism is usually not prominent: some individuals have a meningo-encephalitis.
- *Focal neurological signs.* Hemiparesis or memory loss (usually indicative of temporal lobe involvement) is not uncommon.
- *Seizures* are common; some are complex partial in nature.
- *Raised ICP* and signs of brain shift (📖 p.438).
- *Predisposing factors:* immunocompromised patient.

Management

1. Antibiotic therapy

If there is any suspicion that the illness is meningitis, start antibiotics (📖 p.356). It is not necessary to await CSF analysis.

2. Specific antiviral therapies

Aciclovir has dramatically reduced mortality and morbidity in HSV encephalitis. Most clinicians therefore give it in suspected encephalitis without waiting for confirmation that the pathogen is herpes simplex.

- *Aciclovir* 10mg/kg IV (infused over 60min) every 8h (reduced dose in renal insufficiency) is given for 10–14 days.
- *Ganciclovir* 2.5–5.0mg/kg IV (infused over 60min) every 8h should be given if cytomegalovirus is a possible pathogen (more likely in renal transplant patients or those with AIDS). Treatment is usually for 14–28 days depending upon response.

3. CT scan: scan all patients prior to LP

In a patient with focal neurological signs, focal seizures, or signs of brain shift a CT scan must be arranged urgently. CT may not demonstrate any abnormalities. In herpes simplex encephalitis there may be low attenuation areas, particularly in the temporal lobes, with surrounding oedema. MR imaging is more sensitive to these changes.

4. Lumbar puncture

- *Measure opening pressure.* CSF pressure may be raised (>14cm CSF) in which case the patient must be observed closely at 15-min intervals.
- *Analysis of CSF* usually reveals a lymphocytic leukocytosis (usually 5–500/mm^3) in viral encephalitis, but it may be entirely normal. The red cell count is usually elevated. PCR on CSF is sensitive and specific. CSF protein is only mildly elevated and glucose is normal.

5. Further investigations

- *Serology:* save serum for viral titres (IgM and IgG). If infectious mononucleosis is suspected a monospot test should be performed.
- *EEG:* should be arranged even in those without seizures. There may be generalized slowing and, in herpes simplex encephalitis, there may be bursts of periodic high-voltage slow wave complexes over temporal cortex.

Complications

Neurological observations should be made regularly. Two complications may require urgent treatment.

- ***Raised ICP*** 2° to cerebral oedema may require treatment with dexamethasone (see 📖 p.376). There is some experimental evidence that steroids may potentiate spread of herpes virus, so dexamethasone should not be given prophylactically without a specific indication. In the acute situation, if there is evidence of brain shift, mannitol may be used (see 📖 p.373). Another cause of raised ICP is haemorrhage within necrotic tissue. Perform a CT if there is any deterioration in the patient and discuss with neurosurgeons.
- ***Seizures*** may be difficult to control but are treated as seizures of any other aetiology.

Causes in UK

- Herpes simplex
- Varicella zoster
- Coxsackie
- Cytomegalovirus (in immunocompromised)
- Mumps
- Epstein–Barr virus
- Echovirus.

Box 6.7 Management key points: viral encephalitis

- ***Antiviral therapies:*** aciclovir without waiting for confirmation of HSV: 10mg/kg IV infused over 60min, tds (reduced dose in renal insufficiency) for 10–14 days. Ganciclovir if CMV is a possible pathogen (renal transplant patients or in AIDS).
- ***Antibiotics*** if there is any suspicion of meningitis. Do not delay treatment because of investigations (i.e. CT and LP).

Head injury: presentation

- Varies from transient 'stunning' for a few seconds to coma.
- A fraction of patients who attend A&E need to be admitted for observation (indications for admission are given in in Box 6.13, p.369).

In the alert patient, determine the following.

- ***Circumstances surrounding injury*** Was it caused by endogenous factors, e.g. loss of consciousness whilst driving? Or exogenous factors, e.g. another driver? Was there extracranial trauma?
- ***Period of loss of consciousness*** This relates to severity of diffuse brain damage.
- ***Period of post-traumatic amnesia*** The period of permanent memory loss after injury also reflects degree of damage (NB: period of retrograde amnesia or memory loss for events prior to injury does not correlate with severity of brain damage).
- ***Headache/vomiting*** Common after head injury but if they persist raised ICP should be considered (p.372).
- ***GCS score.***
- ***Skull fracture present?***
- ***Neurological signs*** Are there any focal neurological signs?
- ***Extracranial injury*** Is there evidence of occult blood loss?

The drowsy or unconscious patient needs the following:

- ***Urgent assistance from senior A&E staff and anaesthetists.***
- ***Protection of airway*** The patient who has deteriorating level of consciousness or is in coma should be intubated because hypocarbia and adequate oxygenation are effective means of reducing ICP rapidly. If the patient is neurologically stable and protecting their airway, intubation may not be necessary. Assume there is a cervical spine injury until an XR (of all 7 cervical vertebrae) demonstrates otherwise.
- ***Hyperventilation*** The pattern of breathing should be noted (p.436). Hyperventilation of intubated patients with the aim of lowering P_aCO_2 is controversial: consult an intensivist.
- ***Support of circulation*** Hypotension should be treated initially with colloid. If persistent or severe, exclude a cardiac cause (ECG) and occult haemorrhage (e.g. intra-abdominal).
- ***Treatment of seizures*** Diazepam 5–10mg IV/rectally which may be repeated to a maximum of 20mg. If seizures continue, consider IV phenytoin (see p.390).
- ***Rapid survey of chest, abdomen, and limbs.*** Looking for a flail segment or haemo/pneumothorax, possible intra-abdominal bleeding (if there are any doubts peritoneal lavage may be required), limb lacerations, and long bone fractures.
- ***Brief history*** Should be obtained from ambulance crew or relatives. The patient may have lost consciousness just before the injury, e.g. due to subarcahnoid haemorrhage, seizure, or hypoglycaemia. The tempo of neurological deterioration should be established.
- ***Guidelines for performing skull X-rays and CT scans*** are on p.366.

Box 6.8 Symptoms following head injury

Symptoms associated with minor head injury

Headache, dizziness, fatigue, reduced concentration, memory deficit, irritability, anxiety, insomnia, hyperacusis, photophobia, depression, and general slowed information processing.

Symptoms associated with moderate to severe head injury

As for minor head injury, but also:

- *Behavioural problems* include irritability, impulsivity, egocentricity, emotional lability, impaired judgment, impatience, anxiety, depression, hyper- or hyposexuality, dependency, euphoria, aggressiveness, apathy, childishness, and disinhibition.
- *Cognitive impairment* includes deficits of memory, difficulty in abstract thinking, general slowed information processing, poor concentration, slow reaction time, impaired auditory comprehension, reduced verbal fluency, anomia, and difficulty planning or organizing.

Head injury: assessment

Examination

Rapid neurological assessment should take only a few minutes

- The level of consciousness must be noted with GCS score (📖 p.432).
- Note the size, shape, and reactions of pupils to bright light.
- Resting eye position and spontaneous eye movements should be observed. If the latter are not full and the patient unresponsive, test oculocephalic and/or oculovestibular responses (📖 p.440).
- The doll's head manoeuvre should not be attempted if cervical spine injury has not been excluded.
- Test the corneal reflex (cranial nerves V and VII).
- Motor function should be assessed (see 📖 p.432); any asymmetry should be noted.
- Look for features suggesting brain shift and herniation (📖 p.438).

Head and spine assessment

- The skull should be examined for a fracture. Extensive periorbatal haematomas, bruising behind the ear (Battle's sign), bleeding from the ear, and CSF rhinorrhoea/otorrhoea suggest a basal skull fracture. Look for facial (maxillary and mandibular) fractures.
- Only 1% of patients will have a skull fracture. This greatly increases the chances of an intracranial haematoma (from 1:1000 to 1:30 in alert patients; from 1:100 to 1:4 in confused/comatose patients). NB: potentially fatal injuries are not always associated with skull fracture.
- *Consider* the possibility of spinal cord trauma. 'Log-roll' the patient and examine the back for tenderness over the spinous processes, paraspinal swelling, or a gap between the spinous processes. The limbs may have been found to be flaccid and unresponsive to pain during the neurological assessment. There may be painless retention of urine.

Box 6.9 Indications for skull X-ray

- History of high-impact injury
- ↓level of consciousness
- Amnesia
- Nausea/vomiting
- Neurological signs/symptoms
- CSF/blood from nose/ear
- Scalp bruising/swelling
- Suspected penetrating injury
- Difficulty in clinical assessment (e.g. alcohol, drugs, very young/elderly)
- Seizures
- If GCS <12/15, arrange an urgent head CT.

Box 6.10 Things to look for on skull X-rays

- Linear skull fracture
- Depressed skull fracture (requires elevation if depressed by more than the vault thickness)
- >3mm shift of a calcified pineal (if present)
- Integrity of craniocervical junction
- Fluid level in sphenoid sinus.

Box 6.11 Definite indications for CT scan*

- Skull fracture and persistent neurological dysfunction
- Depressed level of consciousness and/or neurological dysfunction (inc. seizures)
- Coma after resuscitation
- Suspected compound fracture of vault or base of skull (e.g. CSF leak)
- Skull fracture
- Confusion/neurological disturbance persisting >12h
- Seizure
- Significant head injury requiring general anaesthaesia.

*Adapted from *Report of the Working Party on the Management of with Head Injuries* (1999). Royal College of Surgeons of England, London.

Box 6.12 Things to look for on C-spine films

- Check all 7 C-spine vertebrae and C7-T1 junction are visible
- Check alignment
  - Anterior and posterior of vertebral bodies
  - Posterior margin of spinal canal
  - Spinous processes

A step of >25% of vertebral body suggests facet joint dislocation

- Check contours
  - Outlines of vertebral bodies
  - Outlines of spinous processes

Look for avulsion fractures, wedge fractures (>3mm height difference between anterior and posterior body height)

- Check odontoid
  - Open mouth and lateral views
- The distance between ant. arch C1 and odontoid should be <3mm disc space and odontoid
  - Disc spaces
  - Space between anterior C3 and back pharyngeal shadow >5mm suggests retropharyngeal mass (e.g. abscess or haematoma from fracture of C2)
- Check soft tissues

Head injury: immediate management

- After resuscitation, *take blood* for *FBC, G&S, U&Es, ABGs* and if the circumstances of injury are not clear or there is a suspicion of drug intoxication, *toxicology screen*.
- Indications for admission (Box 6.13).
- *Subsequent* management depends upon the pace of events and the clinical situation. >40% comatose patients with head injury have intracranial haematomas and it is not possible definitively to distinguish between these patients and those who have diffuse brain injury and swelling on clinical examination alone.
- *Urgent CT scan*. This is the next step in most patients who have depressed level of consciousness or focal signs (see 🕮 Box 6.11, p.367). The speed with which this needs to be arranged depends upon the tempo of neurological deterioration (relative change in GCS score, 🕮 p.432) and/or the absolute level of consciousness (GCS <8). If CT scanning is not available at your hospital you must discuss with your regional neurosurgical centre.
- *Treatment of raised ICP* is discussed on 🕮 p.372; corticosteroids have no proven benefit. Discuss with your neurosurgical centre. In a rapidly deteriorating situation it may be necessary to proceed directly to surgery. It may be decided to hyperventilate and to give mannitol (1g/kg over 10–15min or ~250mL of 20% solution for an average adult) and furosemide (20–40mg IV) while obtaining an urgent CT scan.
- *Surgery* may be indicated for extradural (🕮 p.378), subdural (🕮 p.382), and possibly some intracerebral haemorrhages (🕮 p.380) and complex head wounds such as compound depressed skull fractures.
    - A general rule is urgent evacuation is required of extradural haematomas which produce mid-line shift of 5mm or more and/or 25mL in calculated volume.
    - If the extradural haemorhage is considered too small to warrant surgery on a CT scan performed within 6h of injury, the scan should be repeated after a few hours irrespective of whether there has been a deterioration in the patient's condition.
- *Non-operative management*. Brain contusion may be evident as areas of ↑ or ↓ density but CT is not a sensitive way to detect 1° diffuse brain injury. Effacement of the cavity of the third ventricle and of the perimesencephalic cisterns suggests raised ICP but the absence of these signs is not to be taken as an indicator or normal ICP. Many centres therefore proceed to ICP monitoring (🕮 p.804) although this is a controversial subject.
- Points for patients being discharged, Box 6.14.

Box 6.13 Indications for admission following head injury

- Confusion
- Abnormal CT scan
- ↓level of consciousness (<15/15)
- Clinical or radiological evidence of skull fracture
- Neurological signs or severe headache + vomiting
- Difficulty in assessment (e.g. alcohol, drugs, very young/elderly)
- Concurrent medical conditions (e.g. clotting disorders, diabetes)
- Poor social circumstances/living alone.

NB: very brief loss of consciousness or post-traumatic amnesia is not an absolute indicator for admission but each patient needs to be assessed on their own merits.

Box 6.14 If patients are discharged they should be sent home with

- A responsible adult who will be with them over the next 24h
- A head injury card which describes potential signs and symptoms (e.g. undue sleepiness, headache, vomiting, or dizziness) of delayed neurological dysfunction.

Head injury: further management

The aim of subsequent management is to minimize 2° injury to the brain other than intracranial haematomas (see Box 6.15). Management may be better undertaken at a neurosurgical centre and if this is arranged the guidelines in Box 6.15 should be followed for transfer.

The principles of management are

- ***Regular and frequent neurological observation*** If there is deterioration consider whether there may be a 2° cause of brain injury contributing to this (see Box 6.16). If there are new signs of raised ICP, declining level of consciousness, or signs of transtentorial herniation (📖 p.438), the patient requires intubation and hyperventilation if this has not already been performed. Mannitol may be started or a repeat bolus may need to be given (see 📖 p.373) and repeat CT scanning may be necessary.
- ***Regular monitoring of BP, blood gases, electrolytes, urinary output*** Pre-emptive treatment of a decline in any of these may prevent neurological deterioration. Hypotension is commonly due to sedative agents and/or hypovolaemia. But fluid therapy needs to be conducted with care because overgenerous administration may exacerbate raised ICP. Monitor CVP.
- ***Prompt treatment of seizures*** (📖 p.390).
- ***Nasogastric tube*** to administer nutrition and drugs including ranitidine 150mg bd for prophylaxis against gastric ulceration.
- ***A bowel regimen*** of stool softeners should be started.

Before transfer to Neurosurgical Unit[1]

- Assess clinically for respiratory insufficiency, shock, and internal injuries.
- Perform CXR, ABG estimation, cervical spine XR.
- Appropriate treatment might be to:
  - Intubate (e.g. if airway obstructed or threatened)
  - Ventilate (e.g. cyanosis, P_aO_2 <7.9kPa, P_aCO_2 >5.9kPa)
  - Commence IV fluids carefully
  - Give mannitol, after consultation with neurosurgeon
  - Apply cervical collar or cervical traction.
- Patient should be accompanied by personnel able to insert or to ETT, to initiate or maintain ventilation, to administer O_2 and fluids, and to use suction.

Box 6.15 Indications for neurosurgical referral (and/or urgent CT head scan) following head injury*

- Recent intracranial lesion seen on CT
- Persisting coma (<9/15) after initial resuscitation
- Confusion which persists for >4h
- Progressive focal neurological signs
- Seizure without full recovery
- Depressed skull fracture
- Definite or suspected penetrating injury
- CSF leak or other sign of a basal skull fracture
- Urgent CT indicated but no local facilities available

*Adapted from *Report of the Working Party on the Management of with Head Injuries* (1999). Royal College of Surgeons of England, London.

Box 6.16 Causes of secondary brain injury[2]

Systemic
- Hypoxaemia
- Hypotension
- Hypercarbia
- Severe hypocapnia
- Pyrexia
- Hyponatraemia
- Anaemia
- DIC

Intracranial
- Haematoma (extradural, subdural, or intracerebral)
- Brain swelling/oedema
- Raised ICP
- Cerebral vasospasm
- Epilepsy
- Intracranial infection

References

1. Mendelow AD andTeasdale G (1991). In Swash M and Oxbury J, eds. *Clinical Neurology*, Section 14, p. 698.

2. Miller JD (1993). Head injury. *J Neurol Neurosurg Psychiat* **56**: 440–7.

Raised intracranial pressure (ICP)

Presentation

Normal ICP in adults is 0–10mmHg at rest. Treatment is required when it exceeds 15–20mmHg for >5min. Symptoms and signs suggestive of raised ICP include

- ***Headache and vomiting*** worse in mornings; exacerbated by bending.
- ***Focal neurological signs*** may occur if there is a space-occupying lesion and in some metabolic conditions (e.g. liver failure). But there may also be false localizing signs, e.g. VIth cranial nerve palsy.
- ***Seizures*** may occur with space-occupying lesions, CNS infection, or metabolic encephalopathies associated with raised ICP.
- ***Papilloedema*** is present only if there is CSF obstruction.
- ***Impaired level of consciousness:*** from mild confusion to coma.
- ***Signs of brain shift***[1] may accompany decreasing level of consciousness. They are discussed with examination of brainstem function (📖 p.337 and p.436).
- ***Late signs:*** bradycardia and hypertension.

Causes

- Head injury → intracranial haematoma/brain swelling/contusion
- Stroke (haemorrhagic, major infarct, venous thrombosis)
- Metabolic (hepatic or renal failure, DKA, hyponatraemia, etc.)
- CNS infection (abscess, encephalitis, meningitis, malaria)
- CNS tumour
- Status epilepticus
- Hydrocephalus (of any cause)
- Idiopathic ('benign') intracranial hypertension.

Assessment of severity

- GCS (📖 p.432)
- Signs of brain shift and brainstem compromise (📖 p.438).

Management

1. Stabilize the patient
2. Consider active means of reducing ICP
3. Attempt to make a diagnosis
4. Treat factors which may exacerbate raised ICP
5. Observe for signs of deterioration and attempt to reverse them
6. Consider specific therapy.

What follows is the management for stabilizing a patient presenting acutely with raised ICP and may not be appropriate for many patients with a long progressive history of deterioration.[1]

Stabilize the patient

- ***Open the airway*** by laying the patient on their side. Give O_2. Measure *ABGs*. Intubation and mechanical ventilation may be necessary because of respiratory compromise. It may also be necessary to reduce ICP by hyperventilating the patient (see next section) to keep P_aCO_2 between 3.3–4.0kPa (25–30mmHg).

- ***Correct hypotension*** Volume expansion with colloids or infusions of inotropes needs to be conducted with careful and frequent monitoring of CVP and/or PAWP. In general, patients with raised ICP should be fluid restricted to 1.5–2.0L/day. So if volume expansion is required it should be kept to the minimum required to restore BP.
- ***Treat seizures*** (📖 p.390).
- ***Examine rapidly*** for signs of head injury (📖 p.364). If the patient is hypotensive, examine carefully for any occult site of bleeding. If there is a rash, consider the possibility of meningococcal meningitis; take blood cultures and give antibiotics (📖 p.356).
- Take blood for *glucose* (this may be raised in diabetic ketoacidosis or hyperosmolar non-ketotic states, it may be very low in liver failure), *U&Es* (biochemical assessment of dehydration and renal function, potassium for susceptibility to dysrhythmia, hyponatraemia from inappropriate ADH, or hypernatraemia from aggressive diuretic-induced dehydration), *LFTs, albumin, clotting studies and ammonium* (to assess liver function), *FBC*, and *blood culture*.

Measures to reduce ICP

The value of ICP monitoring is a controversial subject. Irrespective of whether or not your patient's ICP is monitored, the following interventions should be considered.

- ***Elevate head of*** *bed* to ~30° (once cervical spine injury has been excluded) to promote venous drainage.
- ***Hyperventilation*** so that P_aCO_2 is kept between 3.7–3.9kPa will promote cerebral vasoconstriction and lower cerebral blood volume: this requires intubation and paralysis. It will also lower the BP and may compromise cerebral circulation. In patients with liver failure this is no longer recommended. Discuss with your local ITU.
- ***Mannitol:*** 0.5–1g/kg over 10–15min (~250mL of 20% solution for an average adult) reduces ICP within 20min and its effects should last for 2–6h. *Furosemide* 20–40mg IV may be given with mannitol to potentiate its effect. If required further boluses of smaller doses of mannitol (0.25–0.5g/kg) may be given every few hours. U&Es and serum osmolality should be monitored as a profound diuresis may result. Serum osmolality should not be allowed to rise over 320mOsm/kg.
- ***Corticosteroids*** are of benefit in reducing oedema around space-occupying lesions (📖 p.376) but are not helpful in the treatment of stroke or head injury. Dexamathasone is given as a loading dose of 10mg IV. It may be followed by 4–6mg q6h PO/via NG tube.
- ***Fluid restriction*** to 1.5–2.0L/day. U&Es must be checked frequently.
- ***Cooling*** to 35°C reduces cerebral ischaemia.
- ***Avoid/treat hyperglycaemia*** because it exacerbates ischaemia.

Reference

1. Posner JB *et al.* (2007). *Plum and Posner's Diagnosis of Stupor and Coma* (Contemporary Neurology 71). Oxford University Press, New York.

Raised ICP: further management

Attempt to make a diagnosis

Often the history makes the diagnosis obvious and usually raised ICP is a 2° diagnosis. If a history is not available, focal neurological signs or focal seizures suggest an underlying structural cerebral lesion (although such signs may occur with hepatic or renal failure). Meningism raises the possibility of subarachnoid haemorrhage or meningitis.

A CT scan should be performed in all patients suspected of having raised ICP before lumbar puncture is considered.

(Lumbar puncture should be discussed with a senior colleague and/or Neurologist.) Blood sent for analysis on admission may help to detect metabolic causes of raised ICP.

Benign intracranial hypertension (BIH)

BIH is a syndrome of raised ICP in the absence of an intracranial mass lesion or hydrocephalus. Although rarely life-threatening, BIH can cause permanent visual loss due to optic nerve damage. This disorder affects 1 in 100,000 of the population overall, but this increases to 1:5000 obese women of child-bearing age. There is a predominance in women over men (4:1), aged 17–45 years.

Presentation

- Constant but variable headaches
- Visual disturbances (incl. diplopia, visual obscurations, scotoma) ± nausea
- Problems with balance, memory
- Tinnitus
- Neck and back pains
- The presence of focal neurology incl. epilepsy does ***not*** occur in BIH
- Preservation of cerebral function distinguishes BIH from acute viral encephalitis or bacterial meningitis
- Fundoscopy almost invariably shows papilloedema (may be unilateral).

Associations

- Obesity is present in >90%
- Menstrual problems
- Drugs (tetracycline, isoretinoin and etretinate, nalidixic acid, nitrofurantoin, and lithium)
- Oral contraceptive pill
- Steroid withdrawal
- ↑spontaneous abortion.

Investigations

- CT head scan or MRI are usually normal but look at veins for sinus venosus thrombosis
- Lumbar puncture reveals an elevated CSF pressure (>20cm, but may increase in obesity anyway).

Treatments (seek advice)

- Losing weight
- Repeated therapeutic LP every 2–5 days
- Prednisolone (40–60mg/day) is effective in relieving the headache and visual obscuration due to papilloedema. However, steroids are to be avoided long term
- Acetazolamide ± furosemide
- Surgical shunting (lumboperitoneal shunts).

Treat factors which exacerbate raised ICP[1]

- *Hypoxia/hypercapnia.* ABGs need to be measured regularly.
- *Inadequate analgesia, sedation, or muscle relaxation* → hypertension. NB: hypertension should not be treated aggressively. Pain, e.g. from urine retention, may be the cause. Rapid lowering of BP may lead to 'watershed'/'border zone' cerebral infarcts.
- *Seizures* are not always easy to identify in paralysed patients.
- *Pyrexia* increases cerebral metabolism and, as a consequence, cerebral vasodilatation. It also appears to increase cerebral oedema. The cause of pyrexia should be sought but paracetamol (given rectally) and active cooling should be commenced.
- *Hypovolaemia.*
- *Hyponatraemia* is usually the result of fluid overload but may be caused by a syndrome of inappropriate ADH secretion. Treat with desmopressin 1–4mcg IV daily (see 📖 p.536).

Consider specific therapy

- Once a diagnosis is established it may be appropriate to consider surgery in order to decompress brain or insert a ventricular shunt to drain CSF.
- Intracranial infections need to be treated with the most suitable antibiotics.
- Hyperglycaemia (ketotic/non-ketotic) and liver or renal failure have their own specific management (see relevant sections).
- Often, however, there may not be a specific intervention that is appropriate, e.g. contusion following head injury, and management is confined to optimizing a patient's condition whilst awaiting recovery.

Reference

1. Pickard JD & Czosnyka M (1993). Management of raised intracranial pressure. *J Neurol Neurosurg* Psychiat **56:** 845–58.

Intracranial space-occupying lesion

Presentation

- *Symptoms of raised ICP*: headache, nausea, and vomiting (see 📖 p.372).
- *Papilloedema* is present in the minority of cases.
- *Focal neurological symptoms and signs*. These depend upon location of the lesion, its extent and that of surrounding cerebral oedema, and compression of long tract fibres or cranial nerves. Some lesions, particularly those in the frontal lobe, are relatively 'silent' and may produce no signs or simply change in personality.
- *Seizures*.
- *Impaired level of consciousness* ranging from confusion to coma.
- *Signs of brain shift* (📖 p.438) may be present.
- *Fever* suggests an infection. There may be a recent history of ear ache/discharge, tooth ache, foreign travel, or immune compromise.
- *Acute onset of symptoms* suggests the possibility of a vascular event, either 1° or bleeding into another type of lesion, e.g. tumour.

Management

Depends upon the diagnosis. In a comatose individual with known inoperable brain metastases it is usually not appropriate to intervene. On the other hand, if a patient presents for the first time with signs suggestive of a space-occupying lesion the diagnosis needs to be established.

- ***Assess severity:***
  - If comatose, protect the airway and manage as on 📖 p.334.
  - If there are signs of brain shift which suggest impending transtentorial herniation (📖 p.438) give dexamethasone (10mg IV (loading dose), followed by 4–6mg PO or NG q6h), and/or mannitol 0.5–1g/kg over 10–15min (100–250mL of 20% solution for an average adult) and hyperventilate to keep P_aCO_2 between 3.7–3.9kPa. This may be followed by smaller doses of mannitol every few hours (📖 p.373).
  - If the patient is alert and stable it is best to await CT scan and in the interim make regular neurological observations.
- If the patient is ***pyrexial*** or the history is suggestive of ***infection***, blood, sputum, and urine cultures should be sent. An urgent CT scan should be arranged for these cases; CSF analysis may be necessary but lumbar puncture should *not* be performed before the scan or discussion with neurologists/neurosurgeons.
- If a ***vascular event*** is suspected a CT should also be arranged urgently because decompression may be possible.
- ***Seizures*** should be treated. If they are recurrent, the patient may require loading with IV phenytoin. Many neurosurgeons, give oral phenytoin prophylactically to patients (300mg/day; therapeutic levels are not reached for at least 5 days).
- ***Steroid therapy*** is given if it is thought that some of the symptoms/signs are due to tumour-related brain oedema. Give dexamethasone 10mg IV (loading dose), followed by 4–6mg PO or NG q6h. This is a large dose of steroid (NB: dexamethasone 20mg/day equivalent to prednisolone 130mg/day) and urine/blood glucose should be

monitored. Duration of therapy is guided by response to steroid and the patient's general condition.
- ***Neurosurgery/radiotherapy*** may be of some benefit in some individuals: discuss with your regional neurosurgical centre.

Box 6.17 Common causes of intracranial space-occupying lesions

- Cerebral tumour (1°/2°)
- Subdural haematoma
- Intracerebral haemorrhage
- Tuberculoma
- Cerebral abscess
- Extradural haematoma
- Subdural empyema
- Toxoplasmosis (immunocompromised)

Box 6.18 Management key points: intracranial space-occupying lesions

- Protect the airway.
- Establish the diagnosis (urgent CT, followed by LP; if infection is suspected send blood/urine/sputum for culture).
- If there are signs of brain shift which suggest impending transtentorial herniation (📖 p.438): give 20% mannitol (100–250mL of 20% solution for an average adult) and hyperventilate (requires intubation and paralysis) to keep P_aCO_2 between 3.7–3.9kPa.
- Dexamethasone (10mg IV loading dose, followed by 4–6mg qds po/ng): reduces the oedema around the SOL (monitor blood/urine glucose).
- Discuss with neurologists/neurosurgeons regarding possibility of neurosurgery or radiotherapy.
- Treat seizures. If recurrent: load with IV phenytoin. Many neurosurgeons, give oral phenytoin (300mg/day) prophylactically.
- Regular neurological observations.

Practice point

Hemi-sensory loss involving the trunk is likely to be due to a deep lesion involving the thalamus. Complete hemi-sensory loss may be seen in functional disorders, and can be distinguished by placing a tuning fork on each side of the forehead and the sternum. Patients with functional disease report that vibration is less on the affected side, which is anatomically not possible.[1]

Reference

1. Hawkes C (2002). Smart handles and red flags in neurological diagnosis. *Hosp Med* **63**: 732–42.

Extradural haemorrhage

Presentation

There are no specific diagnostic features. Consider the diagnosis in any head-injured patient who fails to improve or continues to deteriorate.

- *Head injury* is almost invariable.
- *Skull fracture* present in over 90% of adult cases.
- *Headache and vomiting* may occur.
- *Impaired level of consciousness.* There may be an initial lucid interval following head injury but extradural haematomas may be present in patients who have been in coma continuously after the injury. Uncommonly, if the cause is a dural venous sinus tear (rather than shearing of a meningeal artery) lucid interval may extend for several days.
- *Seizures.*
- *Contralateral hemiparesis and extensor plantar* may be elicited.
- *Signs of brain shift* (📖 p.438).

Causes

Common

- Head injury → tearing of meningeal artery (commonly middle menigeal)

Rare

- Head injury → dural sinus tear
- Intracranial infection (sinuses, middle ear, orbit)
- Anticoagulants/blood dyscrasia

Assessment of severity

Bilateral extensor plantars or spasticity, extensor response to painful stimuli, and coma are severe effects of an extradural haemorrhage.

Management

Depends upon tempo of presentation. Priorities are:

- ***Stabilize the patient:*** protect the airway; give O_2, support the breathing and circulation. Assume C-spine injury till excluded.
- ***Treat seizures*** (📖 p.390).
- ***Urgent CT scan:***
    - Haematomas with >5mm mid-line shift on CT and/or >25mL calculated volume require urgent evacuation.
    - If the extraduaral haemorrhage is considered too small to warrant surgery on a CT scan performed within 6h of injury, the scan should be repeated after a few hours irrespective of whether there has been a deterioration in the patient's condition.
- ***Closely monitor neurological state (inc. GCS):***
    - If the patient slips into coma and signs of tentorial herniation (📖 p.438) are progressing rapidly, give 1g/kg of 20% mannitol as a bolus and inform on-call surgeons.
    - If there is evidence of brain shift, discuss with neurosurgeons: ICP should be reduced with mannitol (0.5–1.0g/kg 20% mannitol) and hyperventilation.
- ***All patients must be discussed with neurosurgeons*** Neurological impairment is potentially reversible if the extradural haematoma is treated early.

Intracerebral haemorrhage

Presentation

- Headache, nausea, and vomiting of sudden onset is common.
- Focal neurological deficit: the nature of this depends upon location of haemorrhage. Putaminal haemorrhages (~30% of cases) or lobar bleeds (~30% of cases) may lead to contralateral hemiparesis and sensory loss, visual field disturbance, dysphasia (left hemisphere), or spatial neglect (more severe with right hemisphere lesions). In other words, they may present like a middle cerebral artery infarct (p.403) but often there is a greater alteration in the level of consciousness. Thalamic haemorrhages (~10% cases) may result in eye signs (forced downgaze, upgaze paralysis, or skew deviation) as well as contralateral sensory loss and hemiparesis. Cerebellar haemorrhage is dealt with on p.406 and pontine bleeds on p.404.
- Seizures may occur.
- Global neurological deficit with decreasing level of consciousness progressing to coma. There may be signs of brain shift (p.438).
- Hypertension.

Common predisposing factors

- Hypertension (40–50%)
- Anticoagulants
- Metastatic neoplasm: bleeds may occur within lesion
- Drug abuse (alcohol, cocaine, pseudoephedrine, amphetamines).

Assessment of severity

A low GCS (<9), a large-volume haematoma, and the presence of ventricular blood on the initial CT are factors that are predictive of a high mortality rate.

Management

Priorities are:

1. Stabilize the patient: protect the airway, give O_2 if required, support the circulation if necessary or appropriate, commence general measures for treating comatose patient (p.334) if necessary. If there is evidence of raised ICP, it should be reduced.
2. Correct bleeding tendency or effects of anticoagulants.
3. Make a definitive diagnosis with urgent CT scan. Liaise with regional neurosurgery unit early as surgical intervention may be of benefit. Whether aggressive intervention is appropriate should be decided early.
4. If appropriate, intensive care/high dependency ward nursing observations are required for the drowsy or comatose patient if they are not transferred to neurosurgical centre immediately.
5. Surgical decompression may be beneficial: usually for accessible bleeds within the posterior fossa (see p.406), putamen, or thalamus.
6. Patients who have a seizure at the onset of the haemorrhage should receive IV anticonvulsants.

7 BP control: severe hypertension may worsen intracerebral haemorrhage by representing a continued force for haemorrhage and can cause hypertensive encephalopathy. IV labetalol, nicardipine or nitroprusside may be given if the SBP is >170 mmHg.1–3 The target systolic BP should be 150mmHg or slightly less.4 More pronounced drops in BP should be avoided (Avoid lowering SBP to <140mmHg as this may cause ischaemia). Patients should be carefully monitored for signs of cerebral hypoperfusion induced by the fall in BP.

Box 6.19 Management key points: intracerebral haemorrhage

- Protect the airway, O_2, support the circulation if necessary, monitor in ITU
- Make a definitive diagnosis with urgent CT scan.
- Liaise with neurosurgeons: regarding possibility of surgical decompression for accessible bleeds e.g. within the posterior fossa.
- If there is evidence of raised ICP, it should be reduced:
  - 20% mannitol: initial bolus of 1g/kg, followed by infusions of 0.25–0.5g/kg qds. The goal is to achieve plasma hyperosmolality (300–310mosmol/kg) while maintaining an adequate plasma volume.
  - Hyperventilation: requires intubation and paralysis; discuss with local ITU.
- Correct bleeding tendency or effects of anticoagulants.(e.g. with FFP, vitamin K, platelet transfusion).
- Treat the seizure with IV anticonvulsants.
- Hypertension: if SBP >170mmHg, consider IV labetalol, nicardipine or nitroprusside. Aim for target BP of 150mmHg. More pronounced drops in BP should be avoided.

References

1. Lavin P (1986). Management of hypertension in patients with acute stroke. *Arch Intern Med* **146:** 66–8.

2. Phillips SJ and Whisnant JP (1992). Hypertension and the brain. The National High Blood Pressure Education Program. *Arch Intern Med* **152:** 938–45.

3. Caplan LR. (1992). Intracerebral haemorrhage. *Lancet* **339:** 656–8.

4. Ohwaki K *et al.* (2004). Blood pressure management in acute intracerebral hemorrhage: relationship between elevated blood pressure and hematoma enlargement. *Stroke* **35:** 1364–7.

Subdural haematoma

Presentation

- This may present in one of two ways: acute or chronic. Both are usually the result of tearing of bridging veins (between cortical surface and venous sinuses).
- Acute haemorrhage into the subdural space follows head injury and can be impossible to distinguish on clinical grounds from extradural haemorrhage (📖 p.378).
- A chronic haematoma is also preceded in most cases by head injury but this is often so trivial that patients are unable to recollect it.
- Both types of patient may present with:
  - *Skull fracture* (more common in acute cases)
  - *Headache*
  - *Impaired and fluctuating level of consciousness* ranging from mild confusion, through cognitive decline (e.g. impaired memory) to coma. The diagnosis should be considered in any individual, particularly elderly, who presents with intellectual deterioration or 'dementia' of relatively recent onset
  - *Focal neurological signs* (hemiparesis, dysphasia, hemianopia, etc.)
  - *Seizures* occur in a minority of patients
  - *Signs of brain shift* (📖 p.390) or *papilloedema*.

Common predisposing factors

- Head injury: in young or old
- Old age: cortical atrophy stretches bridging veins.
- Long-standing alcohol abuse
- Anticoagulant use.

Assessment of severity

The following are severe effects of a subdural haemorrhage:

- Bilateral extensor plantars or spasticity
- Extensor response to painful stimuli
- Coma.

Management

Depends upon tempo of presentation.

- In suspected ***chronic cases***, a CT scan is required less urgently unless there has been an acute deterioration on a background of steady neurological decline. Chronic haematomas become isodense with brain and are therefore sometimes difficult to distinguish; MRI may be better.
- In ***acute cases***, priorities are
  - Protection of airway, give O_2, support the breathing and circulation as necessary.
  - Liaison with neurosurgical team early.
  - Close monitoring of neurological state (GCS).
  - Consider methods to reduce ICP if raised if the patient slips into coma and signs of tentorial herniation (📖 p.438) are progressing rapidly, give 1g/kg of 20% mannitol as a bolus, inform on-call surgeon, and very urgent CT scan.
  - Treat seizures (📖 p.390).

Box 6.20 Management key points: subdural haematoma

- Protection of airway, O_2.
- Liaison with neurosurgical team early.
- Close monitoring of neurological state (GCS).
- If the patient deteriorates (slips into coma and signs of tentorial herniation progress rapidly): give 1g/kg of 20% mannitol as a bolus, inform on-call surgeon, and arrange urgent CT scan.
- Treat seizures.

Subarachnoid haemorrhage: assessment

Presentation

- ***Headache:*** classically sudden and severe ('thunderclap'), radiating behind the occiput with associated neck stiffness. Often, the time from onset to peak of headache is only a few seconds, but less dramatic presentations are common. Consider the diagnosis in any unusually severe headache, especially if the patient does not have a previous history of headaches and is >40 years. ~4% of aneurysmal bleeds occur at/after sexual intercourse, but most coital headaches are not subarachnoid haemorrhages. 10% of patients with subarachnoid bleeds are bending or lifting heavy objects at onset of symptoms.
- ***Nausea, vomiting, dizziness*** may be transient or protracted.
- ***Impaired level of consciousness:*** there may be initial transient loss of consciousness followed by variable impairment. Patients may present in coma.
- ***Early focal neurological signs*** may occur, especially if there has been a concomitant intracerebral haemorrhage. Third nerve palsy raises possibility of posterior communicating aneurysm.
- ***Seizures*** are uncommon, but subarachnoid haemorrhage in a person known to have fits suggests underlying AV malformation.
- ***Herald bleed:*** Between 20–50% of patients with documented SAH report a distinct, unusually severe headache in the days or weeks before the index bleed.[1] These are often misdiagnosed as simple headaches or migraine, so a high degree of suspicion is required.
- Patients may present with 2° head injury following collapse. Blood seen on CT scanning may be attributed to trauma.

Causes

Common

- Aneurysm (70%)
- AV malformation (5%)
- No known cause in up to 20%

Rare

- Clotting disorder/anticoagulants
- Tumour
- Vasculitis
- Associated with polycystic kidney disease (berry aneurysm)

Assessment of severity (prognostic features)

- ***Hunt & Hess Scale*** allows grading at presentation and thereafter:
  - Grade 1: asymptomatic or minimal headache + slight neck stiffness
  - Grade 2: moderate or severe headache with neck stiffness, but no neurological deficit other than cranial nerve palsy
  - Grade 3: drowsiness with confusion or mild focal neurology
  - Grade 4: stupor with moderate to severe hemiparesis or mild decerebrate rigidity
  - Grade 5: deeply comatose with severe decerebrate rigidity.
- Prognosis is best in Grade 1 (mortality <5%), worst in Grade 5 (mortality 50–70%), and intermediate in between.
- Neurological deterioration following presentation has a worse prognosis. Patients should be re-graded on the Hunt & Hess Scale.

Practice points

- First and worst headache in someone not prone to headaches should suggest subarachnoid haemorrhage
- Thunderclap headache may be due to a ruptured intracranial aneurysm.[2]
- Patients who wake, often at the same time, with severe unilateral orbital pain will usually have cluster headache. Mostly middle-aged males.[2]

References

1. Edlow JA and Caplan LR (2000). Avoiding pitfalls in the diagnosis of subarachnoid hemorrhage. *N Engl J Med* **342:** 29–35.

2. Hawkes C (2002). Smart handles and red flags in neurological diagnosis. *Hosp Med* **63:** 732–42.

Subarachnoid haemorrhage: immediate management[1]

Confirm the diagnosis

- *Urgent high-resolution CT scanning* is required. This will clinch the diagnosis in 95% of patients scanned within 24h. Furthermore, it gives valuable information regarding possible location of aneurysm and may even demonstrate AV malformation. It may also display concomitant intracerebral and/or intraventricular bleeds.
- *Lumbar puncture* is ***not*** usually required, unless CT scan is normal but the history is highly suggestive. It is important to examine the CSF for blood under these circumstances; the presenting event may be a 'warning leak'. Blood in the CSF may result from a traumatic tap. If this is the case there should be diminishing numbers of red cells in each successive tube of CSF (although this is not always reliable). If the blood has been present for >6h, the supernatant should be xanthochromic after centrifugation.
- Once the diagnosis is confirmed, discuss with regional neurosurgeons.
- Transfer Grade 1 and 2 patients as soon as possible. Surgery will prevent rebleeding and although optimal time for operation is debated (2 days versus 7–10 days post bleed), outcome is probably improved by early transfer.
- Surgery on poor prognosis patients is unrewarding; they are usually managed conservatively. However, suitability for surgery should be re-assessed if their condition improves.

Stabilize the patient (Box 6.21)

- *Protect the airway* by laying the drowsy patient in the recovery position. Give O_2.
- Consider *measures to reduce ICP* if signs suggest it is raised (📖 p.372) but avoid dehydration and hypotension.
- *Treat seizures* with usual drugs (📖 p.390) but beware of over-sedation and hypotension.
- *Correct hypotension* if necessary with colloid or inotropes.
- *To avoid hypertension* the patient should be nursed in a quiet room, sedatives may be required, and stool softeners should be given to avoid straining. Once the diagnosis is established, nimodipine is usually given to reduce vasospasm; it helps also to reduce BP.
- *ECG monitoring* and *treat dysrhythmias* if they compromise BP or threaten thromboembolism. Rarely subarachnoid haemorrhage is associated with (neurogenic) pulmonary oedema.
- Take blood for *clotting screen* (if bleeding diathesis suspected) and *U&Es* (biochemical assessment of dehydration, potassium for susceptibility to dysrhythmia, hyponatraemia from inappropriate ADH or hypernatraemia from aggressive diuretic-induced dehydration).

Reference

1. Kopitnik TA and Samson DS (1993). Management of subarachnoid haemorrhage. *J Neurol Neurosurg Psychiat* **56:** 947–59.

Box 6.21 Management key points: subarachnoid haemorrhage

- Protect the airway (lie the patient in the recovery position). Give O_2.
- Correct hypotension (and electrolyte disturbances).
- Treat seizures with usual drugs (but beware of over-sedation and hypotension).
- Discuss with regional neurosurgeons when diagnosis is confirmed (on urgent CT; LP for ?xanthochromia if CT is normal but history is highly suggestive (if the blood has been present for >6h).
- Nimodipine 60mg PO qds.
- Appropriate analgesia (codeine phosphate) and anti-emetics for awake patients.
- Regular neurological observations to detect a deterioration (?2° to cerebral ischaemia, rebleeding or acute hydrocephalus): CT scan should be performed.

Subarachnoid haemorrhage: further management

Specific therapies

- *Nimodipine* is a calcium channel blocker which works preferentially on cerebral vessels to reduce vasospasm (and consequent cerebral ischaemia).[1] It has been shown to reduce morbidity and mortality following SAH. Give 60mg PO (or in the comatose patient) every 4h; IV therapy is costly and requires central venous access.
- *Antifibrinolytics* were introduced to prevent lysis of clot and rebleeding. They have been associated with ↑thrombotic complications and are not advised at present.
- Appropriate analgesia (codeine phosphate 30–60mg every 4 to 6h) and anti-emetics should be given for awake patients.[2]

Observe for deterioration. Attempt to reverse it

Neurological observations should be performed regularly. If there is a deterioration, e.g. lowering of the level of consciousness, a CT scan should be performed. There are several possible mechanisms for deterioration:

- *Cerebral ischaemia* is usually insidious and multi-focal. It may give rise to focal and/or global neurological deterioration. Volume expansion with colloid or induced hypertension with inotropes have been attempted but these procedures have not been properly studied.
- *Rebleeding* may be immediately fatal or lead to apnoea. It is reported that assisted ventilation for 1h may be all that is necessary for spontaneous breathing to return to the majority of apnoeic individuals.[3] Patients who rebleed are at high risk of further bleeding and should be considered for emergency aneurysm clipping.
- *Acute hydrocephalus* may be treated with ventricular drainage. This can lead to dramatic improvement in the patient's condition.

Refer for definitive treatment

Unless the patient has a poor prognosis (see Hunt & Hess Scale, 📖 p.384), they should be cared for at a neurosurgical centre. The complications listed here should be managed by clinicians experienced in treating them.

References

1. Pickard JD *et al.* (1989). Effect of oral nimodipine on cerebral infarction and outcome after subarachnoid haemorrhage: British aneurysm nimodipine trial. *BMJ* **298:** 636–42.

2. Kirkpatrick PJ (2002). Subarachnoid haemorrhage and intracranial aneurysms: what neurologists need to know. *J Neurol Neurosurg Psychiat* **73**(suppl. 1): i28–i33.

3. van Gijn J (1992). Subarachnoid haemorrhage. *Lancet* **339:** 653–5.

Status epilepticus (tonic–clonic)

Presentation

Generalized tonic–clonic status epilepticus is either continuous tonic–clonic convulsions (30min or longer) or convulsions so frequent that each attack begins before the previous post-ictal period ends.

Causes

- Cerebral tumour (1°/2°)
- Intracranial infection
- Hypoglycaemia
- Head injury
- Electrolyte disturbance (low sodium, calcium, or magnesium)
- Drug overdose (e.g. tricyclics)
- Drug withdrawal (e.g. alcohol)
- Hypoxia (e.g. post cardiac arrest)
- Sequela of stroke
- Anti-epileptic non-compliance/ withdrawal

NB: most episodes of status do not occur in known epileptic patients.

Management (Box 6.23)

Priorities

1. Stabilize the patient. Give O_2.
2. Anti-epileptic drug therapy.
3. Attempt to identify aetiology.
4. Identify and treat medical complications.
5. Initiate long-term maintenance therapy if appropriate.

Stabilize the patient

- *Open the airway* by laying the patient on side in a semiprone position with the head slightly lower to prevent aspiration. Usually an oral airway will suffice and ET intubation is rarely necessary.
- *Give O_2.*
- *Correct hypotension* with colloid if necessary. Obtain an ECG if the patient is hypotensive. CVP monitoring may be necessary.
- Take blood for *U&Es, glucose, calcium, magnesium, liver enzymes, FBC (inc. platelets)*; if relevant, blood should also be sent for *toxicology screen* (if drug overdose or abuse suspected) and *anticonvulsant levels.*
- *Thiamine 250mg* IV should be given if alcoholism or other malnourished states appear likely.
- If hypoglycaemia is suspected *50mL of 50% glucose* should be administered IV. Because glucose increases the risk of Wernicke's encephalopathy, thiamine 1–2mg/kg IV should be administered beforehand in any patient suspected of alcohol excess.

Anti-epileptic drug therapy[2]

- A number of agents may be used:
  - Benzodiazepines (diazepam, lorazepam)
  - Phenytoin
  - Fosphenytoin
  - Miscellaneous (general anaesthesia, paraldehyde).
- *Lorazepam* 0.07mg/kg IV (usually 4mg bolus which may be repeated once after 10min). Because lorazepam does not accumulate in lipid

stores and has strong cerebral binding and a long duration of action, it has distinct advantages over diazepam in early status epilepticus.

- Alternatively, *diazepam* 10–20mg IV or rectally, repeated once 15min later if necessary. Intravenous injection should not exceed 2–5mg/min. Diazepam is rapidly redistributed and therefore has a short duration of action. With repeated dosing, however, as peripheral lipid compartments become saturated, there is less redistribution and blood diazepam levels increase. When this happens there is a risk of sudden central nervous and respiratory depression as well as cardiorespiratory collapse.
- With the benzodiazepine, start an infusion of *phenytoin* at 15–18mg/kg at a rate of 50mg/min (e.g. 1g over 20min). NB: 5% glucose is not compatible with phenytoin. The patient should have ECG monitoring because phenytoin may induce cardiac dysrhythmias; pulse, BP, and respiratory rate should also be monitored. IV phenytoin is relatively contraindicated in patients with known heart disease, particularly those with conduction abnormalities.
- If seizures continue, give *phenobarbital* 10mg/kg IV at a rate of 100mg/min (i.e. about 70mg in an average adult over 7min).
- An alternative is *fosphenytoin* given as an infusion of 15mg PE (phenytoin equivalents) at a rate of 100mg PE/min (i.e. about 1000mg PE in an average adult over 10min).
- In refractory status (seizures continuing for 60–90min after initial therapy), the patient should be transferred to intensive care.
    - General anaesthesia with either *propofol* or *thiopental* should be administered.
    - *Paraldehyde* (5–10mL IM) is an alternative but requires glass syringes as it corrodes rubber and plastic.
    - *Treat raised ICP* (📖 p.372).
    - *EEG monitoring* should be commenced.
    - The anaesthetic agent should be continued for 12–24h after the last clinical or electrographic seizure; the dose should then be tapered down.

If treatment is failing to control seizures, consider whether:

- Initial drug dose is adequate.
- Maintenance therapy has been started and is adequate.
- Underlying cause of status epilepticus has been correctly identified.
- Complications of status adequately treated (see 📖 p.392; Box 6.23).
- Co-existing conditions have been identified (e.g. hepatic failure).
- There has been a misdiagnosis: is this 'pseudo status'?

Practice point

Intermittant olfactory hallucinations may indicate a malignant glioma of the anteromedial temporal lobe (uncus) leading to uncinate fits.[1]

References

1. Hawkes C (2002). Smart handles and red flags in neurological diagnosis. *Hosp Med* **63:** 732–42.

2. Shorvon SD (2001). The management of status epilepticus. *J Neurol Neurosurg Psychiat* **70**(suppl. 2): ii22–ii27.

Status epilepticus (tonic–clonic) 2

Attempt to identify aetiology

- A history of previous anticonvulsant use, drug abuse/withdrawal (including alcohol), diabetes, trauma, or recent surgery (e.g. hypocalcaemia post thyroid or parathyroid surgery) is obviously helpful.
- Examine the patient for signs of head trauma, meningism, focal neurological deficit (the seizures may also have some focal characteristics), needle tracks, or insulin injection sites.
- Consider urgent CT scan if head injury may be a precipitant; a lumbar puncture may be necessary if CSF infection is likely.
- Although hypoglycaemia and hypocalcaemia should be corrected promptly, hyponatraemia should be reversed cautiously because of the possibility of precipitating pontine myelinosis.
- See Box 6.23 for key points in management.

Identify and treat medical complications of status

Treatment is required for:

- Hypoxia
- Lactic acidosis
- Hypoglycaemia
- Dysrhythmias
- Rhabdomyolysis
- Electrolyte disturbance (especially hyponatraemia, hypo/hyperkalaemia)
- Hypotension/hypertension
- Raised ICP
- Hyperpyrexia
- Pulmonary oedema
- DIC

These complications are managed as in other contexts.

Initiate long-term therapy (if appropriate)

Some disorders, e.g. hypoglycaemia in a diabetic taking insulin, do not require long-term anticonvulsant therapy, but rather correction of the underlying problem. Other conditions may need anticonvulsant treatment for a short while, e.g. alcohol withdrawal, or indefinitely, e.g. repeated status epilepticus in multi-infarct dementia.

- *Sodium valproate* is now considered first-choice treatment, with *carbamazepine* as an alternative.[1] Initially, sodium valproate should be given 400–600mg/day orally in 3 divided doses (IV therapy can also be given). It should be ↑ by 200mg/day at 3–6-day intervals; the maintenance dose is 20–30mg/kg/day (usual adult dose is 1–2g/day). Carbamazepine should be started at 100–200mg 1–2 times daily; the maintenance dose is 7–15mg/kg/day divided in 2–3 doses (200–800mg/day for adults).
- *Phenytoin* may be continued after IV loading at daily dosages of 5mg/kg (about 300mg for an average adult) either orally or via a NG tube or slow IVI. Dosage should be guided by phenytoin level measurements. Plasma concentration for optimum response is 10–20mg/L (40–80μmol/L). Phenytoin is disadvantageous because it requires monitoring.
- Driving advice, see Box 6.22.

Box 6.22 Driving advice

In the UK, patients should inform the Driving and Vehicle Licensing Agency (Swansea). Driving licences are revoked until the patient has been free of daytime seizures for 1 year, treated or untreated. Drivers of large goods or passenger carrying vehicles usually have those licences revoked permanently.

For current medical standards of fitness to drive go to http://www.dvla.gov.uk/at_a_glance/content.htm

Box 6.23 Management key points: status epilepticus

- Open the airway (Lie the patient on side in a semiprone position with the head slightly lower to prevent aspiration; oral airway if necessary), Give O_2.
- Correct hypoglycaemia (50mL of 50% glucose, give 250mg IV thiamine before glucose if alcoholism or malnourishment is likely) and hypotension.
- Lorazepam (4mg IV bolus, may be repeated once after 10min) or diazepam 10–20mg IV or rectally (may be repeated once 15min).
- In addition to lorazepam start phenytoin at 15/kg at a rate of 50mg/min (e.g. 1g over 20min) with ECG monitoring.
- In refractory status (seizures continuing for 60–90min after initial therapy): General anaesthesia with either propofol or thiopentone with EEG monitoring. Continue the anaesthetic agent for 12–24h after the last clinical or electrographic seizure; the dose should then be tapered down.
- Attempt to identify aetiology: send blood for U&Es, glucose, calcium, magnesium, liver enzymes, FBC (inc. platelets), anticonvulsant levels and if relevant toxicology screen (if drug overdose or abuse suspected).

Reference

1. Smith D and Chadwick D (2001). The management of epilepsy. *J Neurol Neurosurg Psychiat* **70**(suppl. 2): ii15–ii21.

Stroke: overview

Presentation

- Sudden-onset focal deficit of cerebral function is the most common presentation.
- Alternative presentations include apparent confusion (e.g. due to dysphasia or visuospatial impairment), seizures, declining levels of consciousness or global loss of brain function and coma.
- If the symptoms last for >24h (or lead to death) and there is no apparent cause other than a vascular event, the diagnosis is most likely to be a stroke. If the symptoms last <24h and, after adequate investigation, are presumed to be due to thrombosis or embolism, the diagnosis is a TIA.

Causes

- Thrombosis or embolism causing cerebral infarction (~80% cases)
- Primary intracerebral haemorrhage (~15% cases)
- Subarachnoid haemorrhage (~5% cases)
- Cerebral venous thrombosis (1%).

Risk factors

See Box 6.24.

Differential diagnosis

Many conditions may masquerade as a stroke:

- Cerebral tumour (1° or 2°)
- Brain abscess
- Demyelination
- Focal migraine
- Subdural haematoma
- Todd's paresis (post seizure)
- Hypoglycaemic attack
- Encephalitis.

An alternative diagnosis to stroke is more likely in:

- Patients <45 years
- Presence of seizures
- Presence of papilloedema
- Prolonged and/or discontinuous evolution of symptoms.
- Absence of risk factors
- Fluctuating levels of consciousness
- Pyrexia (at presentation)

In general, a stroke commences suddenly and the deficit is at its peak and established within 24h. If the evolution of symptoms is longer or progresses in a stuttering way over days or weeks, a space-occupying lesion must be suspected. If there is a variable depression of consciousness, the diagnosis of a subdural haematoma should be entertained, and pyrexia at presentation should alert one to the possibility of a cerebral abscess.

Seizures occur in 5–10% of strokes at their onset although they are frequent sequelae. Papilloedema would be extremely unusual in arterial strokes but may occur in cerebral venous sinus thrombosis. Consider this diagnosis particularly in patients who may have become dehydrated and young women (particularly during the puerperium) with headache and seizures ± focal signs.

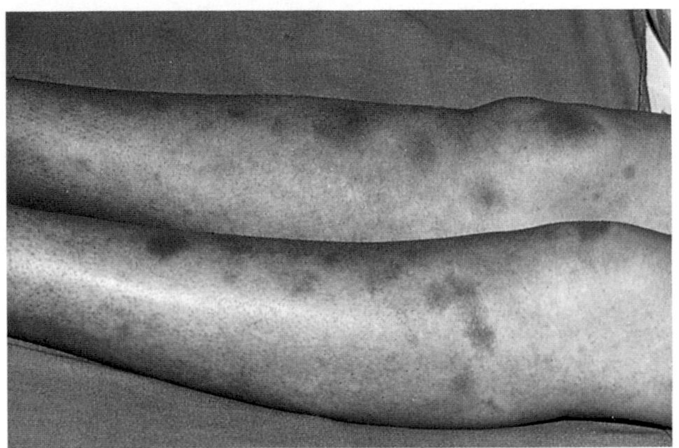

Plate 1 Erythema nodosum. The lesions can be very faint, but are indurated and painful on palpation. The dermatology plates are taken from: Rona M MacKie (2003) *Clinical dermatology*, 5th edn. Oxford University Press, Oxford (with permission) (see 📖 p.448)

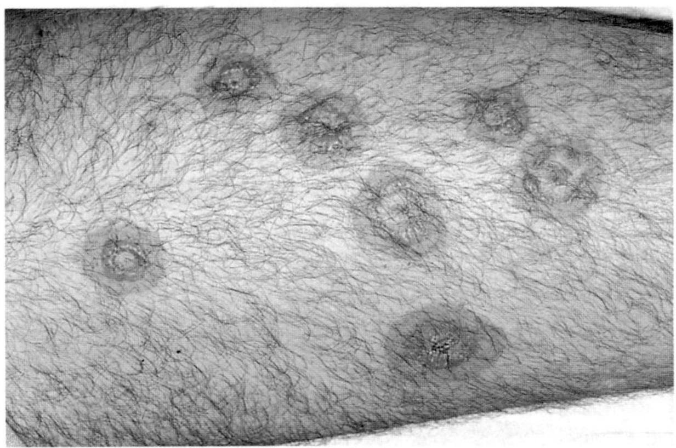

Plate 2 Erythema multiforme on the leg, note the presence of target lesions. The dermatology plates are taken from: Rona M MacKie (2003) *Clinical dermatology*, 5th edn. Oxford University Press, Oxford (with permission) (see 📖 p.654)

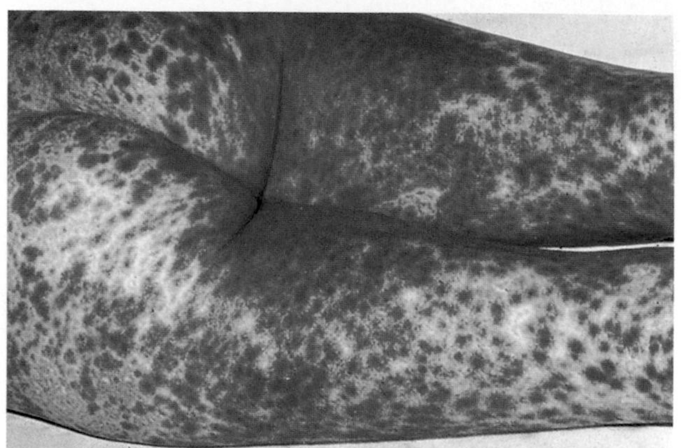

Plate 3 Morbilliform eruption caused by administration of ampicillin to a patient with infectious mononucleosis. The dermatology plates are taken from: Rona M MacKie (2003) *Clinical dermatology*, 5th edn. Oxford University Press, Oxford (with permission) (see 🕮 p.654)

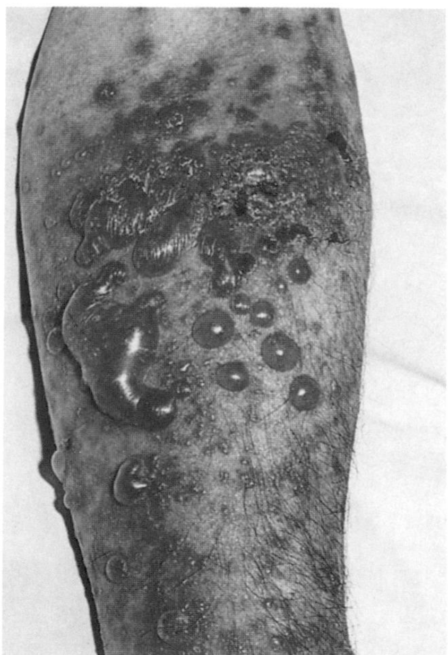

Plate 4 Blisters of bullous pemphigoid. Large, tense, raised lesions are seen on an erythematous eczematized base. The dermatology plates are taken from: Rona M MacKie (2003) *Clinical dermatology*, 5th edn. Oxford University Press, Oxford (with permission) (see 🕮 p.654)

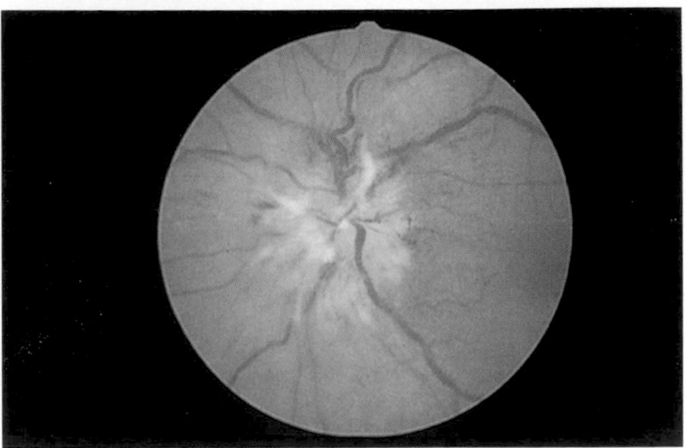

Plate 5 Acute papilloedema. The opthalmology plates are taken from: David L Easty and John M Sparrow (eds) (1999) *Oxford Textbook of Opthalmology*, Oxford University Press, Oxford (with permission) (see 📖 p.372)

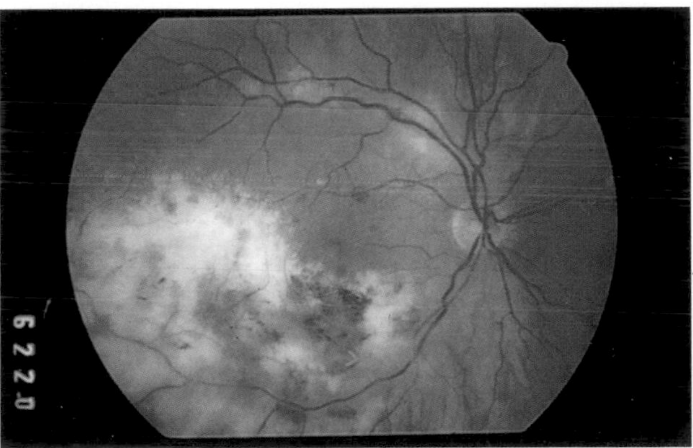

Plate 6 The typical appearance of cytomegalovirus retinitis in a patient with AIDS, characterized by retinal necrosis with an irregular granular border, patchy retinal haemorrhage, and retinal inflammatory sheathing of the retinal vessels.
The opthalmology plates are taken from: David L Easty and John M Sparrow (eds) (1999) *Oxford Textbook of Opthalmology*, Oxford University Press, Oxford (with permission) (see 📖 p.506)

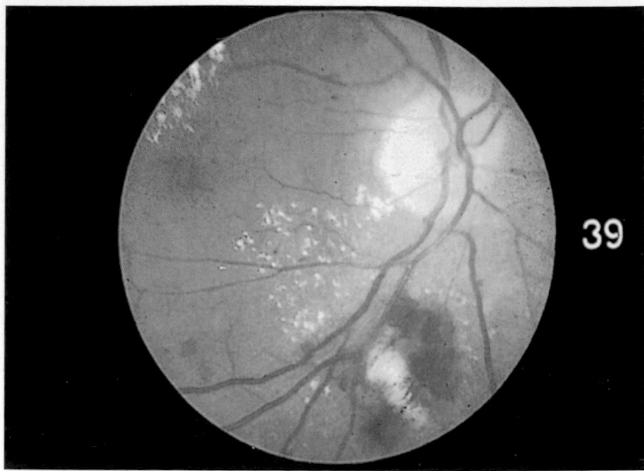

Plate 7 Hard exudates and cotton-wool spots in the right eye. The opthalmology plates are taken from: David L Easty and John M Sparrow (eds) (1999) *Oxford Textbook of Opthalmology*, Oxford University Press, Oxford (with permission) (e.g. diabetes mellitus, Chapter 9)

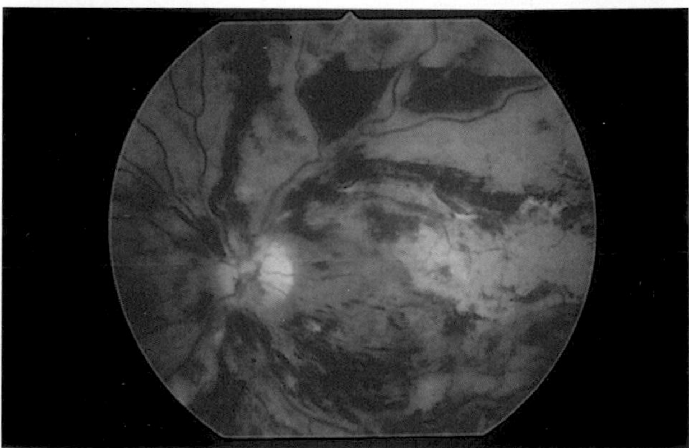

Plate 8 Central retinal vein occlusion with assorted closure of the arterial circulation above the macula. The opthalmology plates are taken from: David L Easty and John M Sparrow (eds) (1999) *Oxford Textbook of Opthalmology*, Oxford University Press, Oxford (with permission) (see 🕮 p.350)

Dissection of the internal carotid or vertebral arteries should always be considered, particularly in younger patients who may have experienced only mild neck trauma. Often, however, there may be no clear history of preceding trauma. Carotid dissection may be accompanied by a Horner's syndrome; vertebral dissection presents with symptoms associated with brainstem stroke.

Box 6.24 Risk factors for stroke

Global
- Increasing age
- Hypertension
- Diabetes
- Family history
- ↑lipids
- Homocysteinaemia

Lifestyle
- Drug abuse (cocaine)
- Smoking
- Oral contraceptive pill
- Hormone replacement therapy
- Diving (Caisson's disease)
- Neck trauma/manipulation

Cerebral
- Cerebrovascular disease
- Berry aneurysms
- Cerebral amyloid
- Cerebral AV malformation

Cardiac
- Atrial fibrillation
- Myocardial infarction
- Left ventricular aneurysm
- Ischaemic heart disease
- Cyanotic heart disease
- Patent foramen ovale
- Endocarditis

Peripheral vascular
- Carotid stenosis
- Pulmonary AV malformations
- Ehlers Danlos
- Type IV (carotid dissection)

Haematological
- Hypercoagulable states
- Polycythaemia
- Sickle cell disease
- Warfarin (haemorrhage)
- Thrombolysis

Stroke: haemorrhage or infarct?

Intracerebral haemorrhage often has an apoplectic onset with a combination of headache, neck stiffness, vomiting, and loss of consciousness of acute onset. Conscious level can be depressed for >24h, there may be bilateral extensor plantar responses, and the BP is more likely to be raised 24h after admission. But although features such as these have been integrated into scoring systems, it is not possible with certainty to differentiate ischaemic from haemorrhagic stroke on clinical grounds alone. A CT scan is required.

When to scan?

All patients suspected of having a stroke should be scanned as soon as possible, at least within 24h of onset. CT is the investigation of choice in the majority of cases because it is better at detecting haemorrhage in the early stages compared with MRI. After the first 24h, and in cases where the stroke is suspected to involve brainstem or cerebellum, MRI is superior. Where the CT scan is normal, diffusion-weighted MRI may reveal areas of cerebral ischaemia or infarction.

Urgent CT should be performed in the presence of:

- Depressed level of consciousness.
- History of anticoagulant treatment or known coagulopathy.
- No available history.
- Features suggesting an alternative diagnosis requiring immediate action, in particular:
  - Subarachnoid haemorrhage (severe headache, depressed level of consciousness, neck stiffness)
  - Subdural haemorrhage (headache, history of minor trauma, progressive or fluctuating signs and symptoms)
  - Space-occupying lesion (depressed level of consciousness, progressive signs, papilloedema)
  - Cerebral infection (headache, fever, neck stiffness, cranial nerve palsies).
- Indications for thrombolysis (Box 6.25) or early anticoagulation.

Brain imaging should always be undertaken before anticoagulant treatment is started.

Stroke: thrombolysis

Box 6.25 Thrombolysis in acute ischaemic stroke

- Hospitals offering thrombolysis for ischaemic stroke, outside a trial, should only do so after specialist staff training and registration with the UK SITS-MOST (Safe Implementation of Thrombolysis in Stroke Monitoring Study) programme.
- The use of thrombolysis for acute ischaemic stroke requires coordination of emergency services, stroke neurology, intensive care, and radiology services.
- Early identification of patients who might benefit from thrombolysis is crucial. Patients should have a neurologic deficit that is sufficiently significant to warrant exposure to the risks of thrombolysis.
- Urgent CT or MRI is mandatory to exclude brain haemorrhage.

Box 6.25 *(continued)*

- IV alteplase may be used in acute ischaemic stroke (MCA or Basilar occlusion) provided that treatment is initiated within 3h of clearly defined symptom onset.
- BP must be <185/110mmHg prior to thrombolysis and must be maintained below 180/105mmHg for 24h after thrombolysis (see 🕮 p.401). The optimal lower end of the range of desired BP is unclear. However avoid excessive BP lowering which may worsen blood flow and cerebral ischemia.
- Inclusion criteria:
  - Clinical diagnosis of acute ischaemic stroke with the onset of symptoms within 3h of commencement of thrombolysis and with a measurable neurological deficit
- Exclusion criteria:
  - History
    —MI, stroke, or head trauma within the previous 3 months
    —Lumbar puncture or arterial puncture at a non-compressible site within previous 7 days
    —Major operation within previous 14 days
    —GI or GU haemorrhage within previous 21 days
    —Any previous history of intracranial bleed
    —Active haemorrhage or acute trauma/fracture
    —Rapidly improving stroke symptoms
    —Seizure at the onset of stroke with post-ictal neurological impairments
    —History suggestive of subarachnoid haemorrhage
    —Pregnancy or breastfeeding
  - Examination
    —Only minor and isolated neurological signs
    —Persistent SBP >185, DBP >110 mmHg, or requiring aggressive therapy to control BP
  - Blood tests:
    —platelet <100,000/mm^3
    —serum glucose <2.8mm/l or >22.2mm/l
    —INR >1.7 if on warfarin; elevated APTT if on heparin.
  - Head CT: evidence of haemorrhage or signs of major early infarct e.g. diffuse swelling of the affected hemisphere, parenchymal hypodensity or effacement of >1/3 of the MCA territory.

Adapted from Report of the Quality Standrads Subcommitee of the American Academy of Neurology (1996). Practice advisory: thrombolytic therapy for acute ischemic stroke – summary statement. *Neurology* **47:** 835–9; and Adams HP *et al.* (2003). Guidelines for the early management of patients with ischemic stroke: A scientific statement from the Stroke Council of the American Stroke Association. *Stroke* **34:** 1056–83.

Stroke: other investigations

Apart from a CT scan, there are some basic tests that most patients suspected of having a stroke should have.

- FBC, to detect polycythaemia, thrombocythaemia, or thrombocytopenia.
- *ESR and CRP*, to screen for vasculitis, endocarditis, hyperviscosity.
- *Electrolytes and calcium* (neurological defect may be non-vascular and caused by hyponatraemia, hypercalcaemia, or renal failure).
- *Glucose* to exclude hypoglycaemia and non-ketotic hyperglycaemia (which can mimic stroke) and diabetes mellitus (a risk factor).
- *Cholesterol* (if taken within 12–24h of stroke).
- *Syphilis serology* (low yield but treatable condition). NB: VDRL (but not TPHA) may be positive in SLE and the 1° anticardiolipin syndrome. TPHA (but not VDRL) is positive in patients previously exposed to non-syphilitic treponemes (e.g. yaws).
- *Prothrombin time/INR* if the patient is taking warfarin.
- *ECG* to determine cardiac rhythm and exclude acute myocardial infarction.
- *Carotid Doppler ultrasound* to exclude high-grade (>70%) stenosis or dissection. This should be performed in patients who would be suitable for carotid endarterectomy or angioplasty. A bruit need not be present!
- *Cardiac echocardiography* may demonstrate the presence of valvular disease or intracardiac clot or may detect some rare causes of stroke such as atrial myxoma or patent foramen ovale.

Young patients, or those without common risk factors for stroke (see 📖 p.395), should be investigated further. Possible tests include

- *Serum protein, electrophoresis, viscosity*. In hyperviscosity syndromes the ESR is usually raised but not always.
- *Autoantibody screen* (particularly for SLE).
- *Haemostatic profile*. In haemorrhagic stroke not apparently 2° to hypertension, measurement of PT, APTT, bleeding time, and fibrin degradation products may be indicated. In cerebral infarcts, blood should be taken for protein S, C, antithrombin III, and anticardiolipin antibodies. APTT may be prolonged in anticardiolipin syndrome. Consider testing for sickle cell in black patients. The Factor V_{Leiden} mutation may be an important risk factor for the development of venous thrombosis.
- *Toxicology screen* on admission sample if drug abuse (e.g. cocaine, pseudoephedrine, or amphetamines) suspected.
- *Urine tests* may detect homocystinuria (without other clinical manifestations) or porphyria. If BP is labile consider phaeochromocytoma and measure urinary catecholamines.
- *CSF analysis* may be necessary if the diagnosis of stroke is not well established, e.g. normal CT scan and no risk factors.
- *Cerebral angiography* is also reserved for cases where the diagnosis is not well established and in those in whom cerebral vasculitis or malformation is suspected.
- *MRI* is more sensitive at detecting small infarcts, cerebral venous thrombosis, and lesions in the posterior fossa. In expert hands magentic resonance angiography may be comparable to conventional angiography.

Stroke: management

Box 6.26 Key points: assessment and management of acute ischaemic stroke

Assessment

- Exclude hypoglycaemia.
- Brain imaging should be undertaken as soon as possible, within 24 hours of onset.
- It should be undertaken as a matter of urgency in patients with:
  - Known bleeding tendency or those on anti-coagulants
  - ↓ level of consciousness
  - Unexplained progressive or fluctuating symptoms
  - Papilloedema, neck stiffness or fever
  - Severe headache at onset
  - Indications for thrombolysis.
- Thrombolysis if indicated (<3 hours from symptom onset) (see 📖 p.397).
- Assess swallowing before giving oral foods, fluid or oral medication on admission. If impaired: specialist assessment of within 24–72 hours of admission.
- Screen for malnutrition

Acute interventions

- Admit to a specialist acute stroke unit for specialist monitoring and treatment.
- Give aspirin (300mg) orally or rectally as soon as possible after primary haemorrhage has been excluded.
- Control hydration, temperature (<37.2°C), blood pressure (see 📖 p.401), maintain O_2 (> 95%), blood glucose (4–11 mmol/l).
- If surgical referral for decompressive craniectomy is indicated*: refer within 24 hours of onset of symptoms and treat within a maximum of 48 hours.
- Maintain adequate nutrition (initiate IV/NG tube feeding if the patient is unable to take adequate nutrition and fluids orally.
- Patients should be mobilized as soon as possible.

Secondary prevention

- Give appropriate advice on lifestyle factors.
- Hypertension persisting for > 2 weeks should be treated (target: <140/85 mmHg; diabetics <130/80 mmHg). Use a thiazide diuretic (e.g. bendroflumethiazide or indapamide) or an ACE-inhibitor (e.g. perindopril or ramipril) or preferably a combination of both, unless there are contraindications.
- Patients who are not on anticoagulation should be taking an aspirin (75mg) plus dipyridamole MR 200mg bd. If aspirin intolerant, use clopidogrel 75mg daily.
- Start anticoagulation in patients with atrial fibrillation (persistent or paroxysmal) unless contraindicated.
- Anticoagulants should not be started until brain imaging has excluded haemorrhage, and not until 14 days have passed from the onset of an ischaemic stroke.
- Treatment with a statin (e.g. 40mg simvastatin) if total cholesterol >3.5 mmol/L unless contraindicated.
- Any patient with a carotid artery territory stroke, and carotid artery stenosis 70-99%, without severe disability, should be considered for carotid endarterectomy.

*Indications for decompressive craniectomy: aged up to 60 years; clinical deficits suggestive of the MCA territory infarction with a score on the National Institute of Health Stroke Scale (NIHSS) of >15; decrease in the level of consciousness to a score of ≥ 1 on item 1a of the NIHSS; signs on CT of an infarct of at least 50% of the MCA territory, or infarct volume >143 cm^2 as shown on MRI with DWI.

Stroke: complications[1]

Cerebral complications

Further neurological deterioration may be caused by the following:

- ***Transtentorial herniation*** (📖 p.438) is the commonest cause of death within the first week and carries a mortality of 80%. It is due to raised ICP (📖 p.372) 2° to cerebral oedema, and in ischaemic stroke is commonest after large MCA infarcts. Corticosteroids do not improve outcome; mannitol and hyperventilation may be useful temporary measures (📖 p.372); surgical decompression may be indicated in large haemorrhages, particularly cerebellar ones.
- ***Haemorrhagic transformation*** occurs in ~30% of ischaemic strokes (and up to ~70% of cardioembolic strokes), usually 12h to 4 days after the event. Neurological deterioration, it is usually due to a mass effect.
- ***Acute hydrocephalus*** due to compression of the aqueduct of Sylvius by oedema or blood may occur. Ventricular shunting may be of value.
- ***Seizures*** complicate ~10% of infarcts and are commonest in large, haemorrhagic, and cortical strokes. They usually respond to monotherapy (e.g. phenytoin).
- ***Inappropriate ADH secretion*** occurs in 10–15% strokes. It may initiate or worsen cerebral oedema and is treated by fluid restriction.
- ***Depression*** occurs in ~50% and may require therapy if it persists.

Systemic complications

- ***Aspiration*** is common. Dysphagia occurs in at least half of all cases of stroke[2], the incidence is higher in those with brainstem involvement or pre-existing cerebrovascular disease. It is often undetected at bedside and usually leads to aspiration. Testing the gag reflex is not a sufficient assessment; swallowing must be observed and if there is any suspicion video-fluoroscopy may be used. Patients should generally be fed upright.
- ***Infection*** is a common cause of death following stroke. Pneumonia (including aspiration) and UTIs are the usual problems.
- ***Fever*** usually occurs as a result of infection or DVT. Occasionally, it is a direct result of cerebral damage.
- ***Venous thromboembolism:*** the incidence of DVT following stroke is comparable to that following hip or knee arthroplasty. PE accounts for up to 25% of early deaths following stroke. The use of prophylactic anticoagulants reduces the incidence of venous thromboembolism but it is associated with an ↑risk of haemorrhagic transformation which may outweigh any benefit. Many physicians use prophylactic LMWH, although the RCP guidelines recommend compression stocking only. In the absence of intracranial haemorrhage, sub-clinical or overt proximal DVT should be treated with standard therapy. Below-knee DVT should be managed with compression stockings and serial USS monitoring for evidence of proximal extension.
- ***Pressure sores*** occur easily unless patients are regularly turned.

Stroke: acute blood pressure control

Box 6.27 Management key points: hypertension in acute ischemic stroke*

In patients not eligible for thrombolysis

- DBP >140mmHg:
  - Aim: 10–15% reduction of BP.
  - Nitroprusside 0.5mcg/kg/min IV infusion as initial dose, monitor BP continuously.
- DBP: 121–140mmHg *or* SBP >220mmHg:
  - Aim: 10–15% reduction of BP
  - Labetalol 10–20 mg IV over 1–2min; may repeat or double every 10min (maximum dose 300mg) *or* nicardipine 5 mg/h IV infusion as initial dose; titrate to desired effect by increasing 2.5mg/h every 5min to maximum of 15mg/h.
- SBP <220mmHg *or* DBP <120mmHg :
  - Observe unless other end-organ involvement (i.e. aortic dissection, hypertensive encephalopathy, acute myocardial infarction, pulmonary oedema).
  - Treat other symptoms (e.g. pain, headache, agitation, nausea, and vomiting) and acute complications of stroke (hypoxia, seizures, ↑ ICP, or hypoglycaemia).

In patients eligible for thrombolysis

- Before thrombolysis:
  - SBP >185mmHg *or* DBP >110mmHg:
  - Labetalol 10–20mg IV over 1–2min, may repeat once
- During and after thrombolysis:
  - Monitor BP every 15min for 2h, then every 30min for 6h, and then every hour for 16h.
- DBP >140 mmHg:
  - Sodium nitroprusside 0.5mcg/kg/min IV infusion as initial dose and titrate to desired BP.
- DBP: 121–140mmHg *or* SBP >230mmHg:
  - Labetalol 10mg IV over 1–2min, may repeat or double labetalol every 10min to a maximum dose of 300mg or give the initial labetalol bolus and then start a labetalol drip at 2 to 8 mg/min *or* nicardipine 5mg/h IV infusion as initial dose.
  - Titrate to desired effect by increasing 2.5mg/h every 5min to maximum of 15 mg/h.
  - If BP is not controlled by labetalol, consider sodium nitroprusside
- DBP 105–120mmHg *or* SBP 180–230mmHg
  - Labetalol 10mg IV over 1–2min; may repeat or double labetalol every 10 to 20min to a maximum dose of 300mg or give the initial labetalol bolus and then start drip at 2 to 8mg/min.

*Adapted from Adams HP Jr *et al.* (2003). Guidelines for the early management of patients with ischemic stroke. **34:** 1056–83.

Reference

1. Oppenheimer S and Hachinski V (1992). *Lancet* **339:** 721–4. 2. Perry L and Love CP (2001). *Dysphagia* **16:** 7–18.

Stroke: secondary prevention[1]

- ***Attempt to modify 'risk factors'*** (see Box 6.24, p.395). Target BP should be below 140/85 (lower in diabetics). There is little to choose between the different classes of drugs: all reduce the risk of further events. Consider statins, esp. in those with coexisting IHD.
- ***Antiplatelet drugs*** Aspirin reduces recurrence of stroke and death from other causes. In the absence of absolute contraindications aspirin (300mg initially for 2 weeks and 75mg od thereafter) should be given immediately after the onset of stroke symptoms if haemorrhage is considered unlikely; otherwise it should be delayed until brain imaging has been performed. Patients should be treated chronically with aspirin (75mg od) plus, dipyridamole MR (200mg bd). If aspirin intolerant, use clopidogrel 75mg daily.
- ***Anticoagulants*** To prevent recurrence of ischaemic stroke, warfarin is superior to aspirin in valvular, non-valvular, and paroxysmal AF but it is associated with ↑risk of major bleeding. The balance of benefit may depend on patient group but generally favours warfarin, particularly in valvular AF. Aim for an INR of 2–3 provided there are no contraindications and regular checks of INR are practicable. There is no consensus on when to initiate warfarin and whether a repeat CT is required to rule out late haemorrhagic transformation. Current practice is to delay the warfarinization for 2 weeks after the event, and to repeat the scan where the infarct is very large, or where there is clinical suspicion of haemorrhagic transformation. There is no place for either UFH or LMWH. In such cases, it is best to discuss management with a senior colleague. IV heparinization should be commenced immediately in patients with proven cerebral venous thrombosis (regardless of presence of haemorrhagic change on CT), and many neurologists would also do the same for carotid/vertebral dissection.
- ***Carotid endarterectomy*** Should be considered in all patients with >70% ipsilesional stenosis. The operation has an appreciable morbidity (including further stroke) and mortality but appears to improve overall prognosis in selected patients. In centres with experience of the procedure carotid angioplasty may be an alternative particularly in patients who are considered poor surgical candidates.
- ***Patent foramen ovale*** Some advocate closure using an endovascular device but there is only anecdotal evidence of its effectiveness. Current prospective evidence suggests that stroke patients with PFOs treated with aspirin or warfarin only do not have an ↑risk of recurrent stroke or death compared with controls.[2]
- ***HRT and the oral contraceptive* pill** Combined HRT increases the risk of ischaemic stroke and should be stopped. The combined, but not the progestagen only, oral contraceptive pill also appears to be associated with an ↑risk of stroke. Switch to a progestagen-only formulation, or alternative forms of contraception.

References

1. Marshall RS and Mohr JP (1993). *J Neurol Neurosurg Psychiat* **56:** 6–16.

2. Homma S et al. (2002). Circulation 105: 2625–31.

Cerebral infarction syndromes

Anterior (carotid territory) circulation

Middle cerebral artery syndrome

- Total occlusion of the middle cerebral artery (usually embolic) leads to contralateral hemiplegia, hemianaesthesia, homonymous hemianopia, and deviation of the head and eyes toward the side of the lesion.
- Left-sided lesions → global dysphasia; right-sided ones are more likely to → unilateral neglect of contralateral space.
- Branch occlusions of the middle cerebral artery are more common and → incomplete syndromes: e.g. occlusion of upper branches → Broca's ('non-fluent' or expressive) dysphasia and contralateral lower face and arm weakness; lower branch occlusion, on the other hand, may cause Wernicke's ('fluent' or receptive) dysphasia.

Anterior cerebral artery syndrome

Occlusion of this artery (often embolic) can lead to paralysis of the contralateral leg, gegenhalten rigidity, perseveration, alien limb syndrome, grasp reflex in the opposite hand, and urinary incontinence.

Posterior circulation

Posterior cerebral artery syndrome

Occlusion by thrombus or embolus may lead to combinations of contralateral homonymous hemianopia/upper quadrantonopia, mild contralateral hemiparesis and/or hemisensory loss, dyslexia, and memory impairment.

Lacunar infarction

Infarcts in small penetrating vessels, often the consequence of hypertension, → a number of syndromes: pure motor stroke or pure sensory stroke, or pure sensorimotor stroke, ataxic hemiparesis (combined cerebellar and pyramidal signs in the same limb).

Prognostic significance[1]

The type of stroke appears to be a significant factor in a patient's prognosis.

- Total anterior circulation infarcts, i.e. infarcts in the carotid territory leading to motor and sensory deficit, hemianopia, and new disturbance of higher cerebral function have the worst prognosis in terms of death or disability.
- Posterior circulation infarcts, PACIs, and lacunar infarcts have better prognoses, although patients with PACI have a high risk of recurrent stroke within 3 months.

Reference

1. Bamford J *et al.* (1991). Classification and natural history of clinically identifiable subtypes of cerebral infarction. *Lancet* **337:** 1521–6.

Brainstem stroke

Presentation

Sudden onset of:

- *Headache*, nausea, vomiting, vertigo.
- *Weakness*: bilateral or unilateral.
- *Sensory symptoms* (e.g. paraesthesiae) may be confined to face and if unilateral, may be contralateral to weakness.
- *Ophthalmoplegia, gaze deviation, or dysconjugate eye movements*. In unilateral pontine lesions conjugate gaze deviation is directed away from the lesion and toward the side of the hemiparesis if there is one. The reverse applies for frontal cortical strokes.
- *Horner's syndrome*.
- *Ptosis* caused by a midbrain infarct in the absence of an accompanying third nerve palsy or Horner's syndrome is always bilateral.
- *Nystagmus*.
- *Hearing loss* caused by damage to the VIIth nerve nucleus or fascicle.
- *Dysarthria or dysphagia*.
- *Ataxia* which may be uni- or bilateral due to dysfunction of cerebellar connections.
- *Impaired level of consciousness* ranges from transient loss of consciousness to coma.
- *Altered pattern of respiration*.

Signs associated with brainstem dysfunction are explained on 📖 pp.434–439. They result because of damage either to the nuclei (including cranial nerve nuclei) within the brainstem, to the cranial nerves, or to the long tracts which traverse and/or decussate within the brainstem. *'Crossed signs'* may occur in brainstem strokes, e.g. part of the lateral medullary/Wallenberg's syndrome consists of loss of pain and temperature sensation from the contralateral trunk and limbs (crossed spinothalamic) and ipsilateral loss of the same sensory modalities from the face (uncrossed trigeminal tract). There are a large number of other eponymous syndromes associated with damage to particular zones within the brainstem. Learning these is not particularly rewarding; better to concentrate on the principles of brainstem anatomy.[1]

Causes

Thrombosis, embolism, haemorrhage, or vertebral artery dissection (especially following neck manipulation).

Assessment of severity

- Reduced level of consciousness and coma carry worse prognosis.
- Extent of brainstem dysfunction may be appreciated from systematic examination of brainstem function (📖 pp.434–439).
- Basilar occlusion carries a very poor prognosis (~80% mortality).

Management

Consult a neurologist. The imaging modality of choice is MRI; this should be performed urgently to rule out other diagnoses. Some centres may consider intra-arterial thrombolysis in patients with basilar occlusion if the patient is referred swiftly. Urgent intervention is required for.

- Metabolic coma with brainstem depression, e.g. opiates (📖 p.720)
- Transtentorial herniation → progressive brainstem compression (📖 p.138)
- Posterior fossa mass with tonsillar herniation → brainstem compression
- Cerebellar haemorrhage with/without brainstem compression (📖 p.438).

Reference

1. Rowland L (1991). Clinical syndrome of the spinal cord and brainstem. In Kandel E *et al.* eds *Principles of Neural Science*, 3rd edn, pp. 711–730. Appleton & Lange, Norwalk, CT.

Cerebellar stroke

Presentation

Triad of headache, nausea/vomiting, and ataxia is the classical syndrome. But it occurs in <50% of cases and, of course, is common in a number of other conditions. Patients present with symptoms and signs[1,2] which are often attributed to brainstem or labyrithine causes. Always consider the possibility of a cerebellar stroke as a serious alternative diagnosis because surgical decompression can be life saving if there is a mass effect within the posterior fossa. If the diagnosis is a possibility, ask for an urgent CT scan, or better still, an MRI.

- ***Headache, nausea/vomiting*** Sudden or progressive over hours to days. Location of headache varies widely
- ***Dizziness or true vertigo*** Occurs in ~30% of cases
- ***Visual disturbance*** Diplopia, blurred vision, or oscillopsia
- ***Gait/limb ataxia*** Most alert patients report or demonstrate this
- ***Nystagmus or gaze palsy***
- ***Speech disturbance*** Dysarthria or dysphonia in ~50% of alert patients
- ***Loss of consciousness*** May be transient but many present in coma
- ***Hypertension.***

Predisposing factors

- Hypertension (>50%)
- Anticoagulants: there is a disproportionately higher risk of cerebellar haemorrhage (cf. intracerebral haemorrhage) in patients taking warfarin
- Metastatic neoplasm.

Assessment of severity

Patients who present in coma, or subsequently develop it, will die unless they receive surgical treatment. There is debate about the prognosis of those who remain alert.

Management

Make a definitive diagnosis with urgent CT scan. (Is there a haemorrhage/infarct? Is there distortion of fourth ventricle and aqueduct with dilatation of lateral ventricles?) Liaise with regional neurosurgery unit early.

Priorities

1. Stabilize the patient and protect the airway. See 'coma' 📖 p.332
2. Correct bleeding tendency or effects of anticoagulants
3. Intensive care/high dependency ward nursing observations if patient is not transferred to neurosurgical centre immediately
4. Definitive surgical decompression if necessary and possible.

References

1. Dunne JW *et al.* (1987). Cerebellar haemorrhage--diagnosis and treatment: a study of 75 consecutive cases. *Quart J Med* **64:** 739–54.

2. Editorial (1988). Cerebellar stroke. *Lancet* **i:** 1031–2.

Transient ischaemic attacks (TIAs)

Presentation

Sudden-onset focal deficit of cerebral function or monocular blindness resolving within 24h. The symptoms should have developed within a few seconds and if several parts of the body (e.g. face, arm, leg) are involved they should have been affected simultaneously without any 'march' or progression.

- ***Symptoms of carotid TIA*** Hemiparesis, dysphasia, or transient monocular blindness (amaurosis fugax) (see 🕮 p.403).
- ***Symptoms of posterior circulation/vertebrobasilar TIA*** Bilateral or alternating hemiplegia or sensory symptoms, crossed motor/sensory signs (ipsilateral face, contralateral arm, trunk or leg deficit), quadriplegia. Sudden bilateral blindness. 2 or more of vertigo, diplopia, dysphagia, ataxia, and drop attacks if they occur simultaneously.
- ***Symptoms of uncertain arterial territory origin*** Hemianopia alone or dysarthria alone.
- ***Symptoms not acceptable as TIA*** Syncope, loss of consciousness or confusion, convulsion, incontinence of urine or faeces, dizziness, focal symptoms associated with migrainous headache, scintillating scotoma.

Causes

Thrombosis or embolism (see 🕮 Box 6.24, p.395 for risk factors).

Differential diagnosis

Many conditions may appear at first to be a TIA, e.g.

- Cerebral tumour (1° or 2°)
- Brain abscess
- Demyelination
- Focal migraine
- Subdural haematoma
- Todd's paresis (post seizure)
- Hypoglycaemic attack
- Encephalitis.

Investigation

In patients with a suspected TIA in whom vascular territory or pathology is uncertain, a diffusion-weighted MRI should be performed. If MRI is contra-indicated (i.e. pacemaker, sharpnel, some brain aneurysm clips and heart valves, metal fragments in eyes, severe claustrophobia) CT scanning should be used.

Management

The objective is to prevent recurrence or complete stroke. The risk of stroke must be assessed using a validated scoring system such as ABCD^{2}*.

ABCD^{2}* is a prognostic score to identify people at high risk of stroke after a TIA. It is calculated based on:

A age (≥ 60 years, 1 point).
B blood pressure at presentation (≥140/90mmHg, 1 point).
C clinical features (unilateral weakness, 2 points or speech disturbance without weakness, 1 point).
D duration of symptoms (≥60 minutes, 2 points or 10–59 minutes, 1 point). The calculation of ABCD^{2} also includes the presence of diabetes (1 point). Total scores range from 0 (low risk) to 7 (high risk).

Box 6.28 Management key points: TIAs

- Exclude hypoglycaemia.
- If history is compatible with TIA: start Aspirin 300mg.
- Specialist assessment and investigation within 24 hours if ABCD^{2} ≥4 or in cases of crescendo TIA (≥ 2 TIAs in a week). Specialist assessment and investigation may be performed within 1 week if ABCD^{2} <4.
- Best medical treatment: control of blood pressure, antiplatelet drugs (aspirin 75 mg/day plus dipyridamole MR 200mg bd, or clopidogrel if aspirin intolerant), cholesterol lowering through diet and drugs (statins), smoking cessation.
- If vascular territory or pathology is uncertain: diffusion-weighted MRI (or CT if MRI contra-indicated) within 1 week of symptom onset.
- Carotid imaging if the patient is a candidate for carotid intervention within 1 week of symptom onset.
- If level of symptomatic carotid stenosis is 70%–99%: carotid endarterectomy within 2 weeks.

Reference

Johnstone, JC, Rothwell PM, Nguyen-Huynh, MN *et al.* (2007) Validation and refinement of scores to predict very early stroke risk after transient ischaemic attack *Lancet* **369:** 283.

Confusional states and delirium: assessment

Up to 10% of acute medical admissions are complicated by acute confusion or delirium. The hallmark of *acute confusional states* is disorientation in time and place, impaired short-term memory, and impaired consciousness level. Typically, the patient is drowsy with a poor attention span and slowed mentation. In *delerium*, there are, in addition, disorders of perception such as hallucinations (seeing or hearing things not there) or illusions (misinterpreting shadows seen or sounds heard) and these may produce restlessness, agitation, and hyperactivity.

The main priority is to identify the cause of any treatable or life-threatening condition. Only a small minority (<10%) of patients will have a primary neurological disorder and commonly there are multiple factors that may apply; these patients carry a good prognosis.

Assessment

- Assess the mental state: check for disorientation and memory impairment with the mini-mental test. An anxiety state can usually be distinguished by talking to the patient. Vivid hallucinations in the absence of history of mental illness suggests alcohol withdrawal.
- Review the patient's notes and try to obtain history from friends/relatives of previous mental state or episodes of confusion. Patients with dementia are prone to confusion with intercurrent illness.
- Review the drug chart: benzodiazepines and narcotics may cause acute confusion in the elderly. Other drugs that may be involved are steroids, NSAIDs, β-blockers, and psychotropic medications.
- Assess the patient for acute illness: exclude faecal impaction and urinary retention. Relevant investigations are listed in Box 6.30.
- Examine for any focal neurological signs (pupils, limb power, reflexes, and plantar responses).
- In patients with prior high alcohol intake, examine for signs of liver disease, liver 'flap', and possible Wernicke's encephalopathy (nystagmus, ataxia, ophthalmoplegia).

Box 6.29 Mini-mental examination for the elderly

1 Age
2 Time (nearest hour)
3 42 West Street: address for recall at the end of the test (make the patient repeat the address to check)
4 Year
5 Place (name of hospital)
6 Recognition of two people (doctor, nurse, etc.)
7 Date of birth (day and month)
8 Year of World War 1 (or 2)
9 Who is on the throne at the moment?'
10 Count backwards from 20 to 1

Each correct answer scores 1 point. Healthy elderly people score 8.

Box 6.30 Differential diagnosis and investigations

Differential diagnosis	*Investigations*

Systemic disorder
• Sepsis
• Alcohol withdrawal
• Metabolic disorder:
  • ↓ or ↑ glc, Na, or Ca
  • Vitamin deficiency
  • Endocrine disease (thyroid, adrenal cortex)
• Myocardial ischaemia
• Organ failure (renal, respiratory, liver, cardiac)
• Organ failure (renal, respiratory, liver, cardiac).
	• Check urine, blood cultures, WBC, CRP, CXR, U&Es, glc, LFTs, Ca^{2+}, arterial gases, pH, ECG, cardiac enzymes
	• Consider magnesium, amylase, porphyrins, thiamine, B12, folate, TSH, free T4.

Drug toxicity	• Check prescribed medication serum alcohol/drug screen
CNS disorder • Dementia • CVA (esp. non-dominant parietallobe) • Intracranial bleed (SAH, subdural) • Infection (encephalitis, meningitis) • Trauma • Malignancy (1°or 2°) • Post ictal; non-convulsive status • Cerebral vasculitis (SLE, PAN)	• Consider CT scan with contrast, lumbar puncture, EEG, blood cultures, CRP, syphilis serology, Lyme serology
Malignancy	• Check CXR ± CT chest, serum calcium, CT brain

Practice point

Patients who repeatedly protrude their tongue may have tardive dyskinesia.[1]

Reference

1. Hawkes C (2002). Smart handles and red flags in neurological diagnosis. *Hosp Med* **63**: 732–42.

Confusional states and delirium: management

Management (Box 6.31)

- Treat the cause. Nurse in a moderately lit room with repeated reassurance. See if a family member can stay with the patient.
- If the patient is agitated and aggressive, sedation may be necessary. Benzodiazepines may exacerbate confusion: use major tranquillizers (e.g. haloperidol 2–10mg IM/PO or chlorpromazine 25–50mg IM/PO). Observe the effect on the patient for 15–20min and repeat if necessary. In patients with cardiac or respiratory failure, correcting hypoxia may calm the patient by itself. Clomethiazole is indicated for confusion due to alcohol withdrawal (see 🕮 p.414).

Box 6.31 Management key points: acute confusional states

- Nurse in a moderately lit room with repeated reassurance. See if a family member can stay with the patient.
- Sedation if agitated and aggressive (e.g. haloperidol 2–10mg PO/IM. Observe the effect for 15–20min and repeat if necessary. Maximum: 18mg daily).

Identify and treat the underlying cause:

- *Hypoxia*: maintain the airway, O_2.
- *Hypoglycaemia*: 50Ml 50% glucose (remember to give IV thiamine before glucose if malnourishment/alcoholism is likely).
- *Vascular* (intracerebral bleed, infarction or subdural haematoma): see 🕮 pp.376–384, p.380, p.382, p.384.
- *Infection* (intracranial: meningitis/encephalitis; extra-cranial: e.g. pneumonia or UTI particularly in the elderly): antibiotics/antiviral treatments.
- *Trauma*: See 🕮 p.364.
- *Tumours* (and other space-occupying lesions): dexamethasone, liaise with neurosurgeons.
- *Toxic* (e.g. alcohol intoxication/withdrawal or overdoses) or *metabolic causes* (e.g. electrolyte disturbances, renal failure, liver failure, vitamin deficiencies or endocrinopathies): correct the underlying cause; liaise with the appropriate specialist teams.
- *Inflammatory* (cerebral vasculitides): liaise with neurologists and rheumatologists.
- *Post-ictal.*

Acute alcohol withdrawal

Minor symptoms may be managed at home by the GP but often a short admission is more effective and allows observation for complications and psychosocial assessment ± rehabilitation.

Presentation

- Initial symptoms include anxiety and tremor, hyperactivity, sweating, nausea and retching, tachycardia, hypertension, and mild pyrexia. These symptoms peak at 12–30h and subside by 48h.
- Generalized tonic–clonic seizures ('rum fits') may also occur during this period, but status epilepticus is unusual. Typically these do not show the EEG characteristics of epilepsy and may be precipitated by flickering lights or other photic stimulation.
- Delirium tremens ('DTs') occurs in <5% of individuals, usually after 3–4 days of cessation of alcohol intake. It is associated with an untreated mortality of 15%. Features include:
  - Coarse tremor, agitation, confusion, delusion, and hallucinations
  - Fever (occasionally severe), sweating, tachycardia
  - Rarely lactic acidosis or ketoacidosis
  - Also look for hypoglycaemia, Wernicke–Korsakoff psychosis, subdural haematoma, and hepatic encephalopathy.

Management

General measures

- Nurse in a well-lit room to prevent disorientation. Rehydrate (IV fluids if necessary; avoid saline in patients with known chronic liver, disease). Monitor urine output.
- Vitamin supplements: IV therapy (e.g. Pabrinex® 2–3 pairs of amps. IV *slowly* 8-hourly; watch for signs of anaphylaxis) for 5 days or oral therapy [thiamine 100mg PO bd, vitamin B tablets (compound strong) 2 tablets tds, and vitamin C 50mg PO bd] for 1 week.
- Monitor blood glucose for hypoglycaemia and treat if necessary.
- Severe hypophosphataemia may complicate alcohol withdrawal and should be treated with intravenous phosphates (polyfusor phosphates) if serum phosphate is <0.6mM (see 🕮 p.547).
- Exclude intercurrent infection (pneumonia, skin, urine).

Sedation

- Long-acting benzodiazepines such as chlordiazepoxide (Librium®) or diazepam (Valium®) are commonly used; lorazepam is not metabolized by the liver and may be used in liver disease.
- Carbamazepine is as effective as benzodiazepines but side effects limit its use. For severe agitation, haloperidol 10mg IM may be used.

Wernicke–Korsakoff syndrome

- Wernicke's disease comprises the triad of ophthalmoplegia (nystagmus, VI nerve palsy), ataxia (cerebellar type), and confusional state. In Korsakoff's syndrome, confusion predominates, often with overt psychosis, amnesia (antegrade and retrograde), and confabulation. Withdrawal symptoms may also occur.

- Diagnosis: reduced red-cell transketolase activity.
- Treat with IV thiamine (see 'General measures') while waiting for results.

Seizures

- Withdrawal seizures are typically self-limiting; if needed, use IV diazepam (Diazemuls®) 10mg over 5min (see 📖 p.390).
- Treat the patient with chlordiazepoxide (rather than clomethiazole or carbamazepine). Phenytoin is less effective but should be added if there is a history of epilepsy or recurrent seizures.

Follow-up

Arrange referral to an alcohol dependence clinic.

Box 6.32 Sedation regimens in delirium tremens: a guide

Chlordiazepoxide	30mg q6h for 2 days
then	20mg daily (divided doses) for 2 days
then	10mg daily (divided doses) for 2 days
then	5mg daily for 2 days.

Start women on 20mg (instead of 30mg) and taper as above. Reduce the dose in liver disease, in elderly, and in slight individuals.

Carbamazepine

As effective as benzodiazepines and no abuse potential.
Start with 200mg/day in divided doses increasing to 400mg/day over the next 2–3 days and taper off by day 8.

Box 6.33 Management key points: acute alcohol withdrawal

- Nurse in a well-lit room to prevent disorientation.
- Rehydrate (IV fluids if necessary; avoid saline in patients with known chronic liver disease).
- Correct electrolyte disturbances (hypokalaemia, hypomagnesaemia and severe hypophosphataemia).
- IV Pabrinex® (2 pairs tds), followed by oral therapy (thiamine 100mg PO bd, vitamin B tablets (compound strong) 2 tablets tds, and vitamin C 50mg PO bd).
- Reducing regimen chlordiazepoxide.
- Treat intercurrent infection (e.g. pneumonia, skin, urine).
- Monitor urine output and blood glucose for hypoglycaemia.

Neuromuscular respiratory failure: assessment

Presentation

A number of disorders of peripheral nerve, neuromuscular junction, or muscle may present with hypercapnic (type II) respiratory failure, or impending failure. There are many differences between these conditions but consider the diagnosis in the presence of the following features:

- *Limb weakness* progressing over hours or days with diminished/no reflexes but no upper motor neuron signs.
- *Muscular tenderness or pain* may be a feature.
- *Facial weakness.*
- *Ptosis.*
- *Bulbar dysfunction* is a particularly ominous sign because it may lead to improper clearance of secretions and aspiration.
- *Paradoxical abdominal movement:* if the diaphragm is paralysed it moves passively into the thorax with the fall in intrapleural pressure produced by expansion of the ribcage in inspiration. As a result, the anterior abdominal wall also moves in (rather than out) during inspiration.
- *Dyspnoea* or *distress in supine position:* if the diaphragm is paralysed movement of abdominal contents towards the thorax is more prominent when the patient lies flat because gravity no longer acts to counteract this passive movement. As a result, the volume of air inspired is reduced. This is a rare but important cause of orthopnoea.
- *Sensory symptoms* may be present with or without glove-and-stocking sensory loss.
- *Autonomic instability* may be a prominent feature of Guillain–Barré syndrome and may lead to cardiac arrest.
- *Pneumonia* in known neuromuscular disease.
- *Respiratory arrest:* a common pitfall is to consider the degree of respiratory distress unimpressive. Peripheral weakness in combination with an expressionless 'myopathic' facies may lead to a false sense of well-being when the patient may in fact be confronting impending respiratory arrest.

Assessment of severity

- The measurement of forced vital capacity (FVC) is *mandatory* (measured with Wright respirometer available from anaesthetic nurse or ICU). Note that O_2 saturations, peak flow rate, and FEV1 *do not correlate* with the degree of neuromuscular impairment.
- FVC <30mL/kg causes impaired clearance of secretions.
- FVC <15mL/kg suggests ventilatory failure and is an indication for immediate intubation and ventilation regardless of other parameters of respiratory function.
- ABGs: hypercapnia occurs relatively late.
- CXR to determine extent of consolidation if there is concomitant aspiration or infective pneumonia. Subtle linear atelectasis is often seen as a direct result of reduced lung volume.

Neuromuscular respiratory failure: investigations and management

Box 6.34 Investigations for neuromuscular respiratory failure

- FBC, U&Es, CPK, ESR, CRP
- Forced vital capacity
- ABGs
- CXR
- NCS
- EMG
- Anti-AChR antibody/Tensilon® test
- CT/MRI scan for brainstem pathology
- Nerve biopsy, muscle biopsy
- Urine/plasma toxin screen (see Table 6.4)

Management

- Assess severity and measure FVC frequently.
- Consider intubation and ventilatory support if in adults FVC <1L or 15mL/kg. Do not use suxamethonium as a muscle relaxant. It may cause a sudden rise in potassium in patients with denervated muscles.
- Liaise with neurologist early. Consider transfer to regional neurology unit if the patient is well and FVC >25mL/kg and stable. If the patient is unwell and FVC <15mL/kg or falling precipitously from a higher level, intubate electively and then consider transfer. All patients should be accompanied by an anaesthetist.
- Investigations (see Table 6.4). Most of these conditions will not come into the differential but it is advised that blood be taken for virology screen and autoimmune profile, and 20mL be saved for retrospective analysis if required.
- ECG monitoring and frequent observation of BP and pulse is required if Guillain–Barré is suspected because there is a high incidence of autonomic instability.
- Consider specific therapies (see Table 6.4) and
    - Guillain–Barré syndrome p.426
    - Myasthenia gravis p.420
    - Botulism p.428
    - Heavy metal intoxication p.694
    - Organophosphate exposure p.694
    - Porphyria
    - Rhabdomyolysis p.294.
- SC heparin prophylaxis for DVT.
- Enteral nutrition should be considered early.

Table 6.4 Neuromuscular respiratory failure

Condition	Investigation	Specific treatments
Central nervous system disease		
Brainstem disease	• MRI scan	• Reduce ICP • Decompress
Spinal cord disease	• MRI scan	• Decompress
Peripheral neuropathies		
GBS (see 🕮 p.426)	• NCS	• IV immunoglobulin • Plasma exchange
Organophosphates	• Red cell cholinesterase • Plasma pseudo-cholinesterase	• Atropine • Pralidoxime
Heavy metals: lead, thallium, gold, arsenic	• Blood and urine levels	• Specific antidote (see 🕮 p.694)
Drugs (e.g. vincristine)		• Stop drug
Malignancy	• Nerve biopsy	• Cytotoxics
Vasculitis (e.g. SLE)	• Nerve biopsy	• Immunosuppressants
Metabolic (porphyria)	• Urinary porphyrins	• Avoid precipitants • IV glu/haematin
Diphtheria	• Throat swab	• Antitoxin
Neuro-muscular junction disease		
Myasthenia gravis	• Anti-AChRAb • Tensilon® test	• Steroids • Plasma exchange
Anti-cholinesterase overdose	• −ve Tensilon® test	• Stop drug
Hypermagnesaemia	• Plasma Mg	• IV calcium
Botulism(see 🕮 p.428)		• Antitoxin
Muscle disease		
Hypokalaemia	• Plasma K^+	• K^+ replacement
Hypophosphataemia	• Plasma PO_4^{3-}	• PO_4^{3-}replacement
Polymyositis	• EMG • Muscle biopsy	• Steroids
Acute rhabdomyolysis (see 🕮 p.294)	• EMG • Muscle biopsy	• VI hydration • Urine alkalinization

Myasthenic crises[1]

Presentation

- ***Generalized weakness*** usually worse proximally, and classically painless and fatiguable. There may be ptosis and diplopia. Reflexes and sensation are normal.
- ***Dyspnoea*** The patient may not at first glance appear very distressed. An expressionless myopathic facies together with weak muscles of respiration may give a false sense of well-being.
- ***Bulbar dysfunction*** is potentially dangerous as it may lead to impaired clearance of secretions and aspiration pneumonia.
- ***Exhaustion and ventilatory failure*** leading to coma.
- ***History*** of penicillamine use (may cause a syndrome identical to idiopathic myasthenia gravis).

Common predisposing factors

Infection, surgery, drugs (see Box 6.35). NB: corticosteroids used to treat myasthenia can initially lead to an acute crisis.

Assessment of severity

- Vital capacity is the most useful indicator. ABGs are not sensitive enough and demonstrate hypercarbia late.
- Bulbar dysfunction.

Cholinergic crisis

It may not be possible on clinical evaluation to distinguish between worsening myasthenia and excessive anticholinesterase treatment (which leads to weakness by producing depolarization block). Consider withdrawing anticholinesterases only after consulting a neurologist. Note that cholinergic crisis is very rare compared to myasthenic crisis.

Management

- Stabilize the patient: protect the airway; intubate and ventilate if necessary. Ensure there are no electrolyte disturbances (↓K^+, ↓Ca^{2+}, ↑Mg^{2+}) or drugs prescribed which exacerbate weakness.
- Consider Tensilon® (edrophonium) test (see Box 6.35). Anticholinesterase treatment may be helpful if cholinergic crisis is excluded. If there is no effect with Tensilon®, reconsider the diagnosis. Withhold all anticholinesterase medications for 72h. The Tensilon® may be repeated at intervals.
- Immunosuppression should be supervised by a neurologist: prednisolone 120mg/day on alternating days produces improvement after 10–12 days, but should be introduced with care because there may be initial worsening of weakness. High-dose steroids are given until remission occurs. Azathioprine (2.5mg/kg) has also been used for maintenance therapy but takes months to have an effect.
- Plasmapheresis is used to remove circulating antibody. It usually involves exchange of 50mL/kg/day over several days. Most centres use IV immunoglobulin (IVIG) therapy instead of plasmapheresis.
- Regular anticholinesterase inhibitor therapy should be directed by a neurologist. Therapy depends upon response but one initial strategy is to commence with pyridostigmine 60mg q4h. This can be given by NG-tube or, if necessary, IM neostigmine can be used instead (1mg neostigmine should be given for every 60mg pyridostigmine).

Box 6.35 Drugs which may exacerbate myasthenia

Antibiotics

- Gentamicin
- Neomycin
- Colistin
- Tetracycline
- Tobramycin
- Clindamycin
- Streptomycin
- Kanamycin
- Lincomycin

Cardiac drugs

- Quinidine
- Propranolol
- Quinine
- Procainamide

Local anaesthetics

- Lidocaine
- Procaine

Anticonvulsants psychotropic drugs

- Phenytoin
- Lithium
- Barbiturates
- Chlorpromazine

Muscle relaxants

- Suxamethonium
- Curare

Analgesics

- Pethidine
- Morphine

Hormones

- Corticosteroids (initially)
- Thyroxine

Others

- Magnesium salts

Tensilon® (edrophonium) test

1. A history of asthma or cardiac dysrhythmias are relative contraindications. Atropine should be drawn up prior to the test in case edrophonium (an inhibitor of acetylcholinesterase) produces a severe cholinergic reaction, e.g. symptomatic bradycardia.
2. Prepare and label two 1-mL syringes: one containing saline, the other 10mg of edrophonium.
3. Select a muscle to observe for the test and ask a colleague to assess its strength prior to the test.
4. Inject, in stages, the contents of either syringe, keeping both patient and colleague blinded to the contents of each syringe. Ask the observer to reassess muscle strength after the contents of each syringe have been injected.
5. Edrophonium should first be given as a bolus of 2mg (0.2mL) and untoward cholinergic effects should be observed for. If it is tolerated the remaining 0.8mL can be given 1min later.
6. Improvement in muscle strength following edrophonium suggests the patient is suffering a myasthenic, not cholinergic, crisis.

Reference

1. Thomas CE *et al.* (1997). *Neurology* **48:** 1253–60.

Spinal cord compression: assessment

Presentation

- ***Back pain*** is usually the first symptom. It often starts weeks before other features and becomes progressively unremitting keeping the patient awake at night. There may also be *radicular pain* which is misinterpreted and leads to a long and unrewarding search for the cause of chest or abdominal pain.
- ***Sensory symptoms*** such as paraesthesiae or a sensation of limb heaviness or pulling may then occur.
- ***Sensory loss*** may be apparent as a sensory level on testing. It is wise to test for pin prick (spinothalamic function) and joint position sense/ vibration sense (dorsal column function): anterior or posterior portions of the cord may be selectively compressed. 'Sacral sparing' refers to preservation of sensation in (usually) S3–S5 dermatomes; it is a relatively reliable sign of an intramedullary lesion (see Box 6.36) which initially spares laterally placed spinothalamic tract fibres subserving sacral sensation. Note that a sensory level only indicates the lowest possible level of the lesion: it may well be several segments higher.
- ***Weakness*** is often first described as clumsiness but soon progresses to clear loss of power.
- ***Autonomic dysfunction:*** if the sympathetic pathways are involved, especially in high thoracic or cervical lesions, hypotension, bradycardia, or sometimes cardiac arrest may occur. This may be triggered by noxious stimuli such as pain, urinary tract infection, or abdominal distension caused by constipation or bladder outflow obstruction.
- ***Sphincter dysfunction*** commences as hesitancy or urgency of micturition and may progress to painless urinary retention with overflow. Constipation is another consequence of cord compression.
- ***Fever*** should alert one to the possibility of an infectious cause.
- ***Respiratory failure*** occurs with high cervical cord compression and is one cause of acute neuromuscular respiratory paralysis (📖 p.416).
- ***Conus medullaris lesions*** compress the sacral segments of the cord and → relatively early disturbance of micturition and constipation, impotence, reduced perianal sensation and anal reflex; rectal and genital pain occurs later. Plantar responses are extensor.
- ***Cauda equina lesion:*** lesions at or below the first lumbar vertebral body may compress the spinal nerves of the cauda equina leading to a flaccid, areflexic, often asymmetric paraparesis. Lumbosacral pain occurs early; bladder and bowel dysfunction appear relatively late. A sensory level is found in a saddle distribution up to L1 (corresponding to roots carried in cauda equina).
- ***Combined conus and cauda lesions*** produce a combination of lower and upper motor neuron signs.
- ***General examination***: remember that likeliest cause is malignant compression from metastatic disease. Perform a careful examination, including breast, testicles, and thyroid if appropriate.

Assessment of severity

The degree of weakness, sensory loss, and sphincter dysfunction are useful indicators of severity.

Box 6.36 Causes of non-traumatic spinal cord compression

- Tumours:
  - *Primary*: intradural + extramedullary: schwannoma, meningioma; intradural + intramedullary: astrocytoma, ependymoma.
  - *Metastatic (usually extradural)*: breast, prostate, lung, thyroid, GI tract, lymphoma, myeloma
- Infection: staphylococcal abscess, tuberculoma, infected dermoid
- Prolapsed intervertebral disc (central)
- Cyst: arachnoid, syringomyelia
- Haemorrhage
- Skeletal deformity: kyphoscoliosis, achondroplasia, spondylolisthesis.

Spinal cord compression: management

This depends on the diagnosis and the condition of the patient. If the diagnosis is unknown it is imperative to make it swiftly and discuss the case with the regional neurosurgical centre. If the patient is known to have neoplastic disease and malignant compression is very likely, urgent radiotherapy is first-line therapy in most but not all cases. In some patients with disseminated disease it may not be appropriate to make any intervention apart from analgesia. Always consult a senior oncologist.

- Plain XRs of the spine should be obtained immediately. These may show vertebral collapse, lytic lesions, or sclerosis. Perform a CXR to look for malignancy.
- MRI or CT myelography is the next investigation of choice. This should be arranged urgently. If facilities are not available locally, discuss with regional neurosurgical Centre.
- The use of steroids is an important component of the initial management of epidural spinal cord compression. However the optimal dose and schedule remain uncertain. Some experts recommend a bolus of dexamethasone 10mg IV, followed by 16mg/day orally in divided doses for patients with minimal neurologic symptoms. The dose is gradually reduced once definitive treatment is well underway. In patients with paraparesis/paraplegia, high-dose dexamethasone may be given (96mg IV, followed by 24mg qds for 3 days) and the dose can be tapered over 10 days (halve the dose every 3 days).
- A proton pump inhibitor should be given for gastric protection.
- If the cause of compression appears to be infective (fever, neutrophilia, raised CRP, etc.), blood, sputum, and urine cultures should be sent.
- Monitor haemodynamics and watch for autonomic dysfunction. Control pain and act to prevent constipation.
- If there is bladder dysfunction, urinary catheterization may be necessary. If immobile, start prophylactic subcutaneous heparin (5000U tds).
- If there is high cervical compression or if ventilation appears to be compromised, FVC and ABGs should be measured. The indications for intubation (if this is appropriate) are discussed in 'acute neuromuscular respiratory paralysis' (📖 p.416).
- If a diagnosis is not apparent and immediate neurosurgical action is not indicated discuss with radiology with a view to CT-guided biopsy.
- See Box 6.37 for key points in management of spinal cord compression.

Box 6.37 Management key points: spinal cord compression

- Establish the diagnosis:
  - Spine x-ray: (? vertebral collapse, lytic lesions, or sclerosis)
  - Urgent MRI, CXR (?Malignancy)
  - If the cause appears to be infective (fever, neutrophilia, raised CRP): send blood, sputum, and urine cultures
- Discuss the case with the regional neurosurgical centre and consult a senior oncologist regarding advice for urgent radiotherapy for neoplastic disease and malignant compression.
- Corticosteroids:
  - Patients with minimal neurologic symptoms: a bolus of dexamethasone 10mg IV, followed by 16mg/day orally in divided doses.
  - Patients with paraparesis/paraplegia: dexamethasone 96mg IV, followed by 24 mg qds for 3 days and the dose can be tapered over 10 days. A proton pump inhibitor should be given for gastric protection.
- Control pain and act to prevent constipation.
- Urinary catheterization if there is bladder dysfunction.
- Prophylactic SC heparin if immobile.
- Monitor ABG and FVC In cases of high cervical compression or compromised.
- Monitor haemodynamics and watch for autonomic dysfunction.

Guillain–Barré Syndrome (GBS)

Presentation

- ***Progressive weakness of more than one limb*** in an individual who may recently have experienced a mild respiratory or GI febrile illness. Weakness is as commonly proximal as distal. It is usually symmetrical but may be asymmetrical.
- ***Diminished tendon reflexes/areflexia*** is common.
- ***Sensory symptoms***. Paraesthesiae often precede weakness. Sensory loss is not usually profound although there may be a glove-and-stocking distribution impairment of two-point discrimination, joint position, and vibration sense. If there is a sensory level, spinal cord compression (📖 p.424) should be the diagnosis until proved otherwise.
- ***Limb or back pain*** is a major symptom in ~30%.
- ***Cranial nerve dysfunction*** occurs in 50%. Bulbar function and muscles of mastication are affected in 30%; ocular muscles in 10% of patients.
- ***Ventilatory failure:*** see 📖 p.416.
- ***Autonomic dysfunction*** is common: sweating, tachycardia, sudden swings of BP, dysrhythmias, and cardiac arrest. Bladder or bowel dysfunction occurs but if it is present from the outset or if it is persistent, reconsider the diagnosis.
- ***Miller–Fisher variant:*** ophthalmoplegia (giving rise to diplopia), ataxia, and areflexia without significant weakness or sensory signs. Associated with anti-GQ1b antibodies in the serum.

Causes

GBS probably represents an immune-mediated attack on peripheral nerves. Infections which may precede it include cytomegalovirus, *Campylobacter jejuni*, Epstein–Barr virus, hepatitis B, *Mycoplasma*, and herpes simplex virus.

Assessment of severity

Poor prognostic features on presentation include:

- Rapid onset
- Requirement for ventilation (bulbar compromise, reducing VC, respiratory failure)
- Age >40 years
- Reduced amplitude of compound muscle action potential (<10% of control) and extensive spontaneous fibrillation in distal muscles suggesting denervation (NB: electrophysiological studies may be normal in early GBS)
- Presence of autonomic dysfunction
- Axonal variant (often with preceding *Campylobacter jejuni* infection).

A grading system has been devised to follow a patient's progress:

- Grade 1: able to run
- Grade 2: able to walk 5m but not to run
- Grade 3: able to walk 5m with assistance
- Grade 4: chair/bed bound
- Grade 5: ventilated.

Practice point

Acute onset of bilateral facial palsy is usually due to Guillain-Barré syndrome. Long-standing bilateral facial weakness is usually due to Sarcoid or Lyme disease.[1]

Management

It is important to appreciate that GBS is a diagnosis of exclusion with an extensive differential. The pace at which alternative diagnoses need to be excluded depends upon the history and findings.

The management of the patient with GBS is that of any patient with neuromuscular paralysis, although there are a few important specific measures:

- *Monitor FVC* twice daily
- *Autonomic instability* is a common feature, so ECG monitoring and frequent assessment of BP and pulse is advisable, particularly in any patient with bulbar or respiratory involvement (NB: tracheal suction may lead to bradycardia or asystole)
- *CSF analysis* may be required. CSF protein may be normal initially but characteristically rises markedly and peaks in 4–6 weeks
- *Steroids* are of no benefit in GBS
- *Plasma exchange* is currently the only treatment that is proven to be better than supportive treatment alone. *IVIG* (0.4g/kg for 5 days) has never been adequately compared with placebo and is as effective as plasma exchange and is currently the standard treatment. Therapy should not be commenced without prior discussion with a neurologist.
- *DVT prophylaxis.*

Prognosis

Around 65% are able to resume manual work, 8% die in the acute stage (usually from autonomic dysfunction or PE), and the remainder are left with residual disability. The prognosis is worse in those with more severe disease.

Box 6.38 Management key points: Guillain-Barré syndrome

- The management of GBS is that of any patient with neuromuscular paralysis.
- Monitor FVC twice daily.
- Autonomic instability is a common feature (monitor ECG, BP, and PR).
- Plasma exchange.
- IVIG (0.4g/kg for 5 days) appears to be as effective as plasma exchange.
- Therapy should not be commenced without prior discussion with a neurologist.
- DVT prophylaxis.

Reference

1. Hawkes C (2002). Smart handles and red flags in neurological diagnosis. *Hosp Med* **63**: 732–42.

Botulism

Presentation

Botulism is caused by exotoxins of *Clostridium botulinum*. There are 3 syndromes: food-borne, SC drug users wound, and infantile. The latter two causes are rare and will not be discussed here. The most common form of botulism is food-borne with outbreaks usually attributed to canned food. Patients present with symptoms usually within 18h of ingestion of the toxin (Box 6.39):

- *Sore throat, fatigue, dizziness, blurred vision.*
- *Nausea, vomiting, constipation.*
- *Rapidly progressive weakness* often beginning in the extraocular and/or pharyngeal muscles and descending symmetrically in severe cases to give upper and lower limb paralysis and respiratory failure (see 🕮 pp.416–419).
- *Paraesthesiae* may occur but there are no sensory signs.
- *Parasympathetic dysfunction* causes a dry mouth, ileus, and dilated non-reactive pupils in an alert patient. This pupillary response may help to distinguish botulism from other neuromuscular disorders; however, in most cases the pupils remain reactive.

Wound botulism is similar, except GI upset does not occur.

Assessment of severity

Limb weakness and ventilatory failure are indicators of severe disease. Patients with these features have a worse prognosis, as do patients >20 years, and those who have ingested type A toxin.

Management

- Assess severity, *measure FVC frequently*, and attempt to exclude other important causes of neuromuscular failure (see 🕮 p.416). In particular, a *Tensilon® test* should be performed to exclude myasthenia gravis (🕮 p.421); *nerve conduction* should be normal but it is important to exclude Guillain–Barré syndrome (🕮 p.426); *electromyography* is frequently abnormal in botulism (decrement of compound muscle action potential at slow rates of repetitive stimulation of $3s^{-1}$ and facilitation of motor response at rapid rates of $50s^{-1}$). Serum and stool should be assayed for toxin and *C. botulinum*.
- *General management* is described elsewhere (🕮 pp.416–419).
- *Specific treatment:* if botulism is suspected 10,000U of trivalent (A, B, E) antitoxin should be administered IV immediately and at 4-hourly intervals. Approximately 20% patients have minor allergic reactions to this and require corticosteroid and antihistamines as for anaphylaxis (for supplies outside normal working hours contact Department of Health Duty Officer (UK), tel: 020 7210 3000).
- *Guanidine hydrochloride* (an acetylcholine agonist) may be of benefit in some patients (35–40mg/kg/day orally in divided doses).

- Gastric lavage, emetics, cathartics, and enemas may be used with caution to accelerate elimination of toxin from the GI tract. The first 2 interventions are contraindicated if bulbar weakness is present; magnesium-containing cathartics should not be used as there is a risk that magnesium may enhance toxin activity.

Box 6.39 Pathophysiology of botulism

Preformed botulinum toxin is a potent presynaptic blocker of acetylcholine release at the neuromuscular junction, post-ganglionic parasympathetic terminals, and autonomic ganglia. There are 6 antigenically distinct toxins (A–F) but only A, B, and E appear to be associated with human illness.

Tetanus

Presentation

Tetanus is caused by the effects of exotoxins produced by *Clostridium tetani*. It occurs after *C. tetani* spores have gained access to tissues. The wound may be very trivial and in 20% of cases there is no history or evidence of injury. Incubation of spores may take weeks but most patients present within 15 days with:

- *Pain and stiffness of jaw.*
- *Rigidity and difficulty in opening mouth:* trismus or 'lockjaw'.
- *Generalized rigidity of facial muscles* leading to the classical risus sardonicus or clenched teeth expression.
- *Rigidity of body musculature* leading to neck retraction and spinal extension.
- *Reflex spasms* are painful spasms elicited by stimuli such as pressure or noise. These usually occur 1–3 days after the initial symptoms and are potentially very dangerous as they may endanger respiration and precipitate cardiorespiratory collapse.
- *Convulsive seizures.*
- *Autonomic dysfunction* with both sympathetic (sweating, hypertension, tachycardia, dysrhythmias, hyperpyrexia) and parasympathetic (bradycardia, asystole) involvement.

Cause

Exotoxin blocks inhibitory pathways within the CNS.

Assessment of severity

Rapidly progressing features and the onset of spasms signify worse disease and prognosis.

Management

- *Assess severity.* In severe spasms/respiratory failure ventilation will be required. Otherwise patients should be nursed in a quiet, dark room (to reduce reflex spasms) under close observation. Sedation with diazepam may be necessary but beware of respiratory depression.
- *General management* as discussed on 📖 p.416.
- *Specific treatment:* human hyperimmune globulin 3000–10,000U IV or IM should be given to neutralize circulating toxin. This will not ameliorate existing symptoms but will prevent further binding of toxin to CNS. Penicillin IV (1.2g qds), or alternatively tetracycline 500mg qds, should be prescribed to treat *C. tetani*.
- *Wound care and debridement as appropriate:* swabs should be sent for culture but often do not grow the organism.
- *Prophylaxis in patients who have previously been immunized:* for any wound, give a booster dose of tetanus toxoid if the patient has not received a booster in the last 10 years. If the wound appears dirty and infected, or the patient has never been immunized/cannot recall/unable to give history, give human antitoxin (250U IM) in addition to toxoid.

Glasgow Coma Scale (GCS)

Developed to assess depth and duration of impaired consciousness in a standard fashion. The total is out of 15 (see table opposite); the worst possible score is 3 (which even the dead can achieve). The scale has a high rate of inter-observer agreement and GCS score is one useful way of monitoring conscious level.

Eye opening

- If spontaneous, indicates brainstem arousal mechanisms are probably intact, but the patient need not be aware of their surroundings.
- Eye opening to speech is not necessarily a response to a verbal command to open the eyes; any verbal approach, e.g. calling the name of the patient, may elicit this.
- Eye opening to pain is best tested by using a stimulus in the limbs because supra-orbital or styloid process pressure can lead to grimacing with eye closure.

Verbal responsiveness

- An orientated patient knows who they are, where they are, and why they are there; they can recollect the month and year.
- A confused patient will converse but their responses indicate varying degrees of disorientation and confusion.
- An individual with inappropriate speech cannot sustain a conversation; their utterances are exclamatory or random and may consist of shouting or swearing.
- Incomprehensible speech does not consist of any recognizable words but involves moaning and groaning.

Motor response

See Fig. 6.1.

- Patients who obey commands show the best possible motor response but be careful not to misinterpret postural adjustments or the grasp reflex.
- If there is no response to command, a painful stimulus may be applied initially by applying pressure to the fingernail bed. If this elicits flexion at the elbow, pressure may be applied to the styloid process, supra-orbital ridge, and trunk to see if there is localization.
- If pain at the nail bed elicits a rapid withdrawal with flexion of the elbow and abduction at the shoulder it is scored 4.
- If instead it produces a slower flexion of the elbow with adduction at the shoulder, it is considered an *abnormal flexion response* (sometimes called *decorticate posturing*).
- If pain elicits extension of the elbow, adduction, and internal rotation of the shoulder with pronation of the forearm, this is noted as an *extensor response* (sometimes called *decerebrate posturing*).

Prognosis

The GCS is a valuable tool in predicting likely outcome from coma, *but it has limitations* and should not be the only factor used to assess prognosis. Patients with GCS 3–8 generally have far worse prognoses than those with >8. But the cause of coma is also an important predictor, e.g. metabolic coma (especially due to drug intoxication) generally has a better outlook than other causes, irrespective of GCS.

Box 6.40 GCS

Eye opening	
Spontaneously	4
To speech	3
To painful stimulus	2
No response	1
Best verbal response	
Orientated	5
Disorientated	4
Inappropriate words	3
Incomprehensible sounds	2
No response	1
Best motor response	
Obeys verbal commands	6
Localizes painful stimuli	5
Withdrawal to pain	4
Flexion to pain	3
Extension to pain	2
No response	1

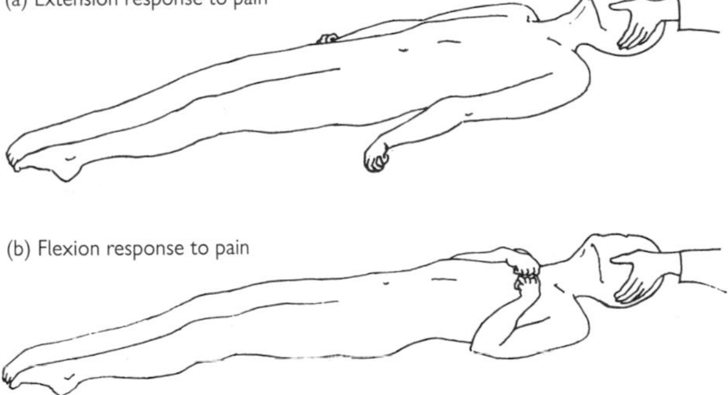

Fig. 6.1 Posturing in coma.

Examination of brainstem function 1

Assessment of brainstem function is vital to the management of coma (📖 p.332), raised ICP (📖 p.372), brainstem strokes (📖 p.404), and brain death (📖 p.442). It is not necessary to have a detailed knowledge of brainstem anatomy. Some simple observations reveal a great deal about function at different levels of the brainstem.

Examination of the eyes

- ***Pupillary reactions*** The size of the pupils and their reactions to bright light should be assessed. This tests the pathway from each eye (IInd cranial nerve) through the superior colliculus (midbrain), its connection to the nearby Edinger–Westphal IIIrd nerve nucleus (also in the midbrain), and efferent parasympathetic outflow of the IIIrd nerve. The pupillary reflex is consensual so light in one eye should elicit constriction of both pupils. Thus observations of the pupillary response can interrogate brainstem function at the level of the midbrain.
- ***Corneal reflex*** This tests the integrity of the afferent pathway (Vth nerve) through to the efferent pathway (VIIth nerve). The corneal reflex is also a consensual reflex. This reflex allows one to interrogate brainstem function at the level of the pons.
- ***Resting eye position*** This may give a useful clue to asymmetric brainstem dysfunction. If the eyes are dysconjugate there must be a disorder of the nuclei of the IIIrd, IVth, or VIth nerves, their connections, or the nerves themselves. Note the IIIrd and IVth nuclei are located in the midbrain, whereas the VIth nucleus is located in the pons.
- ***Spontaneous eye movements*** If there are spontaneous fast (saccadic) horizontal and vertical conjugate eye movements the brainstem mechanism for generating saccades is intact and there is no need to test for the oculocephalic or oculovestibular response because
  - Horizontal saccades require the integrity of the paramedian pontine reticular formation (pons), the IIIrd nerve nucleus, the VIth nerve nucleus, and the medial longitudinal fasciculus connecting these.
  - Vertical saccades require the dorsal midbrain to be intact.
  - Dysconjugate eye movements raise the possibility of unilateral damage to brainstem oculomotor nuclei, their connections, or cranial nerves innervating the extraocular muscles. In this case the resting position of the eyes may also be dysconjugate.
  - A number of oculomotor signs associated with brainstem dysfunction have been identified; none are absolutely specific but they may provide useful clues to site of lesion.[1]

- ***Oculocephalic response*** The 'doll's head manoeuvre' (📖 p.440) should be performed only if cervical injury has been excluded. Both it and caloric stimulation assess the integrity of the vestibulo-ocular reflex which is a three-neuron arc from the semicircular canals via the vestibular nuclei to the IIIrd and VIth nerve nuclei.
- ***Oculovestibular response*** Caloric stimulation (📖 p.440).

Reference

1. Lewis SL and Topel JL (1992). Coma. In Weiner WJ, ed. *Emergent and Urgent Neurology*, pp.1–25. Lippincott, Philadelphia.

Examination of brainstem function 2

The swallowing reflex

This may be tested by injecting 10mL of water in a syringe into the mouth of the patient. Reflex swallowing requires, amongst other things, that the swallowing centre in the reticular formation of the medulla, very close to the solitary nucleus, be intact.

Respiratory pattern (Fig. 6.2)

- This is sometimes useful in localization but often is not.
- *Central neurogenic hyperventilation*, for example, has no localization value. It is rapid, regular deep continuous breathing at ~25/min which is not produced by acidosis or hypoxaemia. Its usefulness is that increasing regularity of this pattern signifies increasing depth of coma and worsening prognosis.
- *Apneustic breathing* (prolonged inspiration followed by a period of apnoea), on the other hand, implies damage to the pons, as does *cluster breathing* (closely grouped respirations followed by a period of apnoea). Damage to the medullary respiratory centres is suggested by *ataxic breathing* and *gasping breathing* (Biot's respirations). The former are characterized by a chaotic pattern of respiration; the latter consist of gasps followed by apnoeic periods of variable duration. Both are usually soon followed by respiratory arrest.
- Shallow, slow breathing may be due to medullary depression caused by drugs, e.g. opiates. *Cheyne–Stokes respiration* may be caused by bilateral deep hemispheric and basal ganglia damage but is more usually due to non-neural causes, e.g. primary cardiovascular or respiratory dysfunction.
- *Long tract signs*. Finally, structural damage to the brainstem may produce long tract signs with dysfunction of descending pyramidal/extrapyramidal tracts or ascending sensory pathways. There may be 'crossed signs' because of decussation of pathways within the brainstem.

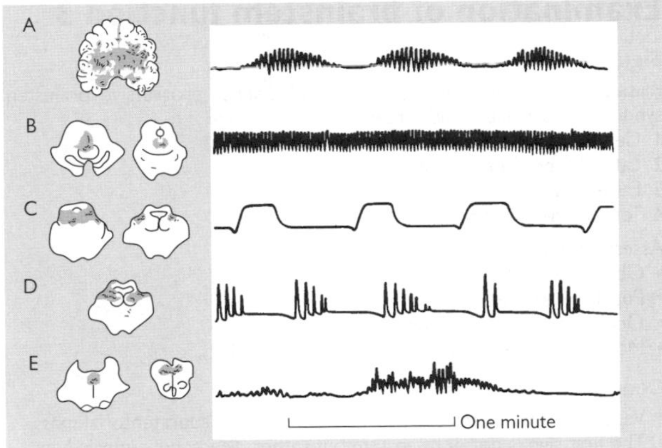

Fig. 6.2 Abnormal respiratory patterns associated with pathologic lesions (shaded areas) at various levels of the brain. (A) Cheyne–Stokes respiration. (B) Central neurogenic hyperventilation. (C) Apneusis. (D) Cluster breathing (E) Ataxic breathing. From Plum F and Posner JB (1980). *The Diagnosis of Stupor and Coma 3rd edn.* FA Davis, Philadelphia, PA, with permission.

Examination of brainstem function 3

Signs of brain shift[1]

Raised ICP may produce a number of distinct progressive brainstem syndromes associated with brain shift:

1 Central herniation syndrome
2 Lateral (uncal) herniation syndrome
3 False localizing signs
4 Tonsillar herniation.

Assessment involves:

- Observation of respiratory pattern
- Pupillary reaction
- Oculocephalic/oculovestibular response
- Motor response at rest or to pain (see 📖 p.432).

Central herniation syndrome

- Vertical displacement of the brainstem due to a supratentorial mass.
- The first sign is not of brainstem but rather *diencephalic* impairment. The patient becomes less alert and there may be Cheyne–Stokes breathing. The pupils are small (perhaps due to hypothalamic sympathetic dysfunction) but reactive. There may initially have been unilateral hemiplegia due to the supratentorial mass. Characteristically in the early diencephalic stage, paratonic resistance (*gegenhalten*) develops in the contralateral limbs and both plantar responses become extensor. Eventually there is a decorticate response to pain (📖 p.432).
- *Midbrain–upper pontine* dysfunction becomes evident with fluctuations in temperature, onset of central neurogenic hyperventilation, apneustic or cluster breathing (see earlier in this section), unreactive pupils which are 'mid-position' and often irregular in shape, loss of vertical eye movements (which may be tested with the doll's head manoeuvre), increasing difficulty in eliciting horizontal oculocephalic and oculovestibular responses which may become dysconjugate (📖 p.440). Motor responses progress from decorticate (flexor) rigidity to decerebrate (extensor) rigidity in response to pain (📖 p.432).
- *Lower pontine–upper medullary* compromise is revealed by often ataxic breathing, fixed mid-position pupils, and failure to elicit oculocephalic and oculovestibular responses. The patient is flaccid at rest; painful stimuli may not elicit any motor response except occasional flexor responses in the lower limbs.
- *Medullary dysfunction* is terminal. Breathing is ataxic or gasping. The *pulse rate may decrease and BP increase* (Cushing response). After a few gasps, breathing stops and pupils often dilate and become fixed.

Lateral (uncal) herniation syndrome

- Due to lesions in the lateral middle fossa or temporal lobe pushing the medial edge of the uncus and hippocampal gyrus over the free lateral edge of the tentorium.
- The first sign is a *unilaterally dilating pupil* (due to compression of the IIIrd nerve at the tentorial hiatus), which is initially sluggish in response to light. This may soon be followed by ptosis and a complete IIIrd nerve palsy with a fixed, dilated pupil. Oculocephalic and oculovestibular responses initially reveal only the palsy, but are otherwise intact.
- *Midbrain* compression by the herniating uncus may follow rapidly (the diencephalic stage of central herniation is by-passed). The patient becomes progressively less alert and slips into coma. The oculocephalic and oculovestibular responses cannot be elicited. A hemiplegia ipsilateral to the expnading supratentorial lesion (due to the opposite cerebral peduncle being compressed at the tentorial edge) develops and soon progresses to bilateral extensor plantar responses. As compression continues both pupils become fixed in mid-position and central neurogenic hyperventilation commences.
- The rostrocaudal progression of signs associated with central herniation then follow with decerebrate/extensor rigidity etc. as already described. Note decorticate/flexor response to pain is not usually seen in uncal herniation because the diencephalic stage is bypassed.

False localizing signs

As they expand, supratentorial lesions may distort intracranial structures and produce signs which appear to help in localizing the 1° lesion but are in fact due to traction 'at a distance'. The most common of these involve cranial nerves V–VIII.

Tonsillar herniation

Sub-tentorial expanding lesions cause herniation of the cerebellar tonsils through the foramen magnum and compress the pons and midbrain directly. A degree of upward herniation through the tentorial hiatus may also occur and lead to compression of the upper midbrain and diencephalon. It may be difficult to distinguish these effects from those produced by supratentorial lesions. One clue is that there is usually a lack of the rostrocaudal sequence of central herniation.

Reference

1. Posner JB *et al.* (2007). *Plum and Posner's Diagnosis of Stupor and Coma* (Contemporary Neurology 71), 4th edn. Oxford University Press, New York.

Oculocephalic and oculovestibular responses

Background

Passive rotation of the head with respect to the trunk stimulates vestibular and neck receptors. In comatose patients with intact brainstems, this leads to reflexive *slow conjugate* eye movements in the direction opposite to head rotation. The contribution of neck proprioceptors (cervico-ocular reflex) is minimal; the most important reflex pathway in the brainstem extends from the semicircular canals to the oculomotor nuclei (VOR). Ice water irrigation of a semicircular canal 'switches off' its contribution to this pathway and leads to unopposed function of the contralateral semicircular canal. The eyes then deviate toward the irrigated semicircular canal. Both the doll's head manoeuvre and caloric tests check the integrity of the VOR; the latter is more sensitive.

Oculocephalic/doll's head response

- The doll's head manoeuvre should not be attempted if there is any possibility of cervical spine injury.
- The patient's head is first rotated laterally from one side to the other. Vertical movements may be elicited by flexion and extension of the head.
- 'Positive' responses are noted if turning of the head elicits *slow conjugate* deviation of both eyes in the direction opposite to head movement (Fig. 6.3).
- Because there is much confusion about what constitutes positive or negative responses, it is best simply to describe what you see.

Oculovestibular/caloric response

- Caloric testing should be performed when the oculocephalic response is abnormal or cannot be performed (e.g. spine fracture).
- The head is then raised 30° above supine and 100mL of ice water is injected into the external auditory meatus using a thin polyethylene catheter.
- A 'positive' response occurs when both eyes move toward the irrigated ear (Fig. 6.3). This may take up to a minute. 5min should elapse before the other ear is tested.

Significance of results

- If the VOR is intact, major brainstem pathology is unlikely.
- If the horizontal VOR is absent but the vertical one is present, there may be a lesion at the level of the pons.
- If both responses are absent, there is either a major structural brainstem lesion (Fig. 6.3) or there is a metabolic disturbance depressing brainstem function (e.g. opiates). Check pupil size and response to light; symmetrically, reactive pupils suggest metabolic coma. Only a few drugs such as atropine, hyoscine, and glutethimide depress brainstem function and produce pupillary abnormalities.

- If dysconjugate eye movements are elicited, a brainstem lesion is likely. Check to see if there is an internuclear ophthalmoplegia.
- It may not be possible to elicit a VOR using the doll's head manoeuvre because the patient has fast, roving saccadic eye movements. These suggest an intact brainstem.

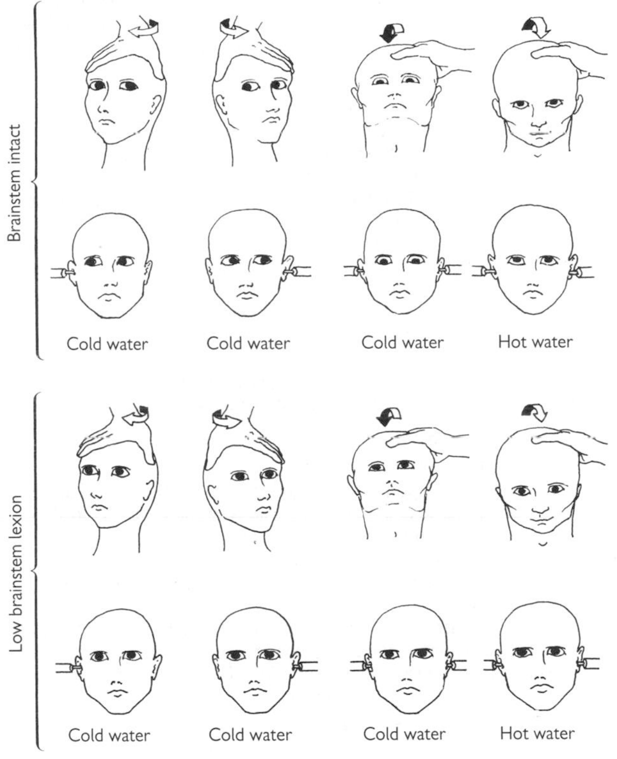

Fig. 6.3 Oculocephalic responses.

Brain death

This is irreversible loss of the capacity for consciousness combined with irreversible loss of the capacity to breathe. Without the brainstem both these functions are lost. But patients with severe, irreversible brain damage who have no brainstem function may survive for weeks or months provided they have a normal circulation and are mechanically ventilated. Criteria for brain death have therefore been developed. It has been shown that patients who fulfil these, even if they are ventilated, will eventually develop cardiovascular collapse.

Preconditions

- There must be no doubt that the patient has irremediable structural brain damage which has been diagnosed with certainty. Usually, this a head injury or intracranial haemorrhage, but it may be anoxia post-cardiac arrest when it is not always possible immediately to be certain that brain damage is irremediable.
- The patient must be in apnoeic coma (unresponsive to noxious stimuli and on a mechanical ventilator) with no spontaneous respiratory effort.
- There must be no possibility of drug intoxication and no paralysing or anaesthetic drugs should have been administered recently. Hypothermia must be excluded as a cause of coma and the core temperature (rectal or external auditory meatus) should be >35°C.
- There must be no significant metabolic, endocrine, or electrolyte disturbance either causing or contributing to coma.

Tests for confirming brain death

All brainstem reflexes must be absent

- Pupils fixed and unresponsive to bright light (they need not be dilated). Paralytic eye drops, ocular injury, and lesions of the IInd/IIIrd cranial nerves may pose problems in this assessment.
- Absent corneal reflexes.
- Absent vestibulo-ocular reflexes on irrigation of each ear in turn with 20mL ice-cold water.
- No motor response within the cranial nerve distribution (eye, face, head) elicited by stimulation of any somatic area (nail bed, supraorbital and Achilles tendon pressure on each side). Purely spinal reflexes, e.g. deep tendon reflexes, may be retained.
- No reflex response to touching the pharynx (gag reflex), nor to a suction catheter passed into the trachea (cough reflex).

Apnoea

- No respiratory movements when the ventilator is disconnected and P_aCO_2 reaches 6.65kPa. (In order to avoid anoxia during this procedure, the patient should be ventilated with 100% O_2 for 10min beforehand; during disconnection, 6L/min 100% O_2 should be delivered via a tracheal catheter. If just prior to disconnection P_aCO_2 is <3.5kPa, give 5% CO_2 in O_2 via the ventilator until this level is reached, usually within 5min.)

The tests must be performed by 2 experienced clinicians and all the above should be repeated after an interval which depends upon the clinical context.

NB: consider the patient a potential organ donor. Discuss with relatives and contact the transplant co-ordinator for your area. Alternatively contact the duty officer for the UK Transplant Support Service (tel: 01179 757575).

Chapter 7

Infectious diseases

Fever in a traveller 1

Assessment

- It is important to obtain a very accurate history of what countries were visited, what areas within those countries, and the activities of the individual whilst they were there (i.e. visits to rural areas or urban travel only, camping versus luxury hotels etc.), together with dates in relation to onset of illness, what drugs were taken, and what were forgotten.
- Do not forget that although the patient has travelled they may have common infections such as pneumonia or pyelonephritis.

Initial investigations

See Box 7.1.

Management

- The epidemiology and drug-resistance patterns of many tropical pathogens are constantly changing and expert advice can be easily obtained from local regional infectious diseases unit. The telephone numbers of the schools of tropical medicine are given on 📖 p.848.
- *Patients should only be sent home if there is no evidence of serious bacterial infection, they are afebrile, and a malaria film is negative. A single malaria film does not exclude malaria and the patient must be reviewed immediately if a further fever occurs.*
- *Isolation.* If there is a history of travel to rural West Africa (particularly rural Nigeria, Sierra Leone, Guinea, or Liberia) and the patient is febrile consider viral haemorrhagic fever (📖 p.468). Discuss the case *immediately* with the regional infectious diseases unit. Only a malaria film and other immediately relevant blood tests should be performed after discussion with the on-site labs. Unless clearly suffering from a haemorrhagic illness, the patient is kept on site until malaria has been excluded and then transferred to a supra-regional high-security infectious diseases unit capable of nursing patients with viral haemorrhagic fevers. If malaria is diagnosed, management can proceed as described on 📖 p.453. All other patients should be nursed in a side room until a diagnosis is established.
- Clinical *rabies* is rare in the UK but should be considered in travellers with severe encephalitis coming from a rabies-endemic area. A more common problem is that patients quite frequently present having suffered an animal bite when travelling in an endemic area. Post-bite prophylaxis can prevent rabies in virtually all cases (see 📖 p.472).
- *TB* should be considered when evaluating all patients, particularly from eastern Europe, the Indian subcontinent, or Africa. TB is a frequent presenting illness in advanced HIV infection, especially in sub-Saharan African patients and may be extra-pulmonary (e.g. TB meningitis, miliary TB, abdominal TB). All patients with TB should be offered HIV testing. Consider drug-resistant TB especially if patient previously treated for TB or has been in prison in eastern Europe.

Box 7.1 Investigations for febrile travellers

• *FBC*	Look for anaemia (malaria, hookworm, malabsorption, leishmaniasis), leucocytosis (bacterial infections, amoebic liver abscess) or leucopenia (malaria, typhoid, dengue fever, acute HIV seroconversion), eosinophilia (helminth/worm infection), thrombocytopenia (malaria, typhoid, dengue fever).
• *Blood films*	Thick and thin films should be examined by a haematologist for malaria. Malaria antigen dipstick tests on blood are now commercially available, quick, and require minimal training.
• *U&Es*	Renal failure may be seen with *P. falciparum*, viral haemorrhagic fevers (📖 p.468), and bacterial sepsis.
• *LFTs*	Jaundice and abnormal liver function are seen with hepatitis A–E, malaria, leptospirosis, yellow fever, typhoid, liver abscesses, and many others.
• *Clotting studies*	Deranged with viral haemorrhagic fevers (📖 p.468), *P. falciparum*, bacterial sepsis, viral hepatitis.
• *Blood cultures*	Mandatory for all febrile patients.
• *Urinalysis*	For leucocytes, nitrites, blood and protein, and a specimen for culture.
• *CXR*	For pneumonia. Raised right hemidiaphragm in amoebic liver abscess.
• *Other investigations to consider*	Serology (hepatitis A, B, C and E), CXR, USS abdomen, sputum MC&S.

Fever in a traveller 2

Presenting feature	Diagnosis to consider
• *Jaundice*	Malaria, hepatitis A, B, C, and E, leptospirosis, yellow fever, typhoid, liver abscess.
• *Splenomegaly*	Malaria, leishmaniasis.
• *Hepatosplenomegaly*	Malaria, schistosomiasis, typhoid, brucellosis, leishmaniasis.
• *Diarrhoea and vomiting*	*E. coli, Salmonella, Shigella, Campylobacter, Giardia, E. histolytica, cholera, V. parahaemolyticus,* viral gastroenteritis.
• *Skin lesions*	Erythema nodosum (TB, leprosy, fungi, post-streptococcal infection).
	Burrows (scabies). See Plate 1.
	Painful nodule with punctum (cutaneous myiasis, i.e. maggots. These need removal).
	Dermatitis (onchocerciasis).
	Ulcers (syphilis, leprosy, leishmaniasis).
	Scabs, eschars (typhus, anthrax).
	Erythema chronica migrans (Lyme disease).
• *Abdominal pain*	With diarrhoea in dysentery, perforation of bowel (typhoid, dysentery), cholecystitis and cholangitis.
• *Haematuria*	Viral haemorrhagic fevers (📖 p.468), schistosomiasis, haemoglobinuria in *P. falciparum.*
• *Meningism/confusion*	Bacterial, viral, fungal, or parasitic meningitis or meningoencephalitis.
• *Bleeding tendency*	Meningococcal septicaemia, haemorrhagic fevers, leptospirosis.
• *RUQ pain ,intercostal tenderness ± R pleural effusion*	Amoebic liver abscess.
• *Pleural effusion*	TB, liver abscess, parapneumonic effusion, empyema.

Malaria: assessment

Malaria: assessment

There are ~2000 cases of Malaria in the UK each year with 1% mortality. The national guidelines can be accessed at: http://www.hpa.org.uk/web/HPAwebFile/HPAweb_C/1194947343507

Organism

- *Plasmodium falciparum* is the causative agent of the most severe and potentially fatal form of malaria.
- *P. vivax*, *P. ovale*, and *P. malariae* may cause chronic, recurrent disease but are not life threatening.
- There are no reliable clinical guides to distinguish each type of infection. The different species can be distinguished by their morphology on a blood film but this needs expert interpretation. Malaria antigen blood dipstick testing can differentiate reliably between *P. falciparum* and *P. vivax*. Mixed infections can occur. If in doubt therapy should be directed against *P. falciparum*.

Symptoms

- Incubation period from 7 days minimum up to 1 year (but usually within 3 months) for *P. falciparum*, up to 2 years for *P. vivax* and *P. ovale*, up to 20 years for *P. malariae*.
- High fever, chills, and rigors followed by sweating. Alternate day fever is described but many patients do not exhibit this.
- Headache is a very common symptom. If associated with impairment in consciousness, behavioural change, or seizure activity, consider hypoglycaemia. Cerebral malaria is defined as unrousable coma (GCS ≤9). Retinal haemorrhages, drowsiness, and other neurological signs may indicate lesser cerebral involvement, which may progress.
- Generalized flu-like symptoms, malaise, and myalgia.
- Abdominal symptoms: anorexia, pain, vomiting, and diarrhoea.

Examination

- No specific features
- Pyrexia in most, but not all cases, often up to 40°C during paroxysms
- Splenomegaly
- Anaemia and jaundice
- Indications of severity (Box 7.2).

Box 7.2 Indicators of severity in *P. falciparum* malaria

- Impaired consciousness or seizures
- Renal impairment (oliguria <0.4mL/kg bodyweight per hour or creatinine >265μmol/L)
- Acidosis (pH <7.3)
- Hypoglycaemia (glucose <2.2mmol/l)
- Pulmonary oedema or ARDS
- Haemoglobin <8g/dL
- Spontaneous bleeding/DIC
- Shock (BP <90/60mmHg)
- Haemoglobinuria (without G6PD deficiency).

Some would also add severe parasitemia (>2%).

Malaria: investigations

All patients should have FBC, U&E, creatinine, LFTs, and blood glucose. In ill patients, blood gases, blood cultures, lactate, and clotting studies should be performed. Urine dipstick/MC&S, stool culture, CXR, and lumbar puncture may be appropriate

- ***FBC*** Anaemia, non-immune haemolysis, leucopenia, and thrombocytopenia suggest *P. falciparum*.
- ***Blood films*** Repeated blood samples over several hours should be examined by an experienced individual if the patient is unwell and malaria not found on the initial blood film. At least 3 films should be examined. A malaria antigen blood dipstick test for *P. falciparum* should also be performed (this is as sensitive as a blood film read by an experienced microscopist). If in doubt, treat for malaria and send the films to a reference laboratory for a definitive opinion. Thick films are more sensitive. Thin films make speciation easier and are used to calculate the parasitaemia.
- ***Parasitaemia*** Mild: <2% parasitaemia, temp. <39°C, and patient ambulant with no complications; severe: >2% parasitaemia or schizonts on film or complications.
- ***G6PD status*** Causes haemolysis in G6PD deficiency.
- ***Glucose*** Hypoglycaemia may occur with *P. falciparum* or IV quinine therapy, especially during pregnancy.
- ***U&Es, LFTs*** Acute renal failure and haemoglobinuria may occur in severe *P. falciparum*. Elevated unconjugated bilirubin, AST, and LDH reflect haemolysis.
- ***Blood cultures*** Even if malaria is confirmed. Other infections such as a Gram-negative septicaemia may also be present.
- ***Head CT scan and LP*** May be required in suspected cerebral malaria to exclude other pathologies.
- ***ABG*** Metabolic acidosis (pH <7.3) indicates severe malaria.

Malaria: management

General measures

- Malaria should be managed in consultation with an infectious disease specialist.
- All cases of falciparum malaria should be admitted to hospital.
- Lower fever with tepid sponging and paracetamol.
- If severe malaria or cerebral malaria admit to HDU/ITU.
- Fits can be controlled with diazepam.
- In severe cases catheterize the bladder to monitor urine output and insert a CVP line to help manage fluid balance, as ARDS can easily be precipitated in these patients. Renal support may be required.
- 2-hourly blood glucose estimations. Regular TPR, BP, urine output.
- Pre-treatment ECG required for IV quinine (causes QT prolongation).
- In severe cases repeat blood films at least twice daily until parasitaemia clearly falling and then perform daily. Daily U&Es, FBC, LFTs.
- Thrombocytopenia is usual and rarely needs support unless platelet count <20 × 10^9/L or bleeding.
- Discuss any severe or complicated malaria with ID unit early. *P. falciparum* acquired on the Thai borders and in neighbouring countries may be quinine resistant and need additional treatment with anti-malarials not generally available (e.g. parenteral artemether or artesunate).
- See 🕮 Box 7.3 p.455.

Malaria: anti-malarial therapy

(For advice in the UK phone London: 020 7387 9300 (treatment); 020 7388 9600 (travel prophylaxis). See *BNF* Section 5.4 for details of other centres.) See Box 7.3 for key points.

P. falciparum

Uncomplicated, non-severe P. falciparum in adults

- Quinine orally, 600mg 8-hourly, reduced to 12-hourly if patient develops severe cinchonism (nausea, tinnitus, deafness). For 5–7 days until afebrile and blood film negative *followed by* either a single dose of 3 tablets of Fansidar® (pyrimethamine and sulfadoxine) or, if Fansidar® resistant (particularly areas of East Africa) or Fansidar® allergic, give doxycycline 100mg bd for 7 days.
- Malarone® (atovaquone/proguanil) and Riamet® (artemether/lumefantrine) have both been licensed for the treatment of non-severe *P. falciparum*. The doses for adults are Malarone®, 4 tablets once daily for 3 days; alternatively, Riamet®, 4 tablets initially, followed by 5 further doses of 4 tablets each given at 8, 24, 36, 48, and 60h .
- Parenteral treatment of malaria should be given if there is parasitaemia >2%, the patient is pregnant, or in patients unable to swallow tablets.

Complicated or severe P. falciparum in adults

- For patients with severe malaria give a loading dose of quinine dihydrochloride IV 20mg/kg in 5% glucose or glucose/saline over 4h (maximum dose 1.4g). After 8h, the patient should be treated with quinine at 10mg/kg infused over 4h (max dose 0.7g) every 8h for 48h. NB: consider using 10mg/kg first dose if recent mefloquine, halofantrine, or Riamet® because of possible toxicity.) Watch carefully for toxicity (QT prolongation). Change to oral regime at 48h and continue quinine 600mg tds until 5–7 days of treatment completed.
- Quinine treatment should be accompanied by a second drug (doxycycline 200mg tds or clindamycin 450mg tds) for 7 days.
- Mefloquine may be effective but resistance is emerging. It is best to contact a malaria expert for advice on the best regimen for the country of origin.
- Chloroquine resistance is widespread. It is not used to treat *falciparum* malaria.

Intensive care management of severe or complicated malaria

- Careful management of fluid balance to optimize O_2 delivery and reduce acidosis.
- Monitoring of CVP to keep right atrial pressure <10cmH_2O, to prevent pulmonary oedema, and ARDS.
- Regular monitoring for hypoglycaemia.
- Consider broad spectrum antibiotics if evidence of shock or 2° bacterial infection.
- Haemofiltration for renal failure or control of acidosis or fluid/electrolyte imbalance.
- Consider medication to control seizures.

Consider exchange transfusion in patients with parasitaemia >10%

- Steroids are not recommended for cerebral malaria.
- Daily blood films until trophozoites cleared.

P. vivax, P. ovale, and P. malariae

- ***Admission*** If the diagnosis is clear and the patient is stable, admission may not be necessary, however many will require admission for short stay. General measures are as described earlier.
- ***Acute therapy*** Chloroquine remains the drug of choice with only very limited resistance reported for *P. vivax*. Give chloroquine: 600mg (base) stat followed by 300mg 6h later and 300mg daily for 2 days.
- ***Radical cure*** Relapse due to persistent hepatic hypnozoite occurs with *P. vivax* and *P. ovale*. Primaquine given after course of chloroquine. Treatment is with primaquine 15mg daily for 14 days. Check G6PD levels before giving primaquine as induces severe haemolysis in these patients, seek advice.
- ***Patient advice*** Avoid contact sports for 1 month because of the risk of splenic rupture.

Box 7. 3 Management key points: malaria

- Admit to ITU if severe or cerebral malaria.
- Monitor blood glucose, temp., PR, BP, urine output, fluid balance.
- Discuss with ID unit. Contact a malaria expert for advice on the best regimen for the country of origin.
  - *P. falciparum:* quinine + Fansidar® (or doxycycline) or Malarone® or Riamet®
  - *P. malariae:* chloroquine
  - *P. vivax*. and. *ovale*: chloroquine: + primaquine (check G6PD levels before giving primaquine).
- Repeat blood films, daily FBC, U&Es and LFTs.
- Other: lower fever with tepid sponging & paracetamol. Control fits with diazepam. Renal support may be required. Thrombocytopenia is usual and rarely needs support unless platelet count $<20 \times 10^9$/L or bleeding.

Infections presenting with fever and rash

Table 7.1 Features of the common childhood exanthems

Rashes table: Features of the common childhood exanthems

Infection	Morphology	Distributioon	Incubation	Associated features	Complications
Varicella (chickenpox)	Clear vesicles on erythematous base (5–12mm), evolving into pustules that burst and crust	Lesions occur in crops, start on trunk and spread peripherally. Mucosal involvement common	10–21 days	Pyrexia 1–2 days flu-like prodrome	Bacterial infection Varicella pneumonia Encephalitis Reactivates as herpes zoster
Measles	Maculopapular, morbilliform	Starts on head and neck spreading peripherally	10–14 days	Coryza, conjunctivitis, cough, lymphadenopathy, Koplik's spots in late prodrome	Otitis media, bacterial pneumonia, measles pneumonia, encephalitis (1:1000), deafness, sub-acute sclerosing panecephalitis(SSPE)
Rubella (German measles)	Pink macular	Progresses from trunk over 2–4 days, may be very mild or absent	14–21 days	Lymphadenopathy especially suboccipital	Arthritis in adults Encephalitis rare
Parvovirus (slapped cheek, erythema infectiosum, fifth disease)	Facial erythema in children. Macular or maculo-papular, morbilliform or annular	Facial rash in children (slapped cheek) Generalized in adults	5–10 days	Lymphadenopathy Arthralgia	Arthritis in adults Foetal loss in pregnancy (hydrops) Anaemia in patients with haemoglobinopathies Cronic infection in immunocompromised

Primary varicella infection (chickenpox)

Chicken pox is an acute infectious disease caused by varicella zoster virus (VZV), usually seen in children <10 years. Reactivation of previous infection can cause shingles (herpes zoster). Chickenpox is highly contagious—infects >90% of those in contact. Incubation period is 10–21 days. Infective period is from 2 days before appearance of rash until all the lesions have crusted (5–6 days). The classical rash is described in 📖 Table 7.1, p.456. Atypical presentations may occur in the immunocompromised host who may have fulminant cutaneous involvement with haemorrhagic chickenpox or conversely can develop systemic involvement with minimal rash.

Complications

Systemic complications are rare in the immunocompetent child but more frequent in adults and the immunocompromised. In the UK chickenpox is responsible for about 20 deaths per year in otherwise healthy adults.

- ***Secondary bacterial infections*** Most frequent complication, 20–50% of hospitalized adults, and responsible for approximately 50% of chickenpox-associated deaths. Super-infections with group A streptococcal septicaemia in children and staphylococcal skin infections (including toxic shock syndrome) or bacterial pneumonia predominate.
- ***Viral pneumonia*** Approximately 1:400 adult cases with 20% mortality. Commoner in smokers. Characterized by cough, breathlessness, and hypoxia with diffuse pneumonitis on CXR.
- ***Hepatitis*** Severe hepatitis rare except in severely immunocompromised. Modest elevation in transaminases is usual.
- ***Encephalitis*** Incidence of 0.1% in adults, 20–30% mortality.
- ***Cerebellar ataxia*** ~1:4000 cases in children, generally self-limited.
- ***Reye syndrome*** Epidemiological association in childhood with concomitant aspirin use.
- ***Congenital varicella syndrome.***

Management

Anti-viral and anti-microbial therapy

- *Immunocompetent children* Anti-viral therapy not indicated. Have a high index of suspicion for bacterial infection if ill enough to require hospitalization.
- *Immunocompetent adult moderately unwell* Within first 24h of the onset of rash may benefit from oral valaciclovir 1g tds, or aciclovir 800mg 5 times per day with reduction in fever and number of lesions.
- *Immunocompetent adult with evidence of pneumonitis* IV aciclovir 10mg/kg q8h and anti-staphylococcal and streptococcal antibiotic cover (e.g. cefuroxime).
- *Pregnancy* Aciclovir is not licensed for use in pregnancy, but appears to be safe and non-teratogenic. Pregnant women are at ↑risk of severe disease and if presenting within 24h of onset of rash, the use of aciclovir should be discussed with an expert.

- *Immunocompromised adult or child* Aciclovir indicated in all cases. If mild disease and minimal immunosuppression, oral therapy with 800mg 5 times per day may be sufficient. In more severe immunosuppression, e.g. post transplant, or any evidence of dissemination, treat with IV 10mg/kg q8h (adult dose).

Prophylaxis for high-risk susceptible patient

- *Hyperimmune immunoglobulin (VZIG also known as varicella zoster immune globulin, VZIG)* is effective in preventing or modifying varicella when given up to 10 days after exposure. VZIG should be given to all susceptible (i.e. absent serum VZV IgG, result usually available within 48h if discussed with lab) immunocompromised individuals as soon as possible after exposure to chickenpox or zoster. VZIG is indicated for VZV IgG-negative pregnant women contacts and should also be given to newborn infants whose mothers have had primary varicella 7 days before to 7 days after the birth.
- Prophylactic aciclovir (taken from days 7–14 after exposure) is also effective in certain groups, but is not licensed for this indication.
- Two live attenuated vaccines are now available in the UK: Varilix® and Varivax®. These are not part of the routine childhood immunization programme. They are currently indicated for vaccination of susceptible health care workers (VZV IgG negative) or for susceptible non-immune adults at risk and others felt to be at ↑risk.
- Pregnant or immunosuppressed susceptible patients (VZV IgG-negative) are at high risk of developing severe disease may be given antiviral drugs e.g. aciclovir and/or VZIG. Contact your local microbiologist/virologist for advice.
- VZIG supplies are limited and tightly controlled. Your consultant virologist or microbiologist should be contacted in the first instance.

Herpes zoster (shingles)

Reactivation from latent virus in the sensory root ganglia. Risk increases with age and immunodeficiency. Vesicular rash developing in crops in a single dermatome, multiple dermatomes, or may be disseminated in the immunocompromised, Up to 20 vesicles are normal in immunocompetent individuals. Suspect immunodeficiency in zoster that is recurrent or affects several dermatomes.

Complications

These are more frequent in immunocompromised patients.

- 2° bacterial infection.
- Post-herpetic neuralgia.
- Eye complications: keratitis occurs in 10% of patients with involvement of the trigeminal nerve (ophthalmic zoster). Rarely there may be retinal necrosis.
- Aseptic meningitis: CSF pleocytosis is common and generally asymptomatic.
- Cerebral angiitis leading to a contralateral hemiparesis.
- Transverse myelitis: mainly in immunocompromised patients.
- Cutaneous dissemination: in excess of 20 vesicles outside of the affected dermatome suggests a high risk of systemic dissemination.
- Systemic dissemination: lung, liver, and brain spread occurs, mainly in immunocompromised patients.

Management

- ***Immunocompetent adult*** Valaciclovir 1g tds, or famciclovir 250mg tds instead of aciclovir (800mg 5 times a day) appears to reduce the duration of post-herpetic neuralgia if given within 48h of onset.
- ***Ophthalmic zoster*** Stain cornea with fluoroscein to detect keratitis; ophthalmology opinion vital if ↓visual acuity or any evidence of eye involvement. If keratitis present treat with topical, aciclovir, or trifluoridine ointment and IV aciclovir or oral valaciclovir or famciclovir.
- ***Uncomplicated zoster in immunocompromised*** Give aciclovir to prevent dissemination. Oral aciclovir, famciclovir, or valaciclovirfor patients with mild immunosuppression (e.g. on long-term steroid therapy). IV aciclovir (10mg/kg q8h) for patients with severe immunosuppression.
- ***Disseminated zoster*** Give IV aciclovir 10mg/kg q8h.

Varicella infection control

Chickenpox is infectious from 48h before the onset of the rash until about 5 days after the onset. Patients should be nursed by immune staff using contact precautions in a neutral- or negative-pressure side room on a ward without immunocompromised patients. Shingles is much less infectious unless it involves the face or other uncovered part of the body.

Meningococcal infection: assessment

Meningococcal meningitis and septicaemia and are severe systemic infections caused by *Neisseria meningitidis*. ~10% of the population carry *N. meningitidis* in their nose or throat but few develop invasive disease. Outbreaks are most common in teenagers, young adults, and crowded environments. Meningism is absent in 30% of cases. It is a notifiable disease.

Rashes

Pupuric lesions are the hallmark of meningococcal septicaemia but several different patterns may be seen either separately or together.

- ***Petechial*** Initially 1–2mm discrete lesions frequently on trunk, lower body, and conjunctivae. Enlarge with disease progression and correlate with thrombocytopenia and DIC, which are poor prognostic signs.
- ***Ecchymoses*** The petechial lesions coalesce and enlarge to form widespread purpura and ecchymoses particularly on the peripheries.
- ***Purpura fulminans*** In extreme cases entire limbs or sections of the body become purpuric and necrotic due to DIC and vascular occlusion.
- ***Maculopapular*** Non-purpuric and easily mistaken for a viral rash occurs early in some patients. May look like flea bites.

Presentation

- ***Predominantly septicaemia*** Symptoms and signs of septicaemia, shock, respiratory distress. May progress from first signs to death within a couple of hours. Purpuric rash almost always develops but may be absent at presentation. Patient often not meningitic. Give antibiotics immediately after blood cultures. Call ICU immediately. Do not perform LP or CT scan.
- ***Predominantly meningitis*** No shock, no respiratory distress. Neurological signs predominate and rash may or may not be present.
- ***Bacteraemia without meningitis or sepsis*** Non-specific flu-like symptoms ± rash. Positive blood cultures. Rash less often present. May develop focal spread such as septic arthritis, pericarditis.
- ***Chronic meningococcaemia*** Low-grade fever, purpuric rash, and arthritis, often confused with gonococcaemia. Sepsis and meningitis do not develop and the illness may last for weeks unless recognized.
- ***Recurrent meningococcaemia*** Suspect immunocompromise, particularly complement deficiency.

Antibiotics

IV 2g cefotaxime or ceftriaxone (see 📖 p.464)

Investigations

- ***Blood cultures*** Immediately. Also take EDTA blood sample for PCR and throat swab. FBC, U&Es, glu, LFT, clotting.
- ***Brain CT scan*** Recent guidelines from the British Infectious Society recommends that an LP can be performed without a head CT in patients with simple meningitis, i.e. not obviously septicaemic and no focal neurological signs and no decrease in conscious level. A CT scan

should be performed prior to lumbar puncture in all cases of meningitis with depressed consciousness (GCS <12 or fluctuating coma score, focal neurology, papilloedema, fits, bradycardia, and hypertension). Give antibiotics before CT scan. Do ***not*** delay treatment. *Do not perform in patients with presumed septicaemia—delays ICU care.*

- ***LP: do not perform in patients with predominantly septicaemia*** (delays their vital immediate management and may be dangerous if DIC). Do ***not*** delay antibiotics beyond 30min (see Box 7.4).

Differential diagnosis of purpuric rash and fever

- Gonococcaemia
- Bacterial septicaemia with DIC
- Haematologic malignancy with sepsis
- Henoch–Schönlein purpura
- In travellers consider:
  - Rocky mountain spotted fever (USA)
  - Viral haemorrhagic fevers (see 🕮 p.468)

Box 7.4 LP findings in meningococcal infections

- Opening pressure: often elevated
- WBC: elevated in ~100%: median 1200 cell/μl, mainly PMN but may be mixed if partially treated
- Protein: elevated in 90%
- Glucose : reduced in 75–80%
- Gram-stain: positive with a negative culture in 10–15%
- Culture: positive in 50–80% of meningitis
- Antigen testing: positive in 50% and correlates with Gram stain
- Meningococcal PCR: positive.

Meningococcal infection: management

Antibiotic therapy (Box 7.5)

- Treatment must be started *immediately* if the diagnosis of *predominantly meningococcal septicaemia* is suspected. If the diagnosis is *predominantly meningitis*, perform LP if no contraindications, but do not delay more than 30min before antibiotics are given.
- If called by a GP then instruct the GP to administer benzylpenicillin 1.2g IM/IV or a third-generation cephalosporin before arranging urgent transfer to hospital.

Treatment

- Cefotaxime 2g qds or ceftriaxone 2g bd.
- If the patient has had definite anaphylaxis or near anaphylaxis to penicillin, then chloramphenicol 25mg/kg 6-hourly (max. 1g qds) may be considered initially.
- If there is a possibility that the patient has pneumococcal meningitis and is severely obtunded start dexamethasone 10mg 6-hourly for 4 days with or just before the first dose of antibiotics: this has been shown to reduce mortality substantially.

Prophylaxis

- Notify the case immediately to the local CCDC.
- CCDC will advise on antibiotic prophylaxis.
- Close contacts only, i.e. household, kissing contacts, close family, institutional contacts (if from a nursing home) etc. in previous 7–10 days.
- Staff members only if involved in resuscitation or ET intubation and suctioning without a mask on.
- Adults: ciprofloxacin 500mg as a single dose (unlicensed indication) or rifampicin 600mg bd for 2 days or ceftriaxone 250mg IM stat.
- Children: rifampicin 10mg/kg bd for 2 days.

Supportive therapy

- Intensive care monitoring is essential in any shocked patient or if significant impairment of consciousness.
- If shocked, urgent fluid replacement, aided by invasive monitoring, is essential. Supportive care for septic shock is discussed on 📖 p.316.
- Treatment of DIC is supportive. Role of drotrecogin alfa (rAPC) is not yet clear: may be contraindicated because of thrombocytopenia, haemorrhage.

Prognosis

- Meningitis without shock: mortality approximately 10%, neurological sequelae uncommon. Coma is a poor prognostic sign.
- Fulminant meningococcaemia: mortality related to organ failure between 20–80%.

Box 7.5 Management key points: meningitis

- Do ***not*** delay treatment because of investigations.
- If called by a GP, instruct the GP to administer benzylpenicillin or a third-generation cephalosporin before arranging urgent transfer to hospital.
- Give cefotaxime 2g qds or ceftriaxone 2g bd. (If there is a history of anaphylaxis to penicillin, chloramphenicol may be used.)
- IV fluids in case of septic shock.
- Monitor shocked patients or those with reduced GCS in ITU.
- If pneumococcal meningitis is suspected and GCS is reduced, consider IV dexamethasone (10mg qds for 4 days with or just before the first dose of antibiotics)
- Notify the CCDC who will advise on antibiotic prophylaxis for close contacts (adults: ciprofloxacin or rifampicin or ceftriaxone; children: rifampicin).

Enteric fever (typhoid)

Enteric fever is a severe systemic infection caused by the bacteria *Salmonella enterica* serovar Typhi and *Salmonella enterica* serovar Paratyphi (Box 7.6). These are usually acquired outside the UK following the ingestion of contaminated food and water.

Presentation

- Non-specific symptoms, e.g. anorexia, myalgia, headache, malaise, fever, chills, and sweats common. Remittent temperature gradually rising during the first week to ~40°C with a relative bradycardia.
- Abdominal pain (30–40%), D&V (40–60%), or constipation (10–50%) may all be seen. Acute abdomen occurs in later stages (perforation of bowel). Splenomegaly (40–60%) and hepatomegaly (20–40%).
- Respiratory symptoms common including sore throat and cough.
- Neurological manifestations including encephalopathy, coma, meningism, and/or seizures are seen in 5–10%.
- Rose spots are 2–4mm erythematous maculopapular lesions, blanch with pressure, and occur in crops of ~10 lesions on upper abdomen lasting only a few hours. Present in 10–30% and easily missed.
- A fulminant, toxaemic, form occurs in about 5–10% of cases with rapid deterioration in cardiovascular, renal, hepatic, and neurological function. In other patients, onset may be quite insidious. In the first 7–10 days after infection bacteraemia occurs with seeding into the Peyer's patches of the gut leading to ulceration and necrosis (weeks 2–3).

Investigations

- ***Initial week of illness*** Normal Hb, ↓WCC or elevated liver enzymes. Blood cultures positive in 80–90%.
- ***2nd–3rd weeks*** ↓Hb, ↑WCC, and ↓platelets due to bone marrow suppression. Blood cultures become negative, urine and stool cultures become positive. Marrow culture positive. AXRs and imaging is indicated if there is abdominal pain.
- ***Serology*** Unhelpful at discriminating active infection from past exposure or vaccination.

Complications

All uncommon with prompt diagnosis and therapy.

- ***Toxaemia*** Acute complications include hyperpyrexia, renal and hepatic dysfunction, bone marrow failure, and myocarditis.
- ***Gastrointestinal*** Late complications due to breakdown in Peyer's patches including GI haemorrhage and perforation.
- ***Metastases*** Meningitis, endocarditis, osteomyelitis, liver/spleen.
- ***Chronic carriage*** 1–3% beyond 1 year.

Management

- ***Supportive care*** If toxaemic admit to ITU. Urinary catheter and CVP line to manage fluid balance. May need renal support.
- ***Antibiotics*** Multiple drug resistance has become a problem and ampicillin can no longer be used for empirical treatment. Quinolones, e.g. ciprofloxacin, 750mg bd orally for 14 days or 400mg bd IV, are currently the agents of choice but resistance has been described and ceftriaxone 2g od is an alternative until sensitivities are known.
- ***Steroids*** Indicated for the severe toxaemic form and have reduced acute mortality although with a small increase in relapses. Give high-dose dexamethasone 3mg/kg followed by 1mg/kg 6-hourly for 8 doses.
- ***Surgery*** Essential for bowel perforation (add metronidazole).
- ***Infection control*** Notify the case to CCDC. Spread is faecal/oral and individuals should not prepare food until follow-up stool cultures (off antibiotics) are negative.
- Consider vaccination.

Box 7.6 Epidemiology of enteric fever

- *Salmonella enterica* serovar Typhi and serovar Paratyphi (less severe) have a widespread distribution including Africa, South America, and Indian sub-continent.
- Incubation period is 7–21 days and it is very rare >1 month after return from an endemic area.
- Untreated mortality 10–15%; with adequate therapy mortality is less than 1% in the UK.
- Relapse rate 1–7%.
- Chronic carrier state: ↑ incidence in elderly, immunocompromised, and with gallstones. Ampicillin or amoxicillin (4–6g/day + probenicid 2g/day) or ciprofloxacin (750mg bd) for 4 weeks will clear 80–90% of patients, falling to 20–50% if the patient has gallstones. Cholecystectomy may eradicate carriage, but not usually indicated if carriage is asymptomatic.

Viral haemorrhagic fevers

Viral haemorrhagic fevers (VHF) are a group of illnesses caused by several different families of viruses (Table 7.2). The incubation period is 3–21 days. Some cause relatively mild disease e.g. dengue fever, whereas others can cause severe life-threatening disease e.g. Ebola and Marburg viruses. VHF are endemic in areas of Africa, south America, and Asia and should be considered in febrile travellers returning from endemic areas.

Many patients with suspected VHF will turn out to have malaria, but when suspected, their management should always be discussed with infectious disease specialist.

Table 7.2 Characteristics of some viral haemorrhagic fevers

Disease	Clinical features	Outcome/management
Dengue fever (serotypes I–IV) Tropical/sub-tropical zones, Americas, Caribbean, Oceania, Asia, Africa Transmission: mosquito–man Huge epidemics Incubation: 3–15 days (usually 4–7 days)	*First exposure:* high pyrexia, headache, joint pains, maculopapular rash on trunk, ↓WCC and ↓platelets *Second exposure to different serotype:* Dengue haemorrhagic shock in 15–25% cases	Isolation not required Mortality low in non-shock cases Treatment supportive Serological diagnosis (acute and convalescent sera) PCR useful in first 5 days of illness only
Yellow fever Tropical Africa, Central and South America *Transmission:* mosquito–human *Incubation:* 3–14 days	Severe cases: headache, myalgia, high fever, and vomiting 3–4 days. 1–2 days later symptoms return with jaundice, haemorrhage, and renal failure, relative bradycardia, leucopenia, DIC, and abnormal liver function	Standard blood/body fluid isolation, advise staff on vaccination Case fatality 5–20% Treatment supportive Diagnosis by PCR and serology

Disease	Clinical features	Outcome/management
Lassa fever Rural districts of West Africa (esp. Sierra Leone, Guinea, Liberia, Nigeria) *Transmission:* rodent–man–man *Incubation:* 3–21 days Possibly 300,000 cases/year in West Africa Ebola virus Rural areas of Central, East, (and possibly West) Africa in outbreaks affecting up to a few hundred people Transmission: person–person Incubation: 2–21 days Marburg virus similar	Fever, pharyngitis, retrosternal pain, and proteinuria Haemorrhagic complications 20–30% of those admitted. Fever, headache, joint pains, sore throat, abdominal pain, and vomiting. Maculopapular rash. Haemorrhagic manifestations common 3–4 days after onset	Refer suspected cases to high-security isolation facility *Mortality:* 1–2%, rising to 15–20% in haemorrhagic cases Ribavirin effective treatment and prophylaxis. Diagnosis by PCR and serology Refer suspected cases to high-security isolation facility. Case fatality 50% Treatment supportive Diagnosis by PCR and serology
Congo-Crimean haemorrhagic fever (CCHF) CCHF is a serious tick-borne viral disease. It is a zoonosis (disease acquired from animals), and infects a range of domestic and wild animals. CCHF virus is endemic in many countries in Eastern Europe, the Middle East, Africa, and Asia. Outbreaks have recently been recorded in Russia, Turkey, Iran, Kazakhstan, Mauritania, Kosovo, Albania, Pakistan, and South Africa.		
Hanta virus Hantaviruses are rodent-borne, zoonotic (acquired from animals) viruses. They cause two serious infections in humans; 'haemorrhagic fever with renal syndrome' (HFRS) and 'hantavirus pulmonary syndrome' (HPS). There are several different Hantaviruses; some are present in Europe and Asia, while others occur in North and South America.		

- Dengue fever is commonly imported into the UK (estimated at 100–150 cases/year) and presents with fever, headache, and rash. Cases of the other haemorrhagic fevers are imported only once every few years.
- Recognition is important because Lassa, Ebola, Marburg, and CCHF have been transmitted to healthcare workers of patients (including laboratory staff). Discuss suspected cases urgently with specialist high-security infectious diseases centres regarding investigation and possible transfer.
- Suspected cases include patients with the onset of their fever within 21 days of leaving an endemic area, particularly if a malaria film is negative.
- Limit local haematological investigations to an absolute minimum if one of these 4 VHFs is suspected (but *always* perform malaria testing).

Rickettsial infections

- These present with fever, headache, and rash and should be included in the differential diagnosis of febrile travellers. Recognition is important because the rickettsial illnesses have significant mortality if left untreated. Isolation is not necessary. Incubation is about 5–14 days.
- *R. conorii* and *R. africae* are probably the two commonest of the group to be imported into the UK, usually from Africa, but *Rickettsiae* are widely distributed across the world.
- Molecular and direct immunofluorescent diagnostic techniques are not widely available, so treatment has to be given on clinical suspicion. Serology is not positive until the 2nd week of the illness at the earliest and may take 3–4 weeks to become positive (and may be modified by treatment).
- First-line treatment is with doxycycline 100mg bd × up to 7 days (other tetracyclines, chlorampenicol, or quinolones have also been used).

Table 7.3 Rickettsial infections

Disease	Clinical features
Typhus group	
Epidemic typhus: *Rickettsia prowazeki*	Fever, severe headaches, maculopapular rash on trunk spreading to extremities. Complications include pneumonitis, encephalitis and myocarditis
Murine typhus: *Rickettsia typhi*	*R. typhi* less severe than *R. prowazekii*
Spotted fever group	
Boutonneuse fever: *Rickettsia conorii* African tick typus: *Rickettsia africae* (plus others)	Fever, severe headache, eschar (black scab with surrounding erythema) at site of bite, sparse papular rash
Rocky mountain spotted fever (N America): *Rickettsia rickettsiae*	Fever, headache, confusion and neck stiffness, joint pains, malaise. Macular rash starts at wrists and ankles spreading to trunk, may be petechial or purpuric. Similar to meningococcal septicaemia. Mortality 30% untreated
Scrub typhus	
SE Asia: *Orientia tsutugamishi*	Eschar, painful regional lymphadenopathy, fever, headache, malaise, maculopapular rash in 60%

Q fever

Coxiella burnetii is a disease of rural areas (reservoirs in sheep and cattle) and transmitted by inhalation of infectious particles in dust, contact with infected carcasses (e.g. in abattoirs) and by tickbites.

- ***Presentation:*** non-specific symptoms, fever, myalgia, malaise, sweats; dry cough and features of atypical pneumonia; hepatitis; PUO and splenomegaly.
- ***Investigations:*** patchy CXR shadowing (lower lobes), hepatic granulomata. Complement fixation tests identify antibodies to phase 1 antigens (chronic infection, e.g. endocarditis 📖 p.96) and Phase 2 antigens (acute infection). *Treat* with oral doxycycline (to try to prevent chronic infection) ± co-trimoxazole, rifampicin, or quinolone

Human bites

- ***Superficial abrasions:*** clean the wound. Re-dress the area daily.
- Give tetanus prophylaxis as needed. Check hepatitis B status and immunize if necessary (see 📖 p.256). HIV counselling and urgent PEP if indicated (see 📖 p.513). HCV has also been transmitted by human bite, so appropriate follow-up needed (there is no HCV PEP).
- Have a low threshold for admission to hospital and IV antibiotic therapy: the human mouth contains a number of aerobic and anaerobic organisms that may produce aggressive necrotizing infection, particularly if the 'closed' spaces of the hand or feet are involved.
- ***Antibiotic therapy:*** all wounds that penetrate the dermis require antibiotics. Aerobic and anaerobic cultures should be taken prior to treatment with antibiotics. A suggested regimen is co-amoxiclav 500/125mg tds PO (or IV cefuroxime and metronidazole). Consult your local microbiologists.
- ***Facial bites:*** cosmetically significant bites should be referred to a plastic surgeon. Puncture wounds should be cleaned thoroughly and treated with prophylactic antibiotics (as described earlier). Patients should be instructed to re-open the wound and express any purulent or bloody material 3–4 times a day for the first few days.
- ***Hand bites:*** should be referred to the orthopaedic team; exploration is recommended. Clean the wound thoroughly. Give the first dose of antibiotics IV and subsequent doses PO unless there are signs of GI upset.

Non-human mammalian bites

- General management is as for human bites (see 📖 p.471). Clean the wound, swab for aerobic and anaerobic culture, tetanus prophylaxis as needed, and prophylactic antibiotics (see 📖 p.471). Rabies prophylaxis (vaccine *plus* rabies-specific immunoglobulin) should be considered in all cases if the bite occurred outside the UK, or if the bite was from a bat *within* the UK, or from an animal in a quarantine facility. For up-to-date advice and supplies of vaccine and immunoglobulin contact the duty doctor, Virus Reference Division, Health Protection Agency, Colindale, London NW9 5HT (Tel. 020 8200 4400). See http://www.hpa.org.uk/infections/default.htm.
- *Rabies* is transmitted by infected saliva inoculated through the skin or by inhalation of aerosolized virus (from infected bats). Presenting features are a viral prodrome followed by parasthesiae and fasciculations. Agitation, confusion, muscle spasms, localized paralysis, and brainstem dysfunction follow. There is no effective treatment once symptoms appear; prevention is essential.
- *Rabies vaccine* should be given prophylactically (in the deltoid) to those at risk of bites from infected animals (vets, animal handlers, field workers, UK bat handlers) as well as frequent travellers to endemic areas.
- Some Old World monkeys, particularly rhesus and cynomolgus macaques are infected with simian herpes B virus (causes a similar illness in monkeys as HSV does in humans). It can be transmitted by bite and saliva and has caused fatal disseminated infection in humans. If the bite is from a macaque from a colony clear of the virus, consider starting valaciclovir 1g tds × 14 days pending further investigation.

Infections in intravenous drug users

Skin and soft tissue infections are common in IVDUs and may be severe e.g. *Clostridium novyi* infections. Deep vein thromboses and infected clots may occur. *Staphylococcus aureus* bacteraemia and right-sided endocarditis are serious complications. In the UK many are HCV positive, but the minority are HIV and HBsAg positive. *S. aureus* bacteraemia and septicaemia is common. Patients with murmurs should have echocardiography to investigate possibility of endocarditis. Multiple round lung infiltrates (± lysis) are characteristic of tricuspid endocarditis with septic emboli.

Necrotizing fasciitis

- Necrotizing fasciitis is a rare infection of the subcutaenous tissues that tracks along fascial planes. It is usually caused by group A streptococci but may also bc polymicrobial. Urgent surgical debridement is the mainstay of treatment. Samples should be sent for urgent Gram stain and culture /as well as sensitivity testing. Empiric antimicrobial therapy usually includes IV clindamycin (reduces toxin production) and co-amoxiclav.
- Patient usually extremely unwell.
- Erythematous, exquisitely tender area, sometimes with underlying crepitus. XR may show gas in subcutaneous tissues.
- Mainstay of treatment is *urgent* debridement of all necrotic tissue by senior surgeon. Further imaging prior to theatre merely delays procedure without providing further therapeutic information.
- Often polymicrobial.
- Clindamycin seems to be an important component of any antimicrobial therapy. One suggested treatment regime is ciprofloxacin 400mg bd IV, clindamycin 600mg qds IV, benzylpenicillin 1.2–2.4g 4-hourly.
- Patients usually require daily debridement in theatre followed by reconstructive surgery.

Severe acute respiratory syndrome (SARS)

- SARS is severe respiratory illness caused by SARS coronavirus. It was first reported in China in 2002 and spread worldwide before being contained in 2004. The re-emergence of SARS remains a possibility.
- This is a new coronavirus infection in man with a high transmission rate to close respiratory contacts, particularly healthcare workers. Also probable transmission by faeco-oral route and fomites. Causes fever, myalgia, and variable pneumonic illness with rapid deterioration in 2nd week of illness. Very low morbidity in pre-adolescents. High mortality in patients >60 years.
- Strict isolation and rigorous enforcement of infection control essential.
- Epidemic waned July 2003, but may reappear.
- Treatment as yet undefined. High-dose steroids may be of some benefit in severely ill. Ribavirin is probably of no value.
- See http://www.who.int/csr/sars/en/index.html

Bioterrorism

- Possible agents of bioterrorism include anthrax (*Bacillus anthracis*), botulism (*Clostridium botulinum*), brucellosis (*Bacillus anthracis*), glanders/melioidosis (*Burkholderia mallei, Burkholderia pseudomallei*), plague (*Yersinia pestis*), Q fever (*Coxiella burnetti*), small pox, tularaemia (*Francisella tularensis)* and VHF.
- There is increasing awareness of the possibility of a deliberate release of biological and chemical agents. Historically plague, *Salmonella* spp. and anthrax have all been used, as have nerve gases and biological toxins. The most recent large-scale releases have been Sarin gas (a nerve gas) on the Tokyo underground in 1995, and anthrax spores (as white powder in the mail) in the USA in 2001.
- Releases are likely to be either airborne or food and water contamination.
- Clues that a deliberate release may have occurred would be the unexpected appearance of an infection outside its normal range (e.g. anthrax in a city), an infection appearing in a patient unlikely to contract the disease, or a sudden cluster of patients with the same pattern of symptoms. 'White powder' incidents also continue to cause concern.
- Any suspicion of a deliberate release should be communicated urgently to the consultant microbiologist and the CCDC (Consultant in Communicable Disease Control). Specific guidelines on diagnosis, management and prophylaxis can be found on the HPA website: http://www.hpa.org.uk/infections/topics_az/deliberate_release/menu.htm
- Current organisms of particular concern include smallpox, plague, tularaemia, melioidosis, botulism, glanders (an infectious disease caused by the bacterium *Burkholderia mallei*), and VHS although other agents may be involved.
- See Table 7.4.

Table 7.4 Characteristics of some bioterrorism agents

Agent	Clinical	Person to person transmission risk	Treatment	Prophylaxis
Smallpox	Initially macules, then deep vesicles predominantly on peripheries (of chickenpox superficial vesicles predominantly on trunk)	Yes	Supportive	Vaccination (post-exposure vaccination effective)
Plague	Likely to be pneumonic with severe sepsis in inhalational plague	Yes	Gentamicin, streptomycin, ciprofloxacin	Ciprofloxacin, doxycycline
Tularaemia	Likely to be flu-like or pneumonic with sepsis in inhalational tularaemia	Very low possibility, but respiratory precautions advisable	Gentamicin, ciprofloxacin	Ciprofloxacin, doxycycline
Anthrax—inhalational	Sepsis, haemorrhagic medistinitis (widened mediastinum), may be minimal pneumonitis	Highly unlikely	Ciprofloxacin, doxycycline	Ciprofloxacin, doxycycline, vaccination
Anthrax—cutaneous	Necrotic ulcer with marked surrounding oedema	Highly unlikely	Ciprofloxacin, doxycycline	Ciprofloxacin, doxycycline, vaccination
Anthrax—white powder incident	Necrotic ulcer with marked surrounding oedema	Highly unlikely	Ciprofloxacin, doxycycline	Ciprofloxacin, doxycycline, vaccination
		If powder contains anthrax spores then highly infectious. Controlled decontamination essential		Ciprofloxacin, doxycycline, vaccination

Meliodosis	Likely to present as septicaemic illness, but spectrum of illness		Ceftazidime, meropenem	
Botulism	Multiple cranial nerve palsies, other palsies. No alteration in conscious level	No	Antitoxin given on clinical suspicion?	
VHFs	Haemorrhagic illness with fever	Yes	Ribavirin for lassa and CCHF	Ribavirin for lassa and ?CCHF
Nerve gases	Anticholinesterase inhibitors, salvation, bronchorrhoea, sweating, bronchospasm, bradycardia, abdominal cramps, diarrhoea, meiosis, muscle fasciculation, weakness, respiratory paralysis, tachycardia, hypertension, emotional lability, confusion, ataxia, convulsions, coma, central respiratory depression	Yes—if clothing contaminated (transcutaneous absorption)	Supportive, atropine, pralidoxime, diazepam	

Chapter 8

Emergencies in HIV-positive patients

Emergency presentations of HIV infection

Patients with human immunodeficiency virus (HIV) infection may present with:

- HIV-related or HIV-unrelated problems
- Toxicity related to anti-HIV therapy
- Patients presenting with 1° HIV infection (seroconversion).

It is important to recognize and diagnose HIV infection in individuals in whom this has been previously unrecognized, and identify patients who may have been exposed to HIV and who may need treatment.

Where there is local expertise in the management of HIV infection, it is recommended that care is provided in consultation with the appropriate team. It is essential to consult with specialists before prescribing any specific treatments.

General principles

- The use of combination antiretroviral therapy is very successful. HIV is now considered to be a chronic manageable disease. Successful antiretroviral therapy significantly increases the CD4 count and reduces the risk of opportunistic complications. HAART reduces HIV RNA load to undetectable levels (e.g. <50 copies/mL plasma) in >95% patients.
- Patients with known or suspected HIV infection should be investigated and managed aggressively.
- Unusual opportunistic infections and malignancies are common and may occur simultaneously or sequentially.
- Toxicity from antiretroviral therapy may present to acute medical services.
- Drug interactions with antiretroviral therapy are common.
- Common diseases still affect HIV-positive individuals but may present atypically.
- All patients should have a full examination including a careful examination for unusual rashes, skin lesions and lymphadenopathy as well as the mouth. Examination of the mouth can reveal a great deal of information regarding the level of immunity (e.g. oral thrush, hairy leucoplakia suggests reduced immunity and ↑risk of severe opportunistic infection; Kaposi sarcoma suggests ↑risk of visceral KS).
- ***Indicator diseases*** that should alert the clinician to investigate for HIV include TB, candidiasis, cryptococcosis, cryptosporidiosis, cytomegalovirus infections, KS, toxoplasmosis (see 🕮 Table 8.1, p.486).
- Always consider HIV in patients from sub-Saharan Africa.
- The acute physician may be the first to consider HIV in previously undiagnosed patients.

Box 8.1 Key points: acute presentations of HIV-positive patients

- Common diseases still affect HIV patients but may present atypically.
- Think of unusual opportunistic infections and malignancies.
- Always consider toxicity from antiretroviral therapy.
- Many drugs interact with antiretroviral therapy.

Factors influencing presentation in HIV disease

Degree of immunosuppression

- The normal CD4 count is 500–1500 x 10^6 cells/mm^3 and gradually decreases during the course of HIV infection.
- The CD4 count is used as a guide to a patient's susceptibility to complications of HIV infection (see Fig. 8.1). For example, *Pneumocystis jiroveci* (formerly known as *P. carinii*) pneumonia (PCP) is uncommon with a CD4 count >200.

Patients (who are aware of their HIV status) are usually familiar with these measures and are likely to be aware of their most recent results.

Risk group and predisposition to different complications

HIV in the UK is predominantly seen in specific patient groups, and the incidence of HIV-related complications varies between these groups.

- Homosexual men have a higher incidence of Kaposi's sarcoma than other Caucasians.
- Injecting drug users are more likely to be co-infected with hepatitis C, and to develop sepsis related to injecting.
- Individuals of African or Asian origin are more likely to present with TB (which may be atypical and/or extra-pulmonary in presentation).
- Individuals of African origin are more likely to experience cryptococcal infection.

Travel history

Many infections in the HIV-infected patient represent reactivation of latent pathogens and a comprehensive travel history is helpful in the differential diagnosis, particularly for individuals presenting with pyrexia.

- Histoplasmosis: travel to central America and the eastern USA.
- Coccidiomycosis: travel to the SW USA and parts of South America.
- Penicillinosis: travel to countries in SE Asia and Indonesia.
- Strongyloides hyperinfection: previous travel in the tropics.
- Leishmaniasis: travel in Mediterranean and tropics.

Antiretroviral therapy

- Patients who respond well to antiretroviral therapy (i.e. low HIV RNA load with a significant increase in CD4 count) have a markedly reduced risk from opportunistic complications of HIV infection. General medical/surgical conditions should be considered as being equally likely in successfully treated patients, as well as in those with untreated HIV infection with a high CD4 count.
- However, antiretroviral therapy is toxic and may present to the emergency clinician (see 📖 p.510), and caution should be exercised when prescribing other drugs.

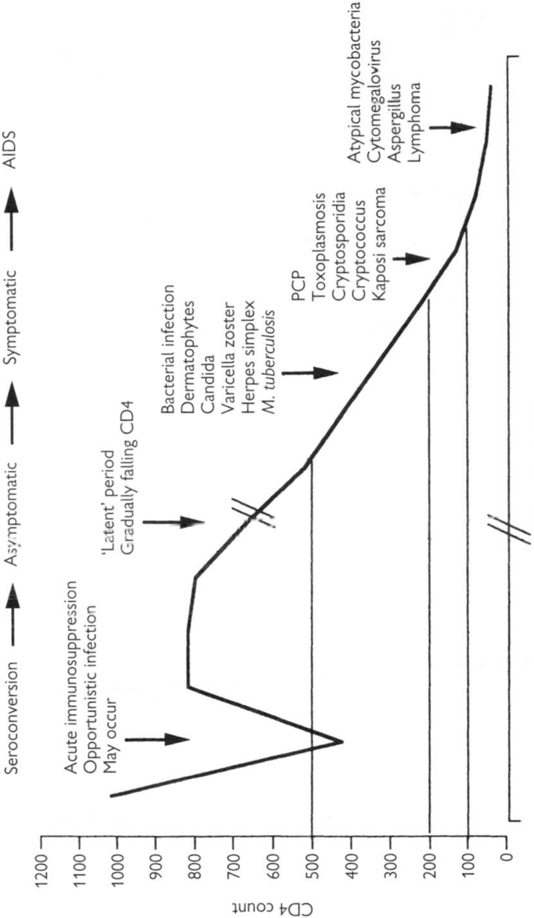

Fig. 8.1 CD4 count is used as a guide to a patient's susceptibility to complications of HIV infection.

HIV testing

In most situations, HIV testing is carried out with informed consent by GUM/STI clinics, in primary care, or as part of routine antenatal care. However, the presentation of individuals with potentially HIV-related complications or at potential risk of previous HIV exposure to the emergency clinician provides the opportunity to diagnose infection. Whilst most choose to have an HIV test within the confidential setting of a specific HIV-testing service, any healthcare provider should possess the essential skills for appropriate discussion of HIV testing. HIV testing should no longer be exceptional but should be considered with informed consent in all patients with clinical indicator diseases or presentations

Pre-test discussion

The following issues should be included in a 'pre-test' discussion:

- Rationale for testing.
- Benefits of knowing status.
- When and by whom the result will be given.
- 'Window period' of infection (i.e. may take up to 3 months from exposure for HIV antibody test to become positive).
- Confidentiality: a negative test may not require disclosure to a GP and does not have implications for insurance/mortgages, etc.; a positive result does not necessarily need to be disclosed to third parties without consent but will have implications for insurance/mortgages.

Post-test discussion

The following principles should be followed in a 'post-test' discussion:

- Giving a positive result should follow the principles of breaking bad news.
- If a result is positive, early referral to an HIV clinician is essential.
- If a result is negative, the window period should be reinforced (particularly in situations where seroconversion is suspected: see 🕮 p.487).
- If a result is negative, the opportunity for future risk reduction should be considered.

HIV testing without consent

It is rarely necessary to test for HIV infection without consent. However, this is justified in the following settings:

- Testing of organ transplantation donors.
- Testing of the unconscious/confused patient where HIV infection is suspected and the management of the patient will be materially changed by knowledge of their HIV status.
- Testing of the unconscious patient who is the 'donor' in a significant needlestick/splash injury. In this situation, testing is justified if the patient is unlikely to regain consciousness for 48h, but should only be performed on a blood specimen that has been previously taken for another purpose.
- Given the potential litigation arising from HIV testing without consent, it is advisable to seek a second opinion (preferably from a physician with HIV experience) that such testing is justified.

Universal HIV testing is recommended in the following settings:

- GUM or sexual health clinics
- Antenatal services
- Termination of pregnancy services
- Drug dependency programmes
- Healthcare services for those diagnosed with TB, viral hepatitis B or C, and lymphoma.

HIV testing should be routinely recommended to the following:

- All patients presenting for healthcare where HIV, including 1° HIV infection, enters the differential diagnosis (see 🕮 Table 8.1, p.486 and 🕮 p.487)
- All patients diagnosed with a STI
- All sexual partners of men and women known to be HIV-positive
- All men who have disclosed sexual contact with other men
- All female sexual contacts of men who have sex with men
- All patients reporting a history of injecting drug use
- All men and women from a country of high HIV prevalence
- All men and women who report sexual contact abroad or in the UK with individuals from countries of high HIV prevalence.

Clinical indicator diseases for adult HIV infection

Table 8.1 Clinical indicator diseases for adult HIV infection

AIDS-defining conditions	Other conditions where HIV testing should be considered
Respiratory: TB Pneumocystis	Bacterial pneumonia Aspergillosis
Neurology: Cerebral toxoplasma Primary cerebral lymphoma Cryptococcal meinigitis PM leucoencephalopathy	Aseptic meningitis/encepahilitis Cerebral abscess Space lesion of unknown cause Guillain–Barré syndrome Transverse myelitis Dementia Peripheral neuropathy
Dermatology: Kaposi's sarcoma	Severe psoriasis Severe seborrhoeic dermatitis Multi-dermal zoster
Gastroenterology: Persistent cryptosporidiosis	Oral candidiasis Oral hairy leucoplakia Chronic diarrhoea (unknown cause) Weight loss (unknown cause) HBV or HCV infection Salmonella, Shigella, or Campylobacter
Oncology: Non-Hodgkins lymphoma	Hodgkin's lymphoma or Castlemans Anal cancer or dysplasia Lung cancer Seminoma Head and neck cancer
Gynaecolgical: Cervical cancer	Cervical or vaginal dysplasia
Haematological	Any unexplained blood dyscrasia
Ophthalmological: CMV retinitis	Any infective retinitis (zoster, toxo-)
ENT	Lymphadenopathy (unknown cause)
Other	PUO or STD Mononucleosis like syndrome

Primary HIV infection (PHI)

PHI (also known as HIV seroconversion illness) is easily overlooked. Intervention may help prevent further spread of HIV (individuals recently infected with HIV are thought to be highly infectious, particularly if unaware of their status).

Risk of recent infection

A significant history of exposure to a potential HIV source within the last 3 months (sexual, percutaneous, or mucocutaneous) in conjunction with any of the features listed here warrants performing specific diagnostic tests for PHI.

Symptoms and signs

- Typically within 2–4 weeks of exposure but can be up to 3 months.
- Flu-like illness (fever, myalgia, headache, lymphadenopathy, retro-orbital pain).
- Maculopapular rash (differential diagnosis of secondary syphilis).
- Pharyngitis/oral ulceration.
- Concomitant sexually transmitted infections (e.g. 1° or 2° syphilis, gonorrhoea, genital ulcer disease).

Laboratory findings

- HIV antibody tests may be negative at the time of seroconversion and an HIV RNA viral load test may be required to confirm the diagnosis.
- Lymphopenia, thrombocytopenia, and raised ALT/AST may occur.

Sequelae of acute immunosuppression

- CD4 count may transiently fall to <200 cells/mm^3 (therefore risk of opportunistic infections, particularly PCP).
- Candidiasis, viral warts, VZV.

Management

- The diagnosis of PHI will enable appropriate partner notification, screening for other STIs, and strategies to reduce onward transmission.
- The utility of antiretroviral therapy in this setting remains controversial and under study.
- New infections may have 1° resistance to one or more antiretroviral agents: knowledge of local resistance rates and patient's resistance profile is needed before initiating antiretroviral therapy.
- Early referral to an HIV specialist is essential.

Acute neurological conditions in HIV-positive patients: assessment

Opportunistic infections and malignancies, the direct effect of HIV itself, and antiretroviral drugs can all cause disease of the central or peripheral nervous system. The presenting features of different conditions are often varied and non-specific and tend to involve the same diagnostic approach and investigations.

Key symptoms and signs

- ***General*** Look for evidence of advanced immunosuppression (see Fig. 8.1, p.483).
- ***Unconsciousness*** Assess and manage as on p.332.
- ***Seizure*** Requires urgent contrast CT or preferably MRI head scan to detect SOL and, if none detected, suitability for diagnostic LP. Consider anti-epileptics but be aware of antiretroviral and other drug interactions (sodium valproate commonly recommended if receiving protease inhibitor or non-nucleoside therapy). Lorazepam is preferable to diazepam for terminating seizures.
- ***Headache*** Elucidate symptoms of raised ICP suggestive of a SOL such as nausea, early morning headache, and ↑intensity on coughing. Distinguish from facial pain caused by dental, sinus, or herpetic neuralgia (check for herpetic rash).
- ***Meningism*** May be reduced or absent due to reduced inflammatory response. Aseptic meningitis can occur during 1° HIV infection (seroconversion illness). With advancing immunosuppression, viral, bacterial, tuberculous, and fungal (cryptococcal) meningitides are more common and may not manifest typical signs of meningism.
- ***Paraparesis*** Consider viral transverse myelitis (HIV, CMV, VZV, or HSV) or cord compression by infection or malignancy. Requires urgent MRI spine and subsequent LP if not contraindicated.
- ***Cognitive impairment*** Wide differential. If associated with any focal neurological signs consider SOL, PML, HIV dementia, late syphilis.
- ***Psychiatric disturbances*** An organic cause is often found. May be a result of antiretroviral drug interactions with antipsychotic and recreational drugs. If aggressive, ensure patient has no access to contaminated sharps.
- ***Peripheral neuropathy*** Typically of gradual onset and caused by certain antiretrovirals or HIV itself.
- ***Myopathy*** Zidovudine (AZT) can cause myopathy or even rhabdomyolysis (check creatine kinase and renal function), arising from mitochondrial toxicity (see p.510). It may also be due to the concomitant use of lipid-lowering agents.
- ***Rapid visual deterioration*** Consider CMV-related retinitis (often apparent on fundoscopy), uveitis, endophthalmitis, and intracerebral causes. Retinal detachment may be a consequence of treatment. Immediate referral to ophthalmologist.

Acute neurological conditions in HIV-positive patients: investigations

Blood tests

- ***Baseline*** (useful if already done—patient will often know results): CD4 cell count, HIV RNA viral load, serology for toxoplasma IgG (positive in >90% of patients with cerebral toxoplasmosis, indicative of risk of reactivation), CMV IgG, serological tests for syphilis (STS).
- ***Routine:*** FBC (low lymphocyte count may give a clue to CD4 depletion), U&Es, LFTs.
- ***Acute:*** inflammatory markers (CRP and ESR), STS, LDH (may be raised in lymphoma), blood cultures (bacterial, mycobacterial (4–6 weeks)). Measure peripheral blood CMV DNA by PCR and cryptococcal antigen (CrAg) if CD4 count <200 cells/mm^3 (positive in >80% with cryptococcal meningitis).

Specific

- ***Stool, urine and throat cultures***. (See Box 8.2 for lumbar puncture).
- ***CXR*** Consider TB at any CD4 count. Para-aortic and hilar lymphadenopathy might suggest MAI or lymphoma.
- ***Contrast CT or MRI scan of head***:
  - Contrast essential, MRI more sensitive than CT (risk of missing brainstem disease, Toxoplasma cysts and PML by CT).
  - Contrast enhancing SOL very likely to be either cerebral toxoplasmosis (typically multiple, with ring enhancement, associated with oedema, at the basal ganglia or grey–white matter interface) or cerebral lymphoma (typically fewer lesions, with irregular enhancement, associated with oedema, periventricular). Poor response to empirical toxoplasmosis treatment suggests lymphoma. Less commonly consider bacterial (e.g. *Streptococcus, Nocardia*), mycobacterial (e.g. tuberculoma), or fungal (e.g. cryptococcoma) lesions. Mycobacterial disease is on the increase especially in 'high risk' populations e.g. patients from endemic TB areas.
  - Meningeal enhancement and hydrocephalus can occur in tuberculous, cryptococcaL, or syphilitic meningitis.
  - PML: non-enhancing, multifocal, subcortical white matter changes. No mass effect.
  - HIV-associated dementia: non-enhancing, diffuse, deep white matter hyperintensities with prominent cerebral atrophy. No mass effect.
  - Viral encephalitis (typically CMV, HSV, VZV) may display variably enhancing confluent changes but often normal.
- ***Brain biopsy*** If disease stage and general prognosis fair, consider performing when no response to empirical treatment.
- ***EEG*** Useful to confirm seizure activity and response to treatment but often non-specific for HIV encephalopathy and opportunistic infections.
- ***Contrast MRI of spine*** The best modality for spinal cord and nerve root imaging.
- ***Nerve conduction studies/electromyogram*** Useful if unusual or treatment-unresponsive sensory or motor symptoms and signs.

Box 8.2 Lumbar puncture

- Arrange for contrast CT or MRI head before any LP and ensure that there are no clotting abnormalities.
- Always measure opening pressure.
- Collect 6–8mL of CSF and divide into 4 universal containers and 1 fluoride tube for glucose (always take paired blood for glucose).
- Bottles 1 and 4 to microbiology for:
  - RBC and WBC estimation
  - Bacterial: microscopy, culture, and sensitivity
  - Mycobacterial: Ziehl–Nieelson microscopy, culture, and consider PCR
  - Viral: PCR for CMV, HSV, VZV, JC virus (PML), EBV (lymphoma)
  - Other: Indian ink microscopy and CrAg (near 100% sensitivity and specificity for neurological cryptococcal disease), fungal culture, and STS.
- Bottle 2 and both fluoride tubes to biochemistry for protein and paired glucose measurement.
- Bottle 3 to cytology (rarely diagnostic) or immunology if indicated.
- Raised CSF cell count and protein (up to 1g/L) can be an incidental finding in asymptomatic HIV infection; conversely, there may be little inflammatory response, e.g. in cryptococcal meningitis.

Acute neurological conditions in HIV-infected patients: treatment

Table 8.2 Treatment for acute neurological conditions in HIV-infected patients

Condition	Possible presentations	Diagnostic tests	Treatment
HIV	Encephalitis or aseptic meningitis Dementia/psychiatric presentation Seizures	Diagnosis of exclusion Brain biopsy diagnostic but not performed for this reason	Highly active antiretroviral therapy (HAART)
Toxoplasmosis	SOL Seizures Confusion Encephalitic illness	90% antitoxo antibody positive but do not discriminate active from inactive disease CT: ring-enhancing lesions Brain biopsy gold standard, perform if no response to empirical therapy	• Sulfadiazine 1–2g IV/PO qds + pyrimethamine 100mg PO od on first day then 75mg PO od + folinic acid 15mg PO od for 4–6 weeks • Clindamycin 1.2g PO/IV qds + pyrimethamine 100mg PO od on first day then 75mg PO od folinic acid 15mg PO od • Atovaquone 750mg PO tds for 21 days • (consider use of dexamethasone to reduce cerebral oedema)
Cryptococcosis	Headache ± meningism SOL (cryptococcoma) Seizures Confusion	CSF: pleiocytosis with low glucose but may be normal in 20–30%. India ink stain, culture, and cryptococcal antigen Serum cryptococcal antigen positive 95%	• Amphotericin 0.25mg–1mg/kg IV od for up to 6 weeks ± flucytosine 100mg/kg PO/IV qds for 2 weeks (liposomal formulations may be used if concerns regarding nephrotoxicity • Fluconazole 400mg bd Daily/regular lumbar punctures to reduce ICP ≤ $20cmH_2O$ is essential.
Mycobacterium	Headache ± meningism	CSF: pleiocytosis with low glucose in most cases ZN stain positive in only 10–20%. CSF culture takes 4–6 weeks	Obtain specialist microbiological advice; initiate therapy with at least 4 agents (preferably including those with CNS penetration, i.e. isoniazid + pyrazi namide) and consider steroids if fits or worsening neurological signs

Nocardia	Headache ± meningism SOL (tuberculoma) Seizures Confusion	Brain biopsy/culture Often co-existing pulmonary disease	Combination of at least 2 of co-trimoxazole, amikacin, streptomycin, imipenem (or meropenem) and minocycline
Cytomegalovirus	Encephalitis Transverse myelitis Polyradiculitis	Viral detection in CSF or neural tissue. PCR, culture, or immunohistochemistry	• Ganciclovir 5mg/kg IV bd for 3 weeks • Valganciclovir 900mg PO bd for 3 weeks • Foscarnet 90mg/kg bd IV for 3 weeks
Varicella zoster	Encephalitis Transverse myelitis Polyradiculitis	Viral detection in CSF or neural tissue. Culture, immunohistochemistry, or PCR	• Aciclovir 10mg/kg IV tds for 10 days • Aciclovir 800mg 5 times daily for 5–10 days • Valaciclovir 1g PO tds for 1 week
Herpes simplex	Encephalitis Radiculitis Seizures	Viral detection in CSF or neural tissue. Culture, immunohistochemistry, or PCR	Aciclovir 10mg/kg IV tds for 14–21 days
PML (JC virus)	Motor dysfunction Cranial nerve palsies Dementia	CSF: anti-JC virus antibodies PCR Brain biopsy White matter MRI/CT changes	HAART
Lymphoma	SOL Malignant meningitis Isolated nerve or spinal cord lesion	CSF cytology Brain biopsy	HAART + chemotherapy (treatment or palliative) + intracranial irradiation

Check BNF for contraindications, cautions, side effects, and interactions

Respiratory emergencies in HIV-positive patients: assessment

Caution: HIV-infected patients presenting with cough warrant a high index of suspicion for Mycobacterium TB or multidrug resistant TB. Such patients should wear a filter mask and be admitted to a side-room. If on a ward with other immunocompromised patients, this should be with negative-pressure isolation facilities.

Key symptoms and signs

- ***General*** Look for evidence of advanced immunosuppression and extra-pulmonary clues to aetiology (e.g. cutaneous KS, neurological signs due to cryptococcosis or retinitis due to CMV). Remember—multiple pathologies can coexist.
- ***Cough productive of sputum*** Purulent sputum suggestive of bacterial or mycobacterial aetiology (incidence of *S. pneumoniae*, *H. influenzae* and TB up to 100-fold higher than in HIV-negative controls). Also consider *S. aureus* (in IVDUs), Gram-negative organisms (e.g. *P. aeruginosa*).
- ***Non-productive cough*** In patients with CD4 cell count <200 cells/mm^3 the main concern is *Pneumocystis jiroveci* (previously *carinii*) pneumonia (PCP, a fungus), which typically has a chronic, progressive history associated with breathlessness (see Table 8.3). PCP can occasionally occur in patients during 1° HIV infection (seroconversion illness) and can be seen in patients despite good adherence to co-trimoxazole prophylaxis. Other causes of non-productive cough include viral URTIs (any CD4 count), KS, lymphoma, and rarely lymphocytic interstitial pneumonitis (any CD4 count but typically raised CD8 cell count with Sjögren's symptoms).
- ***Haemoptysis*** Suggestive of mycobacterial or fungal causes, pulmonary embolus, or KS.
- ***Breathlessness*** If sudden onset, consider pneumothorax (2° to PCP), pulmonary oedema, or PE. If gradual and progressive need to exclude PCP.
- ***Chest pain*** More common in bacterial infections, KS, pneumothorax and pulmonary embolus. HIV-infected patients are more at risk of thromboembolic disease. Pneumothorax may complicate up to 10% of patients with PCP.

Table 8.3 Clinical, laboratory, and CXR findings that may distinguish PCP from bacterial pneumonia

Findings	PCP	Bacterial
CD4 cell count	<200 cells/mm^3	Any
Symptoms	Non-productive cough	Productive cough Purulent sputum
Symptom duration	A few weeks	3–5 days
Signs	Occasionally bilateral fine crackles (usually minimal signs)	Focal lung signs
Laboratory tests	WBC variable	WBC frequently elevated
Chest radiograph findings		
Distribution	Diffuse > focal	Focal >diffuse
Location	Bilateral, perihilar initially	Unilateral, segmental/ lobar
Pattern	Diffuse, interstitial infiltrates	Often lobar or focal consolidation
Cysts	10–15%	5–10% (*Klebsiella*, staphylococcal)
Pleural effusions	Very rare	25–30%

Practice points

- Beware 'normal' CXR: respiratory history is the most important.
- If CD4 count <200 cells/mm^3 and history is compatible, consider PCP as the most likely respiratory infection and start empirical therapy.
- Diagnostic investigations should be done as soon as possible.
- TB is on the increase in the UK.

Respiratory emergencies in HIV-positive patients: investigations

Non-invasive investigations

NB: viral and fungal infections may cause few symptoms and signs—if suspected, request viral PCR or culture and fungal microscopy and culture in addition to the investigations listed here:

- ***Baseline (useful if already done)*** CD4 cell count, HIV RNA viral load.
- ***Radiology*** CXR (see Table 8.4). Other radiology such as ultrasound, CT, or high-resolution CT performed as needed.
- ***FBC*** Leucopenia suggests poor prognosis in bacterial infections and if pre-existing can guide choice of empirical therapy.
- ***U&Es*** Low Na^+ or renal impairment suggests poor prognosis.
- ***LFTs*** Abnormalities suggest disseminated disease or other pathology.
- ***Serology*** For *Legionella*, *Mycoplasma*, and other atypical pathogens.
- ***Cryptococcal antigen*** A test with a >90% sensitivity and >95% specificity for systemic cryptococcaemia.
- ***ABGs*** Hypoxia can occur in any pneumonic process but most characteristic of PCP.
- ***Mantoux test (tuberculin skin testing)*** Results can be misleading or unhelpful as anergy is common. Only used in specific circumstances.
- ***Exercise O_2 saturation*** Significant exercise desaturation very suggestive of a diffuse pneumonitis such as PCP. Useful in patients with 'normal' CXR and SaO_2 >93% at rest.
- ***Lung function tests*** If available these may be useful as impaired gas transfer (KCO) has the same significance as O_2 desaturation.
- ***Blood cultures*** Often positive in *S. pneumoniae* infections. Mycobacterial blood cultures may be useful (4–6 weeks).
- ***Sputum cultures*** For microscopy and culture (incl. mycobacteria).
- ***Induced sputum*** Nebulized hypertonic saline administered by specialist nurse or physiotherapist. Silver stain or immunofluorescence of induced sputum or BAL fluid has a sensitivity of 90% for PCP. Also send samples for microscopy and culture (bacterial and mycobacterial). Do not perform on an open ward.

Invasive investigations

- ***Fibreoptic bronchoscopy*** Usually indicated if no response to treatment or second pathology suspected. Look carefully for KS lesions (transbronchial biopsies not routinely taken as risk of pneumothorax and haemorrhage). Send BAL samples for microscopy (including stains for pneumocystis) and culture (bacterial, fungal, and mycobacterial), viruses, and PCR.
- ***Pleural aspiration*** Cell count, protein, microscopy and culture (bacterial and mycobacterial), cytology, LDH, and pH, pleural biopsy of all significant effusions.
- ***Lung biopsy*** Transbronchial, percutaneous, or open lung biopsy. Seek specialist surgical advice.

Table 8.4 CXR patterns in HIV-associated disease

XR finding	Disease process
Normal	• PCP, viral pneumonia (if hypoxic on exercise)
Focal infiltrate	• Bacterial (*S. pneumoniae, H. influenzae*) • Mycobacteria (TB or MAI) • Fungal organisms (*Cryptococcus, Histoplasma capsulatum, Aspergillus, Candida*) • Patients may have atypical presentations i.e. TB presenting with lower lobe consolidation/pleural effusion instead of upper lobe cavity • *Nocardia* or *Rhodococcus equi* (rare) • Pulmonary KS or lymphoma • PCP (apical if on nebulized pentamidine prophylaxis)
Cavitating	• Bacterial (staphylococcal, streptococcal, *Nocardia*, anaerobes) • Mycobacteria • Fungal organisms • PCP may produce thin-walled cysts (pneumatocoeles)
Pneumothorax	• PCP: occasionally when pneumatocoele ruptures • TB
Diffuse infiltrate	• PCP, classical presentation • Respiratory viruses (RSV, adenovirus, parainfluenza) • CMV (often difficult to decide whether pathogenic role) • Miliary tuberculosis • Fungal organisms • Toxoplasmosis • Lymphocytic interstitial pneumonitis
Pleural effusion	• Bacterial (mainly *S. pneumoniae*) • Mycobacteria (mainly TB) • Lymphoma • Heart failure • KS
Mediastinal lymphadenopathy	• Not a feature of HIV-related lymphadenopathy • Mycobacteria, fungal infection • Lymphoma and KS

Respiratory emergencies in HIV-positive patients: management

General measures

- Monitor pulse, BP, and temperature regularly.
- Pulse oximetry should be used with supplementary O_2 to maintain saturations above 90%.

Assisted ventilation

Being HIV-infected is not in itself a contraindication to assisted ventilation or intensive care. Indeed, many acute respiratory infections requiring such support achieve excellent outcomes. It is the individual's stage of disease and general prognosis that deems such management appropriate or inappropriate, as well as the views of the patient and their next of kin.

Specific treatment of respiratory conditions (Table 8.5)

Contact local microbiology or infectious disease services if uncertain.

Table 8.5 Specific treatment of respiratory conditions

Condition	Dosage, route, frequency, duration
Community acquired pneumonia (CD4 count >200 cells/mm^3)	Co-amoxiclav 600mg tds IV/PO or ceftriaxone 2g od IV for 7 days ± azithromycin 500mg od IV/PO for 3 days
Community-acquired pneumonia (CD4 count <200 cells/mm^3)	If any suggestion of PCP treat as PCP + azithromycin 500mg od/IV PO for 3 days
Pneumocystis jiroveci pneumonia (if PaO_2 <8kPa add prednisolone 75mg od PO for 5 days, then 50mg od for 5 days, then 25mg od for 5 days)	First line: • Co-trimoxazole 120mg/kg in 4 divided doses IV/PO for 21 days Second line: • Clindamycin 600mg–1.2g qds PO/IV + primaquine 15–30mg od PO for 14–21 days • Pentamidine isetionate 4mg/kg od IV for 14–21 days. (3-day 'crossover period' is required if changing from first line to second line) • Atovaquone 750mg PO bd for 21 days
Hospital-acquired pneumonia	• Cefotaxime 1–2g tds IV or ciprofloxacin 500mg bd PO/IV for 7 days + • Azithromycin 500mg od IV/PO for 3 days
IV drug user	Cefotaxime 1–2g tds IV + flucloxacillin 1–2g qds po/iv for 7 days + azithromycin 500mg od IV/PO for 3 days or ceftriaxone + flucloxacillin
Neutropenic patient (duration of treatment guided by microbiologist)	If any suggestion of PCP treat as PCP + • Ceftazidime 1–2g tds IV for 7–14 days + azithromycin 500mg od IV/PO • Piperacillin 4g qds IV + gentamicin (2mg/kg iv loading dose then 3mg/kg IV in divided dose according to levels + azithromycin 500mg od • Ciprofloxacin 500mg–1g bd IV + amoxicillin 2g tds IV + azithromycin 500mg od
KS	HAART ± chemotherapy
Lymphoma	HAART ± chemotherapy

Gastrointestinal (GI) presentations in HIV-positive patients: assessment

Opportunistic infections, malignancies, and antiretroviral drug toxicity can all frequently manifest as symptoms/signs in the GI tract.

Key symptoms and signs

- ***General*** Assess hydration, weight, and nutritional status.
- ***Diarrhoea*** Can be caused by multiple pathogens: both common and opportunistic (see 🕮 Table 8.5, p.499), drug therapy, or advanced HIV per se. The presence of associated symptoms (fever, abdominal pain, blood, *per rectum*) should be established. An awareness of CD4 count will assist in directing management.
- ***Weight loss*** Can be caused by advanced HIV infection, may be the result of chronic diarrhoea/malabsorption, may be the presenting symptom of underlying malignancy or opportunistic infection, or may represent toxicity to antiretroviral therapy (particularly subcutaneous fat loss).
- ***Abdominal pain*** Can be a feature of GI infections (see 🕮 Table 8.5, p.499), biliary tree disease, or pancreatitis—which may be drug induced, notably by nucleoside analogues, particularly ddI (didanosine). Lactic acidosis and hepatic steatosis are rare complications of antiretroviral therapy that may present as vague abdominal pain.
- ***Loin pain/nephrolithiasis*** A well-recognized side effect of indinavir therapy. Stones are unlikely to be seen on plain XRs and usually respond to conservative management with fluid input without need to discontinue the offending agent. With severe episodes (haematuria and confirmed calculi on renal tract investigation) change therapy as there is ↑ risk of further episodes and progressive renal damage.
- ***Jaundice*** May be the result of viral hepatitis (acute or chronic), biliary tract disease, drug-induced hepatitis, or hepatic involvement by other opportunistic infections or tumours. Commonly associated with atazanavir (unconjugated hyperbilirubinaemia).
- ***Dysphagia*** Most commonly caused by candidal infection (oral *Candida* is usually present), and less commonly by ulceration 2° to HSV, VZV, CMV, or idiopathic (aphthous).
- ***Oral lesions*** Oral *Candida* (usually in a pseudomembranous form, appearing as white plaques, but may be erythematous or hyperplastic) and oral hairy leucoplakia (white plaques on the side of the tongue) are common signs in individuals with HIV infection and may be the first presenting features of advancing infection. KS may present as red/purple macules on the palate or gingival margin.

Practice point

There is an epidemic of acute hepatitis C and syphilis in sexually active gay males in the UK. Always test for these organisms if there are concerns or symptoms.

GI presentations in HIV-positive patients: investigations

General investigations

- ***FBC, U&Es, LFTs*** Check for evidence of anaemia, dehydration, hepatic dysfunction.
- ***Blood cultures*** Bacterial GI infections are more likely to be accompanied by systemic infection in the immunocompromised host. Mycobacterial blood cultures (particularly considering atypical mycobacteria in individuals with CD4 counts <100 cells/mm^3).
- ***Amylase*** Check for pancreatitis in individuals with abdominal pain.
- ***Uncuffed serum lactate*** Consider the possibility of lactic acidosis in the unwell patient receiving antiretroviral therapy with non-specific abdominal symptoms. Send to a lab rapidly for an accurate result.
- ***Hepatitis serology*** Consider acute hepatitis A/B in the jaundiced patient and chronic hepatitis B/C in patients with evidence of chronic liver disease. New onset of abnormal LFTs may be due to hepatitis C.

Specific investigations

- ***Stool specimens*** Should be examined/cultured for bacteria and ova, cysts, and parasites. At least 3 stool specimens should be sent. *Clostridium difficile* toxin should be requested in individuals who have taken or are taking antibiotics. In an individual with severe immunosuppression (CD4 <100) and negative conventional stool analysis, examination for microsporidial species should be performed.
- ***AXR*** Look for evidence of toxic dilatation in the patient presenting with diarrhoea/abdominal pain. The major causes are CMV (with CD4 counts <100 cells/mm3) and bacterial infections (*Salmonella, Shigella, Campylobacter*) at higher CD4 counts.
- ***USS*** Look for evidence of hepatic/biliary abnormality in patients with jaundice/abnormal LFTs, evidence of ascites in patients with abdominal distension, and abdominal masses/lymphadenopathy in individuals with opportunistic infections/tumours.
- ***CT scanning*** Look for evidence of masses/lymphadenopathy in individuals with abdominal pain, which may represent involvement by underlying opportunistic infections or tumours.
- ***Upper GI endoscopy*** Look for oesophageal lesions in patients with dysphagia, gastric lesions in patients with abdominal pain. Perform duodenal biopsies in individuals with chronic diarrhoea where no pathogen has been isolated.
- ***Sigmoidoscopy/colonoscopy*** Look for evidence of involvement by opportunistic pathogens/tumours in patients with chronic diarrhoea or abdominal pain. Rectal/colonic biopsies should be performed in patients with chronic diarrhoea where no pathogen has been isolated.
- ***ERCP/MRCP*** Should be considered in individuals with evidence of obstructive jaundice where no cause has been found, or in individuals with chronic abdominal pain looking for any evidence of ascending cholangitis.

GI presentations in HIV-positive patients: management

- General principles of rehydration, analgesia, and nutritional support should apply.
- Specific therapy should be directed towards the suspected/proven underlying cause (see 🕮 Table 8.6, pp. 504–505). Consider empiric treatment with antibacterial agents (ciprofloxacin metronidazole) in the unwell patient with diarrhoea and additional anticytomegalovirus therapy (usually ganciclovir) if the CD4 count is <100 cells/mm^3.
- Antiretroviral therapy should not be discontinued or modified without discussion with an experienced HIV clinician.

Table 8.6 GI pathogens in HIV-positive patients

Pathogen	Clinical presentation	Diagnosis	Treatment
Candida	• Oral: usually white plaques. Usually CD4 <350 • Oesophageal: dysphagia or odynophagia. Usually CD4 <200	• Usually based upon clinical appearance • Can be confirmed by biopsy/culture	• Oral: usually with fluconazole (50mg x 5 days) or 400mg stat • Oesophageal: fluconazole 100mg od x 14 days • Higher doses of fluconazole or alternative agents may be recommended in cases of suspected/proven 'azole' resistance
Salmonella	• Diarrhoea ± fever, abdominal pain, and blood per rectum; Colonic dilatation ±. Any CD4 count	• Confirmed by stool (± blood) cultures • Empiric treatment may be considered in the unwell patient	• Ciprofloxacin 500mg bd x 7–14 days • Cephalosporin if ciprofloxacin intolerant
Shigella	• Diarrhoea ± fever, abdominal pain, and Blood per rectum; Colonic dilatation ±. Any CD4 count	• Confirmed by stool (± blood) cultures • Empiric treatment may be considered in the unwell patient	• Ciprofloxacin 500mg bd x 7–14 days • Trimethoprim if ciprofloxacin intolerant
Campylobacter	• Diarrhoea ± fever, abdominal pain, and Blood per rectum; Colonic dilatation ±. Any CD4 count	• Confirmed by stool (±blood) cultures • Empiric treatment may be considered in the unwell patient	• Ciprofloxacin 500mg bd x 7–14 days • Erythromycin if ciprofloxacin intolerant
Crytosporidia	• May present acutely as 'traveller's diarrhoea' at any CD4 count which usually clears spontaneously, or chronically as watery diarrhoea with CD4 <100	• Demonstration of organism on stool analysis and/or biopsy	• No effective anti-microbial therapy (consider nitazoxanide). Acute crytosporidial infection usually resolves spontaneously; treat chronic infection with HAART

Microsporidia	• Watery diarrhoea in individuals with CD4 <100	• Demonstration of organisms by specific stool analysis or on biopsy/electron microscopy	• Albendazole is beneficial in some studies. Effective HIV treatment results in clinical improvement
Isospora	• Watery diarrhoea in individuals with CD4 <100	• AFB smear of stool	• Co-trimoxazole usually effective
Entamoeba histolytica	• Diarrhoea ± blood and abdominal pain. Any CD4 count	• OC&P of stool	• Metronidazole 500mg tds or tinidazole then diloxanide
Giardia	• Watery diarrhoea. Any CD4 count	• OC&P of stool	• Metronidazole 250–500mg tds for 10 days or tinidazole
Cytomegalovirus	• Oesophageal: dysphagia with ulceration • Gastric/upper GI: abdominal pain • Colonic: diarrhoea ± abdominal pain. Toxic dilatation may occur. • CD4 <100	• Demonstration of organisms by immunocytochemistry of biopsy specimens	• Specific CMV therapy (usually ganciclovir 5mg/kg bd for 3–4 weeks). • Effective anti-HIV therapy should reduce risk of recurrence/other end-organ disease
Herpes simplex	• Oesophageal ulceration, or proctitis/colitis	• Demonstration of organisms on biopsy/culture	• Aciclovir 200–800mg 5x/day or 5mg/kg iv for 2–3 weeks
Herpes zoster	• Oesophageal ulceration	• Demonstration of organisms on biopsy/culture	• Aciclovir 400–800mg 5x/day or 5–10mg/kg iv for 2–3 weeks
Mycobacterium avium complex	• Chronic, watery diarrhoea ± abdominal pain. Usually systemic symptoms (fever, weight loss, pancytopaenia). CD4 <50	• Blood cultures (specific mycobacterial culture: may take several weeks), or demonstration of organisms on biopsy	• 3 agents (usually rifabutin, ethambutol, and clarithromycin or azithromycin) • Effective anti-HIV therapy is associated with clinical response
Clostridium difficile	• Watery diarrhoea. History of antibiotics Any CD4 count	• Stool toxin assay	• Metronidazole 250–500mg qds x 10–14 days • Vancomycin 125mg qds x 10–14 days

Pyrexia of unknown origin

Assessment

- Look for signs/symptoms of focal infection
- Check for neutropenia
- Consider TB
- Consider line sepsis if indwelling IV cannulae
- Consider drug-related fever (detailed drug history, including antiretroviral agents)
- Consider underlying lymphoma
- Detailed travel history essential.

Investigations

- Usual investigation of fever
- Cryptococcal antigen
- Mycobacterial blood cultures (MAI if CD4 <100)
- Consider:
  - CT scan head
  - CT scan chest and abdomen
  - Lymph node biopsy (if significant lymphadenopathy)
  - Bone marrow examination
  - Gallium/white cell scan.

Treatment

- Unless clinically unwell, most clinicians would recommend withholding empiric antimicrobial therapy.
- Specific antimicrobial (or other) therapy should be directed against suspected underlying pathogen/process.

Immune reconstitution inflammatory syndrome (IRIS)

- IRIS may be seen following the commencement of antiretroviral therapy in patients with HIV. It is characterized by an inflammatory response associated with worsening of pre-existing infections. These infections may have been previously diagnosed and treated or may be unmasked by the patient's regained ability to mount an inflammatory response.
- This inflammatory reaction is usually self-limited, particularly when the pre-existing infection is effectively treated. However, long-term complications and adverse outcomes may rarely be seen particularly in patients with neurological involvement.
- The clinical features of IRIS are highly variable. Most patients with IRIS develop symptoms within 7 days to a few months after initiation of antiretroviral treatment.
- In order to reduce the likelihood of IRIS, antiretroviral therapy may be delayed for 1–2 months while treating a known opportunistic infection with the appropriate antimicrobial. Antiretroviral therapy should only be delayed for about 2 weeks in patients infected with *M. tuberculosis* who have a CD4 cell count <100 cells/μL.
- IRIS is generally a diagnosis of exclusion. Possibility of drug reaction or resistance, patient non-compliance and persistently active infection should be excluded first. For example, abacavir hypersensitivity may be confused with IRIS, but symptoms are exacerbated following each dose of abacavir.
- When IRIS is thought to be highly likely, further invasive diagnostic procedures to find an occult infection may be delayed. Start or continue to treat the underlying pathogen in patients with IRIS. Continue antiretroviral therapy in most patients except for cases when presentation of IRIS is life- or organ-threatening. Steroids or NSAIDS may reduce the inflammatory response in some cases. When it is decided to use steroids, prednisolone may be given initially at a daily dose of 1mg/kg (60–80mg) and then tapered while monitoring for recurrence of clinical symptoms over weeks to months.

Dermatological presentations

- Consider drug-related causes (including antiretroviral agents), but do not discontinue antiretroviral agents (unless essential) without discussion with an HIV clinician.
- In particular, patients recently having commenced nevirapine therapy may be at risk of Stevens–Johnson syndrome or toxic epidermal necrolysis, and patients having recently commenced abacavir may be at risk of a hypersensitivity syndrome (see 🕮 p.510).
- Most dermatological complaints can behave atypically and more severely in individuals with HIV infection:
  - Shingles (*Varicella zoster*) may present with multi-dermatomal lesions and/or neurological involvement.
  - Herpes simplex may present with more severe lesions and/or-neurological involvement and requires higher doses of aciclovir than used in immunocompetent patients.
  - Seborrhoeic dermatitis may present more aggressively in the HIV-positive patient and may be recalcitrant to conventional therapy.
  - Early syphilis should be considered in *any* HIV-positive patient with dermatological lesions.

Haematological presentations

Cytopenias may be the result of HIV infection per se, antiretroviral (or other drug) toxicity, or bone marrow involvement by opportunistic infections or tumours.

- Mild–moderate thrombocytopenia is a common finding in the HIV-infected patient; a severe ITP picture is well recognized. Usually responds to antiretroviral therapy, but steroids/immunoglobulin may be required in severe cases.
- Anaemia is a recognized side effect of antiretroviral therapy—notably zidovudine (AZT) therapy.
- Neutropenia is a recognized side effect of zidovudine (AZT), ganciclovir therapy, and occurs more frequently in the HIV-infected patient receiving chemotherapy for malignancy. Standard management of neutropenia should apply.

Antiretroviral toxicity

- Many clinicians are unfamiliar with the agents used to treat HIV infection. They are associated with multiple toxicities, some of which may present to the emergency clinician. Always consider discussing the case with a clinician experienced in use and toxicity of these drugs.
- The key principles of management are to recognize the possibility of iatrogenic illness and to exert caution in management. In order to minimize the risk of development of resistance and to preserve future treatment options, antiretroviral agents can be discontinued with discussion with an HIV clinician. If necessary, the toxic agent is switched and the withdrawal of 1 or 2 of a combination of agents (thus leaving an individual on suboptimal therapy) should be avoided.
- In individuals receiving antiretroviral therapy who present systemically unwell, the possibility of lactic acidosis should always be considered (see 'Mitochondrial toxicity').

Rash and hypersensitivity

- Abacavir hypersensitivity reaction (4%) can present as a fever or maculopapular rash (usually in first 2 months of treatment) often associated with one or more other symptoms or signs (fever; sore throat, GI or respiratory symptoms, laboratory abnormalities). If strongly suspected, abacavir should be discontinued and the patient never re-challenged (risk of fatal hypersensitivity reaction). This decision should be taken by an experienced HIV clinician. Most clinicians now use the HLAB5701 test to predict the likelihood of abacavir hypersensitivity (90% risk).
- Non-nucleoside reverse transcriptase inhibitors (efavirenz and nevirapine): maculopapular rash (~10%) peaking at 2 weeks often associated with abnormal LFTs. Sometimes can be 'pushed through' with antihistamines (cetirizine) but needs close monitoring (associated severe or life-threatening hepatotoxicity not uncommon). Stevens–Johnson syndrome and toxic epidermal necrolysis are well recognized but uncommon side effects of nevirapine (↑risk in ♀). Stevens–Johnson syndrome is commoner in patients who start treatment with high CD4 counts (♀ CD4 ≥250; ♂ CD4 ≥400). Nevirapine should not be used in patients with a high CD4 as it increases risk of Stevens–Johnson syndrome.

Mitochondrial toxicity

Usually attributed to the unwanted inhibition of mitochondrial DNA polymerase gamma by the nucleoside reverse transcriptase inhibitors (particularly stavudine and didanosine). Over months this can lead to mitochondrial dysfunction which can manifest as:

- Lactic acidosis/hepatic steatosis resulting from general mitochondrial dysfunction. If suspected (general malaise, abdominal pain, metabolic acidosis, abnormal LFTs), an uncuffed blood sample should be sent for immediate lactate measurement and if high (>5mmol/L) with associated acidosis the offending drug(s) stopped. This condition can be rapidly fatal and admission to intensive care is occasionally required.
- Acute pancreatitis: particularly associated with didanosine (ddI) (also precipitated by alcohol, gallstones, pentamidine, and some OIs).

- Myopathy (muscle biopsy diagnostic): zidovudine (AZT).
- Antiretroviral-induced peripheral neuropathy: particularly associated with zalcitabine, stavudine, and didanosine.
- Renal tubular acidosis/Fanconi's syndrome has been rarely reported with tenofovir.

Practice point

Always discuss treatment initiation/change with an experienced HIV-clinician.

Metabolic disturbances

Hyperlipidaemia and glucose intolerance (including frank diabetes) have been associated with the use of antiretroviral therapy, particularly the protease inhibitors. The association with premature cardiovascular disease currently remains uncertain but is suggested by some cohort studies. The prescription of statins in this patient group should be made with care given the potential drug–drug interactions; simvastatin is contraindicated in patients receiving protease inhibitors (pravastatin or atorvastatin are preferred).

Haematological toxicity

Nucleoside analogues—particularly zidovudine (AZT)—are associated with haematological toxicity especially anaemia and neutropenia which usually occurs during the first few weeks/months of therapy.

Hepatotoxicity

All of the available antiretroviral agents have been associated with hepatotoxicity, particularly in those individuals coinfected with hepatitis C/B. Nevirapine has been rarely associated with fulminant hepatitis (within the first 6 weeks of therapy). Hepatic steatosis (as part of a syndrome of mitochondrial dysfunction—as outlined earlier) is a well-recognized though rare complication of nucleoside analogue therapy. Most HIV physicians would closely monitor LFTs without discontinuation unless there is evidence of clinical hepatitis or an ALT/AST of >5–10 times the upper limit of normal.

Neurological toxicity

Efavirenz (and occasionally nevirapine) can cause significant neuropsychiatric disease. In the majority of patients this occurs in the first 4 weeks of therapy and can present as mood swings or depression. Treatment is discontinued by 5–10% of individuals, though up to 50% will experience some symptoms of 'muzzy head' or nightmares.

Drug interactions with antiretroviral therapy

The protease inhibitors and non-nucleoside reverse transcriptase inhibitors are metabolized through the cytochrome P450 system and exhibit a wide variety of drug interactions, many of which have potentially serious consequences. It is recommended that co-administration of other P450-mediated agents should be with caution. Further information is available in the *British National Formulary* (BNF) or can be accessed via the Liverpool University website (www.hiv-druginteractions.org).

Post-exposure prophylaxis (PEP)

Evidence that PEP may be effective can be drawn from both animal and vertical transmission studies. The most compelling data are from a case-controlled study of healthcare workers where the administration of zidovudine (AZT) monotherapy was shown to be associated with approximately 80% reduction in HIV transmission.

Most hospitals/emergency departments will have established protocols for the management of PEP (see 🕮 Box 8.3, p.514). However, the following general principles apply:

- The risk of HIV transmission is the product of the risk of the 'donor' being HIV and the risk of HIV infection from the exposure.
- To estimate the risk of the donor being HIV positive, an understanding of the epidemiology of the 'risk group' of the individual is helpful.
  - For example, the risk of a sexually active homosexual man in the UK being HIV-positive is estimated at ~10% in London and 2.5% elsewhere.
  - The risk of an IV drug user being HIV-positive is <5%. The risk of a heterosexual being HIV-positive requires knowledge of the HIV prevalence in the country in which they have been sexually active (as high as 20–50% in some sub-Saharan African countries).

Needlestick/splash injury

The risk of HIV transmission from exposures has been estimated at:

- Needlestick injury: 1 in 300
- Splash injury (to eyes or diseased skin): <1 in 1000.

Factors associated with increased risk include

- ***Donor:*** advanced HIV infection; high viral load
- ***Injury:*** hollow-bore needle; insertion of needle into artery or vein of patient; visible blood on device; deep injury.

Following assessment of the risk, consider PEP.

NB: do not forget that optimal management of sharps injuries includes immediate wound management (bleeding and simple washing) and consideration of exposure to hepatitis B (assess vaccination status and consider accelerated vaccination or immunoglobulin) and hepatitis C.

Sexual exposure

The risk of HIV transmission through sexual exposure is estimated as:

- Unprotected vaginal sex (male to female): 1 in 1000
- Unprotected vaginal sex (female to male): 1 in 1000
- Unprotected anal sex (risk to insertive partner): 1 in 1000
- Unprotected anal sex (risk to receptive partner): 1 in 1000 to 1 in 30
- Oral sex with ejaculation: <1 in 25,000.

Given the potential opportunities for future risk reduction and concerns regarding PEP efficacy, HIV resistance, and drug toxicity in this setting, it is recommended that the decision to administer PEP after sexual exposure is taken in conjunction with clinicians experienced in GUM/HIV medicine.

Box 8.3 PEP

A risk assessment should be carried out first. If the risk of infection is considered significant, PEP should be commenced as early as possible, ideally within 1h and certainly within 72h.

Most hospitals recommend the administration of 3 agents:

- Zidovudine and lamivudine (co-administered as Combivir®, 1 tablet bd) or tenofovir/emtricitabine
- A protease inhibitor (e.g. ritonavir-boosted lopinavir)

Notes

- The administration of PEP is associated with significant side effects. The initial discussion and subsequent follow-up should be under the supervision of a clinician experienced in the use of these agents.
- If the 'donor' is known to be HIV-positive, ask about their antiretroviral therapy history, as this may alter the choice of PEP agents.
- If the 'recipient' is pregnant or taking medications, be aware of the safety of these drugs in pregnancy and potential drug–drug interactions.
- Where possible, the 'donor' in such an injury should be encouraged to test for HIV to allow the discontinuation of PEP where possible. It is permissible to test such a donor for HIV without consent if they are deceased or unconscious (and unexpected to regain consciousness within 48h), though in the latter situation this should be performed on a previous blood specimen (see 🕮 p.484).

Chapter 9

Endocrine emergencies

Diabetic ketoacidosis (DKA): assessment

DKA predominantly occurs in patients with insulin-dependent diabetes (type I). It does not usually occur in non-insulin-dependent diabetes, but is being increasingly recognized in some type II diabetics, esp. Afro-Caribbeans. Remember, patients may be prescribed insulin for poor diabetic control, and yet have non-insulin dependent diabetes.

Clinical features

These include:

- Polyuria and polydipsia; patients become dehydrated over a few days.
- Weight loss, weakness.
- Hyperventilation or breathlessness; the acidosis causes Kussmaul's respiration (a deep sighing respiration).
- Abdominal pain: DKA may present as an 'acute abdomen'.
- Vomiting: exacerbates dehydration.
- Confusion, coma occurs in 10%
- On examination assess state of hydration, ventilation rate, and smell for ketones.

Investigations

- ***Blood glucose*** This need not be high. Severe acidaemia may be present with glucose vales as low as 10mM (e.g. if the patient has recently taken insulin, as this alone is insufficient to correct the acidosis in the presence of dehydration.
- ***ABG*** Assess the degree of acidosis.
- ***U&Es*** Corrected $Na^+ = Na^+ + 1.6 \times$ [(plasma glucose mmol/L − 55)/5.5]
  Assess serum K^+ and renal function
- ***Urinalysis*** Ketones strongly positive (ketones may be present in normal individuals after a period of starvation). NB: captopril and other sulphydryl drugs can give a false positive test for urinary ketones.
- ***FBC*** WBC may be elevated (neutrophilia): a leukaemoid reaction can occur in absence of infection.
- ***Septic screen*** Urine and blood cultures.
- ***Plasma ketones*** See 'Note'.
- ***CXR*** Look specifically for any infection..
- ***Amylase*** May be high with abdominal pain and vomiting in absence of pancreatitis. Acute pancreatitis may occur in ~10% of patients with DKA (often in association with hypertriglyceridemia).
- ***Serum osmolality*** $= 2 \times (Na^+ + K^+)$ + urea + glucose.

Note:

- Diagnosis of DKA requires positive urinary or plasma ketones and arterial pH ≤7.30 and/or serum bicarbonate ≤15mmol/L. Many labs do not measure plasma ketones.
- The elderly patient presenting with a high glucose, relatively normal acid–base balance, and ketones in the urine does not have diabetic ketoacidosis, and may not be insulin dependent.
- Consider other causes of hyperglycaemia/acidosis, e.g. aspirin overdose, and in the elderly consider lactic acidosis.

Common precipitants of DKA

- Infections: 30%
- Non-compliance with treatment: 20%
- Newly diagnosed diabetes: 25%.

Poor prognostic features in DKA

- pH <7.0
- Oliguria
- Serum osmolality >320
- Newly diagnosed diabetes.

DKA: management 1

General measures

- Rehydration and insulin therapy are the mainstays of treatment and should be instigated without delay.
- Site 2 IV cannulae: one in each arm (one for 0.9% saline and one for insulin and later glucose) away from a major vein in the wrist if possible (as this may be required for an AV fistula in patients subsequently developing diabetic nephropathy). Start fluid replacement (see next section).
- Insert a central line in patients with a history of cardiac disease/ autonomic neuropathy or the elderly (see 🕮 p.742).
- Consider an arterial line to monitor ABGs and potassium. If arterial line is not inserted, patients should have venous gases for monitoring pH and bicarbonate rather than repeated ABGs which are uncomfortable.
- Nil by mouth for at least 6h (gastroparesis is common).
- NG tube: if there is impaired conscious level to prevent vomiting and aspiration.
- Urinary catheter if oliguria is present or serum creatinine is high.
- Broad-spectrum antibiotics if infection suspected.
- LMWH (e.g. enoxaparin/dalteparin) should be given as prophylaxis against DVTs.
- The $t_{1/2}$ of IV insulin is short and ***continued*** replacement (IV or SC) is essential.

Fluid replacement

Use normal (0.9%) saline to replace the fluid deficit. The average fluid loss in DKA is 100mL/kg. (The following regimen should be modified for patients with cardiac disease.)

- If hypotensive, give 500mL 0.9% saline IV over 15–20min and repeat until SBP >100mmHg (maximum of 3 doses); then
- 1L 0.9% saline 2-hourly × 3 (plus potassium replacement; see 'Potassium replacement')
- 1L 0.9% saline 3-hourly × 3 (plus potassium replacement; see 'Potassium replacement')
- When blood glucose reaches 15mmol/L, IV glucose is given concurrently with 0.9% saline (through an IV cannula in the other arm): 1L 5% glucose over 8h when blood glucose is 7–15mmol/L and 500mL 10% glucose over 4h when blood glucose is <7mmol/L.
- The use of bicarbonate is controversial. If the pH <7.0, isotonic (1.26%) sodium bicarbonate given at a maximal rate of 500mL (i.e. 75mmol) over 1h is safe. Faster infusion rates cause a paradoxical intracellular acidosis. There is no evidence that the use of bicarbonate in DKA improves outcome.

Potassium replacement

Total body potassium is depleted and the plasma K^+ falls rapidly as potassium shifts into the cells under the action of insulin. Do not give potassium chloride in the first litre or if serum potassium is >5.5mmol/L. All subsequent fluid for the next 24h should contain KCl unless urine output is <30mL/h or serum potassium remains in excess of 5.5mmol/L (See Table 9.1).

Insulin replacement

The only indication for delaying insulin is a serum potassium <3.3mmol/L, as insulin will worsen the hypokalaemia by driving potassium into the cells. Patients with initial serum potassium <3.3mmol/L should receive fluid and potassium replacement prior to insulin.

- Start an IV insulin infusion pump with 50 units of soluble insulin added to 50mL 0.9% saline.
- Insulin is infused at ***fixed rate*** of 0.1u/kg/h. The response to insulin infusion pump is reviewed after 1h. If blood glucose is not dropping by 5mmol/h and capillary ketones by 1mmol/L, the infusion rate is ↑ by 1U/h. The increase in insulin infusion rate may be repeated hourly if necessary to achieve reduction in blood glucose and capillary ketones.
- Monitor blood glucose, capillary ketones and urine output hourly, U&Es 4-hourly, venous blood gas at 0, 2, 4, 8, 12h and before stopping fixed rate insulin regimen, and urinary ketones.
- The fixed rate insulin is continued until capillary ketones <0.3, venous pH >7.3, and venous bicarbonate is >18. At this point if patient is eating and drinking regularly change to SC insulin regimen and stop IV insulin pump 1–2h afterwards. If patient is not eating and drinking, change to IV sliding scale (see Table 9.2).
- Urinary ketones may take a little longer to clear.
- If the patient normally takes long-acting insulin (e.g. glargine or detemir), continue at their usual dose from the day of admission.

Table 9.1 Suggested regimen for potassium supplementation

Plasma potassium (mmol/L)	Amount of K^+ (mmol) to add to each litre of fluid
>5.50mmol/L	nil
2.5–5.5mmol/L	40mmol/L
<2.5mmol/L	60–80mmol/L (seek advice from specialist)

Table 9.2 Example of sliding scale insulin prescription

Blood glucose (mmol /L) (hourly)	Insulin infusion (units/h)
0–4.0	0.5
4.1–7.0	1
7.1–11.0	2
11.1–15.0	3
15.1–20	4
>20.0	6— call doctor

DKA: management 2

Box 9.1 Management key points: diabetic ketoacidosis

- Consider HDU/ICU input, central line, arterial line and urinary catheter if severe acidosis, hypotensive, or oliguric.
- ***Insulin:*** 50U of soluble insulin in 50mL N saline—start at 0.1U/kg/h (~6–7U/h) until capillary ketones <0.3, venous pH >7.30, and venous bicarbonate >18mmol/L. At this point, if the patient is able to eat and drink, change to SC insulin regimen. If not, change to IV sliding scale. Do not stop insulin infusion until 1–2h after regular SC insulin is restarted.
- ***Fluids:*** 500mL 0.9% saline over 15–30min until SBP >100mmHg. Then: 1 L 2-hourly × 3 and 1L 3-hourly × 3. IV glucose is started in conjunction with 0.9% saline when blood glucose reaches 15mmol/L: 1L 5% glucose over 8h when blood glucose is 7–15mmol/L and 500mL 10% glucose over 4h when blood glucose is <7mmol/L.
- ***Potassium*** replacement (start in the 2nd bag of fluid). Adjust amount of potassium added to fluids according to plasma potassium.
- ***Monitor*** blood glucose, capillary ketones and urine output hourly, U&Es 4-hourly, and venous blood gas at 0, 2, 4, 8, 12h and before stopping fixed rate insulin regimen. Monitor phosphate and magnesium daily.
- Broad spectrum antibiotics if infection suspected.
- Thromboprophylaxis.
- NBM for at least 6h (gastroparesis is common).
- NG tube: if GCS is reduced (to prevent vomiting and aspiration).
- There is no strong evidence for the use of IV bicarbonate.
- Refer to diabetes team for patient education.

DKA: complications

Assessment during treatment

Remember, rapid normalization of biochemistry can be detrimental in any patient. It is wiser to be cautious and suboptimal than enthusiastic and dangerous.

- Blood glucose/capillary ketones hourly with lab blood glucose 4-hourly.
- Plasma electrolytes 2h after start of treatment and then 4-hourly. The main risk is hypokalaemia.
- Venous blood gases (for monitoring pH and bicarbonate) at 0, 2, 4, 8, 12h and before stopping fixed rate insulin regimen.
- Some patients may require monitoring on an ECG for T-wave changes during treatment.
- Phosphate levels should be monitored daily during treatment (see below).
- Magnesium levels should be monitored daily (see 'Complications').
- The IV insulin infusion should be continued until 1-2h after the patient is commenced on subcutaneous insulin.

Complications

See Box 9.2.

- Avoid ***hypoglycaemia*** from overzealous insulin replacement.
- ***Cerebral oedema*** occurs mainly in children. It may be precipitated by sudden shifts in plasma osmolality during treatment. Symptoms include drowsiness, severe headache, confusion. Treat as on 📖 p.372. Give IV mannitol 0.5g/kg body weight, repeated as necessary. Restrict IV fluids and move to ITU. Mortality is ~70%; recovery of normal function only 7–14%.
- ***Serum phosphate*** falls during treatment, as it moves intracellularly with potassium. If the phosphate level falls to <0.3mmol/L, give phosphate IV (monobasic potassium phosphate infused at a maximum rate of 9mmol every 12h). Check preparations with your pharmacy. Monitor calcium levels during the infusion.
- ***Serum magnesium*** may fall during insulin therapy. If magnesium levels fall <0.5mmol/L, give 4–8mmol (2mL of 50%) magnesium sulphate over 15–30min in 50mL N saline. Repeat as necessary.
- ***Hyperchloraemic acidosis*** (normal anion gap acidosis in a well-hydrated patient) may be seen with excessive administration of saline and ↑ consumption of bicarbonate. No specific treatment is required.
- Tissue hypoperfusion results from dehydration and may trigger the coagulation cascade and result in ***thromboembolism***. Consider using LWMH (e.g. enoxaparin SC) for prophylaxis.

Box 9.2 Complications of DKA

- Hypokalaemia
- Hypophosphataemia
- Hyperchloraemic acidosis
- Hypoglycaemia
- Cerebral oedema in children
- Thromboembolism.

Hyperosmolar non-ketotic coma (HONK) 1

HONK classically occurs in elderly patients with type 2 diabetes, although is appearing increasingly in younger patients. These patients are also at ↑risk of venous and arterial thromboses.

Presentation

- A history of diabetes is not usually known, and the patient is elderly.
- Insidious onset of polyuria and polydipsia.
- Severe dehydration.
- Impaired conscious level: the degree correlates most with plasma osmolality. Coma is usually associated with an osmolality >440.
- Respiration is usually normal.
- The patient may rarely present with a stroke, seizures, or MI.

Precipitants

- Infection—thorough physical examination is important.
- MI or CVA.
- GI bleed.
- Poor compliance with oral antidiabetic agents or high sugar diet.
- Self neglect or elder abuse.
- Drugs: diuretics, beta blockers, antihistamines.

Investigations

- ***Glucose:*** usually very high (>50mmol/L).
- ***U&Es:*** dehydration causes a greater rise in urea than creatinine (normal ratio of Cr: Ur up to 20:1 μM:mM).
- ***Significant hypernatraemia*** may be masked by the high glucose. The hypernatraemia may appear to worsen as the glucose falls.
- ***ABG:*** relatively normal compared with DKA. A coexistent lactic acidosis considerably worsens the prognosis.
- ***Plasma osmolality:*** calculated by: [2 x (Na^{+}+ K^{+}) + urea + glucose]. Needs to be >350mosm/kg for diagnosis.
- ***FBC:*** polycythaemia and leucocytosis may indicate dehydration or infection respectively.
- ***ECG:*** look for MI or ischaemia.
- ***CXR:*** look for signs of infection.
- ***Urine:*** for urinalysis, MC&S. Remember that ketones may occur in any starved person (glycogen depletion causing a switch to lipid metabolism) but the level will be <5mM. Blood and protein on urinalysis may indicate UTI.
- ***Consider stroke or cerebral infection*** as a precipitant.

Management: general measures

- Airway management for patients with altered level of consciousness. Give O_2 if hypoxic on air.
- Rehydration and insulin therapy are the mainstays of treatment. Fluid replacement should be cautious in the elderly.
- Avoid fluid overload. May need central line insertion for central venous pressure monitoring.
- NBM for at least 6h and insert an NG tube in patients with impaired conscious level to prevent vomiting and aspiration.
- Urinary catheter if there is oliguria or high serum creatinine.
- Anticoagulate with LWMH (e.g. enoxaparin 40mg sc daily).

Fluid replacement

The average fluid lost is 8–10L. This should be replaced cautiously. Remember that 0.9% N saline is hypotonic relative to the patient's serum and is therefore the fluid of choice even with hypernatraemia.

- 1 litre N saline over the first 60min, then
- 1 litre N saline with K^+ (see 🕮 Table 9.1 p. 519) every 2h for 4h, then
- 1 litre N saline with K^+ (see 🕮 Table 9.1 p. 519) every 6h until rehydrated (~48h).
- If the plasma Na is >160mmol/L, 0.45% saline (half N saline) may be given for the first 3L. Hyperglycaemia causes a 'translocational hyponatraemia' by drawing water out of the cells. Reversing the hyperglycaemia with insulin will cause water to move from the extracellular fluid into the cells and increases the serum sodium concentration. Therefore a patient with a normal initial serum sodium concentration will probably become hypernatraemic during therapy with insulin and 0.9% saline. The degree to which this is likely to occur can be estimated at presentation by calculation of the 'corrected' serum sodium concentration (i.e. the serum sodium concentration that should be present if the serum glucose concentration were lowered to normal with insulin.)

  (NB: 'corrected' serum Na = measured serum Na + [the increment above normal in blood glucose (in mmol/L) ÷ 2.3].)
- When blood glucose reaches 15mmol/L, commence 5% glucose infusion, stop IV insulin, and continue to monitor blood glucose.

HONK 2

Insulin regimen

Patients with HONK tend to be more sensitive to the effects of insulin, and so the IV insulin infusion should not exceed 4U/h (IV insulin is usually given at a rate of 2–3U/h). When blood glucose reaches 15mmol/L, commence 5% glucose infusion, stop IV insulin and continue to monitor blood glucose. Reducing the serum glucose acutely below 14mmol/L may promote the development of cerebral oedema. If the patient is eating and drinking regularly, consider starting SC insulin or oral hypoglycaemic agents.

Once the IV insulin infusion is stopped, blood glucose levels may start to rise if the patient has an infection (which may have precipitated the HONK). Sliding scale insulin may need to be started as would be in any poorly controlled diabetic patient with sepsis.

Box 9.3 Management key points: HONK (HHS)

- ***Insulin infusion:*** start IV insulin infusion at 2–4U/h. when blood glucose reaches 15mmol/L, commence 5% glucose infusion, stop IV insulin therapy, and continue to monitor blood glucose. If the patient is eating and drinking normally, consider starting SC insulin or oral hypoglycaemic agents.
- ***IV fluid:*** may require 8–10L in the first 48h. Start with 1L N saline over the first hour, then 1L 2-hourly for 4h, then 1L 6-hourly until rehydrated. If Na^+ >160mmol/L, consider 0.45% saline for the first 3L.
- ***Potassium*** replacement.
- Treat the underlying cause (e.g. antibiotics for suspected infection).
- Thromboprophylaxis (SC LMWH) is essential.
- Monitor fluid balance (insert urinary catheter; may need CVP line insertion)
- Monitor U&Es, glucose and osmolality.
- Refer to the diabetes team for specialist input and patient education.

Hypoglycaemic coma: assessment

- All unconscious patients should be assumed to be hypoglycaemic until proved otherwise. *Always* check a blood glucose using a blood glucose testing strip immediately, and *confirm* with a lab determination.
- The most common cause of coma in a patient with diabetes is hypoglycaemia due to drugs. The longer-acting sulphonylureas such as glibenclamide are more prone to do this than the shorter-acting ones.
- Patients who are *not* known to have diabetes, but who are hypoglycaemic, should have a laboratory blood glucose, and serum saved for insulin and C-peptide determination (insulinoma or factitious drug administration) *before* administration of glucose.

Presentation

Sympathetic overactivity (glc <3.6mmol/L)

- Tachyardia
- Palpitations
- Sweating
- Anxiety
- Pallor
- Tremor

Neuroglycopenia (glc <2.6mmol/L)

- Confusion
- Slurred speech
- Focal neurological defect (stroke-like syndromes)
- Coma.

- Cold extremities.
- Patients with well-controlled diabetes have more frequent episodes of hypoglycaemia, and can become desensitized to sympathetic activation. These patients may develop neuroglycopenia before sympathetic activation and complain of 'loss of warning' (hypoglycaemic unawareness).
- β-lockers blunt the symptoms of sympathetic activation and patients taking these drugs lose the early warning of hypoglycaemia.
- Patients with poorly controlled diabetes develop sympathetic signs early, and avoid these by running a high blood glucose. They may complain of 'being hypo' when their blood sugar is normal or high. They do not require glucose but a period of re-education and resetting of their 'glucostat'.
- Patients who have diabetes following a total pancreatectomy have more frequent and severe episodes of hypoglycaemia ('brittle diabetes') because they lack glucagon producing (α) cells as well as β islet cells.

Investigations

- Blood glucose (testing strips must be confirmed by lab glucose as glucose meters are inaccurate at low levels).
- U&Es (hypoglycaemia is more common in diabetic nephropathy)
- Take blood (clotted, heparin, and fluoride oxalate tubes), *prior* to giving glucose, for insulin and C-peptide levels (send ~20mL blood to the lab for immediate centrifugation if indicated).

Note

- A lab glucose of <2.2mmol/L is defined as a severe attack.
- Coma usually occurs with blood glucose <1.5mmol/L.
- Low C-peptide and high insulin level indicate exogenous insulin; high C-peptide and insulin level indicate endogenous insulin, e.g. surreptitious drug (sulphonylurea) ingestion or insulinoma.

Box 9.4 Causes of hypoglycaemia

Drugs
- Insulin
- Sulphonylureas
- Alcohol
- Salicylates
- Prescription errors (e.g. chlorpropamide for chlorpromazine)
- Others:
  - Disopyramide
  - β-blockers
  - Pentamidine
  - Quinine.

Organ failure
- Hypopituitarism (esp. acute pituitary necrosis)
- Acute liver failure
- Adrenal failure
- Myxoedema
- Rarely CCF or CRF.

Infections
- Sepsis syndrome
- Malaria.

Tumours
- Insulinoma
- IGF-2 secreting.

Hypoglycaemic coma: management

Acute measures (Box 9.5)

- Remember to *take blood* prior to glucose administration (glucose, insulin, C-peptide). See 📖 p.528.
- If there is a history of chronic alcohol intake or malnourishment, give IV *thiamine* 1–2mg/kg to avoid precipitating Wernicke's encephalopathy.
- If patient is conscious and cooperative, give 50g *oral glucose* or equivalent (e.g. Lucozade®, or milk and sugar).
- Give 50mL of *50%* glucose IV if patient is unable to take oral fluids.
- If IV access is impossible, give 1mg of *glucagon* IM. Then give the patient some oral glucose to prevent recurrent hypoglycaemia. Glucagon is less effective in hypoglycaemia due to alcohol.
- Admit the patient if the cause is a long-acting sulphonylurea or a long-acting insulin, and commence a continuous infusion of 10% glucose (e.g. 1L 8-hourly) and check glucose hourly or 2-hourly.

Further management

- Patients should regain consciousness or become coherent within 10min although complete cognitive/neurological recovery may lag by 30–45min. Do not give further boluses of IV glucose without repeating the blood glucose. If the patient does not wake up after ~10min, repeat the blood glucose and consider another cause of coma (e.g. head injury while hypoglycaemic, see 📖 p.364).
- Prolonged severe hypoglycaemia (>4h) may result in permanent cerebral dysfunction.
- Patients on sulphonylureas may become hypoglycaemic following a CVA or other illness preventing adequate food intake.
- Recurrent hypoglycaemia may herald the onset of diabetic nephropathy, as this decreases insulin requirements: insulin is partly degraded by the kidney and sulphonylureas are renally excreted.
- Review patient's current medication, and inspect all tablets from home.
- Consider psychiatric review if self-inflicted.

Liver dysfunction and recurrent hypoglycaemia

- Hypoglycaemia is common in acute liver failure, when coma may occur (as a result of liver failure rather than hypoglycaemia). Severe hypoglycaemia is rare in chronic liver disease.
- In chronic alcoholics it is advisable to administer IV thiamine (1–2mg/kg) before IV glucose to avoid precipitating neurological damage.
- An acute ingestion of alcohol can also suppress hepatic gluconeogenesis.

Box 9.5 Management key points: hypoglycaemia

- If the patient is conscious and cooperative: oral glucose (50–100mL of Lucozade® or 3 glucose tablets). Check blood glucose again in 10min and if still <4 give more fast-acting glucose. Follow with a starchy snack. Do not drive for 45min.
- If patient has reduced level of consciousness: 50mL of 50% glucose IV or if no IV access: 1mg glucagon IM. Monitor blood glucose again in 10min.
- Give a carbohydrate-rich snack when patient able to eat.
- If hypoglycaemia is 2° to sulphonylurea or long-acting insulin, admit for 10% IV glucose per 8h with hourly blood glucose monitoring.
- Look for the cause of hypoglycaemia.
- Do not omit subsequent regular doses of insulin—but doses may need to be reduced.
- Give IV thiamine prior to glucose in alcoholics to reduce risk of precipitating Wernicke's encephalopathy.

Urgent surgery in patients with diabetes

Surgery requires patients to fast for several hours. In addition a general anaesthetic and surgery produce significant stresses on an individual. The hormonal response to stress involves a significant rise in counter-regulatory hormones to insulin, in particular cortisol and adrenaline. For this reason, patients with diabetes undergoing surgery will require an ↑dose of insulin despite their fasting state.

Type I DM (insulin dependent)

- Try to put the patient first on the list. Inform the surgeon and anaesthetist early.
- Discontinue long-acting insulin the night before surgery if possible. If the patient has taken a long-acting insulin and requires emergency surgery, an infusion of 10% glucose (10–100mL/h) can be used, together with an insulin sliding scale.
- Ensure IV access is available.
- When NBM, start IV infusion of 5% glucose with potassium (20mmol/L) at 100mL/h and continue until oral intake is adequate. Remember saline requirements (~100–150mmol Na/24h but increases postoperatively but do not stop glucose infusion (risk of hypoglycaemia).
- Commence an IV insulin sliding scale (see Box 9.3). Measure finger-prick glucose hourly and adjust the insulin infusion accordingly. Aim for 7–11mmol/L.
- Continue the insulin sliding scale until the second meal and restart the normal SC dose of insulin. As IV insulin has a very short half-life (3.5min), this must be continued until the patient's SC insulin is being absorbed; an overlap of 4h is recommended.

Type II DM (non-insulin dependent)

- Discontinue glucose-lowering tablets or long-acting insulin the night before surgery if possible. If the patient has taken their oral hypoglycaemic or insulin and requires emergency surgery, start an infusion of 10% glucose (10–100mL/h) with an insulin sliding scale.
- Check a fasting glucose: if >12mmol/L treat as for Type II as described earlier.
- If the patient's diabetes is normally managed with oral hypoglycaemic agents, these can be restarted once the patient is eating normally. The sliding scale can be tailed off 4h later.
- Diet-controlled diabetics often do not require a sliding scale at the time of surgery but may require IV insulin postoperatively for a short period if blood glucose rises >12mmol/L. This may be tailed off, when eating normally.

Add 50U of soluble insulin to 50mL 0.9% saline and administer by IV infusion. The sliding scale in Table 9.3 is a guide only.

- Adjust the scale according to the patient's usual requirement of insulin (e.g. a patient on Mixtard® 36U/24U requires 60U/24h, i.e. 2.5U/h normally).
- If blood glucose is persistently low (<4mmol/L) decrease all insulin infusion values by 0.5–1.0U/h.
- If blood glucose is persistently high (>13.0mmol/L) increase all insulin infusion values by 0.5–1.0U/h.

Table 9.3 An example of a prescription for sliding scale insulin therapy

Blood glucose (mmol /L) (hourly)	Insulin infusion (U/h)
0.0–2.0	Stop insulin, switch to 10% glucose and call doctor
2.1–4.0	Call doctor
4.1–7.0	0.5 or 1
7.1–11.0	2
11.1–20.0	4
>20.0	Call doctor

Hyponatraemia: assessment

Presentation

- Mild hyponatraemia (Na^+ 130–135mmol/L) is common especially in patients taking thiazide diuretics and is usually asymptomatic. Moderate hyponatraemia (Na^+ 120–129mmol/L) is usually asymptomatic unless it has developed rapidly.
- Severe hyponatraemia (Na^+<120mmol/L) may be associated with disturbed mental state, restlessness, confusion, and irritability. Seizures and coma prevail as the sodium approaches 110mmol/L.

History should focus on drugs, fluid losses (diarrhoea, frequency, sweating), symptoms of Addison's, symptoms or history of cardiac, lung, liver, or renal disease.

Examination should focus on careful assessment of volume status, and in particular should assess whether the patient is hypovolemic, normovolemic, and/or oedematous. Patients should therefore have an assessment of their lying and standing BP, HR, JVP or CVP, skin turgor, and the presence of oedema or ascites.

Patients who are hyponatraemic and hypovolemic are salt depleted.

Investigations

- In addition to U&Es, other tests should be aimed at excluding other causes of hyponatraemia (see 📖 p.536).
- Measure serum osmolarity and compare it to the calculated osmolarity [2 × (Na^++K^+) + urea + glucose]. An increase in osmolar gap is with substances such as ethylene glycol, severe hyperglycaemia, mannitol, etc.
- Spot urine Na^+ estimation combined with clinical assessment of fluid status may help determine the underlying cause:
  - Volume depletion from an extra-renal cause (see 📖 p.536) is normally associated with a low urinary Na^+ (<10mmol/L)
  - Volume depletion with a high urinary Na^+ (>20mmol/L) suggests inappropriate renal salt-wasting (e.g. intrinsic renal disease, hypothyroidism, adrenal insufficiency, diuretics)
  - Fluid overload with a low urine Na^+ (<10mmol/L) is seen in conditions such as CCF, cirrhosis, or nephrotic syndrome where there is sodium retention in response to poor renal perfusion
  - Euvolaemia with high urine Na^+ is seen with SIADH and rarely with severe myxoedema.

General principles

- Assessment of the patient's volume status (neck veins, orthostatic hypotension, cardiac signs of fluid overload, ascites skin turgor) will help in both diagnosis and subsequent treatment.
- Mild asymptomatic hyponatraemia will usually respond to treatment of the underlying cause and no specific therapy is necessary.
- Correction of hyponatraemia should be gradual to avoid volume overload and/or central pontine myelinolysis. Aim to restore the serum

Na^+ to ~125mmol/L actively (IV fluids) and allow to rise gradually after that by treating the underlying cause.

- Seek expert help if serum Na^+ <120mmol/L ± severely symptomatic.
- Patients with cirrhosis and ascites and severe hyponatraemia should have diuretics stopped.
- SIADH or other conditions associated with plasma volume expansion can cause hypouricaemia (↑ renal clearance).

Hyponatraemia: causes

Decreased serum osmolarity

Hypovolaemia (hyponatraemia + hypovolaemia = salt depletion)

Renal losses (uNa >20mmol/L)
- Diuretics
- Addison's disease
- Na-losing nephropathies

Non-renal losses (uNa <20mmol/L)
- GI losses (diarrhoea, vomiting)
- Burns
- Fluid sequestration (e.g. peritonitis, pancreatitis)

Normovolaemic (normal or mildly increased ECV)

SIADH: urine osm. >100, serum osm. low (<260), urine Na^+ >40mmol/L

CNS disorders
Trauma
Stroke /SAH
Malignancy (1°/2°)
Vasculitis (e.g. SLE)
Infection (abscess or meningoencephalitis)

Malignancy
- Lung (oat cell)
- Pancreas
- Lymphoma or leukaemia
- Prostrate
- Urinary tract

Pulmonary disease
- Pneumonia
- TB
- Lung abscess
- Cystic fibrosis
- Lung vasculitis

Drugs (via SIADH±↑ renal sensitivity to ADH or Na >H_2O loss)

Opiates
Haloperidol
Amitriptyline
Cyclophosphamide
Vasopressin

- Thioridazine
- Carbamazepine
- Clofibrate
- Oxytocin

- Chlorpropamide
- Thiazides
- Vincristine

Miscellaneous causes
Severe myxoedema
Psychogenic polydipsia

Oedematous states

Congestive cardiac failure
Severe renal failure
- Cirrhosis with ascites
- Nephrotic syndrome

Normal serum osmolarity
- Pseudo-hyponatreemia (e.g. lipaemic serum, paraprotein >10g/dl)
- Intracellular shift of Na^+ (e.g. hyperglycaemia, ethylene glycol).

Hyponatraemia: management

- ***Exclude pseudohyponatraemia:*** lipaemic serum will be obvious (ask the biochemist). Calculate the osmolar gap to check there are no 'hidden' osmoles (📖 p.536). Always exclude the possibility of artefactual Na^+ from blood taken proximal to an IV infusion.
- The correction in sodium concentration must not exceed 10mmol/L in the first 24h and 18mmol/L in the first 48h. Rapid correction of hyponatraemia must be avoided as it can result in osmotic demyelination known as 'cerebral pontine myelinolysis' (see Box 9.6).
- ***Symptomatic hyponatraemia*** (e.g. seizures or coma) requires a more aggressive initial correction to increase serum sodium concentration (see Box 9.7). Seek expert help early.
- ***If volume deplete (dehydrated)*** start an IV infusion of N saline (0.9% = 150mmol/L Na^+); insert a central venous line if indicated. Monitor fluid output. Catheterize the bladder if there is renal impairment. Watch out for heart failure.
- ***If not dehydrated:*** for patients with moderate SIADH, restrict fluid intake to 750mL/24h. Seek expert help.
- Remember that that giving potassium can raise the plasma sodium levels in a hyponatraemic subject. The increase in sodium concentration caused by concurrent potassium administration should be taken into account to avoid over-rapid correction of hyponatraemia. Any potassium added to the infused solution should be considered as sodium in the equation below (see Box 9.7) i.e. the change in $[Na^+]$ = {fluid $[Na^+$+ fluid $[K^+]$} − serum [Na+]/(total body water + 1).

Box 9.6 Clinical manifestations of osmotic demyelination

- May be delayed 2–5 days
- Often irreversible or only partially reversible
- Dysarthria
- Dysphasia
- Paraparesis or quadriparesis
- Lethargy
- Coma or seizures.

Box 9.7 Management key points: hyponatraemia

- If hypovolaemic: IV 0.9% saline and recheck U&Es.
- If hypervolaemic (congestive cardiac failure, renal failure or cirrhosis): fluid restrict.
- SIADH: water restriction (about 500–750mL/day).
- In severe cases of hyponatraemia presenting with seizures or coma: manage airway, anticonvulsant if fitting; cautious use of hypertonic (3%) saline, preferably via central line in HDU setting.

The increase in [Na+] due to 1L of hypertonic (3%) saline = [513] − [serum Na+]/(TBW* + 1). Calculate the volume of 3% saline needed to increase [Na+] by 0.5–1mmol/L. Aim to increase Na^+ by 0.5–1mmol/L/h in the first 4h. Recheck U& Es 4-hourly. Do not exceed more than 10mmol/L rise in first 24h. 3% saline is usually started at about 50–60mL/h (see equation), and is then slowed down to ~30mL/h.

*TBW (total body water) = wt x 0.6 for ♂ and wt x 0.5 for ♀.

Hypernatraemia

Abnormalities in serum sodium are usually associated with changes in serum osmolality and ECV.

Presentation

Symptoms often relate to severe volume depletion: weakness, malaise, fatigue, altered mental status, confusion, delirium, or coma.

Causes

- Osmotic diuresis (glycosuria) as seen in HONK.
- Diarrhoea/protracted vomiting.
- Burns.
- DI (particularly when patient becomes unwell and unable to keep up with oral fluids).
- Respiratory losses (hot, dry environment).
- Iatrogenic (administration of salt/saline).
- Mineralocorticoid excess (Conn's, Cushings).

The way to determine the cause of abnormal serum Na^+ is by:

- Careful assessment of the ECV (evaluation of neck veins, supine and standing BP, any cardiac signs of fluid overload (e.g. S3, oedema), and skin turgor), in association with
- Measuring the serum and urine osmolality. Serum osmolality may be estimated by $(2 \times (Na^+ + K^+)$ + urea + glucose) but this is inaccurate when there are other osmoles (e.g. ketones, ethanol, methanol, ethylene glycol, renal failure) that contribute.

Serum Na^+>145mmol/L is always associated with hyperosmolarity.

Management

- Avoid rapid and extreme changes in serum sodium concentration. It is safer to change serum sodium cautiously.
- If there is hypovolaemia, start fluid replacement. N saline (0.9%) contains elemental sodium at 150mmol/L. Use this initially to correct hypovolaemia if present, then change to 5% glucose to replace water and slowly correct sodium concentration.
- If the patient is haemodynamically stable encourage oral fluids.
- Monitor electrolytes twice daily initially.

Acute hypocalcaemia

Presentation

- Abnormal neurological sensations and neuromuscular excitability.
- Numbness around the mouth and paraesthesiae of the distal limbs.
- Hyper-reflexia.
- Carpopedal spasm.
- Tetanic contractions (may include laryngospasm).
- Focal or generalized seizures. Rarely extra-pyramidal signs or papilloedema.
- Hypotension, bradycardia, arrhythmias, and CCF.
- Chvostek's sign is elicited by tapping the facial nerve just anterior to the ear, causing contraction of the facial muscles (seen in 10% of normals).
- Trousseau's sign is elicited by inflating a BP cuff for 3–5min 10–20mmHg above the level of SBP. This causes mild ischaemia, unmasks latent neuromuscular hyperexcitability, and carpal spasm is observed. (Carpopedal spasm may also occur during hyperventilation-induced respiratory alkalosis.)

Investigations

- Plasma Ca^{2+}, PO_4^{3-}, and albumin
- Corrected calcium = measured Ca^{2+} + [40 − serum albumin(g/L)] × 0.02
- Plasma Mg^{2+}
- U&Es
- ECG (prolonged QT interval)
- Plasma PTH level
- SXR (intracranaial calcification esp hypoparathyroidism).

Management

- The aim of ***acute*** management is to ameliorate the acute manifestations of hypocalcaemia, and not necessarily to return the calcium to normal.
- For frank tetany, 10mL of 10% calcium gluconate (diluted in 100mL N saline or 5% glucose) can be given by slow IV injection over 10min. *NB: 10mL of 10% calcium chloride (9mmol) contains ~4-fold more calcium than calcium gluconate.* Calcium gluconate is preferred as it causes less tissue necrosis if it extravasates. IV calcium should never be given faster than this because of the risk of arrhythmia. This initial treatment with IV calcium gluconate is followed with a slow infusion of calcium gluconate: add 100mL of 10% calcium gluconate to 1L N saline or 5% glucose. Start infusion at 50mL/h and titrate to maintain serum calcium in the low-normal range.
- Post parathyroidectomy, mild hypocalcaemia normally ensues, requiring observation only. In patients who have parathyroid bone disease however, 'hungry bones' may cause profound hypocalcaemia shortly after the parathyroids are removed. This may cause a severe and prolonged hypocalcaemia which requires prolonged treatment.
- Chronic hypocalcaemia is best managed with oral calcium together with either vitamin D or, if the cause is hypoparathyroidism or an abnormality in vitamin D metabolism, a form of hydroxylated vitamin D such as alfacalcidol or calcitriol.

- If magnesium deficiency is present, add 20mL (~40mmol) of 50% magnesium sulphate solution to 230mL N saline (10g/250mL). Infuse 50mL of this (equivalent to 2g $MgSO_4$, 8 mmol) over 10min, and at 25mL/h thereafter.

Box 9.8 Causes of hypocalcemia

- Vitamin D deficiency—more common in Asians
- Hypoparathyroidism:
  - Post-parathyroid, thyroid, or neck surgery
  - Primary (autoimmune)
  - Neck irradiation
- Chronic renal failure: hyperphosphataemia and reduced renal hydroxylation to active vitamin D.
- Pseudo-hypoparathyroidism (PTH resistance—Albright's hereditary osteodystrophy)
- Developmental agenesis of the parathyroids (DiGeorge syndrome).
- Loss of Ca^{2+} from circulation:
  - Extravascular deposition
  - Acute pancreatitis
  - Hyperphosphataemia (renal failure, tumour lysis syndrome)
  - Osteoblastic metastases (e.g. prostatic)
- Intravascular binding:
  - Citrate (massive blood transfusion)
  - Foscarnet (anti-CMV drug)
  - Acute respiratory alkalosis
- Magnesium deficiency
- Sepsis
- Burns
- Fluoride intoxication
- Chemotherapy (e.g. cisplatin).

Practice point

If hypocalcaemia is difficult to correct, check for magnesium deficiency.

Box 9.9 Management key points: hypocalcaemia

- If symptomatic: 10mL 10% calcium gluconate (diluted in 100mL N saline or 5% glucose) over 10min (with cardiac monitor).
- Follow with a slow infusion: 100mL 10% calcium gluconate in 1L N saline or 5% glucose; start infusion at 50mL/h and titrate to maintain serum calcium in the low-normal range.
- Monitor plasma calcium twice daily.
- Correct magnesium deficiency if present.
- Seek expert help regarding oral calcium and vitamin D replacement.

Hypercalcaemia

- The free (ionic) plasma Ca^{2+} concentration is dependent on both arterial pH (increases with acidaemia due to ↓ protein binding of ionized calcium) and plasma albumin.
- Corrected Ca^{2+} = measured Ca^{2+} + [40 − serum albumin(g/L)] × 0.02 (e.g. If measured Ca^{2+} = 2.10mM and albumin = 30g/L, the corrected Ca^{2+} = 2.10 = [(40 − 30) x 0.02] = 2.30mM).
- Most ITUs can now measure ionized calcium.

Presentation

- Routine biochemical screen in an asymptomatic patient.
- ***General:*** depression (30–40%), weakness (30%), tiredness, and malaise.
- ***GI:*** constipation, anorexia; vague abdominal symptoms (nauseas, vomiting), weight loss.
- ***Renal:*** renal calculi (if long standing); nephrogenic DI (20%); type 1 RTA; pre-renal failure; chronic hypercalcaemic nephropathy, polyuria, polydipsia, or dehydration.
- ***Neuropsychiatric:*** anxiety, depression, and cognitive dysfunction; coma or obtundation.
- ***Cardiac:*** hypertension, cardiac dysrhythmias.

Urgent treatment is required if

- Calcium >3.5mmol/L
- Clouding of consciousness or confusion is present
- Hypotension
- Severe dehydration causing pre-renal failure.

Management

- *Rehydrate* patient with *IV N saline* (0.9%). Aim for about 3–6L/24h depending on fluid status (CVP), urine output and cardiac function.
- If patient does not pass urine for 4h, pass a urinary catheter, and a central venous line to monitor CVP.
- *Diuretics:* once patient is rehydrated, continue N saline infusion and add *furosemide* 20–40 mg every 2–4h. The usual dose is 20 mg every 4h (i.e. with each litre); however some patients need a larger dose to avoid pulmonary oedema. Patients need to have potassium added to all the bags to avoid hypokalaemia with this protocol. Continue monitoring CVP carefully to prevent either fluid overload or dehydration.
- Monitor electrolytes, especially K^+ and Mg^{2+} which may fall rapidly with rehydration and furosemide. Replace K^+ (20–40mmol/L of saline) and Mg^{2+} (up to 2 mmol/L saline) intravenously.
- If this fails to reduce plasma Ca^{2+} adequately (Ca^{2+} still >2.8mM) then the following measures should be considered:
    - *Bisphosphonates* inhibit osteoclast activity thereby causing a fall in plasma Ca^{2+}. Administer *pamidronate* at 30–60 mg IV over 4–6h. (As a general rule give 30mg over 4h if Ca^{2+} is <3 mmol/L or for all patients with significant renal impairment, 60mg over 8h if Ca^{2+} is 3–4 mmol/L.) Ca^{2+} levels begin to fall after 48h and remain suppressed for up to 14 days. *Zoledronic acid* has a shorter infusion time (15mins) and is said to more effective with a longer duration of action.
- *Salmon calcitonin* 400IU q8h. This has a rapid onset of action (within hours) but its effect lasts only 2–3 days (tachyphylaxis).

- *Steroids* (prednisolone 30–60mg PO od): most effective in hypercalcaemia due to sarcoidosis, myeloma or vitamin D intoxication.
- *Familial hypocalciuric hypercalcaemia:* elevated Ca^{2+}, N 24h urinary Ca^{2+}. This causes few symptoms (mild fatigue or lethargy). The PTH may be raised but the patients do not respond to parathyroidectomy.

Box 9.10 Causes of hypercalcaemia

- 1° (or tertiary) hyperparathyroidism (85% of cases)
- Malignancy:
  - Humoral hypercalcaemia (PTHrP related)
  - Local osteolytic hypercalcaemia (e.g. myeloma, metastases)
- Hyperthyroidism (present in 15–20% of patients)
- Granulomatous disorders (sarcoidosis)
- Drug related:
  - Vitamin D intoxication
  - Theophylline toxicity
  - 'Milk-alkali' syndrome
  - Thiazide diuretics
  - Lithium (mild, present in 50% patients on long-term lithium, as lithium stimulates the parathyroids)
- Immobilization (Paget's disease)
- Benign familial hypocalciuric hypercalcaemia
- HTLV-1 infection may present with severe hypercalcaemia
- Phaeochromocytoma (part of MEN type II), acromegaly
- Adrenal failure
- Rhabdomyolysis (calcium may be high or low)
- Congenital lactase deficiency

Box 9.11 Investigations for hypercalcaemia

- Plasma Ca^{2+}, PO_4^{3-} and Mg^{2+}
- U&Es
- LFT
- CXR
- Plasma PTH level
- 24-h urinary Ca^{2+}.

Box 9.12 Management key points: hypercalcaemia

- Discontinue exacerbating medications.
- IV fluids: 3–6L N saline in the first 24h. Monitor fluid balance/CVP.
- Once rehydrated, continue N saline infusion and add furosemide 20–40mg every 2–4h. Add potassium to all the bags to avoid hypokalaemia with this protocol.
- If rehydration fails to correct symptoms or Ca^{2+} still >2.8mmol/L or known underlying malignancy at the outset, give a bisphosphonates: IV pamidronate 30mg over 4h if Ca^{2+} <3mmol/L or significant renal impairment, 60mg over 8h if Ca^{2+} >3mmol/L.
- Consider steroids (prednisolone 40–60mg PO od) if hypercalcaemia is 2° to sarcoidosis, hypervitaminosis D, or myeloma.

Hypophosphataemia

Plasma phosphate is normally 0.8–1.4mmol/L. Hypophosphataemia is common, and often unrecognized by clinicians. Most intracellular phosphate is present as creatine phosphate or adenine phosphates (e.g. ATP), and in RBC the predominant species is 2,3-diphopshoglycerate. Hypophosphataemia does not necessarily indicate phosphate deficiency; similarly phosphate deficiency may be associated with normal or high plasma phosphate concentrations. See Box 9.13 for causes of hypophosphataemia.

Box 9.13 Causes of hypophosphataemia

Modest (0.4–0.75mmol/L)

- ↓dietary intake
- Vitamin D deficiency
- Chronic liver disease
- Hyperparathyroidism
- ↓absorption (e.g. phosphate binding antacids)
- Hyperaldosteronism
- Diuretics
- Fanconi's syndrome.

Severe (<0.4mmol/L)

- Respiratory alkalosis or ventilation
- Treatment of DKA
- Alcohol withdrawal
- Acute liver failure
- Refeeding syndrome
- Hungry bones (post parathyroidectomy)
- Lymphomas or leukaemias
- Neuroleptic malignant syndrome.

Presentation

- Most cases of severe hypophosphataemia occur in very sick patients (often in an ITU). *Occasionally seen in asymptomatic patients.*
- Coincident Mg^{2+} deficiency exacerbates PO_4^{3-}, depletion and vice versa.
- Modest hypophosphataemia has no effect, but warrants investigation. Severe hypophosphataemia (<0.4mmol/L) may cause symptoms and requires treatment.
- See Box 9.14 for manifestations of severe hypophosphataemia.

Box 9.14 Manifestations of severe hypophosphataemia

- Myopathy (involving skeletal muscle and diaphragm)
- Rhabdomyolysis
- Cardiomyopathy
- Erythrocyte dysfunction
- Leukocyte dysfunction
- Metabolic acidosis
- CNS dysfunction (encephalopathy, irritability, seizures, paraesthesia, coma)
- Respiratory failure
- Reduced platelet half-life
- Mineral mobilization.

Treatment

- Phosphate repletion should generally be reserved for patients with sustained hypophosphataemia. Give oral effervescent Phosphate-Sandoz® 2 tabs tds or potassium phosphate IV (9–18mmol/24h).
- Excessive phosphate replacement may cause hypocalcaemia and metastatic calcification; monitor Ca^{2+}, PO_4^{3-}, K^+, and other electrolytes. Potassium phosphate (20–30 mEq/L) can be added to replacement fluids and infused over several hours. Aggressive IV phosphate therapy can cause hypocalcaemia with seizures and tetany. Serum phosphate and calcium levels should be monitored during phosphate infusion.

Addisonian crisis: assessment

Adrenocortical insufficiency may be subclinical for days or months in otherwise well individuals. Stress, such as infection, trauma, or surgery, may precipitate an Addisonian crisis with cardiovascular collapse and death if the condition is not suspected (see Box 9.15). Crises may also occur in patients with known Addison's disease on replacement hydrocortisone if they fail to increase their steroid dose with infections.

Presentation

- Hypotension and cardiovascular collapse (shock).
- Faintness, particularly on standing (postural hypotension).
- Anorexia, nausea, vomiting, and abdominal pain.
- Hyponatraemia.
- Dehydration (thirst may not be apparent because of the low sodium).
- Diarrhoea in 20% of cases.
- Symptoms of precipitant: fever, night sweats (infection); flank pain (haemorrhagic adrenal infarction); etc. Note signs/symptoms of other endocrinopathies.
- Non-specific: weight loss, fatigue, weakness, myalgia.
- Hyperpigmentation suggests chronic hypoadrenalism.
- Psychiatric features are common and include asthenia, depression, apathy, and confusion (treatment with glucocorticoids reverses most psychiatric features).

Malignant secondaries

Present in the adrenals of a high percentage of patients with lung cancer, breast tumours, and malignant melanomas. Adrenal failure will only occur when over 90% of the gland is replaced by metastases.

Adrenal haemorrhage

This may complicate sepsis (meningococcal septicaemia, the Waterhouse–Friderichsen syndrome), traumatic shock, coagulopathies, and ischaemic disorders.

- Severe stress substantially increases the arterial blood supply to the adrenals. However the adrenal gland has only 1 or 2 veins, making it vulnerable to venous thrombosis.
- Blood tests: a precipitous drop in haemoglobin, hyponatraemia, hyperkalaemia, acidosis, uraemia, and neutrophilia.
- The *Waterhouse–Friderichsen syndrome* is the association of bilateral adrenal haemorrhage with fulminant meningococcaemia. Adrenal haemorrhage is also seen with other Gram-negative endotoxaemias such as *Diplococcus pneumoniae, Haemophilus influenzae* B and DF-2 bacillus infections.

Hypopituitarism

As there is no mineralocorticoid deficiency (the release of which is renin, not ACTH dependent), the salt and water loss and shock are less profound than in 1° Addison's disease.

Drugs

Rifampicin, phenytoin, and phenobarbital accelerate the metabolism of cortisol and may precipitate Addisonian crisis in partially compromised individuals, or in those on a fixed replacement dose. Most adrenal crises precipitated by rifampicin occur within 2 weeks of initiating therapy.

Box 9.15 Recognized causes of adrenal failure

- Autoimmune adrenalitis (70%)
- TB of the adrenals (10–20%)
- Malignant secondaries in the adrenal glands
- Adrenal haemorrhage incl. meningococcal septicaemia
- Diseminated fungal infection (histoplasmosis, paracoccidioidomycosis)
- Hypopituitarism
- Drugs: metyrapone or aminoglutethimide can precipitate adrenal failure. Other drugs (see Box 9.16) may cause relative adrenal insufficiency
- Congenital conditions
- Adrenoleucodystrophy
- Congenital adrenal hyperplasia
- Familial glucorticoid deficiency.

Box 9.16 Causes of relative adrenal insufficiency

- Drugs:
    - Metyrapone or aminoglutethimide
    - Ketoconazole
    - Etomidate
    - Rifampicin, phenytoin,
    - and phenobarbital
    - Trilostane
    - Megestrol acetate.
- HIV
- Severe sepsis
- Burns
- Acute or chronic liver failure.

Practice points

- ~50% of patients with autoimmune adrenalitis have 1 or more other autoimmune disorders such as polyglandular autoimmune syndrome type 1 or 2.
- Never forget Addison's disease in a sick patient when the diagnosis is unclear.

Addisonian crisis: management

Investigations

- ***U+Es*** Hyponatraemia and hyperkalaemia (rarely>6.0mmol/L). High urea:creatinine ratio indicative of hypovolaemia.
- ***FBC*** Anaemia (normal MCV), moderate neutropenia with a relative eosinophilia/leucocytosis.
- ***Glucose*** Hypoglycaemia (rarely).
- ***Calcium*** May be high.
- ***Cortisol*** Baseline <400nmol/L. In sick patients an expected cortisol is in the range of 1000nmol/L.
- ***ABG*** Mild metabolic acidosis, respiratory failure.
- ***Urine*** MC&S for infection, urinary Na^+ may be high despite hyponatraemia/hypovolaemia.
- ***CXR*** Previous TB, bronchal carcinoma.
- ***AXR*** Adrenal calcification.

Management (see Box 9.18)

- Treatment may be required before the diagnosis is confirmed.
- General measures include O_2, continuous ECG monitoring, CVP monitoring, urinary catheter (for fluid balance), and broad spectrum antibiotics (e.g. cefotaxime) for underlying infection.
- *Treat shock* (📖 p.314): give IV N saline or colloid (Haemaccel®) for hypotension: 1L stat then hourly depending on response and clinical signs. Inotropic support may be necessary.
- Give IV 50% glucose (50mL) if hypoglycaemic.
- If adrenal crisis is suspected, the patient needs glucocorticoids urgently, take blood for cortisol and ACTH measurement or do a short Synacthen® test. The use of *dexamethasone* is now generally discouraged. Hydrocortisone should be administered intravenously (100mg bd initially and reduce dose to maintenance levels (20mg and 10mg daily later). Commencing hydrocortisone can do little harm and may be life saving.
- *Short Synacthen® test* (omit if the patient is known to have Addison's disease): take baseline blood sample (serum) and administer tetracosactrin (Synacthen®) 250mcg IM or IV. Take further samples at 30 and 60min for cortisol assay.
- Continue steroid treatment as IV *hydrocortisone* (200mg stat), then 100mg tds. Change to oral steroids after 72h.
- *Fludrocortisone* (100mcg daily orally) when stabilized on oral replacement doses of hydrocortisone (20mg and 10mg daily).

Prevention

- Patients on long-term steroid therapy and/or known adrenocortical failure should be instructed to increase steroid intake for predictable stresses (e.g. elective surgery, acute illnesses with fever >38°).
- For mild illnesses, if not vomiting, double the oral dose. Vomiting requires IV/IM therapy (hydrocortisone 50mg tds).

- For minor operations or procedures (e.g. cystoscopy) give hydrocortisone 100mg IV/IM as a single dose before the procedure.
- More serious illnesses require hydrocortisone 100mg q6–8h IV/IM until recovered or for at least 72h.
- Double replacement doses when stabilized if on enzyme-inducing drugs.
- See Box 9.17 for equivalent doses of glucocorticoids.

Box 9.17 Equivalent doses of glucocorticoids[1]

Drug	*Equivalent dose (mg)*
• Dexamethasone	0.75
• Methylprednisolone	4
• Triamcinolone	4
• Prednisolone	5
• Hydrocortisone	20
• Cortisone acetate	25

Box 9.18 Management key points: Addisonian crisis

- IV fluids: 1L N saline stat, then hourly according to response.
- Treat hypoglycaemia with 20–50mL IV 50% glucose.
- Steroid replacement: IV in the acute situation. 8mg dexamethasone is preferable if diagnosis is unconfirmed (will not interfere with cortisol assay for Synacthen® testing). If unavailable ***do NOT delay steroids***: give 200mg IV hydrocortisone stat followed by 100mg IV tds for 72h before switching back to oral steroids.
- Maintenance oral dose may need to be higher whilst the patient continues to recover.
- Fludrocortisone 100mcg od when stabilized on oral hydrocortisone replacement (in patients with 1° adrenal failure).
- Advise regarding sick day rules: if still able to eat and drink, double the daily dose. If vomiting, needs IM/IV hydrocortisone 50mg tds. Provide with IM hydrocortisone supply at home and Medicalert bracelet.

Reference

1. *British National Formulary* (1995). Section 6.3.2. Pharmaceutical Press, Royal Pharmaceutical Association of Great Britain, London: p.615.

Myxoedema coma

A common precipitant of coma is the use of sedatives, and subsequent hypothermia, in elderly female patients with undiagnosed hypothyroidism. Myxoedema coma has a high mortality (up to 80%) if inadequately treated.

Presentation

- Altered mental status: disorientation, lethargy, frank psychosis
- Coma (symmetrical, slow-relaxing reflexes, ~25% have seizures)
- Hypothermia
- Bradycardia, hypotension (rare)
- Hypoventilation
- Hypoglycaemia.

Investigations

- ***U+Es*** Hyponatraemia is common (50%).
- ***Glucose*** Hypoglycaemia may occur.
- ***FBC*** Normocytic or macrocytic anaemia (may be a coexistent pernicious anaemia).
- ***CK*** Often elevated due to a myositis.
- ***TFT*** T4 and TSH.
- ***Cortisol*** May be a coexistent adrenal insufficiency.
- ***ABG*** Hypoventilation causing a respiratory acidosis.
- ***Septic screen*** Blood and urine cultures—full examination essential especially in the elderly
- ***CXR*** Pericardial effusion may occur, also as part of septic screen.
- ***ECG*** Small complexes, prolonged QT interval.

Poor prognostic indicators

- ***Hypotension*** Patients with hypothyroidism are usually hypertensive due to high compensatory endogenous catecholamines. Reduced BP indicates possible adrenal failure or cardiac disease. Response to inotropes is poor as patients are usually maximally vasoconstricted.
- ***Hypoventilation*** This is the commonest cause of death in patients with myxoedema coma. The hypoxia responds poorly to O_2 therapy which tends to exacerbate hypercapnoea.

Management

- Transfer the patient to an ICU and monitor closely.
- Mechanical ventilation should be instituted for respiratory failure.
- CVP line. Patients may be hypertensive and hypovolaemic as chronic myxoedema is compensated for by rising catecholamines.
- Hydrocortisone (100mg IV 6–8-hourly) until adrenal insufficiency is excluded.
- Institute thyroid hormone replacement therapy before confirming the diagnosis. No consensus has been reached about optimal thyroid hormone replacement. An accepted regimen includes administration of IV T4: 300–500mcg (depending on patient's age, weight, and risk of

ischaemic heart disease), followed by daily IV doses of 50–100mcg until the patient can take oral T4. If there is no improvement within 24–48h, IV T3 (10mcg 8-hourly) is added and continued until there is clinical improvement and the patient is stable.
- Broad-spectrum antibiotics (e.g. cefotaxime) should be given since bacterial infection is a common precipitant of myxoedema coma.
- Hypothermia should be corrected gently. A space blanket is usually sufficient. Rapid external warming can cause inappropriate vasodilatation and cardiovascular collapse.

Precipitants of myxoedema coma

- Drugs, including sedatives and tranquillizers
- Infection
- Stroke
- Trauma.

Box 9.19 Management key points: myxoedema coma

- Monitor closely in ITU. Mechanical ventilation should be instituted for respiratory failure.
- IV hydrocortisone: 100mg 6–8-hourly until adrenal insufficiency is excluded.
- IV T4: initial dose of 300–500mcg, followed by daily IV doses of 50–100mcg until the patient can take oral T4. If there is no improvement within 24–48h, add IV T3 (10mcg 8-hourly).
- Broad-spectrum antibiotics.
- Appropriate fluid (and glucose) replacement.
- Gentle correction of hypothermia (using a space blanket).

Thyrotoxic crisis: assessment

The term thyrotoxic crisis refers to a constellation of symptoms and signs which together imply a poor prognosis. Thyroid function tests provide no discrimination between simple thyrotoxicosis and thyrotoxic crisis (see Table 9.4). If the diagnosis has not been made, look for clues such as a goitre, or exophthalmic Graves' disease. The presentation may be confused with sepsis or malignant hyperthermia.

Presentation

Cardiovascular symptoms
- Palpitations
- Tachycardia/tachyarrhythmias
- Cardiac failure/oedema.

CNS symptoms
- Anxiety/agitation
- Violent outbursts
- Psychosis/delirium
- Fitting/coma.

GI symptoms
- Diarrhoea
- Vomiting
- Jaundice.

General symptoms
- Fever
- Hyperventilation
- Sweating
- Polyuria.

Rarely, patients may present with an apathetic thyroid storm, and lapse into coma with few other signs of thyrotoxicosis.

Precipitants of thyrotoxic crisis

- Thyroid surgery/general surgery
- Withdrawal of antithyroid drug therapy/radioiodine therapy
- Thyroid palpation
- Iodinated contrast dyes
- Infection
- Cerebrovascular accident/PE
- Parturition
- DKA
- Trauma or emotional stress.

Investigations

- Thyroid function tests (most labs can perform an urgent TSH/free T4 if needed)
- U&Es (?dehydration)
- Calcium (may be elevated)
- Glucose (may be low)
- FBC
- Liver function tests (?jaundice)
- Blood and urine cultures
- CXR (?pulmonary oedema or evidence of infection)
- ECG (rate, ?AF).

Table 9.4 Assessment of severity of a thyrotoxic crisis

Temp (°C) Score	Pulse	Cardiac failure	CNS effects	GI symptoms	
Apyrexial	<99	Absent	Normal	Normal	0
>37.2	>99	Ankle oedema	—	—	5
>37.8	>110	Basal creps.	Agitation	Diarrhoea, vomiting	10
>38.3	>120	Pulmonary oedema	—	—	15
>38.9	>130		Delirium	Unexplained jaundice	20
>39.4	>140		—	—	25
>40			Coma, seizure	—	30

- Add the scores for each column.
- Add an extra 10 points if atrial fibrillation is present.
- Add 10 points if there is a definable precipitant.
- A total score of over 45 indicates thyroid crisis; a score of 25–44 indicates impending crisis.

Thyrotoxic crisis: management

Patients with a thyrotoxic crisis or impending crisis

- Admit the patient to intensive care.
- *Fluid balance*: CVP monitoring is essential to avoid precipitating or worsening cardiac failure. In patients with arrhythmias, the CVP will not accurately reflect left-sided pressures and pulmonary artery pressure monitoring should be considered. GI and insensible (pyrexia and excessive sweating) fluid losses may exceed 5L/day and must be replaced.
- Fever should be treated with *paracetamol* and aggressive *peripheral cooling techniques*. Dantrolene has been occasionally used to control hyperthermia in thyrotoxic crisis. Do not use salicylates which will displace T4 from TBG and can hence worsen the storm.
- *β-block* the patient with propranolol 60–80mg q4h PO or 1mg IV (repeated every 10min as necessary) with cardiac monitoring. Propranolol also inhibits peripheral T4 to T3 conversion. Fever, tachycardia, and tremor should respond immediately. An alternative is esmolol (15–30mg as a bolus followed by 3–6mg/min).
- If β-blockade is contraindicated (e.g. asthma), guanethidine (30–40mg PO 6-hourly) can be used.
- *Treat precipitating factors* such as infection (e.g. cefuroxime 750mg IV tds).
- High-dose *antithyroid drugs*. Propylthiouracil (600mg loading dose then 200–300mg q4h PO/NG) is more effective than carbimazole (20mg 4-hourly), at it inhibits peripheral T4 to T3 conversion.
- *Hydrocortisone*: 100mg 6-hourly. This also inhibits conversion of T4 to T3.
- Enoxaparin 20mg/day SC should be given to very sick patients at risk of thromboembolism.
- Once organification of iodine has been blocked by antithyroid drugs, iodine can be used to inhibit thyroxine release from thyroid gland (Wolff–Chaikoff effect). *Lugol's iodine* contains 5% iodine and 10% potassium iodide in water. Give 1mL every 6h. *Do not give Lugol's iodine until at least 1h after the antithyroid drugs have been given.* Any iodine given prior to antithyroid medication may increase thyroid hormone stores. Continue iodine-containing preparations for a maximum of 2 weeks (lithium is an alternative to iodine in allergic patients).
- *Monitor glucose levels* 4-hourly and administer glucose 5–10% as required. Hepatic glycogen stores are readily depleted during thyroid storm.

Continuing treatment

- Response to treatment is gauged clinically and by serum T3 levels.
- Stop iodine/potassium iodide/lithium and β-blockers when controlled.
- Consider definitive treatment (e.g. surgery or radioactive iodine).
- Treat atrial fibrillation in the usual way (📖 p.72). Higher doses of digoxin may be required as its metabolism is ↑. Amiodarone inhibits peripheral T4 to T3 conversion.

Box 9.20 Management key points: thyrotoxic crisis

- Monitored closely in HDU/ICU.
- IV fluids.
- Paracetamol, peripheral cooling techniques.
- Antiarrhythmic drugs.
- Propylthiouracil (PTU) 600mg loading dose, then 200mg 4-hourly PO/NG
- ***Propranolol*** 60–80mg 4-hourly PO (or 1mg IV, repeated every 10min as necessary). Caution should be taken with complicating cardiac failure.
- ***Hydrocortisone*** 100mg IV qds (inhibits peripheral T4 to T3 conversion).
- ***Lugol's iodine*** 1mL qds at least 1h after first dose of PTU (to block thyroid hormone synthesis first before blocking thyroid hormone release) for a maximum of 14 days (followed by definitive treatment).
- Treat precipitating factors such as infection.
- Thromboprophylaxis.
- Monitor blood glucose.

Pituitary apoplexy

Presentation

Pituitary infarction may be *silent*. Apoplexy implies the presence of symptoms. The clinical manifestations may be due to leakage of blood/necrotic tissue into the subarachnoid space or rapid expansion of a suprasellar mass and pressure on local structures. This may be the presenting symptom of the pituitary tumour (see Box 9.21).

- Headache occurs in 95% of cases (sudden onset; variable intensity).
- Visual disturbance occurs in 70%, (usually bitemporal hemianopia).
- Ocular palsy (40%) causing diplopia, unilateral or bilateral.
- Nausea/vomiting.
- Meningism (common).
- Hemiparesis or rarely seizures.
- Fever, anosmia, CSF rhinorrhoea, and hypothalamic dysfunction (disturbed sympathetic autoregulation with abnormal BP control, respiration, and cardiac rhythm) are all described, but are rare.
- Altered mental state, lethargy, delirium, or coma.
- Symptoms of preceding pituitary tumour.
- Acute hypopituitarism.

Clinically, pituitary apoplexy may be very difficult to distinguish from subarachnoid haemorrhage, bacterial meningitis, midbrain infarction (basilar artery occlusion), or cavernous sinus thrombosis. Transient neurological symptoms are common in the preceding few days.

The clinical course is variable. Headache and mild visual disturbance may develop slowly and persist for several weeks. In its most fulminant form, apoplexy may cause blindness, haemodynamic instability, coma, and death. Residual endocrine disturbance (panhypopituitarism) invariably occurs.

Investigations

- ***U&Es*** Hyper- or hyponatraemia may occur.
- ***Endocrine function tests (save clotted blood)*** Cortisol, TFT, prolactin, GH, IGF-1, LH, FSH, The short Synacthen® test is unreliable in the first 2–3 weeks.
- ***CT head*** Pituitary cuts with IV contrast will reveal a tumour mass or haemorrhage 24–48h after onset.
- ***MRI (Gd enhanced with pituitary views)*** May be more informative in the subacute setting.

Management

- Stabilize the patient (Airway, Breathing, Circulation).
- Hydrocortisone 100mg IV should be given if the diagnosis is suspected after the blood samples above have been collected.
- Monitor U&Es and urine output for evidence of DI.
- Patients with macroprolactinomas may respond to dopamine agonists.
- *Neurosurgical decompression* may be indicated (seek neurosurgical review). Obtundation and visual deterioration are absolute indications for neurosurgery. Patients without confusion or visual disturbance generally do well without surgery.
- Assess pituitary function once the acute illness has resolved and treat as necessary. A TSH in the normal range may be inappropriate if the T4 is low in pituitary disease, but this may occur in the sick euthyroid state characteristic of many seriously ill patients.

Box 9.21 Causes of apoplexy in patients with pituitary adenomas

- Spontaneous haemorrhage (no obvious precipitant, the commonest)
- Anticoagulant therapy
- Head trauma
- Radiation therapy
- Drugs (e.g. bromocriptine or oestrogen)
- Following dynamic tests of pituitary function.

Hypopituitary coma

Hypopituitarism does not become evident until 75% of the adenohypophysis is destroyed, and at least 90% destruction is required for total loss of pituitary secretion. Complete loss of hormone secretion can rapidly become life threatening and requires immediate therapy. In a mild or incomplete form, hypopituitarism can remain unsuspected for years.

Presentation

In the absence of stress, patients with severe hypopituitarism may have few symptoms or signs. A general anaesthetic or infection may precipitate hypoglycaemia and coma, due to the combination of a lack of GH, cortisol, and thyroxine, all of which have a counter-regulatory effect on insulin. See Box 9.23 for causes of panhypopituitarism.

Clues from the history include:

- Known pituitary adenoma.
- Recent difficult delivery: pituitary infarction following postpartum haemorrhage and vascular collapse is still the commonest cause of hypopituitarism. Features include failure of lactation (deficiency of prolactin and oxytocin), failure of menstruation (lack of gonadotrophins), non-specific features, e.g. tiredness, weakness, loss of body hair, and loss of libido (due to ACTH deficiency, hypothyroidism, and gonadotrophin deficiency).
- Men may give a history of impotence, lethargy, and loss of body hair.
- Women report loss of menstruation.

Examination

- Examination of the comatose patient is discussed on 📖 p.332.
- Examine specifically for 2° sexual characteristics and physical signs of myxoedema.
- Consider other causes for coma (📖 p.332.)

Investigations

- General investigations for patients in coma are discussed on 📖 p.332.
- Take blood for baseline cortisol, ACTH, thyroid function, LH, FSH, prolactin, and GH.
- Short Synacthen® test must be performed to test for adrenocortical reserve (📖 p.550.)
- LHRH and TRH test may be performed at the same time as the short Synacthen® test but are rarely necessary.
- Defer formal pituitary function testing until the patient is stable.
- CT scan of pituitary (tumour or empty sella).
- MRI scan may give additional information.

Management

- General measures are as for any patient in coma (📖 p.332.)
- Give IV N saline to restore BP if the patient is in shock.
- Give glucose if the patient is hypoglycaemic.
- Hydrocortisone 100mg IV should be administered if the diagnosis is suspected and continued (100mg IV tds–qds).

- Start liothyromine (10mcg bd) ***after*** hydrocortisone is started.
- Investigate and treat any precipitating intercurrent infection.
- If the patient fails to improve, consider other causes for coma. (See 📖 p.332.)
- Long term, the patients will require replacement with hydrocortisone, thyroxine, testosterone or oestrogen/progesterone, and GH.

Box 9.22 Causes of panhypopituitarism

Pituitary

- Mass lesion (adenoma, cyst)
- Pituitary surgery or irradiation
- Infiltration (haemochromatosis)
- Infarction (Sheehan's)
- Apoplexy (haemorrhage)
- Empty sella syndrome
- Trauma e.g. fractured skull base.

Hypothalamic

- Mass lesion (metastases e.g. breast, lung; craniopharyngioma)
- Radiotherapy
- Infiltration (sarcoid, histiocytosis)
- Infection (TB).

Phaeochromocytomas: assessment

- Phaeochromocytomas are catecholamine-producing tumours usually involving one or more adrenal glands. ~10% are bilateral, ~10% are extra-adrenal (usually around the sympathetic chain—paragangliomas) and ~10% are malignant. They usually secrete AD or NA. A small proportion secretes DA, when hypotension may occur.
- Most are diagnosed during routine screening of hypertensive patients (they are found in only 0.1% of hypertensives). Pure AD-producing tumours may mimic septic shock due to AD-induced peripheral vasodilatation (β_2-receptors).

Presentation

- Classically a triad of episodic headaches, sweating, and tachycardia.
- Hypertension (mild to severe sustained or uncontrolled paroxysmal hypertensive episodes) and orthostatic hypotension (low plasma volume). 50% have sustained elevated BP and 50% have paroxysmal elevations.
- Anxiety attacks, tremor, palpitations, cold extremities, and pallor.
- Cardiac dysrhythmias (incl. AF and VF) and dilated cardiomyopathy
- Hypertensive crises may be precipitated by β-blockers, tricyclic antidepressants, metoclopramide, and naloxone.
- Unexplained lactic acidosis.
- Triggers for hypertensive crises include surgery (particularly manipulation of the tumour itself), opiates and contrast media.
- See Box 9.24 for other causes of sympathetic overactivity.

Investigations (Box 9.23)

- 2–3 24-hour urine collections for measurement of catecholamines (adrenaline, noradrenaline and dopamine) and if available metanephrine and normetanephrine.
- Urine should be collected in acid-containing bottles and kept refrigerated as catecholamines are more stable at low pH and low temperature.
- Urinary creatinine and volume should be measured to verify an adequate (i.e. 24-h) collection.
- In patients who are at high risk for phaeochromocytoma (i.e. familial syndromes or previously surgically cured phaeochromocytoma or paraganglioma), plasma free metanephrine and normetanephrine should be measured if available (higher sensitivity: ~99%).
- Certain drugs (e.g. tricyclic antidepressants, levodopa, prochlorperazine) should be tapered and discontinued at least 2 weeks before any biochemical tests.
- Catecholamine secretion may be appropriately ↑ in stress or illness (e.g. stroke, MI, congestive cardiac failure, obstructive sleep apnoea and head injury).

- If the biochemical results are abnormal, imaging with CT or MRI of the abdomen/pelvis is required to locate the tumour. Caution: radiocontrast can cause catecholamine release.
- 123-I-meta-iodobenzylguanidine (MIBG) is taken up by adrenergic tissue. An MIBG scan can detect metastases or tumours not detected by CT or MRI.
- *Plasma catecholamines* should be collected from an indwelling cannula placed over 30min previously in a supine patient. Samples need to be taken directly to the lab (on ice) for centrifugation.
- *Selective venous sampling* may be used to localize extra-adrenal tumours.

Box 9.23 Investigations for suspected phaeochromocytoma

- U&Es (↓K^+,↑urea)
- Glucose (↑)
- Urinary catecholamines and fractionated metanephrines
- Plasma catecholamines in high-risk patients
- CT scan or MRI of adrenals
- MIBG scan.

Box 9.24 Other causes of sympathetic overactivity

- Abrupt withdrawal of clonidine or β-blockers.
- Autonomic dysfunction e.g. Guillain–Barré syndrome or post-spinal cord injury
- Stress response to surgery, pain, panic, or acute illness.
- Sympathomimetic drugs:
  - Phenylpropanolamine (decongestant)
  - Cocaine
  - MAOI plus tyramine-containing foods (cheese, beer, wine, avocado, bananas, smoked or aged fish/meat).

Phaeochromocytomas: management

Patients are usually volume depleted at presentation, and should be rehydrated prior to initiation of β-blockade, otherwise severe hypotension may occur. β-blockade alone may precipitate a hypertensive crisis, and must never be given prior to adequate α-blockade. Labetalol is predominantly a β-blocker and should not be used alone. Long acting α-blockers prevent escape episodes.

- Adequate fluid replacement with CVP monitoring.
- Acute hypertensive crises should be controlled with *phentolamine* (2–5mg IV bolus, repeated as necessary every 15–30min). Alternatively start an infusion of nitroprusside (0.5–1.5mcg/kg/min, typical dose 100mcg/min).
- Preparation for surgery
  - Initiate oral α-blockade: *phenoxybenzamine* 10mg daily increasing gradually to 40mg tds. Monitor BP closely. Tumour β-stimulation may produce excessive vasodilatation and hypotension requiring inotropic support. Recent studies have shown that prazosin or doxazosin are equally effective and are being used increasingly.
  - When the BP is controlled with phenoxybenzamine, add propranolol 10–20mg tds.
  - Invasive monitoring—pulmonary artery (Swan–Ganz) catheter and arterial line—is mandatory.
- Hypotension commonly occurs intraoperatively when the tumour is removed, and this should be managed with blood, plasma expanders, and inotropes as required. Inotropes should only be used when the patient is appropriately fluid replete. Expansion of intravascular volume 12h before surgery significantly reduces the frequency and severity of postoperative hypotension. Angiotensin II should be available as an alternative inotrope for cases of resistant hypotension.

Autosomal dominant conditions with a high risk of developing phaeochromocytoma include:

- *Neurofibromatosis (Von-Recklinghausen disease)*: neurofibromata, café au lait spots, Lisch nodules (iris hamartomas), and axillary freckling.
- *Von-Hippel Lindau disease:* cerebellar haemangioblastomas, retinal haemangiomas and other neoplasms including hypernephroma.
- *Multiple endocrine neoplasia types 2a* (hyperparathyroidism and medullary thyroid carcinoma) *and 2b* (medullary thyroid carcinoma, bowel ganglioneuromatosis, hypertrophied corneal nerves, Marfanoid habitus).

Polyuria

Definition: >3L urine per day.

Presentation

- Confusion (hyponatraemia or dehydration)
- Coma
- Proteinuria on screening
- Depression or other psychiatric manifestations
- Renal stones.

Causes

- Excessive fluid intake
- Endocrine dysfunction (DM, DI, hypercalcaemia)
- Hypokalaemia
- Intrinsic renal disease (polycystic kidneys, analgesic nephropathy, medullary cystic disease, amyloidosis) or renal recovery from ATN.
- Post-obstructive uropathy e.g. after catheterization of patient in chronic retention.
- Post-renal artery angioplasty
- Drugs (furosemide, alcohol, lithium, amphotericin B, vinblastine, demeclocycline, cisplatinum).

History

- Duration and severity (nocturia, frequency, water consumption at night)
- FH of DM, polycystic kidneys, renal calculi
- Drug history (see 'Causes')
- Renal calculi (hypercalcaemia)
- Weakness (low potassium), depression (hypercalcaemia)
- Psychiatric history
- Endocrine history (menses, sexual function, lactation, pubic hair)
- Other significant pathology (e.g. causes of amyloid).

Investigations

- U&Es (renal disease, hypokalaemia)
- Glucose
- Calcium, phosphate, and alkaline phosphatase
- Plasma and urine osmolality: a U:P osmolality of <1.0 indicates DI, intrinsic renal disease (incl. low K^+), or hysterical drinking
- AXR (nephrocalcinosis)
- Lithium levels if appropriate
- Dipstick protein and quantification if indicated.

Management

- Assess fluid status (JVP, BP, postural drop, weight charts, CVP).
- Strict fluid balance and daily weights.
- CVP line may be necessary.
- Measure urinary sodium and potassium (random spot samples will give an indication of the loss of sodium or potassium initially, and if losses are great, accurate timed samples of <6h are possible).

- Replace fluid losses as appropriate to maintain a normal homeostasis, using combinations of saline and glucose.
- Monitor potassium, calcium, phosphate, and magnesium daily or twice daily if necessary.
- If lithium toxicity is present, see 📖 p.716.
- Avoid chasing fluids. At some point a clinical judgement has to be made to stop replacing urinary losses with IV fluids to allow the patient to reach their 'normal equilibrium'. Once the patient is optimally hydrated and is able to drink freely, then avoid replacing fluids IV to allow physiological homeostasis to occur.
- If DI is suspected, arrange a water deprivation test (see Box 9.25).

Box 9.25 Water deprivation test

- Stop all drugs the day before the test; no smoking or caffeine.
- Supervise the patient carefully to prevent surreptitious drinking.
- Empty the bladder after a light breakfast. No further fluids PO.
- Weigh the patient at time 0, 4, 5, 6, 7, 8h into the test (stop the test if >3% of body weight is lost).
- Measure serum osmolality at 30min, 4h, and hourly until end of test (check that the plasma osmolality rises to >290mosmol/kg to confirm an adequate stimulus for ADH release).
- Collect urine hourly and measure the volume and osmolality (the volume should decrease and the osmolality rise; stop test if urine osmolality >800mosmol/kg as DI is excluded).
- If polyuria continues, give desmopressin 20mcg intranasally at 8h.
- Allow fluids PO (water) after 8h. Continue to measure urine osmolality hourly for a further 4h.

Interpretation

- *Normal response:* urine osmolality rises to >800mosmol/kg with a small rise after desmopressin.
- *Cranial DI:* urine osmolality remains low (>400mosmol/kg) and increases by >50% after desmopressin.
- *Nephrogenic DI:* urine osmolality remains low (<400mosmol/kg) and only rises a little (<45%) with desmopressin.
- *Primary (psychogenic) polydipsia:* urine osmolality rises (>400mosmol/kg) but is typically less than the normal response—often difficult to diagnose.

Malignant hyperthermia

Malignant hyperthermia is a drug- or stress-induced catabolic syndrome characterized by excessive muscular contractions, a sudden rise in body temperature, and cardiovascular collapse. The incidence is ~1:15,000, with a 30% mortality. The cause is unknown, but may involve abnormal calcium homeostasis in skeletal muscle cells. The condition seems to be inherited in an autosomal dominant manner with variable penetrance.

Box 9.26 Drugs precipitating malignant hyperthermia

- Halothane
- Succinylcholine
- Methoxyflurane and enflurane
- Cyclopropane
- Phencyclidine
- Ketamine

Halothane and succinylcholine account for 80% of cases

Box 9.27 Drugs considered safe in malignant hyperthermia

- Barbiturates
- Nitrous oxide
- Diazepam
- Opiates
- Pancuronium
- Tubocurare.

Diagnosis

- Malignant hyperthermia most commonly presents in patients in their early 20s. The early signs are muscular rigidity, sinus tachcardia and SVTs, ↑ carbon dioxide production, and hypertension.
- Hyperthermia occurs late, and may be rapidly followed by hypotension, acidosis, and hyperkalaemia, which gives rise to ventricular tachycardia.
- The condition almost always occurs perioperatively.
- The differential diagnosis includes phaeochromocytoma, thyrotoxic crisis, narcotic-induced hyperthermia in patients taking MAOIs, and drug-induced hyperthermia (caused by cocaine, phencyclidine, amphetamine, LSD, tricyclics, and aspirin), and certain infections such as malaria.
- Plasma CPK is high.

Treatment

The aim of therapy is to decrease thermogenesis, and promote heat loss.

- *Dantrolene:* 1–2.5mg/kg intravenously every 5–10min to a maximum dose of 10mg/kg. The dantrolene should then be continued at a dose of 1–2 mg/kg (IV or orally every 6h for 2 days).
- Stop any anaesthetic agent.
- External cooling by submersion is helpful. All administered fluids should be chilled.
- Procainamide should be given to all patients to prevent ventricular dysrhythmias (increases uptake of calcium and may reduce hyperthermia).
- Hypotension should be treated with saline or colloids with isoprenaline. Dopaminergic and α-adrenergic agonists reduce heat dissipation and should be avoided.
- Some authorities advocate prophyalctic anticonvulsants as seizures are common.
- See Box 9.26 for drugs precipitating malignant hyperthermia.
- See Box 9.27 for drugs considered safe in malignant hyperthermia.

Neurolepetic malignant syndrome

The neuroleptic malignant syndrome results from an imbalance of dopaminergic neurotransmitters following neuroleptic drug use. The incidence is ~0.5% in patients taking neuroleptic drugs. This syndrome is clinically distinct from malignant hyperthermia (see 📖 p.568); it is not an allergic reaction. The mean age of onset is 40 years. The mortality is ~10%.

Box 9.28 Drugs associated with the neuroleptic malignant syndrome

- Haloperidol
- Phenothiazines
- Metoclopramide
- Loxapine
- Tetrabenazine
- Thioxanthenes
- Withdrawal of levodopa or amantadine.

Clinical features

- Muscular rigidity incl. dysphagia, dysarthria early (96%)
- Extra-pyramidal signs (pseudo-parkinsonism), tremor (90%)
- Oculogyric crisis
- Catatonia: muteness (95%)
- Altered consciousness or coma
- ↑serum CPK/AST (97%)
- Pyrexia (rarely >40°C) follows onset of rigidity.

The syndrome can occur within hours of initiating drug therapy, but typically takes ~1 week. It can also occur following a dosage increase of a well-established drug.

Complications

- Rhabdomyolysis (📖 p.294)
- Renal (15%) and hepatic failure
- Fitting is rare
- Cardiovascular collapse
- DIC
- Respiratory failure.

Differential diagnosis

- Malignant hyperthermia (📖 p.568)
- Heat stroke
- Other causes of catatonia
- Thyrotoxic crisis (📖 p.554)
- Phaeochromocytoma (📖 p.562)
- Drug-induced hyperthermia (caused by cocaine, LSD, phencyclidine, amphetamine, tricyclics, and aspirin).

Management

- Withdrawal of causative agent
- Dantrolene (1–2mg/kg every 6h up to a maximum 300mg/day)
- Paralysis and ventilation (curare, pancuronium)
- Bromocriptine, amantadine, levodopa (increase dopaminergic tone and reduce rigidity, thermogenesis, and extra-pyramidal symptoms).

Chapter 10

Haematological emergencies

Blood transfusion reactions

Assessment

Table 10.1 Blood transfusion reactions: assessment

Presentation	Causes	Timing
Shock (major haemolysis) Lumbar pain, headache Chest pain, SOB Rigors, pyrexia Urticaria, flushing Hypotension Oliguria Haemoglobinuria Jaundice DIC	Red cell antibodies ABO incompatibility Other antibodies	Immediate (min/h)
Shock (septic) Rigors, pyrexia Hypotension Oliguria DIC	Bacterial contamination	Immediate (min/h)
Fever Isolated pyrexia Rigors	White cell antibodies Recipient cytokines	Early (30–90 min)
Allergic reactions Urticaria Pyrexia Rigors Facial oedema Dyspnoea	Donor plasma proteins (more common with plasma or platelets)	Early (min/h)
Circulatory overload Breathlessness Cough	Rapid transfusion	Early (h)
Transfussion-related acute lung injury (TRALI) Non-cardiogenic pulmonary oedema Pyrexia Cough Breathlessness CXR changes	Donor white cell antibodies (rare)	Early (min/h)
Delayed haemolysis Pyrexia Anaemia Jaundice	Minor red cell antibodies	Late (7–10 days)
Delayed thrombocytopenia Purpura Mucosal bleeding	Platelet antibody (commonly anti-Pl^{A1})	Late (2–10 days)

Table 10.1 (*contd*)

Presentation	Causes	Timing
Infection	Hep. B, C, non A/B/C CMV, EBV, HIV Toxoplasmosis Malaria, syphilis	Late (days/months)

Management

The main problem encountered in practice is differentiating a (common) rise in temperature during a blood transfusion from (the rare but potentially lethal) major transfusion reactions. The common patterns of reactions are outlined in Table 10.1

Pointers to a severe reaction include:

- Symptoms: does the patient feel unwell?
- Pattern of temperature: a *rapid* rise in temperature to >38°C is common in minor reactions.
- Hypotension or tachycardia.

Management

Isolated pyrexia	• Slow transfusion • Give paracetamol • Finish transfusion if no progression of symptoms.
Urticarial reaction	• Slow transfusion Give chlorpheniramine 10mg IV/PO Complete transfusion if no progression of symptoms • Rarely, patients need hydrocortisone 100mg IV.
Shock *Anaphylaxis* *ABO incompatibility* *Septic shock*	• Stop transfusion and give O_2 • Give adrenaline 0.5–1mg SC and consider repeating every 10min until improvement. Contact duty anaesthetist and ITU • Give chlorphenamine 10mg IV colloids (also consider crystalloid, inotropes) • Monitor fluid balance. Take blood: FBC, U&Es; full coagulation screen (for DIC); repeat cross-match and Coomb's test; return donor blood • Urine: bilirubin, free Hb.
Circulatory overload (see 📖 p.87)	• O_2, furosemide IV (40–120mg) • Nitrate infusion (0–10mg/h).
TRALI	• Life-threatening. Treat as ARDS (📖 p.198).
Delayed haemolysis	• Report to blood bank • Repeat cross-match and Coombs test Transfuse with freshly X-matched blood.
Thrombocytopenia	• Immune mediated: treat with Pl^{A1}-negative transfusions, high-dose IV IgG, steroids, and plasmapheresis (dilutional ↓platelets seen if >5U transfused).

Report any serious or haemolytic reaction to haematologist.

Sickle cell crisis: presentation

A small percentage of sufferers with sickle cell disease have recurrent crises, and repeated hospital admissions. There is an unwarranted tendency to attribute this to a low pain threshold, or to 'dependence' on opiates, rather than to severity of disease. Analgesia should never be denied to patients. This group of patients has the highest rate of serious complications and mortality as a result of their severe disease.

Painful (vaso-occlusive) crisis

- This is the most common presentation in adults and children.
- Severe/excruciating pain is felt at one or more sites, especially long bones (small bones in children), back, ribs, sternum.
- There may be associated pyrexia (usually <38.5°C), tenderness, local warmth and swelling, or there may be no objective features.
- Haemolysis may be ↑ (↑bilirubin, fall in Hb), but is not a good correlate.
- *There are no reliable clinical markers for severity of crisis.*

Chest crisis

- The commonest cause of mortality.
- Vaso-occlusion of pulmonary microvasculature results in reduced perfusion and local infarction.
- May be heralded by rib/sternal pain.
- May be precipitated by a chest infection, pregnancy, and in smokers.
- Symptoms (which may be minor initially) include pleuritic chest pain, breathlessness.
- Signs are variable (often minimal) but can progress rapidly; usually reduced air entry at lung bases.
- CXR shows uni/bilateral consolidation, usually basal.
- P_aO_2 is often markedly reduced.

Cerebral infarction

- Usually in children <5 years, rare in adults.
- Presents as acute stroke.
- High risk of recurrence.

Splenic/hepatic sequestration

- Usually in children <5 years.
- RBCs trapped in spleen and/or liver, usually causing organomegaly.
- Causes severe anaemia; circulatory collapse.

Aplastic crisis

- Usually in children, young adults.
- Mainly caused by parvovirus infection, exacerbated by folate deficiency.
- Sudden fall in Hb, reduced reticulocyte count.

Haemolytic crisis

- Often accompanies painful crises.
- Fall in Hb; ↑reticulocyte count.

Cholecystitis/cholangitis/biliary colic

- Pigment stones common due to haemolytic anaemia.
- Can be misinterpreted as vaso-occlusive crisis.

Priapism

- Prolonged, painful erections due to local vaso-occlusion (1–24h long).
- Major crisis often preceded by 'stuttering' priapism episodes.
- May result in permanent impotence.
- This is a urological emergency. On-call urologists should be informed on the patient's arrival in casualty.

Sickle cell crisis: management

General measures

Control pain

- Oral analgesia (dihydrocodeine/NSAIDs) may be sufficient for minor crises.
- Usually parenteral opiates are necessary, often in high doses (depending on previous opiate use). Start low and review in 1h, titrating to response, e.g.
  - Morphine 5–40mg im every 2h
  - Diamorphine 5–25mg SC every 2h.
- Failure to control pain using these regimens usually indicates the need for a continuous opiate infusion, or a PCA pump. Some patients prefer pethidine but there is a risk of seizures as the drug metabolites accumulate.
- Supplementary analgesics, such as diclofenac 50mg tds PO, may have a small additional benefit.

Ensure hydration

- IV crystalloids are preferred, but venous access may be a problem.
- Aim for an input of 3–4L/day with close monitoring of balance.
- Fluids can be oral where venous access problematic.

Give oxygen

- Not of proven benefit (except in chest crises), but often provides symptomatic relief.
- Monitor O_2 saturations on air and O_2; falling sats may be early indication of chest crisis.
- In a severe chest crisis, CPAP/full ventilation may become necessary. Transfer to ITU early.

Give folic acid

Give 5mg PO od (continue long term in all patients).

Review sources of sepsis

- Infections are frequent (at least partly due to hyposplenism).
- Penicillin prophylaxis and vaccination (pneumococcal, HIB, meningococcal, influenza) does reduce the incidence, but some penicillin resistant organisms are emerging.
- If an infective precipitant, or component, of the crisis is suspected, start 'blind' antibiotics (e.g. cefuroxime 750mg IV tds) after infection screen.
- Consider less common sources of sepsis (e.g. osteomyelitis, mycobacterium, etc).

Give thromboprophylaxis

LMWH prophylaxis should be used routinely.

Investigations

- *FBC* Hb (?fall from steady state) WCC (neutrophilia common).
- *Reticulocytes* Raised in haemolysis, reduced in aplastic crisis.
- *HbS%* Can guide transfusion requirements.
- *Blood cultures* If pyrexial.
- *Stool cultures* If diarrhoea + bone pain (?salmonella osteomyelitis).
- *CXR* Regardless of symptoms.
- *Pulse oximetry* ± ABGs if hypoxic.
- *Bone XR* ?osteomyelitis (persisting pain, pyrexia, or bacteraemia). ?avascular necrosis (chronic hip/shoulder pain).
- *Viral serology* If aplastic crisis (?parvovirus).
- *X-match* If transfusion/exchange indicated (see 'Exchange transfusion'). Consider extended red cell phenotyping prior to transfusion.

Exchange transfusion

This is performed by venesection of 1–2U, with fluid replacement (N saline, 1L over 2–4h) followed by transfusion of X-matched blood. If a larger exchange is required, or fluid balance is precarious, the exchange can be performed on a cell separator. Aim for Hb between 7–9g/L in either case; *a higher Hb can increase blood viscosity and precipitate further sickling*. In severe crises, red cell exchange should be repeated until the HbS% is <40%.

Indications for urgent exchange transfusion

- Chest crisis
- Cerebral infarction
- Severe, persisting painful crisis
- Priapism.

Box 10.1 Management key points: sickle cell crisis

- ***Analgesia:*** oral dihydrocodeine/NSAIDs for minor crises; usually need parenteral morphine (10–40mg IM 2-hourly) or diamorphine (10–25mg SC 2-hourly). If these fail use continuous opiate infusion, or a PCA pump.
- ***IV fluids***: aim for an input of 3–4L crystalloids/day.
- ***Oxygen*** for symptomatic relief. CPAP/full ventilation/ITU care in a severe chest crisis.
- ***Folic acid:*** 5mg PO od.
- ***Antibiotics*** if an infective precipitant is suspected (start 'blind' antibiotics e.g. cefuroxime 750mg IV tds after infection screen).
- ***Exchange transfusion*** (see 'Exchange transfusion').

Bleeding disorders: general approach

Presentation

- Normal haemostasis requires the interaction of platelets, fibrin from the clotting cascade, and the microvasculature. An abnormality of any of these components may present as easy bruising, purpura, or spontaneous or excessive bleeding.
- Muscle haematomas or haemarthroses suggests clotting factor deficiencies (e.g. haemophilia) whereas purpura or bruising suggests abnormalities of platelet function.
- Mucosal haemorrhage (acute GI bleed) may occur without any haemostatic abnormalities, e.g. due to peptic ulcer disease.
- If a coagulation or platelet abnormality is uncovered on 'routine' testing, examine the patient for occult bleeding (e.g. iron-deficient anaemia, fundal haemorrhages).

Causes

These can be divided into:

- Coagulation abnormalities
- Platelet abnormalities (too few or dysfunctional)
- Microvascular abnormalities.

Investigations

All patients should have:

- Coagulation screen (PT, APTT, fibrinogen)
- FBC and film
- U&Es
- LFTs
- X-match.

Where appropriate consider:

- Bleeding time
- Platelet function tests
- Bone marrow aspirate and trephine
- Autoantibody screen
- Specific coagulation factor levels
- Acquired factor inhibitors.

Management

General measures

- Avoid non-steroidal medications, especially aspirin.
- Never give IM injections.
- Avoid arterial punctures.
- Enlist expert help with invasive procedures. Use internal jugular rather than subclavian route for central line insertion.
- Examine skin, oral mucosa, and fundi for evidence of fresh bleeding.
- Restore circulatory volume with IV colloid/crystalloid if there is haemodynamic compromise and consider blood transfusion.

Specific therapy

- Look for any local cause for the bleeding (e.g. oesophageal varices, vascular damage causing epistaxis, chest infection causing haemoptysis) that may be amenable to treatment.
- Stop any drug that may be exacerbating bleeding (see 🕮 Box 10.2).
- Correct coagulation abnormalities if appropriate (see 🕮 p.582).
- Correct platelet abnormalities if appropriate (see 🕮 p.586).

Box 10.2 Drugs that may cause bleeding disorders

Coagulation abnormalities

- Heparin
- Coumarins (e.g. warfarin)
- Thrombin inhibitors (argatroban, hirudin).

Thrombocytopenia

Immune

- Heparin
- Quinine
- Penicillin
- H_2-receptor antagonists
- Thiazide diuretics.

Non-immune

- Cytotoxic chemotherapy
- Chloramphenicol
- Primaquine
- Alcohol.

Abnormal platelet function

- Aspirin, NSAIDs
- Clopidogrel
- Antibiotics (e.g. piperacillin, cefotaxime)
- Dextran
- SSRIs
- Alcohol.

Abnormal microvasculature

- Corticosteroids.

Abnormal coagulation 1

Common causes

- Anticoagulants
- Liver disease
- DIC
- Massive transfusion.

Rarer causes

- Haemophilia A, B
- von Willebrand's disease:
  - Acquired factor VIII inhibitors
  - Amyloid (acquired Factor X deficiency)
  - α_2-plasmin inhibitor deficiency
- Vitamin K deficiency:
  - Obstructive jaundice
  - Small bowel disease.

Diagnosis

See Table 10.2.

Table 10.2 Diagnosis of abnormal coagulation

Defect	Interpretation	Consider
↑PT	Extrinsic pathway defect	Warfarin, liver disease, vitamin K deficiency
↑APTT	Intrinsic pathway defect	Heparin, haemophilia, von Willebrand's disease, lupus anti-coagulant (anti-phospholipid syndrome)
↑PT and APTT	Multiple defects (usually acquired)	Liver disease, DIC, warfarin
↑TT	Abnormal fibrin production	Heparin effect, fibrinogen defect, excess FDPs (which interfere with reaction)
↑PT, APTT, TT	Multiple (acquired) defects	Deficient or abnormal fibrinogen or heparin. Reptilase time* will be normal if due to heparin
↓Fibrinogen	Excess consumption of clotting factors and fibrinogen	Consumptive coagulopathy (but not necessarily full DIC), severe liver disease
↑FDPs	↑Fibrin(ogen) degradation	The exact interpretation depends on the lab test used. Some do not distinguish between fibrin and FDPs. Some are more specific to fibrin degradation (e.g. D-Dimers) and are therefore suggestive of widespread clot formation and breakdown (i.e. DIC)
↑Bleeding time	Abnormal platelet function	von Willebrand's disease (↑APTT), congenital or acquired platelet dysfunction (see table p.685). Consider platelet function studies
The lupus anticoagulant usually confers a pro-thrombotic rather than a bleeding tendency.		

*Reptilase is a snake venom not inhibited by heparin. It converts fibrinogen to fibrin.

Abnormal coagulation 2

Management

Options are:

- *Fresh frozen plasma*: indicated for treatment of acute DIC with bleeding, improving haemostasis in decompensated liver failure and emergency reversal of warfarin therapy if no prothrombin complex concentrate available. Give approx. 15ml/kg i.e. 4–5 units (approx. 200 ml/unit). Watch for signs of fluid overload and give IV furosemide if necessary.
- *Vitamin K*: Phytomenadione 5–10mg IV slowly (daily for 3 days) if deficiency is suspected. 2–5mg IV/PO will improve over-warfarinization in 6–12h. 0.5–1mg for minor adjustment.
- *Protamine sulphate* (1mg IV neutralizes 100iu heparin) is rarely used in practice. Stopping a heparin infusion will normalize an APTT in 2–4h.
- *Cryoprecipitate or fibrinogen concentrate* should be considered if the fibrinogen is below 500g/L.
- *Factor concentrates* can be used in the treatment of isolated factor deficiencies, e.g. haemophilia. Concentrates of Factors II, VII, IX, and X are also available in some centres for specific reversal of warfarin effects (prothrombin complex concentrate).
- *Antifibrinolytics* are used occasionally for the treatment of life-threatening bleeds following thrombolytic therapy or major surgery (e.g. cardiac surgery or prostatectomy) and in certain conditions associated with hyperplasminaemia (e.g. acute promyelocytic leukaemia, certain malignancies. Give tranexamic acid 0.5–1g slow IV injection tds.
- *Miscellaneous* Desmopressin and oestrogens are occasionally used for haemophilia and renal failure.

Circulating inhibitors of coagulation

Lupus anticoagulant

- Causes prolonged APTT but predisposes to thrombosis, not bleeding (antiphospholipid syndrome).

Acquired haemophilia

- Elderly patients presenting with severe bruising and prolonged APTT
- Discuss with haematologists.

Abnormal platelets

Causes

Thrombocytopenia

Increased platelet consumption
- Immune:
  - Idiopathic (ITP)
  - Drug induced
  - SLE
  - HIV related
- Non-immune:
  - Massive transfusion
  - Hypersplenism
  - DIC, TTP.

Reduced platelet production
- Myelosuppressant:
  - Drugs, alcohol
  - Viral infections
- Marrow infiltration/failure
- B12 or folate deficiency
- Inherited disorders (rare).

Abnormal platelet function
- Drugs (e.g. aspirin)
- Uraemia
- Liver disease
- Myeloproliferative disorders
- Myelodysplasia
- Dysproteinaemia (e.g. myeloma)
- Inherited disorders (rare):
  - Glanzman's disease (GP Ia deficiency)
  - Bernard–Soulier (GP IIb/IIIa deficiency)
  - Chediak–Higashi syndrome (abn. platelet granules).

Investigations
- ***Peripheral blood film:*** evidence of haemolysis (?DIC ?TTP), or marrow infiltration.
- ***Coagulation screen:*** ?DIC.
- ***Autoantibody screen:*** associated autoimmune diseases.
- ***Bone marrow aspirate:*** ↑ megakaryocytes generally indicates peripheral consumption; ↓ or abnormal megakaryocytes suggest a marrow problem.
- ***Antiplatelet antibodies:*** rarely indicated.
- ***Platelet function tests:*** for bleeding in the presence of adequate platelet numbers on the blood film.
- ***Low platelets*** ($<20 \times 10^9$/L) may cause spontaneous bleeding and require platelet transfusion ± treatment for the underlying cause.
- ***Moderately low counts*** ($20–140 \times 10^9$/L) will rarely cause spontaneous bleeding, unless there is an associated clotting abnormality (e.g. DIC) or a 1° marrow defect, with production of defective platelets (e.g. myelodysplasia). Transfuse only if there is continued bleeding or in preparation for major surgery.
- ***High counts*** ($500–1000 \times 10^9$/L) may also indicate a 1° production problem, with abnormal platelets (e.g. myeloproliferative disorders). (NB: moderately raised platelet count is a normal response to bleeding and is also seen in chronic inflammation.)

Management

This depends on the platelet count and severity of bleeding.

Immune-mediated thrombocytopenia

- Platelet transfusions are usually ineffective as sole therapy and rarely indicated unless severe bleeding or urgent surgery required.
- Prednisolone (1mg/kg od) is standard first-line treatment for adult ITP.
- Immunoglobulin 0.4g/kg/day IV infusion for 5 days (or 2g/kg/day for 1 day): this usually works quicker than steroids, but the effect only lasts 2–4 weeks. Start the infusion very slowly, as anaphylactic reactions (fever, urticaria, bronchospasm, and hypotension) are not uncommon.

Acute DIC/massive transfusion

Give platelet transfusions to maintain platelet count >75 × 10^9/L (for chronic DIC, transfuse only for active bleeding).

Surgery

- Depends on the surgery but generally aim for platelet count >50 × 10^9/L.
- For CNS surgery or multiple trauma, aim for count >100 × 10^9/L.

Reduced platelet production (chronic, stable)

If no bleeding, transfuse if count <10 × 10^9/L.

TTP/heparin-induced thrombocytopenia

Platelet transfusions are contraindicated. Discuss all cases with the haematologists.

Platelet transfusion

- A single unit is either a pool of several buffy coats or platelets from a single donor from aphoresis.
- The number of platelets in a unit is <240 × 10^9 which is sufficient for most indications unless there is ongoing consumption (e.g. severe DIC).
- If no consumption, the platelets survive 2–5 days in circulation.

Anticoagulant therapy

Warfarin

- Warfarin overdose (accidental or deliberate self-harm) results in a prolonged PT (and thus INR).
- Risk factors for significant bleeding include poor control, local lesion (e.g. peptic ulcer, angiodysplasia of the colon), high level of anticoagulation (INR >2.5), co-existent haematological abnormality (e.g. thrombocytopenia, myelodysplasia, etc.).

Management

- Moderate warfarin overdose (INR 5–8) without overt bleeding does not usually require specific treatment and patient may be managed as an outpatient. Withhold warfarin until the INR falls to the therapeutic range. Try to identify the cause (incorrect tablets, alcohol binge, etc.).
- Asymptomatic patients with INR >8 are usually given vitamin K as the risk of severe bleeding is high. Withhold warfarin and give 2mg of phytomenadione (IV preparation but absorbed well orally also) if INR <12, or 5mg phytomenadione if INR >12. Repeat INR the next day to confirm reduction. Reintroduce warfarin when INR <5.
- Bleeding in patients on warfarin requires urgent correction of clotting. Prothrombin complex concentrate (purified factors II, VII, IX, and X) is the preferred treatment for life-threatening bleeding. Discuss with haematologists. Also give vitamin K 5–10mg IV (less if only minor bleeding). Identify and treat the local lesion from which the patient is bleeding. FFP (15mL/kg) should only be used if prothrombin complex not available.

Heparin

Risk factors for bleeding include age, recent surgery or trauma, renal or liver failure, malignancy, APTT ratio >3, coexistent haematological abnormality.

Management

- *Stop heparin:* the APTT usually normalizes in 3–4h.
- *Protamine sulphate* (1mg IV neutralizes 100U heparin) may be used; halve the dose if heparin has been turned off 1h previously.
- *LMWHs* are thought to have fewer bleeding complications. However, their plasma half-life is longer and they are less effectively reversed with protamine. Treatment of overdose is as described earlier, but note that the APTT is normal on LMWH.
- *Heparin-associated thrombocytopenia:* see 🕮 p.587.

Bleeding with fibrinolytic therapy

Risk factors for bleeding with fibrinolytic therapy are given on 📖 p.22.
Severe haemorrhage should be managed with:

- ***Supportive measures*** (colloid and blood transfusion).
- ***Cryoprecipitate or fibrinogen concentrate*** transfusion as a source of fibrinogen.
- ***Tranexamic acid*** (0.5–1g slow IV injection, tds) should also be given.

Bleeding in liver disease

The liver is involved in the synthesis of Factors II, VII, IX, and X (the vitamin K-dependent factors), the non-vitamin-K dependent factors (e.g. factor V), as well as the clearance of 'activated' coagulation factors, fibrin molecules, and tPA. The abnormalities most commonly found are:

- ***Obstructive jaundice:*** prolonged PT (vitamin K deficiency)
- ***Acute liver failure:*** prolonged PT and later prolonged APTT and TT (DIC)
- ***Cirrhosis:*** prolonged PT, APTT, and TT; low fibrinogen and/or dysfibrinogenaemia; raised FDPs, ↓ clearance of tPA; low platelets (hypersplenism, DIC ± marrow dysfunction).

Management

Treatment is required for active GI bleeding or as prophylaxis for surgery or liver biopsy.

- Give *vitamin K* 10mg IV slowly (single dose).
- *FFP transfusion* is more effective.
- Consider prothrombin complex concentrate (purified Factors II, VII, IX, and X) for life-threatening bleeding. Contact the haematologists.

Bleeding in uraemia

Uraemia results in both platelet dysfunction (impaired aggregation, adhesion, and activation) and endothelial dysfunction.

Management

- The treatment of choice is haemodialysis.
- Other measures that have been shown to be effective include:
  - Cyroprecipitate infusion
  - Desmopressin (📖 p.592)
  - Conjugated oestrogens
  - Blood transfusion or erythropoietin to raise the haematocrit to >0.25.

Massive transfusion/cardiopulmonary bypass

- Dilutional thrombocytopenia and coagulopathy usually occur once red cell concentrates equivalent to approximately 2 blood volumes have been transfused. With cardiopulmonary bypass, the extracorporeal circuit further damages the native platelets and depletes coagulation factors.
- Abnormalities include ↑PT, ↑APTT, ↑FDPs, ↓fibrinogen.
- Post-transfusion thrombocytopenia is a distinct disorder seen 8–10 days following transfusion and is due to a platelet-specific antibody (see 🕮 p.574).

Management

Treatment should be discussed with the haematology team and involves platelet transfusion to keep platelet count >75 × 10^9/L (or >100 × 10^9/L for CNS lesions/multiple trauma), FFP (4–5U) if PT or APTT >1.5 × control, and cryoprecipitate (10–15U) if fibrinogen <500g/L.

Haemophilia and related disorders 1

Haemophilia A	X-linked recessive deficiency of Factor VIII (↑APTT; ↓Factor VIII activity)
Haemophilia B	X-linked recessive deficiency of Factor IX (↑APTT; ↓Factor IX activity)

Clinical presentation depends upon the degree of factor deficiency:

- Patients with <1% activity have a serious bleeding diathesis. Most are on home therapy.
- Patients with 1–5% activity are moderately affected; spontaneous bleeding is rare but should be treated as severe haemophiliacs when they do.
- Patients with 5–40% factor activity rarely bleed unless there is trauma or surgery.

Acute presentations

- ***Acute haemarthroses*** often occur at sites of previous bleeding, particularly if this has led to degenerative joint disease. Ankles, knees, hips, elbows are the most common sites. Symptoms include local tenderness, warmth, and swelling, and may take days or weeks to resolve.
- ***Intramuscular bleeds*** can cause a compartment-type syndrome, leading to ischaemic necrosis and contracture. Iliopsoas bleed causes entrapment of femoral nerve and produces the triad of groin pain, hip flexion, and sensory loss over femoral nerve distribution. The pain may radiate to the abdomen and mimic appendicitis.
- ***Intracranial bleeding*** is infrequent, but is still a common cause of mortality. It often follows minor head injury. Prognosis of intracerebral haemorrhage is generally poor. Extradural and subdural haemorrhage have a better prognosis.
- ***Bleeding post-trauma:*** classically there may be initial period of haemostasis; bleeding then becomes persistent or intermittent over days/weeks.
- ***Haematuria/ureteric clot colic*** is rare in haemophilia. Usually there is no detectable underlying abnormality of renal tracts.
- ***Problems relating to coexistent HIV or hepatitis B/C infection*** are now the commonest cause of mortality, due to infected Factor VIII administered during the 1980s.

Investigations

Generally, acute investigations are not necessary for simple joint and muscle bleeds in a known haemophiliac. Consider:

- ***USS:*** for muscle haematomas (e.g. iliopsoas bleed)
- ***CT scan:*** history of head trauma, headache, abnormal neurology
- ***Factor VIII levels:*** if bleed is severe and treatment is necessary
- ***Factor VIII inhibitor titre:*** if refractory bleeds/history of inhibitor development.

von Willebrand disease

- Autosomal dominant (Type I with varying expression, Type 2), or recessive (Type 3).
- Reduced levels or abnormal function of vW factor, which normally promotes platelet adhesion and protects factor VIII from destruction (hence ↓factor VIII activity in severe disease).
- Less severe than the haemophilias, with haemarthroses and muscle bleeds being rare. Mucocutaneous bleeding (e.g. epistaxis, prolonged bleeding from cuts, heavy menstrual bleeding) and post-traumatic bleeding are the main problems.

Haemophilia and related disorders 2

Most patients contact their haematologist directly unless they bleed when away from home. Be guided by your local haematologist.

General measures

- ***Rest*** of the affected part and ice packs may be of benefit.
- ***Analgesia:*** avoid IM injections. Oral analgesia (e.g. dihydrocodeine) for minor bleeds; IV injections or infusions of high-dose opiates may be necessary. Use of NSAIDs is controversial.

Moderate or severe haemophiliac

- Treat with IV Factor VIII concentrate.

Mild haemophiliac

- Factor VIII deficiency only: mild or moderate bleeds should be treated with DDAVP. Severe bleeds or those not responding to desmopressin: treat with IV Factor VIII concentrate.
- Factor IX deficiency only: treat with Factor IX.

von Willebrand disease

- ***Mild and moderate bleeds:*** Type I—treat with desmopressin + tranexamic acid. Type 2—usually requires vW factor concentrate (typically an intermediate purity factor VIII preparation).
- ***Severe bleeds:*** treat with vW factor concentrate and for type 3 vW disease consider platelet transfusions.

NB: All CNS and perispinal bleeds are regarded as severe.

Factor VIII replacement

See Table 10.3.

- Minor bleeds may respond to a single, slow, IV bolus of factor VIII.
- Major bleeds: 12-hourly treatments (8-hourly in severe bleeding) with frequent monitoring of Factor VIII levels, pre- and post-treatment.
- Patients with *Factor VIII inhibitors* present a particular problem. This can sometimes be circumvented by the use of other products (e.g. FEIBA or recombinant activated factor VIII).

Factor IX replacement

See Table 10.3.

- Plasma half-life is longer than Factor VIII, and once daily administration is sufficient (twice daily in severe bleeds).
- Avoid overdosage of Factor IX as it is highly thrombogenic.

Desmopressin

- *Indications*: mild–moderate haemophilia A, especially in children, vW disease Type 1 and some Type 2.
- *Dosage*: 0.3mcg/kg in 100ml N saline IV over 30min; may be repeated 8–12h later. Alternatively can be given subcutaneously at the same dose or intranasally (300mcg for an adult). Peak haemostatic effect in 60–90min.

- Monitor pulse and BP closely: side effects include flushing, hypotension, tachycardia, headache, and nausea, rare reports of MI (caution in patients >60 years or with cardiac history). Temporary fluid restriction may be necessary (especially in children) due to ADH effects and risk of hyponatraemia.

Tranexamic acid

- Give with desmopressin in vW disease or mild haemophilia A. Most useful in mucosal bleeds. Avoid in renal tract bleeding (may cause clots).
- Dosage: 1g PO qds (adults). Mouthwash 4.8% q10 min for oral bleeding.

Cryoprecipitate

- Give for severe bleeding in vW disease if vWF concentrate is not available and bleeding not responding to desmopressin and tranexamic acid.
- Dosage: 10–20U (bags) for 70kg adult.

Table 10.3 A rough guide for Factor VIII and IX replacement

Condition	Desired factor level (IU/dL)	Dose of Factor VIII (IU/kg)	Dose of Factor IX (IU/kg)
Mild/moderate bleeds	50	25	65 = BeneFix® 40 = Replenine®
Major/life-threatening bleeds	100	50	130 = BeneFix® 80 = Replenine®

e.g. A 70-kg man with a minor bleed who is known to have haemophilia B and usually receives BeneFix® should receive 65 × 70 = 4550 units (round to the nearest vial = 4500U).

Combined thrombotic and haemorrhagic disorders

A group of disorders in which the pathways of haemostasis become deregulated, leading to microthrombus formation, platelet consumption, and, to a variable extent, clotting factor consumption. The exact pathogenesis varies, but in each case microthrombi cause organ damage, and thrombocytopenia and depleted clotting factors results in bleeding. This coexistence of thrombosis and bleeding makes management very difficult.

Disseminated intravascular coagulation (DIC)

An inappropriate activation of the coagulation pathways leading to:

- Depletion of clotting factors, causing *prolongation of PT and APTT.*
- Widespread thrombin activation, causing *increased TT and reduced fibrinogen.*
- Formation of microthrombi, leading to *end-organ damage.*
- Destruction of RBCs in fibrin mesh, causing *microangiopathic haemolysis.*
- Consumption of platelets; *thrombocytopenia* increasing the bleeding tendency.
- Activation of thrombolysis (*raised FDPs*) and further bleeding.

The 'full house' of abnormalities does not need to be present initially, as the process is a progressive one. For causes see Box 10.3.

Management

- *Treat the underlying cause* (60% have underlying sepsis).
- Supportive measures such as correction of shock, acidosis, and hypoxia may lead to an improvement in the coagulopathy.
- Transfuse blood to correct anaemia. Massive transfusion may exacerbate coagulopathy by dilution of coagulation factors and platelets.

Product replacement

- In acute DIC consider:
    - FFP (15mL/kg, i.e. 4–5U) if PT or APTT >1.5 × control.
    - 1U platelets if platelet count <50 × 10^9/L or <100 × 10^9/L and rapidly falling.
    - Cryoprecipitate (10–15U) or fibrinogen concentrate if fibrinogen <500 g/L.
- Activated protein C concentrate has been used in non-randomized trials for severe sepsis and multiorgan failure with some success, but is not yet widely available.
- Plasma exchange may rarely be considered.

Prognosis

In severe acute DIC overall mortality is high. Obstetric complications have the best prognosis if managed expediently. There is little evidence that measures to prevent thrombosis (heparin, antithrombin III) or prevent thrombolysis improve the general prognosis.

Box 10.3 Causes of DIC

Common

- Gram –ve septicaemia
- *S. aureus* sepsis
- Meningococcal septicaemia
- Malaria (esp. *falciparum*)
- Disseminated malignancy
  - Mucinous adenocarcinomas
  - Prostatic carcinoma
- Liver failure

Rarer

- Incompatible blood transfusion
- Severe trauma/burns
- Acute promyelocytic leukaemia:
  - Obstetric emergencies
  - Abruptio placentae
  - Amniotic fluid embolism
  - Retained dead fetus
  - Severe pre-eclampsia
- Anaphylaxis (e.g. snake bites)
- Hypoxia
- Haemangioma.

Thrombotic thrombocytopenic purpura (TTP) and haemolytic-uraemic syndrome (HUS)

Patients with classic TTP have been found to have an antibody against a metalloproteinase (ADAMTS-13) which cleaves very large multimers of vW factor. These then accumulate and cause microthrombi and thrombocytopenia. The clinical picture tends to vary with age, renal abnormalities being more common in children and neurological problems in adults, but with considerable overlap. In other similar thrombotic microangiopathies and HUS, the 1° event appears to be endothelial damage causing microthrombus formation and end-organ damage. For causes see Box 10.4.

Presentation

- TTP commonly occurs suddenly in a young or middle-aged woman, or following a viral infection
- Fever
- Anaemia (haemolytic picture: associated with jaundice and haemoglobinuria)
- Thrombocytopenia with purpura; significant bleeding is rare
- CNS (confusion, headache, meningitic symptoms, aphasia, visual disturbance, fits, coma, paralysis, psychoses—often fluctuating)
- Renal involvement (oliguria, anuria, haematuria) often mild initially
- HUS is often preceded by gastroenteritis or URTI.

Investigations

• FBC	Anaemia with thrombocytopenia. Moderate leukocytosis with left-shift
• Blood film	Fragmented RBCs, polychromasia, thrombocytopenia
• Clotting	Usually normal
• U&Es	In adults, creatinine sloe to rise over a few days; rapid deterioration more common in children
• LFTs	↑Bili (unconjugated). ↑LDH (from haemolysis)
• Haptoglobins	Decreased
• Urinalysis	Proteinuria frequent; haematuria, haemoglobinuria
• Stool	Culture, especially for *E. coli* strains.

Box 10.4 Associations of TTP and HUS

Recognized
- HIV infection
- SLE
- Normal pregnancy
- Drugs (OCP, ciclosporin)
- Gastroenteritis (esp. with *E coli*, type 0157: H7 in children)

Controversial
- Coxsackie B infection
- *Mycoplasma*
- Malignancies
- Bee stings
- Radiotherapy.

Microangiopathic haemolytic anaemia

Management of HUS and TTP

- Refer to specialist unit (renal and/or haematology).
- While arranging urgent plasma exchange, solvent detergent-treated pooled plasma is currently recommended for TTP in the UK.
- Plasma exchange: aggressive regimen (40mL/kg/day) with FFP results in improvement (and possibly cure) of TTP in many patients. Tail only after remission obtained.
- Steroids used with plasma exchange may be effective.
- Dialysis (haemodialysis or peritoneal dialysis) is used for acute renal failure (usually children).
- Broad-spectrum antibiotics: unproven benefit, but seem sensible given infectious aetiology in some patients.
- Blood transfusion to correct anaemia.
- Platelet transfusion *contraindicated*; exacerbates thrombosis and may worsen the situation.
- Aspirin may be used once platelet count is $>50 \times 10^9$/L.
- Prophylactic LMWH is recommended when platelet count $>50 \times 10^9$/L and solvent detergent-treated pooled plasma product is being used.
- Refractory TTP may respond to high-dose steroids, vincristine, or ciclosporin. Rituximab is increasingly being used.

Prognosis

- Children/predominant HUS picture: 5–30% mortality. Renal impairment and hypertension is common in survivors.
- Adults/predominant TTP picture: 90% mortality if untreated; most die in first few days. With aggressive and early plasma exchange, mortality is now <15%, but relapses are frequent.

Heparin-associated thrombocytopenia

- An idiosyncratic reaction seen in 1–2%. Much less common with LMWHs.
- Type I: mild and transient seen in the first week, often resolving spontaneously with continued therapy.
- Type II: late onset thrombocytopenia seen 5 days to 2 weeks after starting therapy and is caused by an IgG autoantibody that results in platelet activation, and thromboembolic events in 40% if untreated.
- Bleeding is rare at presentation but will be ↑ because of the need for alternative anticoagulant therapy.
- Consider the diagnosis if the problem demanding heparinization does not resolve or worsens while the patient is on heparin (e.g. propagation of DVT) or a new thrombotic event takes place in a heparinized patient, in association with a >50% fall in platelet count.

Management

As for heparin induced thrombocytopenia and thrombosis.

- Stop heparin immediately. Do not wait to see what happens to the platelet count.
- An alternative anticoagulant (e.g. lepirudin or danaparoid) is usually indicated as the risk of thrombosis persists for up to 30 days after stopping heparin.
- LMWHs can have a cross-over effect, and perpetuate the problem.
- Do not start a coumarin (e.g. warfarin) until an alternative anticoagulant has been instated and the platelet count has normalized.
- Do not give platelets to treat thrombocytopenia, as this can lead to further platelet activation and thrombosis.

Acute leukaemias: presentation

Types of acute leukaemia

Acute lymphoblastic leukaemia (ALL)

- In acute leukaemia, the traditional FAB classification is slowly being replaced by the WHO classification which includes cytogenetic data so as to provide more clinical and prognostic information.
- Usually precursor B-cell, occasionally precursor T-cell in origin; also Burkitt's or biphenotype (FAB L1-3).
- Mainly children and young adults.

Acute myeloid leukaemia (AML)

- Traditional FAB classification (M0–M7).
- WHO classification includes AML with characteristic genetic abnormalities, AML with multilineage dysplasia and AML with MDS, therapy-related.
- Mainly adults, including elderly.

Acute leukaemias may occur de novo or may transform from chronic myeloid leukaemia (to 70% AML, 30% ALL). Myelodysplastic syndromes can also evolve into AML.

Poor prognostic factors

- Increasing age
- High white cell count at presentation
- Prior myelodysplastic syndrome
- Philadelphia chromosome positive acute leukaemia (20% in adult ALL, 5% in children)
- Depends upon subclassification of leukaemia on basis of morphology, chromosomal abnormalities, and cell surface markers.

Presentation

Red cell problems

Anaemia: caused by replacement of normal erythropoiesis by leukaemia cells; also by bleeding due to low platelets or deranged clotting. The MCV is usually normal or high, unless blood loss is predominant.

White cell problems

- *High blast count*: may cause 'leucostasis' (crudely, sludging of white cells in small vessels), causing respiratory impairment, myocardial ischaemia/ infarction, renal impairment, acute confusion, stroke, fits, migraine.
- *Leukaemia-related phenomena*: pyrexia, malaise, muscle and joint pains.
- *Neutropenia*: 2° to marrow infiltration by leukaemic cells.

Platelet problems

- *Thrombocytopenia* due to myelosuppression by leukaemic infiltrate.
- Existing platelets may have sub-normal function. Risk of bleeding increases if platelets are $<10 \times 10^9$/L or $<20 \times 10^9$/L if there is concomitant sepsis or coagulation abnormality.

Coagulation problems

Range from a *prolongation of PT to DIC:* may be due to sepsis, or the effects of leukaemia itself, esp. acute promyelocytic leukaemia (M3).

Priorities

1 Stabilize the patient.
2 Treat immediate problems, e.g. bleeding, sepsis.
3 Confirm diagnosis (morphology, cytogenetics, and flow cytometry).
4 Define treatment strategy.

Acute leukaemias: management

Stabilize the patient

- ***Airway*** Stridor may be 2° to mediastinal obstruction in certain cases of leukaemia, mainly T-ALL. If present, call anaesthetist immediately and arrange transfer to ITU.
- ***Breathing*** Breathlessness may be due to infection (including atypical organisms), leucostasis (high WCC), severe anaemia, cardiac failure (leucostasis, severe sepsis), pulmonary haemorrhage. Give O_2: where possible, use pulse oximeter to monitor O_2 saturation, avoiding arterial puncture with thrombocytopenia.
- ***Circulation*** Shock is usually 2° to sepsis, but consider the possibility of blood loss if low platelets/clotting abnormalities, or cardiac failure from leucostasis:
  - Restore circulatory volume.
  - Give broad-spectrum antibiotics immediately (after blood cultures) if sepsis suspected (see 📖 p.610).
- ***Refer to a haematologist urgently***

Treat immediate problems

- ***Infection*** Until the blood film has been reviewed by a haematologist, assume the patient is neutropenic, and treat all infections aggressively (see 📖 p.610).
- ***Bleeding:***
  - Transfuse X-matched blood (CMV-negative blood if available). Caution if high WCCs.
  - If platelets $<20 \times 10^9$/L, give 1U of platelets. If there is active bleeding and platelet count $<50 \times 10^9$/L give platelets.
  - If prothrombin time prolonged ($>1.5 \times$ control), give 4–5U FFP.
  - If fibrinogen <500g/L, consider cryoprecipitate in addition.

Transfusion in the presence of a high WCC is dangerous, and can precipitate the complications of leucostasis.

- ***High WCC*** Discuss with haematologists. May require urgent leucopheresis, preferably in an ITU setting.

Confirmation of diagnosis

- Take a full history, looking for possible aetiological factors. Length of illness (was there a preceding chronic condition, e.g. myelodysplasia?). PMH (?Down syndrome, radiation/chemotherapy exposure). Occupation (?exposure to irradiation, benzenes, other mutagens). Family history (rare familial syndromes, e.g. Fanconi's anaemia).
- Examine the patient, looking for accessory clues to diagnosis (?lymphadenopathy in ALL, hepatosplenomegaly, gum hyperplasia in M5 monocytic leukaemias) and identifying potential sites for infection (dental caries, skin lesions, etc.)
- Final confirmation then rests upon a bone marrow aspirate, with samples being sent for morphology, chromosome analysis, and cell surface markers.

Acute leukaemias: treatment

The treatment of acute leukaemia depends upon the type of leukaemia, and involves several courses of chemotherapy, taking months or even years to complete. The prognosis has improved in recent years and depends upon the exact diagnosis. 80% of children with ALL are now cured whereas only around 30% of adults with AML are cured. The impact of the diagnosis on often young patients and their families is devastating, and extensive time is needed in discussion. Before embarking on chemotherapy, the following must be considered.

Sperm banking

Almost all forms of chemotherapy carry a high incidence of subsequent infertility. When desired by the patient, every attempt must be made to provide for banking of sperm collection prior to starting chemotherapy. Unfortunately in practice the presence of leukaemia itself often makes sperm non-viable, and the need to start treatment precludes repeated collections.

Discussion about side effects

Patients need to be warned about hair loss, sterility, emesis (less of a problem with current antiemetics, but varies with individual), infections, bleeding, mucositis, etc. Patient-orientated literature is available on acute leukaemia and chemotherapy, and may be helpful.

Other considerations

- LP (?CNS involvement). Indicated in:
  - ALL (essential because of high risk of CNS relapse)
  - AML if high WCC at presentation
  - Any neurological symptoms/signs.
- HLA typing of patient/siblings may be considered, with a view to possible bone marrow transplant in the future. This is usually, however, left to a later stage, once the patient has achieved clinical remission. The age limit for sibling allogenic transplants has steadily been pushed up with the ↑ expertise in reduced intensity transplants.
- CMV status should be determined, and CMV-negative products administered to CMV-negative patients throughout their treatment, especially if bone marrow transplantation is an option.

Prior to commencement of chemotherapy

- Commence allopurinol 24h in advance. Rasburicase is used if there is a high risk of tumour lysis syndrome (200mcg/kg IV od for 5–7 days).
- Prescribe regular antiseptic mouthwashes, to be used 4–5 ×/day in conjunction with antithrush prophylaxis (nystatin suspension, amphotericin lozenges, or oral fluconazole).
- Ensure adequate hydration aiming for 3L/day input.
- Give an antiemetic before chemotherapy, and at regular intervals during treatment with chemotherapy. Appropriate regimens include:
  - ondansetron 4–8mg IV/PO bd
  - metoclopramide 10–20mg IV/PO plus dexamethasone 2–4mg IV/PO 4–8-hourly.

Early complications of bone marrow transplantation (BMT)

Always contact and refer the patient back to their BMT centre.

The morbidity and mortality following BMT (especially allogeneic BMT) is high, particularly within the first 100 days. The patients are very reliant on close medical and nursing surveillance to ensure that they do not perish from preventable/treatable causes. Patients may occasionally present outside of their transplant unit overnight or at weekends. They will be vulnerable to all kinds of infections: bacterial, viral, fungal, and protozoal. Even if the neutrophil count as normal, treat the patients as being neutropenic, and they will have poorly functioning lymphocytes and low antibody production. This section is a guide to some of the problems encountered.

Acute graft-versus-host disease

This causes skin rashes either localized (e.g. to palms) or widespread. The rash is typically non-itchy. There may be upper or lower GI symptoms (severe watery diarrhoea) and liver dysfunction (deranged LFTs). Mild GVHD of 1 site may be acceptable but consider early treatment (usually high-dose methylprednisolone) for widespread GVHD or diarrhoea. Always discuss with the transplant centre.

Fever

See 📖 p.610.

Upper GI symptoms (mucositis, vomiting)

Symptomatic management including adequate analgesia (e.g. opiates) and H2-antagonists or PPIs. Search for an infectious cause (mouthwash and swabs for HSV and Candida). Antiemetics usually required: lorazepam 1–2mg q8–12h; metoclopramide 10–20mg q6–8h; or ondansetron 4–8mg q12h.

Diarrhoea

Rehydrate. Monitor strict fluid balance. Stool culture (green watery diarrhoea suggests GVHD). May require early biopsy and steroids if large volume diarrhoea. Discuss with transplant centre.

Abnormal LFTs (drugs, GVHD, veno-occlusive disease)

Supportive measures: monitor fluid balance, coagulation tests, renal function; adjust drug doses accordingly. Search for an infectious aetiology. Veno-occlusive disease presents as hepatomegaly, jaundice, and weight gain. Liver ultrasound with doppler of the hepatic and portal veins (reversed hepatic-portal flow seen in veno-occlusive disease). Discuss with the transplant centre.

Interstitial shadowing on CXR

These may be diffuse or localized and associated with varying degrees of fever, breathlessness, and hypoxia.

Causes

Pulmonary oedema (fluid overload, cardiac failure due to chemo/radiotherapy, non-cardiac (ARDS)—related to sepsis or drug toxicity); infection (bacterial, viral (esp. CMV), fungal, Pneumocystis); thromboembolic; GVHD; pulmonary haemorrhage; idiopathic.

Management

Supportive treatment: O_2, diuretics (if pulmonary oedema) and ventilatory support. CXR changes often minor if neutropenic and so consider high-resolution CT early. Cover for infectious causes with broad-spectrum antibiotics, antifungal agents, or occasionally antiviral agents (if viral RTI is suspected). PCP is unusual if the patient is on co-trimoxazole prophylaxis. Consider bronchoscopy.

Early complications of BMT

- Skin rash
- GI complications
  - Nausea and vomiting
  - Mucositis
  - Diarrhoea
- Abnormal LFTs
- Haemorrhagic cystitis
- Interstitial shadowing on CXR
- Cardiovascular complications
  - Cardiac failure
  - Hypertension
  - Endocarditis
- Deteriorating renal function
- CNS complications.

Complications of BMT

Cardiac failure

- Cardiac toxicity may be 2° to high-dose cyclophosphamide, total body irradiation, and/or previous anthracycline exposure.
- Transient ST- and T-wave abnormalities and LV dysfunction on Echo are seen in up to 30% following conditioning prior to BMT.
- Overt cardiac failure may be seen with repeated high-dose steroid therapy that is required for episodes of GVHD.

Management

Standard therapy with diuretics and ACEI.

Hypertension

Very common in the early days post BMT and due to ciclosporin therapy ± renal impairment.

Treatment

Calcium antagonists (e.g. nifedipine SR, 10–20mg PO bd).

Deteriorating renal function

Causes

- Drug therapy (ciclosporin A, amphotericin, aminoglycosides, chemotherapy, aciclovir, allopurinol).
- Pre-renal (dehydration, shock, bleeding).
- Tumour lysis syndrome (see 🕮 p.617).
- TTP (see 🕮 p.598).

Haemorrhagic cystitis

Frequency, dysuria, and haematuria; commonly related to cyclophosphamide (caused by acreolin, a metabolite), but also seen with anthracyclines, cytosine arabinoside, etoposide, adenovirus, and BK virus infection. Prevent with mesna (see data sheet for dose).

Management

Supportive therapy with blood and platelet transfusion and hydration is usually sufficient. Discuss with urologists if severe as more specialist intervention such as bladder irrigation may be required.

CNS complications

Symptoms

May include seizures, drowsiness/confusion, focal neurological signs, stroke.

Causes

- Metabolic (↓Mg^{2+}, ↓Ca^{2+}, hypoxia, liver failure, renal failure)
- Infection: bacterial, viral (e.g. HSV), fungal (esp. *Aspergillus), Toxoplasma, Cryptococcus*
- Drug toxicity. Ciclosporin can cause tremor, confusion, and seizures
- Intracranial haemorrhage
- Cerebral infarction (embolic)
- Relapse of disease

- TTP (see 📖 p.598)
- Steroid psychosis.

Investigations

FBC and film, LDH, CT scan, LP (after correcting clotting and platelets), blood cultures, serology, Mg^{2+} and Ca^{2+} levels, Echo.

Management

Specific therapy for underlying cause.

The febrile neutropenic patient 1

- Neutropenia (in this context) may be defined as a total neutrophil count of <1 × 109/L, regardless of total WCC.
- Significant infections are usually associated with a fever; and a 'spike' to 38°C is regarded as warranting action. Severely ill patients and those on steroids may not, be able to mount a fever; signs such as tachycardia or hypotension should be considered serious.
- The site of infection is not usually obvious; potential sites include chest, Hickman, or other central line (or inflammation around exit site of line), mouth, perianal area/perineum, urine, or skin.

Organisms

Common

- Gram-positive (60%):
  - Coagulase I –ve staphylococci—*S. epidermidis*
  - Streptococci—viridans streptococci
- Gram-negative (30%):
  - *Escherichia coli*
  - *Klebsiella* spp.
  - *Pseudomonas aeruginosa*

Other (10%)

- *Staphlococcus aureus*
- *Corynebacterium jekium*
- *Acinetobacter* spp.
- Mixed infections
- Anaerobes
- Fungal infections :
  - *Candida* spp.
  - *Aspergillus fumigatus*
- Viral infections (VZV, CMV):
  - *Pneumocystis jirovecii*

- A microbiological diagnosis is reached in only ~40%.
- Coagulase –ve staphylococci: Hickman or other IV lines.
- Viridans streptococci: mucositis ± previous exposure to quinolones.
- Fungal infections: occur after prolonged and profound neutropenia, previous antibiotic therapy, underlying lung disease (pulmonary aspergillosis), stem cell transplantation or prolonged immunosuppression.

Basic microbiological investigations

- ***Blood cultures*** taken from Hickman line and by venepuncture. This allows line infections to be differentiated from bacteraemias.
- ***Culture of urine and faeces*** including stool for *C. difficile*. C. diff toxin.
- ***Cultures from other suspected sites***, e.g. line exit sites, sputum, skin lesions, throat.
- ***Viral serology***: less useful, as a rising titre is often necessary to diagnose infection. Viral detection (e.g. viral PCR-CMV, respiratory viruses such as RSV, influenza and parainfluenza), where possible, may be more helpful in an acute situation.
- ***Line tips***: rush to laboratory. Do not allow to dry out on ward bench or insert into throat swab medium.

Important points

- *Antibiotic therapy should never be delayed to await further assessment of clinical progress, or lab results.*
- Neutropenic patients may not show a localized response to infection. The most common presentation is that of a fever of unknown origin.

- A pyrexia lasting >48h, despite IV antibiotics, usually requires some alteration to the antimicrobial regimen. Consider fungal infection.
- ***Platelet requirements increase with sepsis:*** neutropenic patients are commonly also thrombocytopenic: keep platelet count above 20×10^9/L.
- Thrombocytopenia also demands care with invasive procedures. Central lines and urinary catheters should be inserted with platelet cover, and *arterial puncture is best avoided* (use pulse oximetry).

The febrile neutropenic patient 2

Immediate management

Given the caveats on 📖 p.610, the stabilization of a septic neutropenic patient is similar to that of any other septic patient.

- O_2, IV colloid, crystalloid, and inotropes should be administered as is appropriate to the patient's clinical condition.
- CVP readings may be taken from existing central lines to assess the patient's hydration status, but, with Hickman lines in particular, the readings are frequently not accurate, and should be interpreted in the context of the clinical assessment.

Antimicrobial regimen

When in doubt, take microbiological advice; use hospital policy. Regimens for empirical therapy are based on broad-spectrum, bactericidal antibiotics. Monotherapy is hardly ever appropriate, even when an organism has been isolated: the patient may well have more than one infection. A typical policy is shown in Box 10.5. See Box 10.6 for causes of failure to respond to empirical antibiotics.

Box 10.5 Empirical antibiotic therapy for febrile neutropenia

First line	• Tazocin® 4.5g IV tds (or meropenem 500mg IV qds if penicillin allergic) *plus* • Gentamicin 7mg/kg IV od (guided by levels)
Second line	• Vancomycin 1g IV bd (guided by levels) *or* • Teicoplanin 400mg IV od (bd for first 24h) if line infection is suspected
Third line	Consider amphotericin if fever not settling after 72h esp. in patients with long periods of neutropenia (e.g. AML or BMT patients). Discuss with local haematologists and microbiologists

Notes

- Doses of *vancomycin and gentamicin* will need to be adjusted according to serum levels.
- Add *metronidazole* 500mg IV q8h to first- or second-line regimens if fever persists and anaerobic infection possible (mucositis).
- Add *amphotericin*: most units use the lipid formulations Abelcet® or Ambisome® for proven (or possible) fungal infection. Variconazole is used first line if *Aspergillus* is likely. Caspofungin for *Candida*.
- The *change from first- to second-line therapy* should be considered under the following circumstances:
  - Persistent pyrexia >48h (or less if the patient's condition markedly deteriorates)
  - A new spike of temperature once the fever has settled on first-line antibiotics (suggesting emergence of another, resistant organism)
  - Rising CRP in the face of apparently appropriate antibiotics.

- Choice of *third-line antibiotics* is often more arbitrary, and combinations should again be discussed with the microbiologists. Duration of neutropenia is an important factor, as fungal infections become more likely the longer the period of neutropenia.

Particular situations

- *Infections of the mouth, perianal area, or elsewhere in the GI tract:* consider adding *metronidazole*.
- *Suspected line infections*: ensure good Gram-positive cover (*vancomycin or teicoplanin*).
- *Diarrhoea after prolonged antibiotic therapy:* suspect *C. difficile*; consider empirical oral *vancomycin* or *metronidazole* while awaiting stool toxin detection/culture results.
- Orophyrangeal mucositis due to *reactivation of herpes simplex virus* is common. It is effectively treated with *aciclovir*; the main complication is bacterial super infection.
- *Pyrexias associated with a normal CRP* virtually exclude bacterial or fungal infection as a cause of the fever.
- *Deteriorating renal function*: avoid nephrotoxic agents, particularly in combination (e.g. vancomycin, liposomal formulation of amphotericin, gentamicin).
- *Systemic candidiasis* may be manifest only as fever unresponsive to antibiotics: blood cultures are rarely positive; signs of local invasion, (e.g. endophthalmitis) are seen in a minority. Have a high index of suspicion and treat aggressively with amphotericin or fluconazole.
- *Invasive aspergillosis* presents as fever, abnormal CXR and dyspnoea, or sinusitis (invasive disease of sinuses). There is extensive local tissue destruction with cavitating lung lesions or bone destruction of sinuses. HRCT of lungs should be done urgently. Treat aggressively with IV liposomal amphotericin or voriconazole.
- *GCSF* may shorten a period of neutropenia and may be used for certain patients. Discuss with the haematologists.

When selecting an antimicrobial regimen, it is worthwhile reviewing all recent microbiology results, including skin swabs (axilla, groin, perineal). Review past microbiology for resistant organisms that may need to be covered (e.g. MRSA, VRE, resistant *Pseudomonas*, *E. coli* or *Klebsiella*).

Box 10.6 Causes of failure to respond to empirical antibiotics

- Wrong microbiological diagnosis. Consider infection with fungi, viruses, protozoa, mycobacteria.
- Line-associated fever.
- GVHD (also possible with liver transplantation).
- Drug fever.
- Inadequate antibiotic doses.
- Underlying disease (e.g. relapse).

Infections in the transplant patient

Infectious diseases are a major cause of mortality and morbidity following both solid organ and bone marrow transplantation, related to the immunosuppression (and in the case of BMT, the innate immuno-incompetence in the neutropenic and early engraftment phases).

Different pathogens are typically implicated in infections depending on the degree of immunocompetence of the patient:

- The neutropenic patient (see 📖 p.610)
- The non-neutropenic transplant patient.

Cell-mediated immunity may be impaired for several months after bone marrow (and solid organ) transplantation. This predisposes to viral (CMV, HSV, adenovirus) and protozoal (*Pneumocystis jirovecii*, toxoplasmosis) infections.

- ***Cytomegalovirus infections:*** *see* 📖 p.615.
- *Suspected* **Pneumocystis pneumonia:** treat with *high-dose co-trimoxazole*; (0.96–1.44g q12h IV); consider urgent bronchoscopy/BAL if patient fit enough.
- ***Toxoplasmosis:*** usually due to reactivation of latent infection. Presents as intracranial space-occupying lesion, meningoencephalitis, or diffuse encephalopathy. Seizures and focal neurological signs are common. Treatment is with *pyrimethamine and sulphonamides*.
- ***Other viral infections:***
  - *HSV* commonly produces localized infection and dissemination is rare but recognized to produce encephalitis and pneumonia: Treat with *high-dose aciclovir* IV.
  - *VZV* reactivation is frequently seen and most infections are mild; encephalitis and pneumonitis are usually fatal. Treat with *high-dose aciclovir* (10mg/kg IV q8h). Disseminated VZV can present as central abdominal pain with little or no obvious rash.
  - *Adenovirus* infection produces an interstitial pneumonitis similar to CMV and may disseminate.

Cytomegalovirus (CMV) infections in transplant patients

- Also see 📖 Table 8.2, p.492.
- May be acquired from the reactivation of previous CMV infection in recipient, due to immunosuppression.
- May be acquired from the bone marrow from a CMV-positive donor or CMV-positive blood products. (*All BMT recipients should receive CMV-negative blood products if they are CMV IgG negative prior to BMT.* CMV IgG-positive recipients can receive unscreened blood product).
- Occur more commonly in allogenic and unrelated donor transplants, due to the greater immunosuppression.

Presentation of acute CMV infections

- Fever of unknown origin.
- Positive CMV-PCR or antigenaemia (detected by routine CMV-antigen testing, blood, and urine).
- Graft failure/myelosuppression (anaemia, thrombocytopenia, leucopoenia).
- Interstitial pneumonitis: deteriorating O_2 saturation, with widespread bilateral interstitial opacities on CXR.
- Enteritis (oesophagitis, gastritis, colitis): pyrexia, diarrhoea.
- Hepatitis.
- Retinitis

Immediate management

- Ensure adequate respiration; consult anaesthetists and consider CPAP/ventilation early if O_2 requirements are increasing, or the patient is becoming exhausted.
- Inform haematologist responsible for patient's care.
- Take blood for CMV-PCR or antigen, culture, and antibody testing.
- Send urine sample for CMV antigen.
- If CMV is strongly suspected, commence ganciclovir treatment immediately. Otherwise, consider:
  - Bronchoscopy/BAL if pulmonary infiltrate (send washings for CMV antigen)
  - Upper GI endoscopy and biopsy.

Treatment

- *Ganciclovir* should be commenced at 2.5mg/kg IV tds.
- Side effects of ganciclovir include nephrotoxicity, and myelosuppression/graft failure, which may be difficult to distinguish from the effects of CMV itself.

Hyperviscosity syndrome

Causes

Increased cellularity

- Polycythaemia (1° or 2°)
  - Haematocrit. 50–60%
- Leucocytosis (acute leukaemias)
  - WCC >50–100 × 10^9/L.

Raised plasma proteins

- Waldenstrom's macroglobulinaemia
  - IgM paraprotein level >30g/L
- Myeloma usually IgA subtype
  - Paraprotein level >80g/L.

Presentation

Most patients develop symptoms when serum viscosity reached 5–6 centipoises (normal <1.8).

General features

- Muscle weakness
- Lethargy, headache
- Mental confusion, proceeding to coma
- Visual disturbance
- Congestive cardiac failure
- Fundoscopy:
  - Engorgement and sludging in the veins
  - Haemorrhage, exudates
  - Papilloedema.

Specific features

The predominant symptoms vary with the underlying cause.

- *Raised paraprotein:*
  - Bleeding/purpura: platelet dysfunction and factor deficiency
  - Neuropathies
  - Renal impairment
  - Cardiac conduction abnormalities.
- *Leucostasis:*
  - Myocardial ischaemia/infarction
  - Pulmonary infiltrates.
- *Polycythaemia:*
  - Peripheral ischaemia
  - Transient ischaemic attacks/strokes
  - Myocardial infarction.

Management

Arrange urgent intervention (same day) depending on cause.

- ***Polycythaemia:***
  - Venesect 1–2U
  - Replace with N saline
- ***Leukaemia:*** leucopheresis or chemotherapy
- ***High paraprotein:*** plasmapheresis.

Tumour lysis syndrome

A syndrome of metabolic abnormalities and renal impairment that can occur within hours or days of commencing chemotherapy, due to rapid lysis of tumour cells. It is most likely to occur with bulky, highly chemosensitive lymphoproliferative disease (e.g. T-ALL and Burkitt's lymphoma). Seen less commonly in other lymphomas, high blast-count leukaemias, and some germ-cell tumours.

Features

- Hyperuricaemia ± urate nephropathy and oliguric renal failure.
- Hyperkalaemia (K^+ 6 mmol/L or 25% increase from baseline) especially with progressive renal impairment.
- Hyperphosphataemia.
- Hypocalcaemia (<1.75mmol/L) and hypomagnesaemia (due to rising phosphate).
- Cardiac arrhythmias (2° to ↑K^+, ↓Ca^{2+}, and ↓Mg^{2+}).
- Weakness, twitching, tetany (hypocalcaemia).
- Severe metabolic acidosis (renal failure).

Prevention

- Start *allopurinol* 300mg od (or bd) 48h prior to chemotherapy if renal function is normal.
- Rasburicase should be considered for high-risk patients such as Burkitt's, high WCC ALL and patients with LDH > 2× normal. Standard dose is 0.2mg/kg IV od for 5–7 days. A starting dose of 3mg is often effective.
- *Hyperhydrate*: vigorous hydration is important and a fluid load of 3L/m^2/day should be given to those patients who can tolerate it. A urinary catheter should be used to monitor output. *Leucopherese* if high peripheral blast count.
- Continue IV fluids during therapy, giving furosemide to maintain diuresis (> 100mL/m^2/h).
- Urine alkalinization (with sodium bicarbonate to keep urinary pH >7.0) helps promote urate excretion but this is difficult to achieve in practice.

Management

- Emergency treatment of hyperkalemia.
- Exclude bilateral ureteric obstruction by ultrasound.
- Alkalinize the urine (📖 p.728) if hyperuricaemia is present. Stop as soon as urate levels normal.
- Avoid calcium supplements except if there is neuromuscular irritability.
- Monitor U&Es, PO_4^{3-}, Ca^{2+}, and urate at least twice daily for the first few days of treatment.
- Strict fluid balance measurements, with urinary catheter if necessary.
- Indications for haemodialysis/intensive care:
  - Rising K^+, creatinine, or PO_4 in spite of measures discussed earlier
  - Metabolic acidosis
  - Fluid overload or oliguria in spite of diuretics.

Hypercalcaemia of malignancy

See 📖 p.544.

- Urgent intervention required if Ca^{2+} >3mmol/L
- NB: true Ca^{2+} = measured Ca^{2+} + [(40 − albumin) × 0.02].

Causes

- Bony metastases: probable local cytokine effect
- Myeloma: secretion of an osteoclast-activating factor
- Secretion of PTH-related peptide (non-small-cell lung cancer).

Presentation

Nausea, vomiting, drowsiness, confusion, nocturia, polyuria, bone and abdominal pains, constipation.

Management

- Hydration: 3–6L over 24h, continuing for 4–5 days. In the past, loop diuretics (e.g. furosemide) were given routinely once fluid repletion had been achieved to further increase urinary calcium excretion. This has fallen out of favour due to the availability of drugs such as the bisphosphonates and the potential fluid and electrolyte complications resulting from excessive diuresis such as hypokalaemia, hypomagnesaemia, and even volume depletion if the diuretic-induced losses are not replaced. However, patients who are unable to excrete the administered salt because of renal insufficiency are at risk of fluid overload and should receive furosemide.
- Following overnight hydration recheck $Ca^{2+}$and albumin. If symptoms persist, and/or Ca^{2+} remains >3mmol/L, give pamidronate disodium IV. A maximum of 90mg over 4h. It can be given as an infusion of 60mg/h. Suspected or established renal failure maximum rate 20mg/h. Pamidronate is well tolerated; however there is a small incidence of transient fever and flu-like symptoms.
- For myeloma, consider prednisolone 30–60mg PO daily.

Superior vena cava obstruction

Presentation

Awareness of fullness of head and tightness of collar, symptoms exacerbated by bending down, syncope, breathlessness, facial suffusion and oedema, engorgement of veins in neck, arms, and upper thorax.

Causes

- Usually bronchogenic carcinoma (± 2° thrombosis of SVC)
- Other tumours, including lymphoma, more rarely.

Management

- FBC and film, U&Es, Ca^{2+}, albumin
- CXR, Doppler USS of neck veins if diagnosis uncertain
- Heparin, providing platelet count and clotting function are normal
- Arrange urgent radiotherapy (within 24h).

Massive mediastinal mass

Presentation

Dry cough, stridor and dyspnoea, especially on lying flat.

Causes

- ALL (especially T-ALL with high WCC)
- High-grade non-Hodgkin's lymphoma
- Hodgkin's disease
- Germ cell tumour.

Management

Histological diagnosis (or cytological from pleural effusion if present):

- General anaesthetic carries considerable risk
- Definitive treatment (radiotherapy or chemotherapy)
- Consider prednisolone 1mg/kg/day if urgent treatment is required.

Chapter 11

Rheumatological emergencies

Acute monoarthritis: presentation

An acute monoarthritis should always be treated as septic arthritis until proved otherwise. Failure to treat septic arthritis is a medical disaster. 50% of cartilage proteoglycan is lost within 48h; bone loss is evident within 7 days; mortality of *S. aureus* arthritis is 10%.

Presentation

- Hot, swollen red joint
- Joint line tenderness
- Restricted range of movement
- Systemic features of fever and malaise.

Assessment

Look for any risk factors for infection

- Diabetes mellitus
- Immunodeficiency state (monoarthritis is rare in AIDS)
- Underlying structural joint disease (e.g. rheumatoid arthritis or other deforming arthropathy, prosthesis)
- Sexual impropriety, IV drug abuse (predisposes to sacroileitis and acromioclavicular joint infection)
- TB needs to be considered in at-risk populations.

Ask for risk factors for gout

- Alcohol
- High-purine diet (protein, e.g. meat)
- Drugs (e.g. thiazides, furosemide, ethambutol)
- High cell turnover states (e.g. lymphoma, polycythaemia, psoriasis).

Examine for evidence for multi-system disease

- Rash
- Ocular involvement
- Oro-genital ulceration
- GI symptoms
- Renal involvement
- Pulmonary manifestations.

Conditions that mimic monoarthritis

- Bone pain or fracture close to a joint
- Tendinitis (especially at the wrist)
- Bursitis (commonly olecranon or pre-patellar bursae; no joint line tenderness)
- Neuropathic pain
- Soft tissue pain.

Box 11.1 Differential diagnosis of a monoarthritis

Traumatic

- Traumatic synovitis
- Haemarthroses
  - Fracture
  - Haemophilia
  - Ruptured anterior cruciate ligament.

Non-traumatic

Infective

- *Staphylococcus aureus*
- *Neisseria gonococcus*
- *Staphylococcus albus*
- Streptococcal
- Gram-negative rods.

Crystals

- Uric acid (gout)
- Calcium pyrophosphate (pseudogout)
- Hydroxyapatite— usually a monoarthritis (shoulder) in elderly patients.

Monoarticular presentation of

- Rheumatoid arthritis
- Seronegative arthritis (e.g. reactive (Reiter's), psoriasis)
- SLE.

Miscellaneous

- Pigmented villonodular synovitis
- 2° deposits
- Osteosarcoma.

Practice point

Always assume an unexplained monoarthritis is due to sepsis until proved otherwise.

Acute monoarthritis: investigations

Synovial fluid analysis

Aspirate the joint to dryness (see 📖 p.802) and send fluid for:

- *WBC* Fluid may be placed in EDTA tube.
- *Microbiology* Fluid into sterile container and a sample into blood culture bottles and for AFBs.
- *Polarized microscopy* For crystals; fluid into sterile container.

Take blood for

- *Blood cultures*
- *FBC* WBC high in infection and crystal arthritis.
- *CRP/ESR* Elevated with an inflammatory arthritis. Elevated ESR and normal CRP suggest SLE.
- *U&Es, LFTs* May be impaired with sepsis.
- *Glucose* ?Diabetic.
- *Uric acid* ?Gout.
- *Clotting* Bleeding diathesis causing haemarthrosis.
- *Immunology* RF, ANA, anti-dsDNA, complement levels (?RA or SLE).

XR the joint

- Chondrocalcinosis suggests pseudogout. But *not* helpful in the early diagnosis of a septic arthritis as the appearance may be unchanged for up to 2 weeks in infection.

Sepsis screen

- Cervical, rectal, and throat swabs.

Aspirate any cutaneous pustules for Gram stain in patients with suspected gonococcal infection.

Box 11.2 Indications for synovial fluid aspiration in casualty

- Suspected septic arthritis
- Suspected crystal arthritis
- Suspected haemarthrosis
- Relief of symptoms by removal of effusion in degenerative arthritis.

Box 11.3 Contraindications to joint aspiration

- Overlying sepsis
- Bleeding diathesis.

Septic arthritis

The commonest pathogen in the UK is *Staphylococcus aureus* (70%). *Neisseria gonorrhoea* is a common cause in the young sexually active population. Other important causes include *Streptococcus*. *Haemophilus influenzae* should be considered in children.

Management

- Admit and inform orthopaedic team.
- Aspirate the joint to dryness (see Boxes 11.2 and 11.3 for indications and contraindications for aspiration). Prosthetic joints should be aspirated by the orthopaedic team—liaise with them and consider early arthroscopy to facilitate effective joint washout especially if inflammatory markers are slow to fall.
- Strict rest for the joint (bed rest); no weight bearing on infected joints.
- Analgesics (NSAIDs). Consider adding a PPI if history of dyspepsia.

Antibiotics

- Initially IV for 2 weeks, then oral for a further 4 weeks.
- Emperically start with flucloxacillin 1g q6h and benzyl penicillin 1.2g q4h. For penicillin allergy use vancomycin and clindamycin. In young children use cefotaxime to cover *H. influenzae*.
- (NB: aminoglycosides are not effective in the acid pH of an infected joint; erythromycin penetrates the synovial fluid poorly.)
- Review antibiotics when microbiology available.
- For gonococcal arthritis, treat with IV benzylpenicillin 1.2g q4h for 7 days and then PO amoxicillin 500mg tds for 10 days. Remember to trace and treat contacts (liaise with GU medicine team).

Box 11.4 Management key points: septic arthritis

- Analgesics.
- Aspirate the joint to dryness.
- Antibiotics (initial empirical treatment): IV flucloxacillin (1g qds) and benzyl penicillin (1.2g q4h). For penicillin allergy use vancomycin and clindamycin.
- Review antibiotics when microbiology available.
- Liaise with the orthopaedic team.
- Strict rest and no weight bearing on the affected joint.

Crystal arthropathy

Management

- May usually be managed as an outpatient (Box 11.5).
- Bed rest.
- Analgesics. *NSAIDs*, e.g. diclofenac SR 75 mg bd or indometacin (150mg in 2 to 3 divided doses). Use cautiously in the elderly, patients with peptic ulceration, or patients with cardiac failure, renal, or liver disease.
- *Colchicine* is a good alternative if NSAIDs are contraindicated. Give 1mg initially followed by 0.5mg no more frequently than every 4h until pain relieved or vomiting or diarrhoea occur. Maximum 6mg per course; Course not to be repeated within 3 days.
- Rheumatology consultation if symptoms fail to settle; *Intra-articular steroid* injections may be given in patients who can't take NSAIDS or colchicine (e.g. those with renal failure) and only have 1 or 2 actively inflamed joints. The diagnosis of acute gout should be confirmed and septic arthritis must be excluded before giving steroids.
- *Systemic steroids* may be given in patients who cannot take NSAIDs or colchicine and in whom intra-articular steroid injection is not an option because of polyarticular disease. Oral prednisolone (20–40 mg per day) may be given for 1–2 days and then tapered over 7–10 days. Rebound attacks may occur when steroids are withdrawn. In patients who cannot receive oral medications, SC ACTH may be used.
- Both allopurinol and probenecid are contraindicated during acute gout as both may prolong symptoms. However, once treatment with an antihyperuricaemic drug (allopurinol or probenecid) has been started, it should not be interrupted during an acute attack.
- They may be started for prophylaxis when the acute attack has settled if the patient has had >3 attacks of acute gout in 1 year, if tophi are present, or serum uric acid levels are high. Initiation of these drugs should be accompanied by either a NSAID or colchicine (0.5mg bd or tds) for the first 2–4 weeks.

Box 11.5 Management key points: acute gouty arthritis

- May be managed as an outpatient.
- Bed rest.
- Analgesics: NSAIDs, e.g. diclofenac or indometacin (150mg in 2 or 3 divided doses.)
- Colchicine if NSAIDs are contraindicated. (1mg initially followed by 0.5mg no more frequently than every 4h until pain relieved or vomiting or diarrhoea occur; Maximum 6mg per course.)
- If symptoms fail to settle: intra-articular steroids may be given when only 1 or 2 joints are affected. (Septic arthritis must be excluded first.)
- Oral prednisolone may be given in patients who cannot take NSAIDs or colchicine and have polyarticular disease (30–50mg/day for 1–2 days and then tapered over 7–10 days). Septic arthritis must be excluded first.

Polyarthritis

Presentation

- Pain
- Stiffness (esp. early morning)
- Loss of function
- Joint inflammation.

Differential diagnosis

- Rheumatoid arthritis
- Seronegative arthritis:
  - Psoriatic arthropathy
  - Reactive arthritis
  - Ankylosing spondylitis
  - Enteropathic arthritis
- Systemic lupus erythematosus
- Crystal arthropathy:
  - Chondrocalcinosis
  - Gout
- Infections:
  - Viral
  - Bacterial.

Miscellaneous

- Sarcoid: associated with erythema nodosum (20%), and a transient RA like polyarthritis or acute monoarthritis.
- Behçet's syndrome: polyarthritis (± erythema nodosum) with painful orogenital ulceration and iritis.
- Familial Mediterranean fever: occurs in Middle Eastern individuals with recurrent attacks of fever, arthritis (usually monoarticular), abdominal or chest pain (pleurisy).
- Transient polyarthritis may be associated with SLE, bacterial endocarditis (see 🕮 p.96), para-infectious, Reiter's, reactive arthritis, and Henoch–Schönlein purpura.

Investigations

- Aspirate a large affected joint and analyse synovial fluid (see 🕮 p.802
- Blood cultures if appropriate
- FBC with differential count
- CRP and/or ESR
- Biochemical profile (U&Es, LFTs, urate) and glucose
- Bone profile (looking for hyperparathyroidism)
- Rheumatoid factor, ANA, anti-dsDNA (RA and SLE)
- Anti-CCP antibodies (a marker for erosive arthritis)
- Complement levels
- Viral serology
- XRs (may show chondrocalcinosis typically knees and wrists, or early changes of rheumatoid arthritis with periarticular osteoporosis).

Management

General measures

- Bed rest: rest for the affected joints.
- NSAIDs, e.g. indometacin 50mg tds (or diclofenac 75mg bd) adjusting dose according to symptoms and response (caution in elderly patients, patients with dyspepsia, asthmatics, and patients on anticoagulants).
- IM methylprednisolone (80–120mg) will settle most acute flares of RA/inflammatory arthritis. Exclude infection first.
- Consider specific treatment of underlying condition.
- Consider the need for physiotherapy and exercise regimens to reduce long-term disability.

Box 11.6 Disease Associations of Autoantibodies

Antibody	*Association*
Rheumatoid factor inflammatory	Rheumatoid arthritis and many disorders
ANA	SLE and many autoimmune disorders
Anti-dsDNA	SLE
ENA	Extractable nuclear antigen consists of • RNP • Ro (SSA) • La (SSB) • Anti-am • Anti-centromere • SCL-70 • Jo-1 • Anti-cardiolipin
RNP	MCTD SLE
Ro (SSA)	Primary Sjögrens, SLE
La (SSB)	Primary Sjögrens
Anti-sm	SLE, chronic active hepatitis
Anti-centromere	Limited systemic sclerosis
SCL-70	Systemic sclerosis (diffuse)
Jo-1	Polymyositis
Anti-cardiolipin	SLE, antiphospholipid syndrome

Rheumatoid arthritis

Clinical features

- Typically young women (♀:♂, 3:1).
- Symmetrical polyarthritis involving the small joints of the hands and feet.
- May present as a relapsing or persistent monoarthritis.
- All synovial joints are involved. Signs most common in hands, feet, knees but remember synovial joints of spine (and atlantoaxial joint/ligaments) and larynx (aryetenoid joints).
- Extra-articular manifestations: vasculitis, subcutaneous nodules, lymphadenopathy, peripheral neuropathy, anaemia (normochromic normocytic, Fe deficiency, drug-induced aplasia, haemolytic), ocular involvement, pleurisy, pericarditis, pulmonary fibrosis.

Management

- General measures as before (📖 p.628).
- Early steroids reduce long-term joint destruction.
- Symptomatic treatment with NSAIDs.
- Early use of disease-modifying antirheumatic drugs (DMARDs) reduces long-term joint damage. Most commonly methotrexate, but others such as hydroxychloroquine, sulfasalazine, leflunomide, gold, penicillamine, azathioprine, and ciclosporine may be used.
- Biological therapies are increasingly used, e.g. anti-cytokine therapies such as the tumour necrosis factor alpha (TNF-alpha) blockers (etanercept and infliximab), B-cell depletion, and IL-6 blockade.

Seronegative arthritides (spondyloarthropathies)

Psoriatic arthropathy

Clinical features

- May present as an asymmetrical large- or small-joint oligoarthritis, symmetrical polyarthritis, or clinical picture similar to Rheumotoid arthritis (RA) or anky losing spondyletis (AS). Joint destruction may be extensive (arthritis mutilans).
- Look for rash (scalp, behind ears, umbilicus, natal cleft), nail changes (pitting, onycholysis, ridging).

Management

- Treatment is as for rheumatoid arthritis with NSAIDs as the mainstay.
- Avoid chloroquine as this precipitates psoriasis.

Reactive arthritis

Clinical features

- Typically young sexually active individual with oro-genital ulcers (painless), conjunctivitis (which may progress to iritis), rash (soles—keratoderma blenorrhagica).
- May occur following non-specific urethritis or infection with *Shigella*, *Salmonella*, *Yersinia*, or *Campylobacter*.

Treatment

- NSAIDs are the main therapy.
- See 📖 p.623 for Reiter's syndrome.

Practice point

Marked morning joint pain or stiffness is most likely to be due to rheumatoid arthritis.

Reactive arthritis

Clinical features

- Comprises a triad of seronegative arthritis, non-specific urethritis, and conjunctivitis.
- Skin lesions are psoriasiform (keratoderma blenorrhagicum) with brown macules progressing to pustules on the soles and palms.
- The arthritis begins ~2 weeks after infection and the lower limb joints are most commonly affected (asymmetrical) and resolves over months; occasionally the skin lesions and arthritis progress to typical psoriatic arthropathy.
- It may be associated with a sterile urethral discharge and mild dysuria. Erosive lesions may affect the penis (circinate balanitis) or mouth.
- Rarely progresses to give aortic incompetence, heart block, pericarditis.

Treatment

NSAIDs, and sometimes steroids are the mainstay of therapy.

Ankylosing spondylitis

Clinical features

- Enquire about axial skeleton involvement (lower lumbar back pain with early morning stiffness).
- Peripheral joint involvement (~40%), uveitis (📖 p.352), anaemia of chronic disease, and progressive immobility may be found.

Management

- NSAIDs for pain.
- Exercise to try to prevent progressive immobility.
- Sulfasalazine may be tried for joint disease.
- Methotrexate and biologic therapies are emerging treatments.
- Refer to a rheumatologist for long-term management.

Enteropathic arthritis

- Large joint arthritis often coincides with active IBD.
- Arthritis may predate the onset of intestinal symptoms; often there are other extra-intestinal manifestations (e.g. erythema nodosum and iritis).
- Treatment of colitis improves arthritic symptoms.

Infections

- ***Viral***: rubella, parvovirus B19 (common, often presents with a generalized rash), and HIV seroconversion may present with polyarthritis.
- ***Bacterial:*** *Gonococcus* (rash, tenosynovitis, sexually active), *Staphylococcus* (immunosuppressed with septicaemia and seeding to several joints), infective endocarditis (vasculitic lesions, heart murmur).
- ***Treatment***: see 📖 p.445.

Vasculitis

The term vasculitis denotes an inflammatory reaction with destructive change of blood vessel walls. The vasculitides are classified into *primary* and *secondary* types.

Classification

Box 11.7 Primary systemic vasculitis (simplistic classification)

	Primary	Secondary
Large arteries	Giant cell arteritis, Takayasu's arteritis	Aortitis 2° to RA or syphilis
Medium arteries	Polyarteritis nodosa, Kawasaki	Infection, e.g. HBV
Small and medium arteries	Churg-Strauss, Wegener's, microscopic polyangiitis	Vasculitis 2° to RA, SLE, systemic sclerosis, drugs, or HIV
Small vessel	Henoch-Schonlein purpura, hypersensitivity vasculitis	Drugs, HCV or HBV infection

Box 11.8 Causes of secondary vasculitis

- Infective endocarditis
- Malignancy
- Rheumatoid arthritis
- Systemic lupus erythematosus
- Cryoglobulinaemia (strongly associated with hepatitis C)
- Drug reaction

Organ involvement varies with the type of vasculitis but commonly includes skin, joints, kidneys, lung, and nervous system

Presentation

- Arthralgia or arthritis, myalgia
- PUO
- Generalized systemic illness, e.g. weight loss, malaise
- Rashes: splinter haemorrhages, nail fold infarcts, purpura, livedo, nodules
- Renal disease: haematuria, proteinuria, hypertension, renal failure (Box 11.9)
- Lung disease: haemoptysis, cough, breathlessness, pulmonary infiltrates (Box 11.9)
- Neurological disease: mononeuritis multiplex, sensorimotor polyneuropathy, confusion, fits, hemiplegia, acute cerebral syndrome.

Box 11.9 Vasculitides affecting lungs or kidneys

Causes of lung haemorrhage and renal failure

- Goodpasture's syndrome
- Wegener's granulomatosis
- Microscopic polyarteritis
- Systemic lupus erythematosus
- Leptospirosis

Causes of renal failure only (no lung haemorrhage)

- Anti-GBM disease
- Small vessel vasculitis
- Secondary vasculitis
- Medium vessel vasculitis (rare)

Box 11.10 Patterns of ANCA

c-ANCA (anti-neutrophil α-proteinase 3)
Wegener's granulomatosis
Microscopic polyarteritis

p-ANCA (anti-myeloperoxidase or elastase)
Microscopic polyarteritis
Churg–Strauss syndrome

Atypical ANCA
Ulcerative colitis (also x-ANCA)
Sclerosing cholangitis

ANCA tests need to be interpreted in the clinical context. ANCA positive tests are seen in infection, malignancy, and a wide range of connective tissue disorders. A negative ANCA does not exclude any of the above.

Systemic lupus erythematosus (SLE)

Assessment

This is a chronic autoimmune disorder characterized by the production of a wide range of autoantibodies against both intracellular and cell surface antigens, though most often with ANA. It commonly affects young women (1:3000 in the UK) and is 10× more common in West Indian black patients.

Patients with SLE may present to A&E in 1 of 2 ways:

1. Known diagnosis of lupus having become acutely unwell. Clinically one has to determine whether their symptoms reflect disease activity, an underlying infection which may precipitate a flare up of the disease, or an unrelated condition.
2. As a presenting diagnosis; the attending physician should be alert to the varied presentations of lupus.

Clinical features

- ***Constitutional (90%)*** Fever, malaise, weight loss.
- ***Musculoskeletal (90%)*** Arthralgia, myalgia, myositis,deforming arthropathy (Jaccoud's) 2° to ligament and capsular laxity, aseptic necrosis 2° to steroid therapy.
- ***Cutaneous (80–90%)*** Butterfly rash, photosensitive rash, discoid lupus, Raynaud's phenomenon, purpura, scarring alopecia, livedo reticularis, urticaria.
- ***Haematological (75%)*** Thrombocytopenia, anaemia (normochromic normocytic, Coombs +ve in 15%), leucopenia and lymphopenia.
- ***Neuropsychiatric (55%)*** Depression, psychosis, fits, hemiplegia, cranial nerve lesions, ataxia, chorea, aseptic meningitis/encephalitis.
- ***Renal (50%)*** Glomerulonephritis, nephritis or nephrotic syndrome, proteinuria, hypertension.
- ***CVS or RS (40%)*** Pleurisy, pericarditis, pleural or pericardial effusion, Libman–Sacks endocarditis, shrinking lung syndrome
- ***Aphthous ulcers (40%).***

Urgent investigations

- ***FBC*** Anaemia, ↓WCC, and ↓plts
- ***U&Es, creatinine*** Renal failure
- ***ESR*** Elevated with disease activity
- ***CRP*** Typically normal. ↑ suggests infection
- ***APTT*** Prolonged if there is an 'anti-cardiolipin' antibody (IgG or IgM)
- ***Blood cultures*** Infection-induced flare-ups
- ***Urine*** Dipstick for proteinuria or haematuria, microscopy for casts, culture for infection
- ***CXR*** Infection or pleurisy
- ***ABG*** Hypoxia with infection.

Practice point

SLE is often characterized by a high ESR and a normal CRP.

Other investigations

- ***Immunology*** ANA, DNA, ENA, ACA, complement levels.
- ***LFTs*** Usually normal.
- ***Viral*** PCR for cytomegalovirus.
- ***Urine*** 24-h collection for creatinine clearance and protein excretion; urine protein/creatinine ratio.

Points to note

- Immunology:
  - >95% are ANA +ve (dsDNA antibody is almost pathognomonic of SLE).
  - Anti-dsDNA antibody titre may correlate with disease activity
  - Low complement levels correlate with disease activity (and renal involvement).
  - 40% are rheumatoid factor positive.
- Pneumococcal and meningococcal infections are more common in patients with SLE as a consequence of either hereditary or acquired deficiencies of the components of the complement pathway.
- Immunosuppressive therapy renders patients susceptible to the usual range of opportunistic infections including pneumocystis, cytomegalovirus, and mycobacteria.
- Chest and urine are the commonest sources of infection in clinical practice.
- Patients with disease activity classically have an elevated ESR but a relatively normal CRP.

An elevated CRP should alert you to look for an underlying infection.

Management

- ***Prednisolone*** 30–60mg od.
- Additional ***immunosuppressive therapy*** such as pulsed methylprednisolone, azathioprine, or cyclophosphamide should be given on consultation with a rheumatologist.
- ***Antibiotics*** if infection is suspected (e.g. cefotaxime) which will treat most chest or urinary tract infections. If the source is known then antimicrobial therapy can be more rationally prescribed.
- ***Hydroxychloroquine*** (200mg/day) may be added if there is cutaneous or joint involvement.

Wegener's granulomatosis and microscopic polyarteritis nodosa (PAN) 1

- Both of these small vessel vasculitides may present to casualty with acute renal failure (rapidly progressive glomerulonephritis).
- Wegener's granulomatosis classically involves the upper and lower respiratory tracts and the kidneys.

Clinical features

- ***Systemic features*** Fever, malaise, weight loss.
- ***Upper respiratory*** Nasal discharge, nose bleeds, sinusitis, collapse of the nasal bridge, deafness (all suggest a diagnosis of Wegener's).
- ***Lower respiratory*** Shortness of breath, haemoptysis, cavitating lung lesions.
- ***Kidneys*** Nephritis with deranged renal function, haematuria, proteinuria, and active urinary sediment.
- ***Musculoskeletal*** Myalgia, arthralgias.
- ***Neurological*** Both peripheral and central.
- ***Ask about smoking*** Strongly associated with lung haemorrhage.

Urgent investigations

- ***FBC*** Anaemia, neutrophil leucocytosis, thrombocytosis. Raised eosinophil count suggests Churg–Strauss syndrome.
- ***Renal function*** Impaired renal function or acute renal failure.
- ***LFTs*** Low albumin (nephrotic syndrome). Elevated AST, ALT, and ALP with hepatitis.
- ***CK and AST*** Elevated due to myositis.
- ***PT and APTT*** Prolonged with widespread vasculitis and DIC.
- ***ESR and CRP*** Elevated.
- ***Blood cultures*** Sepsis.
- ***ABG*** Hypoxia (haemorrhage or infection), metabolic acidosis (renal failure).
- ***Urine*** Dipstick for blood or protein, microscopy and culture 24-h collection for creatinine clearance and protein excretion.
- ***Sputum*** Culture (infection often precipitates lung haemorrhage).
- ***Calcium/phosphate*** Low corrected calcium and high phosphate suggest chronicity.
- ***CXR*** Shadowing seen in lung haemorrhage or infection; cavitating lesions typically occur in Wegener's granulomatosis.
- ***USS of the kidneys*** If in renal failure to exclude obstruction.

Wegener's granulomatosis and microscopic PAN 2

Immunology

- *c-ANCA* — Positive (see 'Points to note')
- *ANA, anti-dsDNA* — To exclude SLE
- *RF*
- *Complement levels*
- *Anti-GBM antibody* — A positive test suggests 1° anti-GBM disease such as Goodpasture's syndrome, in which there is rapid progressive glomerulonephritis and lung haemorrhage
- *Cryoglobulins* — To exclude as a 2° cause of vasculitis
- *Hepatitis serology* — Hepatitis B and C.

Miscellaneous investigations

- *ECG* — Baseline ± changes of hyperkalaemia if ARF is present
- *Lung function tests* — Measurement of KCO (↑ with lung haemorrhage)
- *Echo* — To rule out unsuspected indolent IE (2° cause of vasculitis)
- *XR sinuses* — Commonly involved in Wegener's
- *Renal biopsy* — Histological diagnosis (light/immunofluorescence/EM).

Management

Involve specialists early, rheumatology and renal.

Emergency management

- Patients commonly die from hypoxia (pulmonary haemorrhage, pulmonary oedema), arrhythmias (2° to electrolyte abnormalities), and concomitant infection.
- Ensure adequate *oxygenation* and consider ventilation if necessary.
- Assess *fluid balance* and monitor urine output carefully.
- Consider *invasive haemodynamic monitoring* (CVP, arterial line, Swan–Ganz catheter).
- Patients with nephritis may be volume overloaded with *pulmonary oedema*. Treat with IV furosemide (80–120mg; high doses may be required), GTN infusion, venesection, or haemodialysis or haemofiltration.
- *Correct electrolyte abnormalities*: hyperkalaemia (see 🕮 p.288).
- Consider urgent haemodialysis or haemofiltration in patients with ARF or hyperkalaemia (consult renal physicians).
- Treat precipitating infections empirically with *cefotaxime* until a pathogen is identified.
- Treat underlying vasculitis:
  - High-dose prednisolone (60mg/day)
  - Cyclophosphamide (only after renal or rheumatological opinion)
  - Plasmapheresis (renal units).

Points to note

- The ANCA test provides a rapid screening test and shows high sensitivity for patients with small vessel vasculitis.
- Patients with Wegener's granulomatosis are classically c-ANCA positive (cytoplasmic pattern of immunofluorescence, antibody against elastase I), whilst patients with microscopic polyarteritis may be either p-ANCA (perinuclear pattern of immunofluorescence, antibody against myeloperoxidase) or c-ANCA positive. A negative ANCA does not however preclude the diagnosis of a small vessel vasculitis.
- Underlying infection especially infective endocarditis and chronic meningococcaemia should always enter the differential diagnosis of a patient with small vessel vasculitis.
- An infectious episode such as an upper respiratory tract infection often will precipitate the presentation of a small vessel vasculitis.

Cryoglobulinaemia

Cryoglobulins are immunoglobulins that precipitate at low temperatures and dissolve on re-warming. They precipitate in the superficial capillaries or outside vessels in the coldest part of the skin to produce microinfarcts or purpura. Cryoglobulinaemia occurs in several conditions:

- Essential cryoglobulinaemia implies the absence of an identifiable cause.
- Renal disease is associated with all 3 types, and is thought to involve immune-complex pathways.
- Mean age, 42–59 years.♂:♀, 2:3.

Type 1 monoclonal

- Type 1 cryoglobulinaemia, or simple cryoglobulinaemia, is the result of a monoclonal immunoglobulin, usually IgM or IgG.
- Associated with myelo- or lymphoproliferative disease.
- Heavy proteinuria, haematuria, and renal failure may occur (membranoproliferative glomerulonephritis).
- Serum C4 and C1q are low.

Type 2 (mixed monoclonal) and type 3 (mixed polyclonal)

- Type 2 and type 3 cryoglobulinaemia (mixed cryoglobulinaemia) contain RFs (often IgM). These RFs form complexes with the fragment, crystallizable (Fc) portion of polyclonal IgG. The actual RF may be monoclonal (in type 2 cryoglobulinaemia) or polyclonal (in type 3 cryoglobulinaemia) immunoglobulin.
- Type 2 is associated with immune complex vasculitis and 50% have evidence of renal disease. Many cases are associated with HCV infection.
- Type 3 mixed polyclonal is associated with SLE, and systemic infections (post-streptococcal nephritis, leprosy, and syphilis). Renal involvement is also seen.

Clinical features

- Renal involvement (haematuria, proteinuria, renal failure)
- Raynaud's phenomenon
- Purpura (esp. legs)
- Arthralgia and fever
- Confusion and weakness (2° to hyperviscosity)
- Hepatosplenomegaly (probably a manifestation of underlying aetiology).

Management

- There is no specific treatment.
- Plasmapheresis and immunosuppressive therapy may be tried.

Giant cell arteritis (temporal arteritis)

- The commonest type of 1° large vessel vasculitis in clinical practice with an incidence of 1:10000. This is typically a disorder of the elderly (mean age 70 years, with a ♀:♂ ratio of 2:1).
- The diagnosis is made clinically (see Box 11.11) and is supported by an elevated acute phase response (ESR, CRP, and thrombocytosis), and temporal artery histology.
- The classical pathological description is of a segmental granulomatous pan-arteritis but in the early stage changes may be confined to thickening of the internal elastic lamina associated with a mononuclear cell infiltrate.

Investigations

- ***FBC*** Normochromic anaemia, thrombocytosis
- ***Biochemistry*** Elevated alkaline phosphatase
- ***ESR*** ESR >50mm in the first hour, 95% of cases
- ***CRP*** Elevated
- ***CXR*** Exclude underlying bronchial carcinoma
- ***Urinalysis*** Exclude haematuria and proteinuria
- ***Temporal artery biopsy.***

Management

- Patients with suspected giant cell arteritis should be started on *high-dose prednisolone immediately*, as delay may result in blindness.
- If GCA is not complicated by visual loss: give 40–60mg of prednisolone. If potentially reversible symptoms persist or worsen, the dose may be increased until symptomatic control is achieved. If the initial dose of prednisolone is 60mg/day it can generally be reduced to 50mg/day after 2 weeks and to 40mg/day at the end of a month. The dose can be reduced every 1–2 weeks by about 10% of the total daily dose. When a daily dose of 10mg, is achieved, the prednisolone taper should be slowed such that patients remain on some prednisolone for 9–12 months (in progressively lower doses). After reaching a daily prednisolone dose of 10mg, further tapering in 1-mg decrements is appropriate. Check Hb, ESR/CRP prior to each reduction in the steroid dose.
- Low dose aspirin (plus PPIs for gastroprotection) is recommended to reduce the risk of visual loss, TIAs, or stroke.
- If visual loss is strongly suspected to be due to GCA: IV pulse methylprednisolone (1g for 3 days) may be given followed by oral prednisolone 1 mg/kg per day (maximum of 60mg/day), as recommended above.
- Because the patients may be on steroids for 1–2 years, consider osteoporosis prevention: encourage adequate dietary calcium and vitamin D intake. Bisphosphonates for either prophylaxis or treatment may also be appropriate.
- All patients should have a temporal artery biopsy performed within 48h of commencing steroids to try to confirm the diagnosis. A normal biopsy does not exclude the diagnosis because of the 'skip' nature of the disease.

Box 11.11 Clinical features of giant cell arteritis

• Headache	90%
• Temporal artery tenderness	85%
• Scalp tenderness	75%
• Jaw claudication	70%
• Thickened/nodular temporal artery	35%
• Pulseless temporal artery	40%
• Visual symptoms (incl. blindness)	40%
• Polymyalgic symptoms	40% (see 📖 p.646)
• Systemic features	40%
• CVA or MI	rare

Practice point

Continuous headache in patients >60 years may indicate cranial arthritis but may be spondylitic.[1]

Reference

1. Hawkes C (2002). Smart handles and red flags in neurological diagnosis. *Hosp Med* **63:** 732–42.

Polymyalgia rheumatica (PMR)

PMR is a clinical syndrome characterized by an acute phase response (high ESR or high CRP) which predominantly affects the elderly Caucasian population, median age of onset 70 years, ♀ >♂, annual incidence approximately 1:2500.

Clinical features

- Proximal muscle stiffness and pain without weakness or wasting (Box 11.12).
- Systemic symptoms of malaise, fever, and weight loss.

Box 11.12 Causes of proximal upper and lower girdle stiffness or pains

• Cervical spondylosis ± adhesive capsulitis	No acute phase response, CPK (N)
• Lumbar spondylosis	
• Osteomalacia	
• Fibromyalgia	
• Hypothyroidism	No acute phase response, ↑CPK
• Polymyositis/dermatomyositis	↑acute phase response, ↑CPK
• Inflammatory arthritis	↑acute phase response

Investigations

• *FBC*	Normochromic normocytic anaemia
• *U&Es, LFTs*	Elevated alkaline phosphatase is common (50%)
• *CPK*	Normal (if high consider polymyositis or hypothyroidism)
• *ESR*	High (>40mm/h initially)
• *CRP*	High
• *Rheumatoid factor*	PMR may be the presenting feature of rheumatoid arthritis
• *CXR*	PMR symptoms may be the presenting feature of a neoplasm.

Treatment

- *Steroids*: prednisolone 15–20mg PO od initially reducing to 5–10mg od over 2–3 months and very slow reduction thereafter. Some patients may require treatment for years.
- Monitor response with symptoms and ESR.

Points to note

- PMR and giant cell arteritis form part of a clinical spectrum of disease and up to 40% of patients with biopsy-proven giant cell arteritis have polymyalgic symptoms.
- Polymyalgic symptoms may be the presenting feature of an underlying neoplasm or connective tissue disease.

- Polymyalgic symptoms should respond dramatically to prednisolone. Failure to respond should alert the clinician to the possibility of an underlying neoplasm or connective tissue disease.

Practice point

Never diagnose PMR in a patient <50 years old.

Back pain

Approximately 5% of all medical consultations in the UK are for back or neck pain. In the majority of patients no definite anatomical diagnosis is made (non-specific back pain) but it is important not to miss the sinister causes of back pain (Boxes 11.13 and 11.14).

Box 11.13 Causes of back pain

Mechanical back pain
- Spondylolisthesis
- Spondylosis
- Intervertebral disc prolapse
- Spinal stenosis (claudication type pain)
- Apophyseal joint disease (exacerbated by lumbar extension, cervical or thoracic rotation)
- Non-specific back pain
- Trauma

Inflammatory back pain
- Rheumatoid arthritis
- Seronegative spondyloarthritides
  - Psoriatic
  - Ankylosing spondylitis
  - Reiter's
  - Enteropathic
  - Behcet's

Referred pain
- Aortic aneurysm
- Pyelonephritis, renal calculus
- Pancreatitis

Box 11.4 Causes of 'sinister' back pain

- Infection (discitis/epidural abscess)
- Malignancy
- Myeloma
- Osteoporotic crush fracture
- Paget's disease

History

Is pain likely to be mechanical, inflammatory, or sinister in origin?
- Mechanical back pain is exacerbated by prolonged sitting or standing, relieved by movement, and precipitated by trauma.
- Inflammatory back pain is characterized by prolonged early morning stiffness and is relieved by exercise.
- Sinister back pain (e.g. malignancy and infection) often leads to pain at night, constant pain, local bony tenderness, and may be accompanied by other systemic symptoms.
- Are there any sensory or motor symptoms? Ask specifically for any change in bowel or bladder function.

Examination

- General: look for evidence of malignancy.
- Spine (palpation for tenderness, muscle spasm, cervical spine flexion, extension, rotation and lateral flexion, thoracic spine rotation, lumbar spine flexion, extension, side flexion, compression of sacroiliac joints.
- Neurological examination looking specifically for absent ankle jerks (slipped disc) or long-tract signs in the legs. S1 nerve root signs and symptoms can be produced by a lesion in the region of the upper lumbar cord (central disc prolapse compressing the S1 nerve root).
- Always do a rectal examination and test perineal sensation.

Practice points

- Back pain at night suggests a sinister cause such as cancer or infection.
- Patients with acute onset of back pain and signs suggestive of a high lesion (e.g. L1–L3/4) may have weak thighs and absent knee jerks, and are unlikely to have a disc lesion and may have a tumour.

Investigations

Patients with back pain occurring at night and patients with neurological signs warrant investigation.

- XRs of spine ± CXR (?malignancy)
- FBC and ESR (elevated with sinister causes of pain)
- Biochemical profile (calcium, alkaline phosphatase, and phosphate)
- Immunoglobulins and protein electrophoresis (?myeloma)
- Acid phosphatase
- PSA
- Bence-Jones protein and urine protein electrophoresis.

Further imaging

- CT or MRI scan (superior to CT for imaging the spinal cord and roots)
- Technetium bone scan for 'hot-spots' (neoplastic or inflammatory).

Management

- Analgesics
- Bed rest
- Physiotherapy
- Appropriate referral to a specialist.

Prolapsed intervertebral disc

Acute postero-lateral herniation of a lumbar disc, usually L4–L5 or L5–S1, is a common cause of acute incapacitating lower back pain. There is often a clear precipitating event (e.g. lifting) and pain may radiate in the distribution of the L5 or S1 nerve root.

Patients should be examined carefully for:

- Paraspinal muscle spasm is often prominent.
- Straight leg raising is typically reduced on the affected side.
- Look for nerve root signs and test sacral and perineal sensation. Always do a rectal examination.
- L5 lesion leads to weakness of extensor hallus longus, ankle dorsiflexion, and ankle eversion, and altered sensation is perceived in the L5 dermatome.
- S1 lesion leads to weakness of ankle plantar flexion, ankle eversion, and a diminished or lost ankle jerk and altered sensation is perceived in the S1 dermatome.
- Neurosurgical emergencies, see Box 11.5.

Treatment

- If the XRs reveal a fracture, refer the patient to the orthopaedic team; severe pain from inflammatory arthritides should be referred to the rheumatologists.
- Majority of patients respond to conservative management.
- Bed rest until the acute pain subsides followed by mobilization and physiotherapy (patients may often be managed at home with instructions to return to the GP or doctor for review in 2–3 weeks).
- Non-steroidal anti-inflammatory agents.
- Physiotherapy.

Box 11.15 Neurosurgical emergencies presenting as back pain

An acute disc prolapse at the L2/3 level may cause bilateral multiple root lesions and may affect bladder and bowel function (caude equine syndrome).

This requires immediate investigation:

- Acute cauda equine compression (see 📖 p.422).
- Acute cord compression (see 📖 p.422).

C_1-esterase inhibitor deficiency (angioneurotic oedema)

This condition may be inherited or acquired, occurring ~1:50,000 in the UK.

Hereditary

- Autosomal dominant inheritance
- Usually presents in the second decade
- Characterized by low serum concentrations of complement components C2, C4, and C_1-inhibitor, but normal C1 and C3 levels.

Acquired

- Paraneoplastic syndrome: autoantibody against C_1-esterase inhibitor
- Characterized by low serum concentrations of complement components C1, C2, and C4.

Clinical features

- Laryngeal oedema (48% of attacks); may be life threatening
- Subcutaneous oedema (91% of attacks) affecting face, buttocks, genitals, and limbs. Usually non-itchy
- Abdominal symptoms: pain, vomiting, and diarrhoea.

Precipitating factors include

- Stress
- Infection
- Pre-menstrual
- Oestrogen-containing contraceptive pill
- ACEIs.

Management

Acute severe attack

- C_1-esterase inhibitor plasma concentrate (an IV infusion of 1000–1500U) usually effective in 30–60min.
- FFP 2–4U may be given if C_1-esterase inhibitor plasma concentrate is not available.

Laryngeal oedema

- If a patient is admitted with laryngeal oedema 60% O_2 should be given immediately, blood gases should be checked, and a senior anaesthetist or ENT surgeon called as intubation or tracheostomy may be required.
- IM adrenaline 0.5–1mL, 1:1000 (see 🕮 p.322).
- Hydrocortisone 200mg IV.
- Chlorphenamine 10mg IV may be administered initially prior to the infusion of C_1-esterase inhibitor.

Prophylaxis

Those with >1 attack per month:

- Tranexamic acid (1–1.5g 2–4 times daily). Effective in 28%.
- Attenuated androgens, e.g. danazol (unlicensed indication).

Chapter 12

Dermatological emergencies

Cutaneous drug reactions

Presentation

- ***Maculopapular erythema*** ± pruritus and scaling. Resolves over 2 weeks when drug is stopped. 46% of cutaneous drug reactions.
- ***Urticaria/angio-oedema:*** accounts for ~25% of drug reactions. Sudden onset of individual pruritic erythematous lesions which resolve within 24h. Angio-oedema may involve mucous membranes and may be associated with life-threatening anaphylaxis (see 🕮 p.322). Aspirin, morphine, codeine act directly in mast cells to liberate histamine in sensitive individuals. Penicillin (and aspirin) can cause an IgE-mediated or IgG complement-fixing allergic reaction. Urticarial eruptions due to serum sickness may persist and have associated systemic symptoms.
- ***Fixed drug eruption:*** characterized by a few well-demarcated painful erythematous lesions which frequently blister often involving the face, hands, forearms, and genitalia. Hyperpigmentation may persist after recovery. Rechallenge may cause recurrent lesions in the same location. Common drugs include sulphonamides, tetracyclines, barbiturates, salicylates, and dapsone. Represents 10% of cutaneous drug reactions.
- ***Photosensitive drug eruptions:*** cutaneous reaction limited to exposed sites with characteristic sparing of covered areas. May be due to either a photoallergic (immune-mediated, e.g. chlorpromazine, sulphanilamide, amiodarone) or phototoxic (non-immune, e.g. tetracyclines, sulphonamides, griseofulvin, naproxen, high-dose furosemide) reaction. Some drugs cause photosensitive porphyria cutanea tarda or photo-onycholysis.
- ***Erythema multiforme/Stevens–Johnson syndrome:*** 10% of drug reactions. Sudden onset of erythematous lesions affecting the skin and mucous membranes. Acral sites are often involved with target or necrotic lesions. Associated with fever, malaise, and sore throat due to mucous membrane involvement (Stevens–Johnson syndrome) and rarely confluent epidermal necrolysis as seen in toxic epidermal necrolysis (see 🕮 p.666). Drugs implicated include salicylates, sulphonamides, penicillin, sulphonylureas, and barbiturates. Stop the drug; give steroids (prednisolone 30mg/day).
- ***Exfoliative dermatitis:*** presents as erythroderma. 4% of drug reactions. Causative drugs include barbiturates, salicylates, penicillin, sulphonamides, and sulphonylureas.
- ***Toxic epidermal necrolysis (TEN):*** in adults TEN is an immunological disease provoked by drug hypersensitivity, but in babies it is due to the direct necrolytic effect of a *Staphylococcal* toxin. It may be caused by many different drugs including penicillins, sulphonamides and other antibiotics, blood products, NSAIDs, and anticonvulsants.

Points to note

- Cutaneous drug reactions usually develop within 1–2 weeks following start of treatment but occasionally present later.
- Development of extensive angio-oedema is associated with a risk of anaphylaxis, hypotension, bronchospasm, oropharyngeal irritation, flushing, or urticaria and acral oedema.
- Patients who present with erythema multiforme or Stevens–Johnson syndrome may develop confluent areas of epidermal necrolysis as seen in toxic epidermal necrolysis (📖 p.666).
- Peripheral blood eosinophilia is rare.
- IV drug administration is more likely to be associated with anaphylaxis.
- Cutaneous drug reactions are more common in HIV disease.

Management

- Severe angio-oedema and anaphylaxis require immediate treatment (see 📖 p.322).
- Seek specialist advice for severe Steven–Johnson syndrome or toxic epidermal necrolysis.
- Stop any responsible drugs and prescribe an alternative if necessary. Hospitalized patients receiving numerous drugs should be assessed carefully and all non-essential therapy discontinued.
- Prescribe oral non-sedating or sedating antihistamines with simple emollients and medium-potency topical steroids. Short courses of systemic steroids may be required in erythema multiforme or Steven–Johnson syndrome.
- Pyrexia may occur with cutaneous drug reactions but underlying infection should always be excluded.
- There should be clinical improvement within a few days: persistent reactions should prompt a search for other causes.
- Although re-challenge with a suspected drug may provide a definitive diagnosis, reactions may be severe and can lead to fatal anaphylaxis or severe toxic epidermal necrolysis.
- Specific RAST can be used to measure serum IgE antibody production in patients with penicillin allergy. However, a negative reaction does not exclude penicillin allergy.
- Skin biopsies can be useful for specific forms of cutaneous drug reactions such as fixed drug eruption and erythema multiforme.

Erythroderma

Presentation

- Erythroderma may be acute or chronic. Acute erythroderma is more likely to present as an emergency.
- There is generalized erythema associated with exfoliation.
- Scaling can be fine (pityriasiform) or coarse (psoriasiform).
- Patients may be febrile or hypothermic because of loss of temperature control mechanisms.
- Chronic erythroderma may be associated with nail dystrophy, diffuse hair loss, and ectropion. Palmo-plantar hyperkeratosis and peripheral lymphadenopathy may be prominent.

Causes

- ***Common:*** eczema, psoriasis, drug reactions
- ***Rare:*** cutaneous T-cell lymphoma, pityriasis rubra pilaris, toxic shock syndrome, Kawasaki disease, sarcoidosis

Investigations

- Monitor FBC, U&Es, albumin, calcium, and LFTs regularly.
- Blood cultures and skin swabs should be performed and sustained pyrexia, hypotension, or clinical deterioration should prompt a search for underlying sepsis.

Management

General measures

- Discontinue all unnecessary medications.
- Nurse in a warm room with regular monitoring of core temperature and fluid balance. Patients should be nursed on a pressure-relieving mattress and/or Lyofoam® if necessary.
- Encourage oral fluids and high calorific food and protein supplements. Nasogastric feeding may be required. Avoid IV cannulae because they can be a source of infection.
- Monitor fluid balance closely: daily weights and clinical examination (as allowed by the exfoliation).

Specific therapy

- The skin should be treated at least 4 times daily with emollients such as 50% white soft paraffin/50% liquid paraffin or Epaderm®.
- A daily bath should be supplemented with emollients such as Oilatum® or Balneum®.
- Oral sedating antihistamines such as hydroxyzine (10–100mg in divided doses) may be used and the dose adjusted according to severity and weight.
- Application of mild or potent topical steroids may be appropriate but liaise with specialist at early opportunity.
- In eczema, systemic treatment with prednisolone, azathioprine, or ciclosporin may be appropriate, and in psoriasis, acitretin, methotrexate or ciclosporin may be required. Liaise with specialist prior to embarking on this approach.

Complications

- Hypothermia
- Infection
- Hypoalbuminaemia
- High output cardiac failure.

Box 12.1 Management key points: erythroderma

- Discontinue all unnecessary medications.
- Nurse in a warm room and on a pressure-relieving mattress and/or Lyofoam® if necessary.
- Monitor core temperature and fluid balance closely (daily weights and clinical examination).
- Fluids: encourage oral fluids.
- Feeding: encourage high calorific food and protein supplements. NG feeding may be required.
- Emollients e.g. 50% white soft paraffin/50% liquid paraffin or Epaderm® at least 4 times daily.
- Daily bath supplemented with emollients such as Oilatum® or Balneum®.
- Topical steroids: liaise with specialist early.
- Oral sedating antihistamines e.g. hydroxyzine.

Practice point

Non-responsive or relapsing eczemic rash should suggest contact dermatitis.

Urticaria

Presentation

- Urticaria presents as erythematous itchy areas of oedema involving the superficial skin as small weals or larger plaques. Lesions present suddenly and often resolve within 24h, although new lesions may develop repeatedly.
- In severe urticaria systemic symptoms may predominate with the development of anaphylaxis characterized by shock and collapse (see 📖 p.322). Features include hypotension, bronchospasm, angio-oedema, and diffuse urticaria.
- Drug sensitivities and reactions to radiographic contrast media are more likely to produce anaphylaxis.
- Extensive urticarial lesions are not the same as anaphylaxis.

Causes

- Bee/wasp stings, drug reactions (penicillin common, aspirin and NSAIDs), contrast media, blood products, food sensitivity such as nuts and shellfish.
- Physical causes of urticaria such as dermographism, pressure, vibration, cold, solar, and cholinergic (heat/exercise).
- Contact urticaria.
- Malignancy and autoimmune disorders such as lupus associated with a functional deficiency of C_1-esterase inhibitor.
- Chronic idiopathic urticaria possibly due to autoantibodies produced against the low affinity IgE receptor.
- Although urticaria may cause angio-oedema, this is distinct from hereditary angio-oedema which does not cause itching or hives.

Diagnostic points

- In patients with chronic urticaria, ask specifically about possible physical causes (e.g. induced by cold, exercise, water, pressure, heat, and rarely light and vibration. Dermographism is the most common form of physical urticaria; briskly stroking the skin with a firm object produces linear weals.
- Contact urticaria usually occurs within minutes after direct contact with various agents such as plants, aeroallergens, foods (such as cheese, eggs, fish) or latex. Contact sensitivity to latex products has a high incidence of anaphylaxis.
- If urticarial lesions persist for >24h a diagnosis of urticarial vasculitis is likely. Such lesions are tender and painful rather than pruritic and may appear bruised. Unlike other forms of urticaria the diagnosis of urticarial vasculitis should be established by histology.
- Patch tests are not indicated in urticaria. Prick tests will indicate if individuals are atopic but are rarely useful in establishing a specific cause of contact urticaria (there is also a risk of anaphylaxis). Total serum IgE levels may be elevated in atopic individuals.

Management

- Anaphylactic reactions require immediate treatment (see 📖 p.322).
  - Lay the patient flat.
  - Secure the airway and give O_2.
  - Give IM adrenaline 0.5mg (0.5mL of 1 in 1000 adrenaline injection) and repeat every 5min according to BP, pulse, and respiratory function. IV adrenaline may be required if the patient is severely ill with poor circulation (see 📖 p.322).
  - Start IV fluids if hypotensive.
  - Give IV hydrocortisone 100–300mg and chlorphenamine 10–20mg. Continue H_1-antagonist (e.g. chlorphenamine 4mg q4–6h) for at least 24–48h; longer if urticaria and pruritus persist.
  - If the patient deteriorates, start IV aminophylline infusion (see 📖 Box 2.4, p.181). Patients on β-blockers may not respond to adrenaline injection and require IV salbutamol infusion.
- Severe acute urticaria with or without angio-oedema is usually not life threatening unless associated with systemic features of anaphylaxis.
  - Give oral antihistamines such as hydroxyzine 25mg or chlorphenamine 4mg.
  - A single dose of prednisolone 50mg orally may be given but should not be continued without specialist advice.
  - When the patient's condition has stabilized, they can be discharged on regular maintenance treatment with an oral non-sedating antihistamine such as cetirizine 10–20mg daily, levocetrizine 5mg daily, desloratadine 5mg daily, or fexofenadine 180mg daily (sedative antihistamines such as hydroxyzine or chlorphenamine are usually not required for maintenance treatment of chronic urticaria).
- Patients with no specific identifiable cause of acute urticaria and all patients with chronic or physical forms of urticaria should be referred for specialist advice.
- Patients with contact sensitivity to latex should use alternatives such as Allergard® gloves, vinyl gloves, or non-sterile copolymer gloves. Such individuals should be warned to use only non-latex polyurethane condoms.

Autoimmune bullous disease

Presentation

- Intact pruritic fluid-filled blisters
- Itchy urticated erythematous plaques (pre-bullous eruption)
- Cutaneous and/or mucosal erosions.

Causes

- ***Common***: bullous pemphigoid.
- ***Rare***: pemphigus vulgaris, pemphigoid gestationes (second/third trimester), dermatitis herpetiformis, pemphigus foliaceus, epidermolysis bullosa acquisita, bullous lupus erythematosus, linear IgA disease, paraneoplastic pemphigus.

Poor prognostic features

- Pemphigus (higher mortality than other bullous disease)
- Age >60 years
- Extensive involvement.

Diagnosis

- Biopsy of a fresh blister for histology and peri-lesional skin should be sent for immunofluorescence studies.
- Send serum for indirect immunofluorescence studies.

Management

Liaise with specialist at an early opportunity.

General measures

- Intact blisters should be aspirated. Examine for new blisters daily.
- Patients should be bathed daily with emollients and if necessary chlorhexidine bath additive in order to prevent 2° bacterial infection. Use diluted potassium permanganate soaks for eroded and weeping areas with non-adherent dressings under stockinette body suit/bandages. Avoid adhesive dressings. Nurse the patient on a Clinitron® bed.
- Give oral antihistamines (e.g. hydroxyzine) for pruritus.
- Potent topical steroids (e.g. Dermovate® cream) should be applied to individual lesions twice daily.
- Prescribe prophylactic sc heparin or tinzaparin for immobile elderly patients.
- Monitor fluid balance carefully and FBC, U&Es, and LFTs.

Specific systemic therapy

Liaise with specialists.

- Refer severe conjunctival disease to an ophthalmologist early.
- Pemphigus requires high-dose immunosuppression (prednisolone 80–100mg/day) but mild disease may require less.
- Bullous pemphigoid, when localized or mild, may respond to potent topical steroids alone (e.g. Dermovate® cream) or can occasionally be controlled with nicotinamide 0.5–2.5g/day and antibiotics (erythromycin or tetracyclines). Extensive disease will require immunosuppression with prednisolone 30–60mg/day and the dosage gradually reduced according to response (i.e. once no new blisters are formed).

- Steroid sparing agents such as azathioprine 50–100mg/day should also be considered for extensive disease, where response to steroids is inadequate.
- For resistant disease consider methylprednisolone, cyclophosphamide, ciclosporin, mycophenolate, intravenous immunoglobulins, chlorambucil, or plasmapheresis.
- Mucosal disease requires regular benzydamine and tetracycline mouth washes with hydrocortisone 2.5mg lozenges for painful erosions. 0.1% tacrolimus in carmellose is currently experimental.
- If condition deteriorates consider 2° bacterial or viral infection of cutaneous or mucosal sites.

Box 12.2 Pemphigus vs. bullous pemphigoid

Pemphigus is characterized by intra-epidermal separation and acantholysis of individual keratinocytes. In pemphigus vulgaris the split is suprabasal while in pemphigus foliaceus the separation is much higher in the epidermis. Penicillamine, captopril, rifampicin, and other drugs rarely induce a pemphigus-like syndrome which is indistinguishable from pemphigus vulgaris. This accounts for <10% of all cases of pemphigus.

Bullous pemphigoid is characterized by a subepidermal split and an inflammatory infiltrate containing eosinophils. Specialist advice is required. Exclude other causes of bullous disease such as porphyrias, drugs (NSAIDs, barbiturates, furosemide), diabetes mellitus, and bullous amyloid. Also consider bullous insect bite reaction and bullous impetigo in the differential diagnosis particularly for localized blisters. Tense blisters on the palms and soles may be due to endogenous eczema (pompholyx) or fungal infection (tinea).

Eczema herpeticum

Presentation

- Patients with atopic endogenous eczema are predisposed to 2° herpes simplex infection. This may occur as a 1° infection following an episode of herpes labialis or after contact with an affected individual.
- Patients present with a sudden deterioration of their eczema characterized by widespread vesiculopustular lesions which are tender and gradually become necrotic. Resolution of the condition produces extensive crusting and exudation.
- Patients are usually pyrexial and toxic with a tachycardia. Cardiorespiratory collapse is unusual.

Management

- The condition can progress rapidly and therefore localized disease should be treated aggressively. Patients should be admitted and early specialist advice is required.
- Refer patients with ocular disease to ophthalmologist urgently.
- Extensive mucosal disease may make oral nutrition difficult and patients may require IV fluids.
- Perform bacterial swabs daily: 2° bacterial infection is common and if present requires treatment with IV antibiotics.
- Topical therapy:
    - Do not use topical steroids.
    - Use simple emollients such as aqueous cream.
    - Chlorhexidine (topical antiseptic) and diluted potassium permanganate (1/10 000) (should be pale pink) as a soak once or twice daily for brief periods to areas of excessive exudation.
- Give oral non-sedating antihistamines.
- Start high-dose IV aciclovir at the earliest opportunity (maximum 10mg/kg/8-hourly). If IV therapy is not possible, give valaciclovir 1000mg tds for 7 days.
- Patients with severe atopic eczema should be advised about prompt treatment of herpes labialis and to avoid contact with herpes simplex.
- Adults with herpes labialis should be advised to avoid contact with children with atopic eczema.

Herpes zoster

See 🕮 p.460.

Generalized pustular psoriasis

Presentation

- Rapid onset of superficial pustules, usually in a patient with typical plaque psoriasis. Pustules may be confluent or pin-point and may be studded around the periphery of typical psoriatic plaques.
- Irritant topical therapies (e.g. potent topical steroids, vitamin D analogues, coal tar, and dithranol preparations) may precipitate generalized pustular psoriasis in patients with 'unstable' psoriasis (hot tender erythematous psoriatic plaques).
- Rarely patients develop generalized pustular psoriasis without a previous history, and similar presentations can occur in pregnancy.
- Pyrexia is often accompanied by systemic symptoms such as malaise, anorexia, and arthralgia. Cutaneous infection with *Staphylococcus aureus* is common and may result in septicaemia.
- Differential diagnosis includes bullous impetigo, toxic epidermal necrolysis, staphylococcal scalded skin syndrome, autoimmune bullous disorders, and in particular subcorneal pustular dermatosis, pustular vasculitis particularly due to herpes simplex infection or drugs, and eczema herpeticum.

Natural history

- There are repeated acute episodes of generalized pustulation associated with pyrexia and systemic symptoms resolving in 5–7 days to produce extensive superficial crusting. Episodes recur every 7–10 days.
- Patients with localized palmo-plantar pustular psoriasis have a mild chronic disease which is not associated with systemic abnormalities.
- Patients with generalized disease may develop ARDS and shock due to release of cytokines or the presence of septicaemia. Elderly patients with generalized pustular psoriasis (Von Zumbusch) have a worse prognosis.

Investigations

- Monitor FBC, U&Es, and LFTs regularly. A neutrophil leucocytosis is invariable. Abnormal LFTs and ↓Ca^{2+} may occur.
- 1° bacterial or viral infection should be excluded by appropriate bacterial and viral swabs. If febrile, take blood cultures.
- Perform ABGs in hypoxic patients or those with an abnormal CXR.

Management

Liaise with specialists at an early opportunity.

- Enforce bed rest; monitor temperature and fluid balance closely.
- Oral fluids with high calorie and high protein input/supplements.

Topical therapy

- The extensive crusting and exudation of the early phase of pustulation can be treated with topical potassium permanganate (1/10,000) soaks.
- For extensive disease, nurse on a Clinitron® bed in a warm room.

- Bathe daily with emollients and antiseptic washes. Treat skin at least 4 times daily with emollients such as 50% WSP, 50% LP, Epaderm®, or aqueous cream.
- Avoid topical steroids, vitamin D analogues, coal tar, and dithranol (may cause severe irritation and exacerbation of the disease).

Systemic therapy

- Give regular oral sedative antihistamines (e.g. hydroxyzine).
- Bacterial infection should be treated with appropriate antibiotics.
- Severe generalized pustular psoriasis may require systemic treatment with retinoids, methotrexate, or ciclosporin: seek specialist advice.

Practice point

Psoriasis rarely becomes secondarily infected.

Toxic epidermal necrolysis (TEN) 1

Presentation

Acute onset of morbilliform or confluent erythema associated with widespread blistering (necrolysis) and skin tenderness.

Diagnostic points

- Necrolysis is used to describe confluent blistering of the skin associated with epidermal separation rather like a large burn. It should be distinguished from discrete intact blisters which are characteristic of autoimmune bullous diseases.
- There may be clinical overlap between toxic epidermal necrolysis and erythema multiforme as seen in the Stevens–Johnson syndrome. Mucocutaneous involvement is common and both oral and conjunctival erosions may be present.
- TEN should be distinguished from the staphylococcal scalded skin syndrome (SSS). The presence of mucosal lesions is invariable in TEN, and distinguishes from SSS. This usually occurs in children or immunosuppressed adults and is associated with the production of staphylococcal toxins. A skin biopsy is diagnostic: in TEN there is full thickness epidermal necrosis, sub-epidermal separation, and a sparse or absent dermal infiltrate while in SSS there is suprabasal epidermal separation with an intact basement membrane.

Causes

- Idiopathic
- Drug induced—sulphonamides and occasionally other antibiotics, anticonvulsants (not described with sodium valproate), NSAIDs.

Adverse prognostic factors

- Age greater than 60 years (25% overall mortality)
- Area of cutaneous involvement >50%
- Blood urea >17mmol/L
- Neutropenia (neutrophil count $<1 \times 10^9$/L)
- Idiopathic aetiology.

Management

The priorities are:

1. Try to identify the cause and treat. Stop drug.
2. Supportive care: fluid balance and nutrition.
3. Prevent complications
4. Eye care
5. Screening and treatment of sepsis.

Identify the cause

- A specific drug is unlikely to be responsible if treatment was started after the onset of erythema, necrolysis, or mucous membrane involvement.
- A drug aetiology should be considered if TEN develops 7–21 days after the first administration of a drug, or within 48h if the drug has caused an eruption in the past.
- If patients are on several different drugs, stop all that may be a cause.

General supportive care

- Patients should be nursed on an air fluid or Clinitron® bed in a side room. A single designated nurse should attend the patient continuously and the room should be kept warm in order to prevent hypothermia.
- Core temperature should be continuously monitored via a rectal probe and a space blanket may be required if the patient is hypothermic because of cutaneous vasodilatation. However, patients frequently also develop hyperthermia which may necessitate temporary cooling of the room with fans.
- Lyofoam® dressings should be used between the patient and bedding in order to ease mobility and skin dressings. Emollients should be applied every 2–4h to all areas or patients can be 'wrapped' to improve ease of handling and reduce sheer forces on the skin. This involves covering the skin with aqueous cream generously, then applying Jelonet®, followed by Soffban® then Coban® (or equivalent) bandages.
- Oral mucosal surfaces should be cleaned every 4–6h and sprayed with chlorhexidine and benzydamine. Mucosal involvement may produce oral erosions or constrictions affecting the oral aperture or pharynx.
- Nasopharyngeal involvement may result in airway obstruction and necessitate ventilation.
- Mucous membrane involvement usually precedes skin necrolysis by several days. GI involvement may be characterized by bleeding and/or a protein losing enteropathy leading to negative fluid and nitrogen balance.
- Monitor fluid balance closely, preferably by daily weights.
- If possible, fluids should be administered orally or via a NG route. Avoid IV lines to reduce the risk of sepsis. 5–7L are often required during the first 24h. A protein- and energy-rich nasogastric feed should be prescribed.
- Daily FBC, U&Es, LFTs, amylase(↓), phosphate(↓), and glucose (hyperglycaemia produces an osmotic diuresis aggravating dehydration)
- CXR should be performed regularly. Pulmonary oedema and ARDS are frequent complications. ABGs should be monitored and if there is deterioration, have a low threshold for admission to ITU and ventilation.
- Prophylactic anticoagulation should be used (SC calcium heparin 5000U tds or enoxaparin 40mg SC od).
- Patients are frequently terrified and in considerable pain. Adequate analgesia and tranquillizers should be administered.
- Post-inflammatory pigmentary changes are common and will gradually resolve.

TEN 2

Prevent complications: infection

- Central venous lines should be avoided if possible. IV lines should be removed as soon as possible in order to reduce infection risk.
- Several cutaneous and mucous membrane sites should be swabbed daily. Culture sputum and urine daily. IV and in-dwelling catheters should be changed frequently and tips sent for culture. Perform blood cultures daily if febrile. Fever is a common feature of TEN and does not always indicate infection.
- Prophylactic antibiotics are only indicated if the risk of sepsis is extremely high such as severe neutropenia or a heavy single strain bacterial colonization of the skin.
- Antibiotics should be started if there is positive blood, urine, or sputum culture or indirect evidence of sepsis such as hypothermia, hypotension, fever, decreasing level of consciousness, reduced urinary output, or failure of gastric emptying.
- Weeping, crusted, and exudative areas of the skin should be treated by local application of potassium permanganate soaks (1:10 000).
- Necrotic epidermis should be carefully removed because it forms a focus for infection. Affected skin that has not become necrotic should not be removed. Topical silver salfadiazine cream should be avoided as this can cause neutropenia when applied to large surface areas.

Prevent complications: ocular involvement

- Corneal scarring and blindness are the commonest sequelae of TEN.
- The cornea should be examined daily by an ophthalmologist and antibiotic or antiseptic eye drops should be applied every 1–2h.
- Synechiae form usually in the second week. These can be separated using a blunt instrument several times a day but this is controversial and the advice of an ophthalmologist is essential.
- Sicca syndrome and visual impairment due to corneal neovascularization may produce corneal scarring and blindness. Symptoms usually develop several weeks after the onset of TEN.

Specific systemic therapy

- There is no controlled evidence that any specific systemic therapy improves prognosis. In particular there is no evidence that systemic steroids are beneficial and adverse effects are numerous. Steroids should not be used as a standard therapy for TEN.
- Early treatment in first 12–24h with ciclosporin (3–4mg/kg/day) or cyclophosphamide (150–300mg per day) are beneficial but neither drug is established as a standard therapy in TEN and these drugs should not be prescribed without specialist advice.
- More recently good results have been obtained with high-dose IVIG therapy used in conjunction with pulsed methylprednisolone. Plasmapheresis may be of benefit in some patients.

Chapter 13

Psychiatric emergencies

Acute confusion: assessment

Acute confusional states, or delirium, are relatively common. They are particularly common in care of the elderly and orthopaedic wards. Acute confusion may occur on a background of chronic cognitive impairment (dementia), and may last for a prolonged period of days or even weeks. Acute confusion may occur as part of a mental illness or be 2° to organic disease (e.g. brain tumour or encephalitis).

Common features of acute confusion

- Rapid onset
- Fluctuation
- Clouding of consciousness
- Impaired recent and immediate memory
- Disorientation
- Perceptual disturbance, especially in visual or tactile modalities
- Psychomotor disturbance (agitation or ↓ movements)
- Altered sleep–wake cycle
- Evidence of underlying cause.

Common causes of acute confusion

- Pain or discomfort (e.g. urinary retention, constipation)
- Hypoxia
- Metabolic disorders (renal failure, liver failure, acidosis, hypercalcaemia, hypoglycaemia) or endocrine disease (thyrotoxicosis, Addison's disease, diabetes mellitus)
- Infection (systemic or localized)
- Cardiac (MI, CCF, endocarditis)
- Neurological (head injury, subdural haematoma, CNS infection, postictal states)
- Drugs (prescribed: benzodiazepines, opiates, digoxin, cimetidine, steroids, anti-parkinsonian drugs, anticholinergics, or recreational: especially stimulants)
- Alcohol or drug withdrawal.

Detection of acute confusion

- The presence or absence of cognitive impairment may help distinguish between organic and functional mental impairment.
- The 10-point Abbreviated Mental Test Score or the 30-point Mini Mental State Examination (see extract in Table 13.1) give a rapid estimate of key cognitive functions.
- Take a clear history from friends or relatives and try to determine whether delirium is superimposed upon dementia.

Practice point

Patients with visual hallucinations usually have organic confusion.

Table 13.1 Mini-mental state evaluation (MMSE) sample

Score	Section	Task
	Orientation	
5	e.g.	What is the date?
	Registration	
3	e.g.	Listen carefully. I am going to say three words. You say them back after I stop. Ready? Here they are… APPLE (pause), PENNY (pause), TABLE (pause), Now repeat those words back to me. (Repeat up to 5 times, but only score the first trial.)
	Language	
2	e.g.	What is this? (Point to a pencil or pen.)
3	e.g.	Please read this and do what it says. (Show examinee the words on the stimulus form.) CLOSE YOUR EYES.
30	Total score	
Score results		
30–29	Normal.	
28–26	Borderline cognitive dysfunction.	
25–18	Marked cognitive dysfunction—may be diagnosed as demented.	
<17	Severe dysfunction—severe dementia.	

Acute confusion: management

- Treat the cause. Always consider alcohol withdrawal (see Box 13.1).
- It is often sufficient to treat the patient conservatively. Nurse in a well lit quiet room with familiar nursing staff or, better still, a familiar person such as a family member.
- Occasionally patients may refuse investigations or treatment. It may be important to go ahead with baseline investigations in order to rule out life-threatening causes for the confusion and this may need to be done under common law (see 📖 p.680).
- If sedation is required, use small amounts of sedatives given orally if possible. Offer liquid preparations if tablets are refused. Parenteral medication may be indicated if patients refuse or are particularly disturbed. See next section for drugs and doses.
- Patients with on-going disturbance may require regular sedation. Regular use of benzodiazepines may induce tolerance and dependence, so this is best avoided.

Sedation for acutely disturbed patients

- Start with haloperidol 2.5–10mg, which can be used in the elderly. Atypical antipsychotics such as risperidone 1–2mg or olanzapine 5–10mg are best avoided in the elderly, but if used, administer at half the usual dose.
- If needed, add lorazepam 1–2mg (0.5–1mg in elderly) but remember that benzodiazepines may exacerbate confusion.
- Some patients, such as those with parkinsonism or those who are neuroleptic naïve, are extremely sensitive to neuroleptics and may develop severe extra-pyramidal side effects. Use low doses of antipsychotic if you are unsure. Dystonic reactions should be treated with anti-cholinergic drugs such as procyclidine.
- If parenteral medications are required, use lorazepam and/or haloperidol (doses as listed earlier). IM diazepam is sometimes used but is erratically absorbed and hence usually avoided.
- Reassess the degree of sedation after 15–20min.
- Patients with heavy sedation require vital signs monitoring every 5–10min for the first hour then half-hourly until they are ambulatory.

Prognosis in acute confusion

Delirium and dementia both carry adverse prognosis. In particular, delirium increases length of hospital stay and is associated with a significant mortality and may lead to residual cognitive impairment. It is important to ensure that cognitive assessment is repeated after the episode prior to discharge as residual deficits may go undetected otherwise.

Box 13.1 Key points: sedation for acutely disturbed patients

- Oral medication:
  - Atypical antipsychotics: risperidone 1–2mg or olanzapine 5–10mg (half doses in the elderly).
  - Alternatively, haloperidol 2.5–10mg or chlorpromazine 25–50mg may be used.
  - Add lorazepam 1–2mg (0.5–1mg in elderly) if needed.
  - If parenteral medications are required use lorazepam and/or haloperidol (doses as described earlier).
- Reassess the patient after 15–20min to assess the effects of the sedation.
- Monitor vital signs every 5–10min for the first hour then half-hourly until they are ambulatory.
- Patients with parkinsonism, or the neuroleptic naïve, may develop severe extrapyramidal side effects. Use low doses initially and treat any dystonic reactions with an anticholinergic drug (e.g. procyclidine).

Acute alcohol withdrawal

Also see 📖 p.414.

Untreated, this carries a risk of seizures, permanent neurological complications, and death. It should be treated as a medical emergency.

Detection of alcohol withdrawal

Early clinical features include anxiety, restlessness, tremor, insomnia, sweating, tachycardia, ataxia, and pyrexia. Withdrawal may be complicated by seizures especially in those with known epilepsy. Delirium tremens can develop, and is characterized by confusion and disorientation, labile mood and irritability, hallucinations (auditory and visual), and fleeting delusions, often very frightening. Untreated, this condition carries a significant risk of death.

Do not forget to screen for Wernicke–Korsakoff syndrome, a complication of acute thiamine deficiency which occurs in chronic alcoholism. Wernicke's encephalopathy presents with acute confusion, ataxia, nystagmus, and ophthalmoplegia ± peripheral neuropathy. Not all of these symptoms need be present. Untreated, a large number of these patients will develop long-term memory problems from Korsakoff syndrome.

Treatment of alcohol withdrawal

- Alcohol withdrawal patients can often be treated as outpatients.
- The indications for inpatient alcohol withdrawal include patients with a history of seizures or delirium tremens, or signs suggestive of delirium tremens or confusion, symptoms of Wermicke–Korsakoff syndrome, severe nausea and vomiting, comorbid mental/physical illness, polydrug misuse, risk of suicide, or unstable home environment.
- Alcohol withdrawal can be treated by chlordiazepoxide or diazepam. If an IV agent is needed use diazepam. B-complex vitamins are required to prevent Wernicke–Korsakoff syndrome. In the first instance, parenteral therapy as Pabrinex® (ampoules 1 and 2, 1–2 pairs daily for 3–5 days IV or IM) togther with oral thiamine (200mg/day), and thereafter oral vitamin supplements should be given.
- Other useful drugs may include:
    - Atenolol or propranolol for hypertension
    - Carbamazepine for seizures
    - Haloperidol for hallucinations: not usually required.

Withdrawal regime

See 📖 p.414.

Aftercare

- Maintenance thiamine or multivitamin therapy is should be given initially.
- Screen for residual cognitive impairment.

- Mobility and occupational therapy assessments before discharge may help if there are problems with the home environment.
- Identify the patient's local drug and alcohol service and encourage the patient to self-refer.
- Some hospitals have alcohol liaison nurses who may be able to assist with counselling or follow-up. Non-NHS organizations include the AA.

Practice point

Sudden onset of confusion, delirium with sweating and shaking, particularly in patients recently hospitalized, may indicate alcohol withdrawal. Check the serum phosphate, as it may be very low (<0.4 mmol/L) in acute alcohol withdrawal, and lead to confusion or profound weakness. It should be treated with IV phosphates to maintain a plasma concentration >0.4 mmol/L.

Dealing with violent patients

Occasionally you may encounter violent patients in medical settings, and assaults on doctors and nurses do happen from time to time. Violence may be a symptom of a disorder (e.g. psychosis, post-ictal, acute confusion), or patients may be violent because of frustration, criminality etc. Diagnosis is key because management is very different.

Predisposing factors

- Delirium
- Dementia
- Epilepsy
- Brain damage (especially temporal or frontal lobes)
- Alcohol intoxication or withdrawal
- Drugs (cocaine, crack, amphetamine, opiate, or sedative withdrawal)
- Acute psychotic episode
- Personality disorder
- Previous violent behaviour in patients with such conditions may give an indication of future risk.

Management

Risks posed by violent patients may be minimized by following some simple rules.

- Do not see patients who may be violent in an isolated room, and do not see them on your own: ask a nurse or other professional to join you.
- Keep yourself between the patient and the door.
- If you are uncomfortable or afraid, end the interview and leave.
- It is usually sufficient to calm the patient down verbally and avoid confrontation.
- On occasion, it is necessary to sedate violent patients. Offer oral medication first, but give IM if necessary. Haloperidol 5–10mg is the drug of choice, with lorazepam 1–2mg if additional sedation is required.
- Restraint may be required, particularly if sedation is needed: security and nursing staff may do this, ± police if necessary.
- If violence is part of an underlying psychiatric disorder liaise with the psychiatric team about current and ongoing management.

Deliberate self-harm

Deliberate self-harm (DSH) is a common presenting complaint to A&E and reason for admission. The severity and sequelae of DSH vary greatly, from superficial cuts to serious overdoses requiring prolonged spells in hospital. Suicide is uncommon, but DSH increases the risk of subsequent suicide (1% of those who commit acts of DSH kill themselves in the next year—100× the general population risk) and 40–60% of suicides have a history of DSH. Assessment of patients who have harmed themselves is important in order to:

- Detect those at risk of subsequent DSH or suicide (Box 13.2)
- Identify patients with significant mental health problems requiring treatment
- Plan aftercare in hospital or in the community.

Assessment by general medical staff

Assessment of DSH is normally done by a psychiatrist, specialist nurse, or social experienced in the field. However, it is important for all staff to be able to make a basic assessment of these patients, because patients may refuse to see a mental health worker or may attempt to leave the ward or department before a detailed assessment can be carried out.

What if a patient wants to leave before they are assessed by a mental health professional?

- You have a duty of care to the patient that includes protecting them as best you can from ongoing risk.
- Try to persuade the patient to stay for an assessment. If they agree, refer to the psychiatric team and ask the nursing staff to monitor the patient.
- If the patient refuses, then you will need to ask them to stay whilst you make your own assessment of risk.
- If they will not stay, and you are concerned, you will need to detain them under common law pending a formal psychiatric assessment.
- If they agree to stay, make your assessment. Do not forget to enquire about past episodes of self-harm and ongoing psychiatric problems, as well as the questions already detailed.
- If, after your assessment, you have concerns that require the patient to see a mental health professional, try to persuade them to stay. If they refuse, consider detaining them under common law pending urgent psychiatric assessment.
- If you are satisfied that the ongoing risk is not of a magnitude that requires them to be detained, then allow them to be discharged but ensure that the GP is informed.
- Detaining patients who will not stay in hospital: see 📖 p.684.
- Guidelines on treatment for patients who are refusing treatment: see 📖 p.682 and 📖 p.683.

Points to remember about DSH

- Risk assessment in older adults or children and adolescents requires specialist input. Always obtain advice in these cases.
- Staff attitudes towards patients who self-harm, especially if they do so frequently, can be very negative. Patients usually notice this. Try and maintain an empathic attitude and to understand what may motivate the behaviour, however difficult this may be.
- Some patients present repeatedly with DSH. These patients may have personality disorders with or without substance misuse, and may be very difficult to manage. Most A&E departments know their frequent attendees well and have strategies in place for particular individuals: always ask.

Box 13.2 Questions to assess suicide risk after an act of self-harm

- Current mood and mood at time of act?
- Any forward planning, final acts, or suicide notes?
- Any precautions against being discovered?
- What was going through their mind at the time of the act?
- Did they mean to die?
- What is their view on having survived?
- What are their thoughts about the future now?
- Have they any feelings now that they wish to harm themselves? Have they made plans?

Practice point

The phrase 'detain under common law' is contentious. While a doctor who acted to prevent a patient from immediate harm, e.g. by stopping an acutely suicidal patient from leaving A&E is unlikely to be criticized and could claim a common law defence of 'necessity' and 'best interests' if he was, there is strictly speaking no power to detain under the common law.

The Mental Health Act and common law

There is frequent confusion about the ability of patients with mental health problems to consent to or refuse medical treatment, and what to do if a patient is acting in a way that will lead to self harm or harm to others.

The Mental Health Act 1983

Different rules apply in Scotland although the principles are the same: seek local advice.

This act allows for the compulsory detention and/or treatment of patients with mental illness and/or mental impairment of a nature and/or degree that requires inpatient treatment against their wishes. Thus patients who need to be in hospital because of a risk to their health and safety or that of others may be detained or brought into hospital if the appropriate people agree that this is necessary.

- Section 2 allows a period of assessment and/or treatment for up to 28 days, and is usually applied to patients presenting for the first time or known patients with a new problem.
- Section 3 (which may also follow a Section 2) allows detention for treatment for up to 6 months.
- Patients have the right to appeal against both Sections 2 and 3. Both sections require opinions from two appropriately qualified doctors and an approved social worker.
- Section 4 allows patients to be brought to hospital with only one medical and social worker opinion, and is only used in emergencies.
- Sections 5(2) and 5(4) apply to hospital inpatients. See next section.
- Section 136 allows patients to be brought by the police to A&E (or a 'designated place of safety') to be assessed by a doctor and a social worker who may make them informal or arrange for a Section 2 or 3.

People may be placed under a section either in the community or in hospital. It is possible to detain a patient on a medical ward and nurse them there if they require medical treatment (see next section).

Common law

- This allows medical practitioners to act in the patient's best interests in emergency situations where they are unable to give consent (e.g. if they are unconscious, or conscious but lack capacity).
- If in an emergency, it is deemed necessary to detain a patient pending assessment or to treat a patient against their will then it is done so under common law.
- Treatment under common law is given in the best interests of the patient if it is carried out to save life or to ensure improvement or prevent deterioration of physical or mental health.

Always document in the notes that you are giving treatment in the patient's best interests under common law.

Practice point

In emergency situations where patients are unable to give consent (e.g. if unconscious, or lacking 'capacity'), medical practitioners can act in the patient's best interests and detain them pending assessment or to treat them against their will, under 'common law'.

Treating patients against their will

The issue of whether and how to treat patients against their will arises surprisingly often. It is frequently presumed that this is due to mental illness although often this is not so.

What to do in this situation

The key to whether or not a patient is able to refuse treatment is whether or not they have capacity to do so. Psychiatrists are frequently asked to assess capacity, but in an emergency this is not always possible.

For a patient to have capacity, they must be able to understand the decision; understand the alternative courses of action—and which would be reasonable; retain memory of decisions and the reasons for them; communicate their intent.

Remember

- Patients may have the capacity to make some decisions and not others.
- Capacity in the same patient may fluctuate over time.

Mental illness or cognitive impairment may impair capacity, but need not do so: there are legal precedents where patients who are mentally unwell have been wrongfully treated against their will. Disagreeing with medical advice does not automatically constitute incapacity.

If a patient does not have capacity and requires emergency treatment, then this may be given against their will under common law (see 📖 p.686).

The law on consent and capacity

- There is no such thing as proxy consent for adults in the UK: a third party cannot make a decision on a patient's behalf, though it is good practice to take their views into consideration.
- The Mental Health Act 1983 does not allow doctors to treat mentally impaired patients against their will for physical problems. Psychiatrists are occasionally asked to 'section' patients in order that they should be treated for a medical condition. Some regard this as legally contentious, even if the physical problem results from the mental problem (e.g. deliberate self-poisoning). The only exception would be where the physical condition is the cause of the mental condition, e.g. detaining and treating a patient with severe confusion 2° to organic illness. The Scottish act allows a broader view of allowable treatments and may well include treatment of self-poisoning (implied in the code of practice), and certainly does include treatment of delirium and starvation syndrome in anorexia for example.
- Different rules apply to children and individuals with advance directives: you must always obtain specialist advice in such cases.
- Treating a patient who has capacity to refuse against their will can constitute a criminal offence. However, you are unlikely to be criticized for taking a decision to give life-saving treatment against a patient's will if you are unsure about capacity. Most people would acknowledge that it better to treat than not to treat in such situations.
- In any situation where you are unsure of what to do, obtain senior advice at an early stage. Some of the medical defence organizations offer legal advice on a 24-h basis.

Patients who do not wish to stay in hospital

Sometimes patients do not wish to stay in hospital. Usually the problem can be discussed and an agreement can be reached between the patient and the medical team. From time to time this is impossible. If a patient is acutely confused, they may not be willing to stay and require physical restraint in order to keep them there. In the case of patients who have harmed themselves, teams may be concerned about the possible risks to the patient if they leave the ward.

What to do in this situation

- Assess the patient. What are the medical issues that require them to stay? Is their wish to leave a symptom or part of an organic illness that needs to be treated?
- Is it possible to reason with the patient and persuade them to stay?
- If not, they may require psychiatric assessment regarding their capacity to decide to leave.
- If the patient tries to leave before psychiatric assessment, they may be detained under common law.
- If the wait for a psychiatric opinion is likely to take a long time (e.g. no psychiatric team on site), it may be necessary for them to be detained. Hospital inpatients may be detained by a nurse under Section 5(4), or by a single doctor under Section 5(2). Patients in A&E departments must be detained under common law.

Detaining a patient in an emergency

Common law

If you believe it is in the interests of the patient not to be allowed to leave, the security staff may be asked to prevent them from doing so. Document that you are doing this under common law. This should take place until a psychiatric opinion may be obtained.

Section 5(2)

- This section allows an inpatient on any ward to be prevented from leaving. It lasts a maximum of 72h and is only a holding measure pending a full Mental Health Act assessment by appropriate doctor(s) and a social worker.
- Any registered medical practitioner may use Section 5(2), not only a psychiatrist. It must be applied by the consultant under whose care the patient currently is or their 'nominated deputy', i.e. a member of their team or whoever is covering their patients out of hours. It is actioned by filling in a Form 12 (these should be available on the ward) which should be delivered to the local Mental Health Act administration office as soon as it is practicable.
- The Section 5(2) expires once the patient has been seen by an appropriately qualified doctor and it is converted to a Section 2 or 3, or is rescinded. If a patient has been placed under Section 5(2), the duty psychiatry team should be informed, as should the mental health duty Social worker, to ensure that the patient is reassessed appropriately and quickly.
- Section 5(2) does not allow you to enforce medical treatment of any kind. This would need to be given under common law if the patient is not consenting.

Section 5(4)

- This section entitles a suitably qualified nurse to hold a patient for up to 6h pending the arrival of a doctor to assess the patient for Section 5(2). It is only used in situations where a doctor cannot arrive quickly, e.g. if they are off site.
- If the doctor decides that the patient needs to be held under Section 5(2), then the 72-h duration of this latter section begins at the time the nurse imposed the Section 5(4). It ends once the patient has been assessed by appropriate mental health professionals regarding further detention or being made informal.
- Sections 5(2) and 5(4) are only applicable to inpatients, not to patients A&E or outpatients. Patients in these areas are detained under common law pending psychiatric assessment.

Practice point

It is best to detain people under common law if you don't think that they should leave the A&E department. You are unlikely to be criticized for this, and you may ensure their safety in the short term.

Mentally ill patients in hospital

Patients with chronic mental illnesses, such as schizophrenia, are at ↑ risk of ill health compared with the general population, and frequently require care from general physicians.

Guidelines for looking after patients with mental illness

- Hospital is frightening for all patients. Mentally ill patients may require a lot of reassurance and explanation about what is happening to them.
- If people are on regular psychotropic medications, then *give them*. They will usually be able to tell you what they take and when. Remember that sudden discontinuation of certain medications, such as lithium and SSRIs, can precipitate mental health crises.
- Some patients are on depot injections, rather than tablets. Find when their next injection is due and, if this falls during their hospital stay, ensure that they receive it.
- If there is a reason for stopping a drug used in psychiatry, you should ask advice. Ideally, this should be from the psychiatrist and prescriber.
- It is good practice to communicate with the mental health team who know the patient, who will probably be based in the community. They will have a consultant and may have a social worker, community psychiatric nurse, or other keyworker who will appreciate knowing that their patient is in hospital.
- Communicate discharge plans to the community team: it may help you to speed the discharge up as community support may already be in place.

Remember, if you are ever unsure about a patient's mental state, it is best to talk to a psychiatrist about it and ask for them to be reviewed if necessary.

Sectioned patients on medical wards

Occasionally, patients who are in hospital under a section of the Mental Health Act 1983 become medically unwell. They may need to be transferred to and cared for on medical rather than psychiatric wards at these times. Please remember the following:

- Patients who are detained are likely to be seriously mentally unwell and therefore prone to becoming disturbed.
- It is acceptable for patients to be detained on a medical rather than a psychiatric ward under their section if that is where they need to be, but you should expect ongoing input from the psychiatric team caring for the patient during their stay.
- Patients who are under a section should be nursed by a mental health nurse at all times, alongside the general ward nurses. If a patient presents particular risks or is very disturbed, >1 nurse may be required.
- Ensure that the psychiatric team looking after the patient are kept informed of the patient's progress, so that their transfer back to the psychiatric unit and their ongoing medical care may be coordinated smoothly.
- Many psychiatric wards have neither the staff nor the equipment to perform even basic procedures (e.g. IV drips, monitoring). Patients going back to these wards need to be well stabilized medically before they return.

Practice points

- Always find out what medication a psychiatrically disturbed patient is taking. It is dangerous to stop certain psychotropic medications.
- New onset of confusion is organic until proved otherwise. Have a low threshold for starting aciclovir or other antiviral therapy until herpes encephalitis is excluded.

Further reading

- Bethlem and Maudsley NHS Trust (1999). *The Maze: Mental Health Act 1983 Guidelines*. Bethlem and Maudsley NHS Trust, London.
- Hughes R (2003). *Neurological Emergencies*, 4th edn. BMJ Books, London.
- Jones R (2001). *The Mental Health Act Manual*, 7th edn. Sweet & Maxwell, London.
- Royal College of Psychiatrists and Royal College of Physicians (2003). *The Psychological Care of Medical Patients*, A Practical Guide, 2nd edn. Royal College of Psychiatrists and Royal College of Physicians, London.
- Taylor D *et al.* (2001). *The Maudsley Prescribing guidelines*, 6th edn. Martin Dunitz, London.
- Wyatt J *et al.* (2006). *Oxford Handbook of Emergency Medicine*, 3rd edn. Oxford University Press, Oxford.

Chapter 14

Drug overdoses

Overdoses: general approach

- Overdoses account for 15% of acute medical emergencies.
- 65% of drugs involved belong to the patient, a relative, or friend.
- 30% of self-poisonings involve multiple drugs.
- 50% of patients will have taken alcohol as well.
- The history may be unreliable. Question any witnesses or family about where a patient was found and any possible access to drugs. Examination may reveal clues as to the likely poison (e.g. pinpoint pupils with opiates) and signs of solvent or ethanol abuse and IV drug use should be noted.

Management

- Priorities are:
  1. Resuscitate the patient
  2. Reduce absorption of the drug if possible
  3. Give specific antidote if available.
- Secure their airway (place in the recovery position) and monitor breathing, BP, temperature, acid–base and electrolytes, and treat seizures or dysrhythmias. Intubate if GCS <8, and not reversible with naloxone. Flumazenil should not be used diagnostically in the unconscious patient (see Box 14.1).
- Take account of any active medical problems that the patient may have, e.g. IV drug users may have concurrent septicaemia, hepatitis, SBE, pulmonary hypertension, or HIV-related disease.
- Measures to reduce gut absorption include:
  - ***Gastric lavage*** is only effective if used up to 1h post OD following a potentially life-threatening overdose. It is contraindicated if corrosive substances or hydrocarbons have been ingested. Protect the airway with ET intubation if conscious level is impaired.
  - ***Activated charcoal*** (50g as a single dose) will adsorb many drugs if given within 1h of ingestion although its effectiveness falls off rapidly thereafter. Drugs *not* adsorbed by charcoal include iron, lithium, salts, alkalis, acids, ethanol, methanol, ethylene glycol, and organic solvents.
  - ***Multiple-dose activated charcoal*** (50g every 4h) may also accelerate whole body clearance of some drugs by interrupting enterohepatic cycling, e.g. phenobarbital, phenytoin, carbamazepine, digoxin, paraquat, dapsone, quinine, and slow-release preparations such as theophylline. Charcoal is rather unpleasant to drink repeatedly and will be more reliably taken if given down a NG tube.
  - ***PEG bowel lavage:*** in whole bowel irrigation, Klean-Prep®, a solution of polyethylene glycol (not to be confused with ethylene glycol!!) is given orally or by NG tube at 2L/h in adults. It is continued until the rectal effluent becomes clear.
  - ***Indications:*** ingestion of sustained-release or enteric-coated preparations of toxic drugs such as calcium channel blockers, lithium. PEG bowel lavage may be used in body packers to hasten passage of packets of illicit drugs.
  - ***Contraindications:*** bowel obstruction, perforation, ileus, or in seriously ill patients e.g. haemodynamic instability.
  - ***Ipecac-induced emesis*** is *no* longer used.

For uncommon overdoses, always seek advice from the National Poisons Unit (listed inside the front cover of the BNF and on 📖 p.849). Advice about poisoning is also available on TOXBASE (http://www.toxbase.org).

Box 14.1 Signs of poisoning in the unconscious patient

Sign	*Consider*
• Hypoventilation	Opiates, ethanol, benzodiazepines
• Hyperventilation	Metabolic acidosis (aspirin, paracetamol), gastric aspiration, carbon monoxide
• Pinpoint pupils	Opiates, organophosphates
• Dilated pupils	Methanol, anticholinergics, tricyclics, LSD
• Bradycardia	β-blockers, digoxin, GHB, diltiazem, verapamil
• Tachyarrhythmias	Tricyclics, anticholinergics, caffeine, theophylline, digoxin
• Hyperthermia	Ecstasy, amphetamines, anticholinergics, SSRIs
• Pyramidal signs, ataxia, hypertonia, hyper-reflexia and extensor plantars	Tricyclics or anticholinergic agents
• Hypertension	Cocaine, amphetamines, ecstasy

NB. Occasionally patients present where poisoning is suspected but not known. Even where the history suggests self-poisoning be aware that serious underlying disease may be present. For example, patients who feel very ill will often self-medicate with aspirin and paracetamol.

Drug overdoses and antidotes

Table 14.1 Drug overdoses and antidotes*

Drug	Action	Antidote/therapy
Antidepressants	Activated charcoal	Diazepam for convulsion Cardiac monitoring
Aspirin	Activated charcoal Gastric emptying if <1h	Alkaline diuresis, haemodialysis
Benzodiazepines	Protect airway	Flumazenil if severe**
β-blockers	Check ABC	Atropine (3mg), glucagon 7mg IM, consider pacing
Calcium antagonists	Calcium gluconate	Anti-cholinergics
Carbon monoxide	Give 100% O_2	Hyperbaric O_2
Cyanide	Give 100% O_2	Sodium thiosulphate dicobalt edentate
Digoxin	Check K^+ and ECG cardiac monitoring	Digibind®, digoxin- binding Ab.
Ethylene glycol	Check acid-base	Infuse ethanol or fomepazole (4 methylpyrazole)
Heavy metals (DMPS)	Ask NPIS (below)	Chelating agents are occasionally recommended
Iron tablets	Charcoal is ineffective	Desferrioxamine
Lithium	Gastric emptying If >4g and <60min	Adequate hydration and dialysis. Activated charcoal is of NO value
Methanol	Check U&Es, glucose	Infuse ethanol, phenytoin for seizures, dialysis if severe
Organophosphorus insectides	Gastric aspiration if <1h Remove clothes and decontaminate	Atropine, pralidoxime, consult NPIS

Table 14.1 *(Cont.)*

Drug	Action	Antidote/therapy
Opiates	Check ventilation	Naloxone
Paracetamol	Activated charcoal if less than 4h	N-acetylcysteine (or methionine)
Paraquat	Activated charcoal	Fuller's Earth (or bentonite or activated charcoal, vitamin E)
Theophylline	Check plasma potassium urgently Cardiac monitoring	Multiple dose of activated Charcoal haemoperfusion

*This table gives an immediate indication of specific therapies that are currently available.

**Flumazenil should not be given in benzodiazepine-dependent individuals or when drugs lowering the seizure threshold e.g tricyclics have been taken in overdose.

NPIS = National Poison Information Service: Telephone UK (+44) (0) 844 892 0111

Amphetamines

This agent (and its cogener methamphetamine) is widely abused for its effects on CNS arousal. A number of its methylenedioxy derivatives (e.g. 'ecstasy' or MDMA) are also available on an illicit basis and have additional hallucinogenic actions (LSD like).

Presentation

Sympathomimetic effects

- Mydriasis
- Hypertension
- Tachycardia
- Skin pallor.

Central effects

- Hyperexcitability
- Agitation
- Talkativeness
- Paranoia (esp. with chronic use).

Complications

- Intracranial (and subarachnoid) haemorrhage: although attributed to its hypertensive effect this can occur after single dose.
- Vasospasm may be seen on angiography ('string-of-beads').
- Ecstasy is associated with a heat-stroke-like syndrome (📖 p.568).

Poor prognostic features

- Hyperpyrexia (>42°C)
- Rhabdomyolysis
- DIC
- Acute kidney injury
- Acute liver failure.

Management

- Sedate agitated patients with a benzodiazepine (e.g. 5–10mg diazepam IV or 1–2mg lorazepam IM/IV). Psychotic patients may require haloperidol (5–10mg IM). Haloperidol may decrease the seizure threshold.
- Monitor core temperature at least hourly initially.
- Seizures should be controlled with diazepam (5–10mg IV stat). New focal signs should prompt urgent CT scanning looking for evidence of intracranial bleeding.
- Significant hypertension (DBP >120mmHg) may respond to sedation with diazepam. If not it should be controlled with IV nitrates, e.g. GTN 1–2mg/h, titrating to response, or IV labetalol if in an HDU.
- Hyperpyrexia requires prompt cooling with tepid sponging or even chilled IV fluids as necessary to keep the rectal temperature <38.5°C. Chlorpromazine (25–50mg IM) will decrease the core temperature but may cause sedation and hypotension. Dantrolene can decrease hyperpyrexia.
- Acidification of the urine can substantially increase drug elimination but can exacerbate electrolyte and pH disturbances and is best avoided.

Antipsychotic drugs

Chlorpromazine, haloperidol, risperidone, olanzapine

All of these drugs have antipsychotic activity with dopamine receptor antagonist activity. Their management is similar.

Presentations

Include deep sleep, coma, extrapyramidal symptoms, abnormal involuntary muscle movements, hypotension, and occasional fitting. Most antipsychotic drugs may cause prolongation of the QT interval and torsade de pointes, but this is most likely with amisupiride.

Management

Includes essential overdose management, symptom-directed and supportive treatment.

- Consider activated charcoal (50g for adults) if the patient presents within 1h of ingestion of a toxic amount.
- Treat hypotension with IV fluids and raising the foot of the bed. Some patients may need an inotropic support.
- Seizures usually respond to diazepam (5–10 mg IV; may be repeated every 15min; max. 30mg) or to phenytoin.
- Cardiac arrhythmias often respond to IV phenytoin (15mg/kg up to 1g total dose), while other antiarrhythmics may be used. IV magnesium sulphate for torsade de pointes.
- Treat extrapyramidal symptoms e.g. acute dystonic reactions with anticholinergic agents e.g. procyclidine (5–10mg IV) or benzatropine mesilate (1–2 mg IV or IM). Benzatropine may not be readily available. These agents are usually effective within 2–5min but may take up to 30min.

Haloperidol

Haloperidol is rapidly absorbed. Peak plasma levels are reached 2–6h after ingestion, with a half-life of 13–35h. Serious toxicity is uncommon. The most common problems are drowsiness and the development of acute dystonic reactions of the type seen with phenothiazines. These include oculo-gyric crises, torticollis, trismus, orolingual dyskinesia, and a feeling that the tongue is swelling. Rarely, hypotension (or conversely hypertension), tachycardia or bradycardia, QT prolongation, ventricular arrhythmias (torsade de pointes), convulsions, hypokalaemia, hypothermia, acute kidney injury and coma may develop. Ventricular arrhythmias have been reported in adults after ingestion of >200 mg haloperidol, and survival has been reported in overdoses up to 1000mg.

Benzodiazepines

Deliberate overdose with this group of compounds is very common. Unless combined with other sedatives (e.g. alcohol or tricyclics) effects of overdosing are generally mild.

Presentation

- Drowsiness
- Slurred speech
- Nystagmus
- Hypotension (mild)
- Ataxia.
- Coma
- Respiratory depression
- Cardiorespiratory arrest (with IV administration)

The elderly are generally more susceptible to cardiorespiratory depression with benzodiazepine overdose.

Management

- If patients present within 1h give 50g activated charcoal. Ensure the patient can protect their airway. No further intervention is usually required for pure benzodiazepine overdoses.
- Flumazenil, a benzodiazepine antagonist, may be used to reverse significant cardiorespiratory depression in severe overdose. *Flumazenil* is given as an IV bolus of 0.2mg. If no response, give further IV bolus doses of 0.3mg and thereafter 0.5mg to a maximum of 3mg until the patient is rousable. Most benzodiazepines have a substantially longer duration of action than flumazenil and an IV infusion of 0.1–0.4mg/h will be needed to prevent early re-sedation.
- Flumazenil should not be used diagnostically in comatose patients where the diagnosis is uncertain, as it may cause fits or death.
- Avoid giving excess flumazenil to completely reverse the effect of a benzodiazepine. In chronic benzodiazepine abusers this can cause marked agitation and may precipitate seizures in patients who have taken an overdose of a combination of benzodiazepines and proconvulsants (e.g. dextropropoxyphene, theophyllines, and tricyclics).

β-blockers

These agents competitively antagonize the effects of endogenous catecholamines. They cause profound effects on AV conduction and myocardial contractility, and their effects are predictable based on their known pharmacology.

Presentation

- Sinus bradycardia
- Hypotension
- Cardiac failure
- Cardiac arrest (asystole or VF)
- Bronchospasm (rare in non-asthmatics)
- Fits (esp. with propranolol).
- Drowsiness
- Hallucinations
- Coma
- Hypoglycaemia (rare)

Prognostic features

- Subjects with pre-existing impaired myocardial contractility are less likely to tolerate an overdose of β-blockers.
- The ECG may provide some indication as to the severity: first-degree heart block occurs with mild overdose; widening of the QRS and prolongation of the corrected QT interval (particularly after sotalol) with moderate to severe overdose.

Management

- Establish IV access.
- Check a 12-lead ECG and then monitor ECG continuously.
- Record HR, BP regularly (at least every 15min).
- Consider *activated charcoal* (50g for adults) if patient presents within 1h of ingestion.
- *Hypotension*: seek expert help early. Treat with IV glucagon (50–150mcg/kg followed by an infusion of 1–5mg/h). This peptide is able to exert an inotropic effect independent of β-receptor activation by raising myocardial cAMP levels. Inotropes such as dobutamine may be used and use of an intra-aortic balloon may provide an adequate cardiac output whilst the drug is metabolized and excreted.
- *Bradycardia*: may respond to atropine alone (3-mg IV bolus). Isoprenaline infusions (5–50mcg/min) may be tried but are often ineffective. If the bradycardia persists and the patient is in cardiogenic shock they may need pacing (📖 pp.752–756).
- *Convulsions*: give diazepam 5–10mg IV initially (📖 p.390).
- *Bronchospasm*: treat initially with high-dose nebulized salbutamol (5–10mg or higher). If nebulized bronchodilators are ineffective, an aminophylline infusion should be used (e.g. 0.5mg/kg/min).
- *Monitor blood glucose* regularly (hourly BMs). If hypoglycaemia develops give 50mL of 50% glucose followed by an IVI of 10% glucose adjusting the rate as necessary.

Calcium channel blockers

Nifedipine and amlodipine

The most important effects are on the cardiovascular system. Dihydropyridine calcium antagonists cause severe hypotension 2° to peripheral vasodilatation. This may be associated with reflex tachycardia. Bradycardia and AV block may be present in severe poisoning.

- Features include nausea, vomiting, dizziness, agitation, confusion and occasionally coma in cases of severe poisoning. Metabolic acidosis, hyperkalaemia, hypocalcaemia, and hyperglycaemia may be present.
- Other reported features include seizures, pulmonary oedema, paralytic ileus, acute pancreatitis, hepatotoxicity, and mesenteric infarction.
- Consider activated charcoal (50g for adults) if the patient presents within 1h of ingestion of a toxic amount.
- Monitor BP and cardiac rhythm. Check U&Es, calcium, glucose and ABGs.
- Perform 12-lead ECG and further ECGs if a slow-release preparation has been ingested or there is a fall in heart rate or BP.
- Asymptomatic patients should be observed for at least 12h after ingestion.
- Correct hypotension by raising the foot of the bed and by giving an appropriate fluid challenge.
- Give atropine for symptomatic bradycardia (1mg for an adult). Repeat doses may be needed.
- In severe cases an insulin and glucose infusion may improve myocardial contractility and improve systemic perfusion. It is particularly useful in the presence of acidosis. Such patients should be managed in an HDU/ITU setting. An infusion of 10–20% glucose should be given with an infusion of insulin at 0.5–1.0U/kg/h. Monitor glucose and potassium.
- If hypotension fails to respond to these steps, consider adrenaline infusion or a combination of dobutamine and noradrenaline. Both regimens may improve cardiac dysfunction and systemic vascular resistance.

Verapamil and diltiazem

- Verapamil and diltiazem have a profound cardiac depressant effect causing hypotension. They also have effects on the AV node causing bradyarrhythmias including junctional escape rhythms, second-degree and complete heart block and asystole. They also cause peripheral vasodilatation.
- Other non-cardiac effects include nausea, vomiting, dizziness, agitation, confusion and occasionally coma in cases of severe poisoning. Metabolic acidosis, hyperkalaemia, hypocalcaemia and hyperglycaemia may be present. Seizures are rare.
- Management is as detailed for nifedipine and amlodipine.

Carbon monoxide

The commonest sources are smoke inhalation, poorly maintained domestic gas appliances and deliberate inhalation of car exhaust fumes. It causes intense tissue hypoxia by 2 mechanisms. Firstly, it interrupts electron transport in mitochondria. Secondly, it reduces O_2 delivery both by competing with O_2 for binding to Hb (its affinity for Hb is 220-fold that of O_2) and altering the shape of the HbO_2 dissociation curve (making it shift to the left).

Presentation

Patients present with signs of hypoxia without cyanosis. Skin and mucosal surfaces may appear 'cherry-red' (most obvious postmortem). Carboxyhaemoglobin (COHb) levels correlate poorly with clinical features. In general, levels of COHb <30% cause only headache and dizziness. 50–60% produces syncope, tachypnoea, tachycardia, and fits. Levels >60% cause increasing risk of cardiorespiratory failure and death.

Complications

These are the predictable result of local hypoxia. Sites at particular risk are CNS, affecting cerebral, cerebellar, or midbrain function, e.g. parkinsonism and akinetic-mutism; the myocardium with ischaemia and infarction; skeletal muscle causing rhabdomyolysis and myoglobinuria; skin involvement ranges from erythema to severe blistering.

Prognostic features

Anaemia, ↑ metabolic rate (e.g. children), and underlying ischaemic heart disease all increase susceptibility to CO. Neurological recovery depends on the duration of hypoxic coma; complete recovery has been reported in young subjects (<50 years) after up to 21h, versus 11h in older subjects.

Management

- An ABG should be taken. Although P_aO_2 may be normal it is essential to measure the COHb concentration. Most ITUs have a carboxyhemoglobinometer. Note: monitoring O_2 saturation with a ***pulse oximeter is unhelpful*** since it will not distinguish HbO_2 and COHb (hence the apparent O_2 saturation will be falsely high).
- Apply a tight-fitting facemask and give 100% O_2. Check a 12-lead ECG and continuously monitor rhythm. Take blood for FBC, U&E, CPK, and cardiac enzymes.
- If the patient is comatose they should be intubated and ventilated with 100% FiO_2 (this reduces the half-life of COHb to 80min cf. 320min on room air). This should also be considered in all patients who are severely acidotic or show evidence of myocardial ischaemia.
- Fits should be controlled with IV diazepam (5–10 mg). The metabolic acidosis is best treated by increasing tissue oxygenation and IV $NaHCO_3$ is best avoided.
- Hyperbaric O_2 will shorten the washout of COHb but access to a hyperbaric chamber makes this difficult. Consider if:
  - The patients has been unconscious
  - If COHb is >30%

  - If there are neurological or psychiatric signs
  - If significant metabolic acidosis.
- Ensure medical follow-up as the neuropsychiatric sequelae may take many weeks to evolve.

Cocaine

Cocaine is rapidly absorbed, when applied intra-nasally ('snorting') or smoked (free-basing 'crack'). Occasionally it presents as massive overdosing when the swallowed packets of illicit, smuggled cocaine rupture. Its subjective and sympathomimetic actions are often indistinguishable from amphetamine.

Presentation

- Hypertension
- Seizures (common)
- Tachycardia
- Skin pallor
- CNS depression (with high doses)
- Ventricular arrhythmias
- Paranoid delusions (chronic use)
- Cardiorespiratory failure.

Complications

- Vasoconstrictor effects on the coronary circulation can cause myocardial ischaemia and infarction even in subjects with normal vessels.
- Cerebrovascular accident.
- Psychotic reactions may occur.

Prognostic features

- The lethal dose of pure cocaine by ingestion is approximately 1g but regular users tolerate larger doses.
- Cocaine can cause seizures in epileptics in 'recreational' doses. Presentation in status epilepticus in non-epileptics implies massive overdose and carries a poor prognosis.
- Rhabdomyolysis, hyperpyrexia, renal failure, severe liver dysfunction, and DIC have been reported and have high mortality.
- Patients with pseudocholinesterase deficiency are thought to be at particular risk of life-threatening cocaine toxicity.

Management

- General measures: establish IV access taking blood for U&Es and CPK. Ensure the airway is clear. If GCS ≤8, consider intubation and mechanical ventilation. Agitation may require diazepam (5–10mg IV). Monitor ECG continuously for arrhythmias.
- Perform a 12-lead ECG for evidence of myocardial ischaemia, infarction or dysrhythmias.
- Narrow-complex tachycardias: if does not settle after treatment with diazepam, give verapamil (5–10mg IV).
- Ventricular arrhythmias: treat with IV 8.4% sodium bicarbonate (50mmol). Lidocaine IV may be used cautiously if no response.
- Monitor core temperature for evidence of *hyperpyrexia*. If necessary, start cooling measures (see 📖 p.568), e.g. tepid sponging, or chilled IV fluids as necessary to keep the temperature below 38.5°C.

Chlorpromazine 25–50mg IM may be useful but may cause sedation and hypotension.

- Significant hypertension (DBP >120mmHg) should be controlled initially with diazepam (5–10mg IV); if it remains high start GTN (IVI of 1–2mg/min, titrating to response). Alternatively, use calcium channel blockers, combined α- and β-blockers (e.g. IV phentolamine) or IV sodium nitroprusside. β-blockers may worsen the hypertension through unopposed alpha effects.
- Chest pain should be treated with diazepam and nitrates (SL or IV). Myocardial MI due to cocaine should be managed conventionally (see 📖 p.36).
- *Seizures* should be controlled with diazepam (10–30mg IV stat and if necessary an IVI of up to 200mg/24h). Presentation with focal seizures after cocaine ingestion usually implies ischaemic or haemorrhage stroke: arrange an urgent brain CT scan.

Cyanide

Poisoning is most commonly seen in victims of smoke inhalation (HCN is a combustion product of polyurethane foams). Cyanide derivatives are, however, widely employed in industrial processes and fertilizers. Children may also ingest amygdalin, a cyanogenic glycoside, contained in kernels of almonds and cherries. Cyanide acts by irreversibly blocking mitochondrial electron transport.

Presentation

HCN gas can lead to cardiorespiratory arrest and death within a few minutes. Onset of effects after ingestion or skin contamination is generally much slower (up to several hours). Early signs are dizziness, chest tightness, dyspnoea, confusion, and paralysis. Cardiovascular collapse, apnoea, and seizures follow. Cyanosis is not a feature. The classical smell of bitter almonds is unhelpful (it is genetically determined and 50% of observers cannot detect it). Pulmonary oedema and lactic acidosis are common in severe poisoning.

Prognostic features

- Ingestion of a few hundred mg of a cyanide salt is usually fatal in adults. Absorption is delayed by a full stomach and high gastric pH (e.g. antacids).
- Patients surviving to reach hospital after inhalation of HCN are unlikely to have suffered significant poisoning.
- Acidosis indicates severe poisoning.

Management

- Do *not* attempt mouth-to-mouth resuscitation. Give 100% O_2 by tight-fitting face mask or ventilate via ET tube if necessary.
- Establish IV access.
- Check ABGs. Lactic acidosis indicates severe poisoning.
- Skin contamination requires thorough washing of the affected area with soap and water.
- If signs of moderate to severe cyanide toxicity are present, give 300mg of dicobalt edetate (Kelocyanor®) IV over 1min, followed immediately by 50mL of 50% glucose. If there is no response in 1min, repeat the dose. Further doses may cause cobalt toxicity. Dicobalt edetate is very toxic and may be fatal in the absence of cyanide poisoning. Alternatively, give sodium nitrite (10mL of a 3% solution) and sodium thiosulphate (25mL of 50% solution). Methaemoglobin levels should be measured if sodium nitrite is given.
- Hydroxocobalamin 5g (Cyanokit®) infused over 15–30min is also available for use when cyanide poisoning is suspected (e.g. smoke inhalation).

Digoxin

Deliberate overdosing with digoxin is unusual. Significant toxicity is, however, a common adverse drug reaction in patients taking digoxin therapeutically (up to 25% of patients in some series). It is particularly common when renal impairment occurs (digoxin is almost totally cleared by the kidneys), and is exacerbated by hypokalaemia.

Presentation

- Nausea, vomiting, confusion, and diarrhoea.
- Visual disturbance (blurring, flashes, disturbed colour vision).
- Cardiac dysrhythmias (tachyarrhythmias or bradyarrhythmias).

Complications

- Hyperkalaemia.
- Cardiac dysrhythmias. The initial effect is usually a marked sinus bradycardia which is vagally mediated. This is followed by atrial tachyarrhythmias (with/without heart block), accelerated junctional rhythms, ventricular ectopy, and finally VT or VF.

Prognostic features

- Digoxin level >10ng/mL and hyperkalaemia represent a severe overdose.
- Susceptibility to digoxin toxicity is ↑ by renal impairment, electrolyte disturbance (↓K^+ or ↓ Mg^{2+}), and hypothyroidism.

Management

- Take blood for a digoxin level (in patients not normally on digoxin, this should be at least 6h post-ingestion) and U&Es.
- Baseline 12-lead ECG and continuous ECG monitoring.
- Gastric lavage should be attempted if seen within 1h of overdose, followed by activated charcoal (50g stat). Activated charcoal (25g) may be repeated every 2h, provided the patient is not vomiting. Sinus bradyarrhythmias and AV block usually respond to atropine (0.6mg IV repeated to a total of 2.4mg). Asymptomatic ventricular ectopics do not require specific treatment.
- Ventricular tachyarrhythmias should be treated with magnesium sulphate (8–10mmol IV).
- Patients with haemodynamic instability, resistant ventricular tachyarrhythmias, or high K^+ require treatment with digoxin-binding antibody fragments (Fab, Digibind®). Dose: (no. of vials) = 1.67 amount ingested (mg). If latter unknown give 20 vials (infused over 30min). The neutralizing dose for patients intoxicated during chronic therapy: (no. of vials) = digoxin level (ng/mL) × wt (kg) × 0.01. Half this dose should initially be given and repeated if there is recurrence of toxicity. Fab therapy will terminate VT in 20–40min. The K^+ and free serum digoxin levels should be monitored for 24h after Fab therapy. A substantial hypokalaemia can develop and not infrequently there is a rebound in digoxin levels which may require administration of additional Fab. In patients with renal impairment this rebound is delayed and monitoring should be extended to 72h.

- Patients with severe renal failure are obviously unable to clear the Fab–digoxin complexes. Plasmapheresis is indicated to clear the bound digoxin.
- If Digibind® is not available, insert a transvenous pacing wire and try to control arrhythmias with a combination of overdrive pacing, DC shock, and drugs (see 📖 pp.760–764).

Ecstasy

Ecstasy, 'E', and 'XTC' are street names for MDMA (methylenedioxy-metamphetamine). Ecstasy may be combined with LSD, ketamine, caffeine, or sildenafil ('sextasy'). Ketamine causes pain-free floating sensations with vivid dreams.

It produces a positive mood state with feelings of ↑sensuality and euphoria. Side effects with chronic use include anorexia, palpitations, jaw stiffness, grinding, of teeth, sweating, and insomnia. It can cause dehydration with hyperthermia, agitation, and fits. Other features include hyponatraemia, cerebral infarction, cerebral haemorrhage, and vasculitis. Most deaths from ecstasy result from disturbance of thermo- and osmoregulation → hyperthermia and ↑plasma osmolality. MDMA also causes life-threatening, cardiac dysrhythmias, abnormal LFTs, acute liver failure, and has been associated with cerebral infarction and haemorrhage.

Severe hyperthermia may occur within hours of ingestion, and often follows intense physical activity. Features include core temperature >40°C, severe metabolic acidosis, muscle rigidity, DIC, and rhabdomyolysis.

Management

Hyperthermia: consider other causes of hyperthermia (📖 p.568). Patients should be treated with dantrolene 1mg/kg up to a maximum of 10mg/kg. Dantrolene inhibits release of calcium from the SR in cells. Rhabdomyolysis should be treated in the usual way (📖 p.294).

Ethanol: acute intoxication

Patients may present either with acute intoxication, withdrawal syndromes, nutritional deficiency syndromes, or chronic toxicity (liver, CNS, peripheral neuromyopathy, etc).

Presentation

Alcohol intoxication results in disinhibition, euphoria, incoordination, ataxia, stupor, and coma. Chronic alcoholics require higher blood ethanol levels than 'social' drinkers for intoxication. Obtain a history from friends or relatives. Examine the patient for signs of chronic liver disease, trauma, or signs of infection.

Complications

- Acute gastritis causes N&V, abdominal plain, and GI bleeding.
- Respiratory depression and arrest, inhalation of vomit (with ARDS), and hypothermia may accompany profound sedation.
- Hypoglycaemia is common and should be excluded.
- Alcoholic ketoacidosis or lactic acidosis.
- Accidental injury, particularly head injury (subdural).
- Rhabdomyolysis and acute renal failure (ARF).
- Infection (septicaemia, meningitis).

Management

- Mild to moderate intoxication usually requires no specific treatment: the need for admission for rehydration and observation depends on the individual patient. Admit all patients with stupor or coma.
- Check the airway is clear of vomitus and the patient is able to protect their airway. Nurse in the recovery position.
- Ipecacuanha, gastric lavage, or charcoal are not indicated.
- Take blood for U&E, CPK, glucose, amylase, and ethanol (and methanol) levels, ABG (acidosis), lactate, ammonia. Analyse, urine (myoglobin, 📖 p.330). Consider the possibility of other drug overdose.
- Monitor closely for respiratory depression, hypoxia, cardiac arrhythmias, and hypotension and withdrawal syndromes (see 📖 p.414 and p.674).
- Check blood glucose. In comatose patients, there is a good argument for giving 25–50mL of 50% glucose immediately for presumed hypoglycaemia because this will usually not cause any harm. Follow with an IVI of 10% glucose if necessary.
- The only concern is that glucose may precipitate Wernicke's encephalopathy in malnourished individuals. Some clinicians therefore favour giving a bolus of thiamine 1–2mg/kg IV beforehand.
- Rehydrate with IV fluids (avoid excessive use of saline in patients with signs of chronic liver disease); monitor urine output.
- Naloxone reduces the effects of alcohol toxicity but is not standard.
- Rarely, haemodialysis is used if intoxication is very severe or in the presence of acidosis.
- After recovery from the acute episode arrange for a psychiatric or medical assessment and follow-up and referral to an alcohol rehabilitation programme if appropriate.
- Alchohol withdrawal and delirium tremens (DTs) see 📖 p.414 and p.674.

Ethylene glycol

Ingestion is usually accidental when ingested as an ethanol 'substitute'; it is present in 'antifreeze'. Ethylene glycol is rapidly absorbed from the gut. Peak concentrations occur 1–4h after ingestion. It is metabolized to glycolaldehyde then to glycolic, glyoxylic, and oxalic acids which are responsible for the majority of its toxic effects. Glycolic acid is cleared by the kidney and is largely responsible for the marked acidosis seen in severe cases. It seems that calcium oxalate monohydrate crystals are the cause of cerebral oedema and renal failure. This metabolic route is blocked by competitive antagonism with ethanol.

Presentation

- Impaired consciousness ('inebriation' without alcohol on breath).
- Seizures and focal neurological signs (e.g. ophthalmoplegias) are seen in the first 24h.
- Loin pain, haematuria, and ATN occur over the next 48h.

Prognostic features

- As little as 30Ml of ethylene glycol can be fatal in adults.
- It is often taken with ethanol which is actually protective by blocking the metabolism of glycol to toxic metabolites.
- Renal failure can be averted if specific treatment is started early.
- Plasma levels of ethylene glycol >500mg/L (8mM) indicate severe overdose.
- The degree of acidosis is the best indicator of likely outcome.

Complications

- Oliguric renal failure (crystal nephropathy)
- Cerebral oedema
- Hypotension
- Non-cardiogenic pulmonary oedema
- Myocarditis.

Management

- Delay in commencing treatment with an antidote will result in a more severely poisoned patient.
- Perform gastric lavage if presenting within 1h of ingestion. This will also enable confirmation that EG has been taken; commercial 'antifreeze' often contains fluorescein which is easily detected with a UV light source (also detectable in urine).
- Establish IV access and take blood for U&Es, glucose, biochemical profile including Ca^{2+}, plasma osmolality, and ethanol and EG levels.
- Check ABGs to assess degree of acidaemia. Calculate anion gap and osmolar gap. Patients will develop a high osmolar gap as they absorb the glycol over the first few hours. Thereafter, as the glycol is metabolized to acids, the osmolar gap will fall while the patient's anion gap will climb and acidosis worsens.
- Microscope a fresh urine sample. Needle-shaped crystals of calcium oxalate monohydrate are pathognomonic.

- Fomepizole is an inhibitor of alcohol dehydrogenase and unlike ethanol it does not cause CNS depression. It is expensive but easier to use than ethanol. It is given as a loading dose of 15mg/kg in 100Ml saline over 30min followed by 12-hourly maintenance doses. Increase frequency of maintenance doses if haemodialysis is needed.
- The half-life of EG is short (3h). If fomepizole is unavailable then an ethanol infusion should be started as soon as possible (see 📖 p.718). The infusion should be continued until plasma EG is undetectable. Infusion of ethanol will cause intoxication.

Indications for dialysis

Severe acidosis (declining vital signs, an EG level >500mg/L) or oliguria requires haemodialysis or peritoneal dialysis (the former is 2–3-fold more effective). Normal renal function is generally restored in 7–10 days although chronic renal failure may follow.

Stages of ethylene glycol toxicity

Typically, after a brief period of inebriation due to the intoxicating effect of ethylene glycol itself, metabolic acidosis develops, followed by tachypnoea, coma, seizures, hypertension, the appearance of pulmonary infiltrates, and oliguric renal failure. Untreated, death from multiorgan failure occurs 24–36h after ingestion.

- ***Stage 1*** (30min to 12h after ingestion): appears intoxicated with alcohol (but no ethanol on breath), N&V ± haematemesis, coma and convulsions (often focal). Nystagmus, ataxia, ophthalmoplegia, papilloedema, hypotonia, hyporeflexia, myoclonic jerks, tetanic contractions and cranial nerve palsies may occur. Metabolic acidosis develops.
- ***Stage 2*** (12–24h after ingestion): ↑respiratory rate, sinus tachycardia, hypertension, pulmonary oedema and congestive cardiac failure develop.
- ***Stage 3*** (24–72h after ingestion): flank pain, renal tenderness, acute tubular necrosis, hypocalcaemia (as a consequence of calcium complexing with oxalate), calcium oxalate monohydrate crystalluria, hyperkalaemia and hypomagnesaemia.

Flunitrazepam

Flunitrazepam is sometimes referred to as the 'date rape' drug. It is used as a short-term treatment for insomnia, as a sedative hypnotic, and a pre-anaesthetic. It has similar effects to diazepam but is ~10× more potent.

Flunitrazepam intoxication leads to impaired judgement and impaired motor skills and can make a victim unable to resist a sexual attack. The combination of alcohol and flunitrazepam has a more marked effect than flunitrazepam alone. Effects begin within 30min, peak by 2h, and can persist for up to 8h. It is commonly reported that persons who become intoxicated on a combination of alcohol and flunitrazepam have 'blackouts' lasting 8–24h following ingestion. Adverse effects of flunitrazepam include ↓BP, memory impairment, drowsiness, visual disturbances, confusion, dizziness, GI disturbances, and urinary retention. Manage as for benzodiazepine overdose.

Gamma hydroxybutyric acid (GHB) or liquid ecstasy

This drug is dissolved in water and consumed until a high is reached. GHB acts as an agonist at GABA receptors in the brain leading to drowsiness, seizures, hypoventilation, and unconsciousness. It acts synergistically with ethanol → CNS and respiratory depression.

Iron

Accidental ingestion is almost exclusively a problem in children. In overdose, iron binding mechanisms are rapidly saturated leading to high concentrations of free iron. The latter catalyses the widespread generation of free radicals which is the basis of the toxic manifestations of iron overdose.

Presentation

- Iron is extremely irritant and causes prominent abdominal pain, vomiting and diarrhoea, haematemesis, and rectal bleeding.
- Usually the initial GI symptoms subside before 2° signs develop 12–24h after ingestion. Hepatic failure, jaundice, fits, and coma are common.
- Very large overdose can cause early cardiovascular collapse and coma.
- In children, 1–2g of iron may prove fatal. Patients alive 72h after ingestion usually make a full recovery.
- Late sequelae of gastric fibrosis and pyloric obstruction have been occasionally reported.

Management

- *Gastric lavage* should be considered following ingestion of >60mg/kg elemental Fe within 1h, provided the airway can be protected. *A plain AXR* may be useful within 2h of ingestion to assess the number of tablets ingested.
- Establish IV access. Take blood for U&Es, LFTs, FBC, serum iron, % saturation.
- If serum iron is between 55–90μmoles/L, repeat after 2h.
- *Parenteral chelation therapy* is indicated if the serum Fe is >90μmol/L (5mg/L) or in shocked patients.
- Give desferrioxamine IV at a rate of 15mg/kg/h for a maximum daily dose of 80mg/kg (i.e ~5h infusion). Desferrioxamine may cause hypotension if infused more rapidly than recommended. Pulmonary oedema and ARDS have been reported in patients treated at >80mg/kg/day for >24h.
- *Dialysis*: haemodialysis is indicated for very high serum iron levels that respond poorly to chelation therapy or if the urine output is not maintained during chelation therapy as the iron-chelate is excreted in the urine.

Lithium

Lithium has a low therapeutic index and accidental toxicity can and does occur much more frequently than deliberate self-administration. Toxicity is commonly precipitated by administration of diuretics or intercurrent dehydration, e.g. following vomiting or a febrile illness.

Presentation

- Thirst, polyuria, diarrhoea, vomiting, and coarse tremor are common.
- In severe toxicity the effects on the CNS generally predominate, with impairment of consciousness, fine tremor, hypertonia, seizures, and focal neurological signs.
- Cardiac arrhythmia and hypotension are seen in very severe poisoning.

Prognostic features

Features of toxicity are usually associated with Li^+ levels of >1.5mmol/L. However, Li^+ enters cells relatively slowly so that the levels taken shortly after a large overdose may be very high with the patient showing few if any signs of toxicity. Levels >4mmol/L will probably require haemo- or peritoneal dialysis. Patients who are lithium-naïve may tolerate higher levels following an overdose.

Management

- Patients presenting within 1h of ingestion of a large overdose should undergo gastric lavage. Many SR preparations are too large to pass up the lavage tube. If SR preparations are involved whole bowel irrigation with PEG is useful. (NB: activated charcoal does not adsorb lithium).
- Check serum Li^+ level (ensure the tube used does not contain lithium–heparin anticoagulant).
- Check U&Es: if hypernatraemia is present check serum osmolality.
- Any diuretic (especially thiazides) or other drug likely to alter renal handling of Li^+ (e.g. NSAIDs) should be stopped.
- Correct any fluid or electrolyte deficits and ensure adequate hydration. Forced diuresis should *not* be undertaken.
- Patients on chronic lithium therapy with levels >4mmol/L or who have neurological features should be haemodialysed. Although Li^+ can be effectively cleared from the extracellular compartment with dialysis, movement out of cells is much slower. Dialysis should be continued until Li^+ is not detected in the serum or dialysate. Levels should be measured daily for the next week in case Li^+ rebounds due to slow release from intracellular stores.

Lysergic acid diethylamide (LSD)

It is the prototypical psychedelic drug. Although its abuse was a feature of the 1960s and early 1970s it has reappeared in the last few years in increasing amounts. It is no longer manufactured for medicinal use but illicit sources are surprisingly pure, i.e. free of adulterants. The preferred route is ingestion although it is occasionally injected and has been reported to be active if snorted.

Presentation

A typical dose of around 100mcg causes:

- Pupillary dilatation
- Sweating
- An acute anxiety state
- Tachycardia
- Depersonalization, visual illusions, and distortion of time

Large doses can cause convulsions, focal neurological deficit (due to vasospasm), and coma.

Complications

- Acute psychosis with visual hallucination, paranoia, or features of mania is well described.
- Very large overdoses have been associated with a mild bleeding disorder due to blockade of 5-HT-induced platelet aggregation.
- Rhabdomyolysis has been reported in the past but appears to have reflected the physical restraints used, i.e. 'straitjackets'.
- Death from even large overdoses is unusual and usually reflects suicide or accidental trauma while under the psychedelic effects of LSD.

Management

- Absorption is likely to be complete by the time symptoms are manifest. Lavage may worsen the behavioural disturbance.
- Most patients will need a quiet side room and verbal reassurance only ('talking down'). The visual illusions fade in 4–8h.
- Agitated patients can be sedated with diazepam (5–10mg IV) or IM lorazepam (1–2mg) and/or IM haloperidol 5–10mg.
- Seizures respond to diazepam IV (5–10mg bolus).
- Development of focal neurological signs should prompt a CT scan and probably cerebral angiography. Occasionally intense vasospasm is seen involving even the intracranial carotids.
- Comatose patients require supportive care (📖 p.332) but generally recover fully in 24h. Aspiration appears to be a definite risk and protection of the airway is particularly important.
- There are no specific antidotes or methods for enhanced drug elimination.

Methanol

Poisoning usually follows ingestion of contaminated alcohol beverages or 'methylated spirits'. Intoxication in industrial settings follows absorption across the skin or lung. Alcohol dehydrogenase metabolizes it to formaldehyde which is oxidized to the toxic formic acid.

Presentation

- Significant ingestion causes nausea, vomiting, and abdominal pain.
- Its effects on the CNS resemble those of ethanol although in low doses it does not have a euphoric effect.
- Visual symptoms present with falling visual acuity, photophobia, and the sensation of 'being in a snow storm'.

Complications

- Up to 65% of patients have a raised amylase but this does not necessarily represent pancreatitis (usually salivary-gland amylase type). If pancreatitis is suspected clinically, measure serum lipase (haemorrhagic pancreatitis has been reported at postmortem).
- Seizures are seen in severe intoxication. CT scanning usually shows cerebral oedema or even necrosis in the basal ganglia.
- Patients with visual symptoms may develop irreversible visual impairment even with aggressive intervention.
- Rhabdomyolysis and acute renal failure.
- Hypoglycaemia.

Prognostic features

- 10mL of methanol can cause blindness and 30mL can be fatal.
- Peak plasma methanol is useful; >0.2g/L (6.25mmol/L) indicates significant ingestion and 0.5g/L (15.6mmol/L) is severe.
- Arterial pH correlates with formate levels; pH <7.2 is severe intoxication.

Management

- Take blood for U&E, CPK, glucose, amylase and ethanol/methanol levels, plasma osmolality, ABG (acidosis). Calculate anion and osmolar gap. Check urine myoglobin.
- *Seizures* are best treated initially with diazepam (5–10mg IV) and subsequently phenytoin (250mg IV over 5min). Exclude hypoglycaemia.
- *Antidotal therapy* should be given to all patients with methanol levels >0.2g/L (6.25mmol/L), patients with a high osmolar gap (>10 mosm Kg H_2O) or metabolic acidosis (pH<7.3), and anyone needing haemodialysis.
- *Fomepizole* is an inhibitor of alcohol dehydrogenase and has the advantage that unlike ethanol it does not cause CNS depression. It is expensive but is easier to use than ethanol. It is given as a loading dose of 15mg/kg in 100mL saline over 30min followed by 12-hourly maintenance doses of 10mg/kg.
- *Ethanol infusion* is an alternative to fomepizole . Give IV as a 10% solution in 5% glucose or N saline (i.e. take 50mL from a 500-mL bag and replace with 50mL absolute ethanol). A loading dose of 7.5mL/kg

of the 10% solution should be given followed by an IVI of 1Ml/kg/h for non-drinkers (regular drinkers, 2 mL/kg/h). Titrate to a plasma ethanol level of 1–1.5g/L (21.7–32.6mmol/L). Continue ethanol IVI until acidosis or systemic toxicity resolves or methanol level is undetectable.

- Metabolic acidosis should be corrected with IV NaHCO3.
- *Haemodialysis* is reserved for those patients with renal failure, any visual impairment, metabolic acidosis not responsive to sodium bicarbonate or a plasma methanol level of >0.5g/L (15.6mmol/L). The ethanol infusion rate should be doubled during dialysis (or ethanol may be added directly to the dialysis fluid).

Isopropanol

Isopropanol is present in car screen wash. As a cause of poisoning with alcohols this is second after ethanol. It has twice the potency of ethanol on the CNS (its major metabolite, acetone, compounds this) and isopropanol-induced coma can last >24h. Effects are seen within 30–60min of ingestion and large overdoses cause coma and hypotension as the major effect. Haemodialysis is indicated if the hypotension fails to respond to IV fluids, vital signs decline, or blood levels are >4g/L (66.7 mmol/L). Monitor for hypoglycaemia and myoglobinuria.

Olanzapine

See 🕮 Antipsychotic drugs, p.697.

Opiates

Overdosing with opiates usually occurs in regular drug users where the most commonly abused agent is diamorphine (heroin). It may be taken intravenously, by skin-popping, smoked, or snorted. A number of other opiates have been similarly abused. Opiates such as dextropropoxyphene and dihydrocodeine (present in combination formulations with paracetamol) are often taken with alcohol by non-addicts with suicidal intent.

Presentation

Pinpoint pupils, severe respiratory depression ± cyanosis, and coma are typical. The depressive effects are exacerbated by alcohol. BP may be low but is often surprisingly well maintained. Although some opiates, e.g. dextropropoxyphene and pethidine, increase muscle tone and cause fits in overdose in general opiates cause marked hypotonia.

Prognostic features

- Non-cardiogenic pulmonary oedema carries a poor prognosis.
- Patients with underlying ischaemic heart disease may be more susceptible to haemodynamic disturbance after naloxone is given.
- Renal impairment reduces the elimination of many opiates and prolongs their duration of action.

Management

- Monitor respiratory rate, depth of respiration, and pulse oximetry. Give O_2 by mask. Monitor ECG continuously for arrhythmias.
- Establish IV access; take blood for U&Es and CPK. If paracetamol + opiate combinations have been ingested measure a paracetamol level (see 🕮 p.722).
- Any patient who is comatose or has respiratory signs requires a CXR (signs of infection, septic emboli, interstitial shadowing).
- The specific antidote is naloxone (a pure opiate antagonist) which should be given IV in boluses of 0.4mg at 2–3-min intervals until the patient is rousable and any evidence of respiratory depression corrected.

Doses of up to 2mg (and above) may be required but if no response is seen at this level then the diagnosis of opiate overdose should be revised.

- The duration of action of naloxone is shorter than many opiates hence an infusion should be started to avoid resedation (starting with 2/3 the dose required to initially rouse the patient per hour and adjusting as necessary). In the case of overdose with long-acting opiates such as methadone infusion of naloxone may be necessary for 48–72h.
- Avoid giving sufficient naloxone to completely reverse the effect of opiates in an opiate-dependent subject. This is likely to precipitate an acute withdrawal reaction. If this occurs and hypertension is marked (DBP >120mmHg) then give diazepam (5–10mg initially IV), and if it persists, commence IV GTN (1–2mg/h, titrating until BP is controlled). NB: marked hypertension, acute pulmonary oedema, and VT/VF have been observed in non-addicts given naloxone to reverse the effects of high therapeutic doses of opiates for pain.
- Convulsions which are opiate induced (usually pethidine or dextropropoxyphene) may respond to IV naloxone. Additional anticonvulsant therapy may be required.
- Pulmonary oedema present on admission requires O_2, CPAP, or mechanical ventilation (📖 p.776). It does not respond to naloxone.
- Rhabdomyolysis and acute renal failure, see 📖 p.294.

Complications

- All opiates can cause non-cardiogenic pulmonary oedema although it is most frequently seen with IV heroin.
- Rhabdomyolysis is common in opiate-induced coma and should be looked for in all cases.
- The substances used to dilute ('cut') illicit opiates may also carry significant toxicity when injected (e.g. talc and quinine).
- IV drug users may develop right-sided endocarditis and septic pulmonary emboli (several localized infiltrates on CXR).
- Ingestion of paracetamol containing preparations (e.g. co-dydramol) may develop renal or hepatic failure.

Important points

- Dextropropoxyphene in combination with alcohol can cause marked CNS depression. Respiratory arrest can evolve rapidly within <30minutes of ingestion. Give naloxone even if the patient is only mildly drowsy. Dextropropoxyphene also causes an acute cardiotoxicity with arrhythmias due to a membrane-stabilizing effect (naloxone ineffective).
- The respiratory depressant effects of buprenorphine are not fully reversed by naloxone. Doxapram has been used in milder cases of buprenorphine overdose as a respiratory stimulant (1–4mg/min) but mechanical ventilation is preferable in severe cases.

Paracetamol: assessment

In therapeutic doses, only a minor fraction is oxidized to the reactive/toxic species (NABQI) which is detoxified by conjugation with glutathione. In overdose, normal metabolic routes become saturated; therefore an ↑ fraction is metabolized via the cytochrome p450 system to toxic metabolites, whose detoxification rapidly depletes hepatic glutathione stores.

Presentation

- Apart from mild nausea, vomiting, and anorexia, patients presenting within 24h of ingestion are generally asymptomatic.
- Hepatic necrosis becomes apparent in 24–36h with right subchondral pain/tenderness, jaundice (and acute liver failure), vomiting, and symptoms of neuroglycopenia (confusion).
- Encephalopathy may worsen over the next 72h.
- Oliguria and renal failure.
- Lactic acidosis: either <12h (very rare) or late (10% of patients with ALF).

Complications

- Acute liver failure (ALF, see 🕮 p.268) with hypoglycaemia, cerebral oedema, and GI bleeding.
- Severe metabolic (lactic) acidosis.
- Pancreatitis (alone or with liver failure).
- Some 10% of patients develop acute renal failure from acute tubular necrosis which may be seen in the absence of liver failure.
- Very rarely patients with G6PD deficiency develop methaemoglobinaemia and haemolysis.

Investigations

- ***Paracetamol*** Measure levels at least 4h post ingestion and plot on the graph in 🕮 Fig. 14.1, p.725. If the time of overdose is not known, measure paracetamol 4h later, but commence N-acetylcysteine if in doubt.
- ***U&Es*** Renal failure generally occurs on day 3.
- ***Glucose*** May fall with progressive liver failure. Give IV glucose (25–50ml of 50% dextrose) if necessary.
- ***FBC*** Thrombocytopenia may be severe In patients with severe overdoses.
- ***LFTs*** Transaminases rise by 24h.
- ***PT*** May be normal despite high transaminases. The PT is the best indicator of the severity of liver failure.
- ***ABGs*** To assess degree of acidosis.

Prognostic features

Fatal overdose may occur with <10g (usually in alcoholics, epileptics, or patients on enzyme-inducing drugs), but usually involves >30g. The cause of death is usually acute liver failure. Chronic alcoholics or patients on phenobarbital or phenytoin are more susceptible to developing hepatotoxicity and nephrotoxicity.

- Refer to a liver unit all patients with acidosis (pH <7.32) and coagulopathy (INR >1.5) (see Box 14.2).
- If renal failure occurs in isolation (no coagulopathy but transaminase levels high), then refer to a renal unit.

Box 14.2 Indications for liver transplantation in paracetamol overdose

- Late acidosis (>36h post overdose) with arterial pH <7.3
- PT >100sec
- Serum creatinine >300μM
- Grade 3 encephalopathy (confused, distressed, barely rousable).

Practice point

Patients with paracetamol OD often develop subconjunctival haematoma due to vomiting, coagulopathy thrombocytopenia.

Paracetamol: management

- Give activated charcoal 50g to patients presenting within 1h of ingestion.
- All patients with a large overdose of paracetamol (>10g) who present 8–24h after ingestion should be treated with NAC until levels are available.
- Mild reactions to NAC occur in 10–15% of patients but can be effectively treated with an antihistamine. NAC can be restarted at a slower rate once the reaction subsides. True allergic reactions are extremely rare.
- Measure paracetamol levels at least 4h post ingestion and ideally 4h later, and plot on the graph in Fig. 14.1.
- All patients on or above the *'normal' treatment line* (and presenting up to 24h after ingestion) should be given NAC (see Box 14.3). Patients who are truly allergic to NAC may be treated with methionine, but this is less effective unless given early.
- Patients on enzyme-inducing drugs (e.g. phenytoin, carbamazepine, rifampicin, phenobarbital, St John's wort) or with a history of high alcohol intake or have low glutathione stores (anorexics, cachexia, AIDS) may develop toxicity at lower plasma levels and should be treated if the level is above the *'high-risk' treatment line* (Fig. 14.1).
- If the initial levels indicate no treatment is necessary, repeat the paracetamol levels 4h later if there is uncertainty about timing of ingestion, drugs delaying gastric emptying or slow-release preparations have been taken.
- Give NAC to all severe overdoses (>10g) that present at within 72h with symptoms or deranged LFTs and PT.
- *Monitor* U&Es, FBC, PT, LFTs, glucose, and ABGs daily. Monitor glucose with blood glucose testing strips at least 6-hourly.
- Give *vitamin K* IV 10mg (as a single dose, in case body stores are deficient) but *avoid giving FFP* unless there is active bleeding. The PT is the best indicator of the severity of liver failure; FFP may only make management decisions (e.g. liver transplantation) more difficult. Patients with encephalopathy or with a rapidly rising PT should be referred to a liver unit.
- Management of *acute liver failure* is discussed on 📖 p.270.

Box 14.3 Specific treatment for paracetamol poisoning

- ***NAC infusion:***
  - 150mg/kg in 200mL 5% glucose over 15min, followed by
  - 50mg/kg in 500Ml 5% glucose over 4h, and finally
  - 100mg/kg in 1L 5% glucose over 16h.
  - Up to 10% of patients have a rash, bronchospasm, or hypotension during the infusion. Stop the IVI and give chlorphenamine (10mg IV).
- ***Oral methionine:***
  - Only use if patient is allergic to NAC. Give 2.5g stat and 3 further doses of 2.5g every 4h.

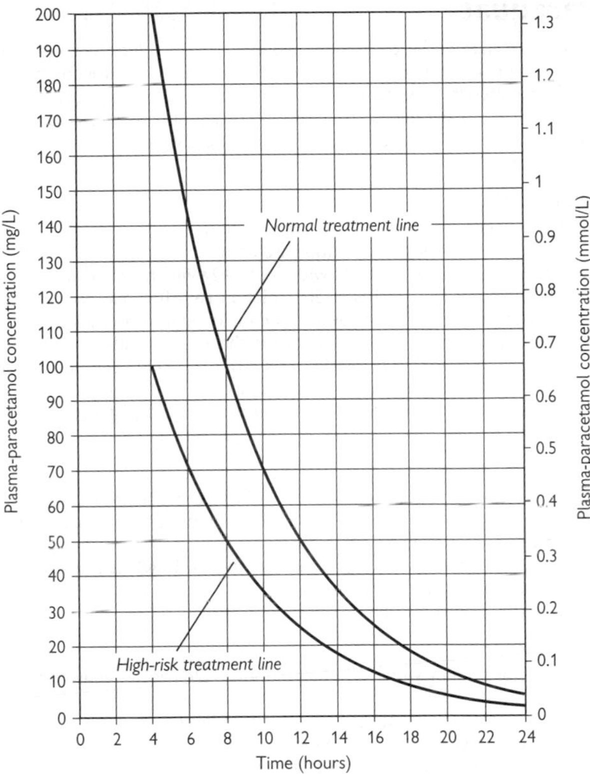

Fig. 14.1 Determining the treatment for paracetamol overdoses. Measure paracetamol levels at least 4h post ingestion and ideally 4h later, and plot on the graph.

Paraquat

This bipyridilium herbicide (Grammoxone® is a 20% solution cf. Weedol® 2.5%) is notoriously toxic in overdose. Children may drink it inadvertantly and horticulturists have occasionally been poisoned through skin splashing. Death is usually due to delayed pulmonary fibrosis and respiratory failure. The mechanism is thought to be due to the generation of cytotoxic oxygen radicals.

Presentation

- N&V are seen within a few hours of ingestion.
- Mouth and oesophageal ulceration are common.
- Oliguric renal failure develops with doses >2g within 12h of ingestion.
- Very high doses (e.g. 50–100mL 20% solution, i.e. >10g) may cause acute dyspnoea with an ARDS-like picture and rapid multi-organ failure.
- Insidious pulmonary fibrosis develops in the 2nd week after exposure (often as the oliguria is resolving). This is not reversible and occasional survivors invariably have a severe handicap.
- Liver failure and myocarditis are also reported and thought to reflect the same free radical-mediated cell damage.

Prognostic features

- The dose ingested is a good predictor of outcome: death has been reported after only 10–15mL of the 20% solution (3g) of paraquat and is universal after 50mL (10g).
- Plasma levels of paraquat e.g. >2mg/L at 4h or 0.1mg/L at 24h are associated with a poor prognosis.
- A low WBC on admission carries a poor prognosis.

Management

- Patients presenting within 1h of ingestion should receive activated charcoal (50–100g).
- Take blood for FBC, U&E, LFT, and paraquat levels.
- Perform a baseline CXR and ABGs.
- Monitor urine output (catheterize if necessary).
- Supplemental O_2 increases toxicity and should be avoided unless required to relieve distressed patients.
- IV fluids (but not a forced diuresis) are indicated when oesophageal ulceration is severe enough to produce dysphagia.
- The use of *haemoperfusion* or *haemofiltration* should be reserved for subjects whose outcome is borderline. It is only in these cases that the very small amounts of paraquat removed by either process (perhaps a few tens of mg) could conceivably affect outcome. Haemodialysis may be needed independently of drug elimination if renal failure develops.
- Attempts should be considered to prevent or slow the process of pulmonary fibrosis.

Risperidone

See 📖 Antipsychotic drugs, p.697 and Haloperidol, p.697.

Salicylates

Aspirin is one of the commonest drugs to be ingested deliberately in overdose. Occasionally poisoning follows the topical application of salicylic acid in keratolytics or ingestion of methyl salicylate ('oil of wintergreen'). Its 1° toxic effect is to uncouple oxidative phosphorylation.

Presentation

- The typical features of moderate salicylate toxicity are sweating, vomiting, epigastric pain, tinnitus, and blurring of vision.
- In adults, there is also an early increase in respiratory rate causing an alkalosis that precedes the later development of a metabolic acidosis (children do not develop the early respiratory alkalosis).
- In severe overdose, the acidosis reduces the ionization of salicylic acid which enhances tissue penetration. In the CNS, this presents as agitation, tremor and fits, coma, and respiratory depression.

Complications

- Disturbance of electrolytes (hypokalaemia and either hyper- or hyponatraemia) and blood glucose (↑ or ↓) are common.
- Pulmonary oedema (non-cardiogenic, ARDS).
- Acute renal failure.
- Abnormal clotting due to hypoprothrombinaemia is very rare.
- Significant GI bleeds are surprisingly infrequent.

Prognostic features

- Therapeutic levels of salicylate are generally <300mg/L (2.2mmol/L). Levels of 500–750mg/L represent moderate OD and >750mg/L (5.4mmol/L) is severe.
    - Children (<10 years) and elderly (>70 years) patients are at higher risk of severe toxicity. Lower threshold for treatment.
- Severe metabolic acidosis is associated with a poor outcome.

Management

- Gastric lavage should be attempted following a large overdose within 1h of ingestion.
- Take blood for U&Es, PT, salicylate, (and paracetamol) level on admission (ideally repeat 4h later to access continued absorption as tablets may adhere to form large masses in the stomach or some preparations are enteric-coated).
- Further doses of oral activated charcoal may be given to patients with rising salicylate levels to prevent late absorption.
- Check arterial blood gases to assess degree of acidosis.
- Monitor blood glucose regularly (lab and/or test strips every 2h).
- Mild or moderate salicylate overdose requires only oral or IV rehydration with particular attention to K^+ supplements.
- Marked signs/symptoms of salicylism or levels >500mg/L need specific elimination therapy (listed in order of use):
    - Urinary alkalinization e.g. 1L 1.26% $NaHCO_3$ over 4h and repeat as necessary to a maximum of ~4L/day to keep urine at pH 7.5–8.5). This may cause hypokalaemia. Check serum potassium every 2–3h.

  Forced alkaline diuresis is no more effective and is potentially dangerous.
  - Haemodialysis is indicated for levels >700mg/L (5.1mmol/L), persistent or progressive acidosis, deteriorating level of consciousness, renal or cardiac failure.
- Pulmonary oedema may indicate either fluid overload or ↑ vascular permeability. Admit to ITU and insert a pulmonary artery catheter for measuring wedge pressures. Non-cardiogenic pulmonary oedema may require CPAP or mechanical ventilation (📖 p.778).

Selective serotonin reuptake inhibitors (SSRIs)

The SSRIs include paroxetine, fluoxetine, citalopram, fluvoxamine and sertraline as well as other drugs.

Presentations

Most SSRIs have similar toxic effects leading to sedation, nausea, vomiting, hepatic dysfunction, sinus tachycardia, ataxia, coma, urinary retention, acute renal failure, dilated pupils, and ECG abnormalities (QT prolongation). The maximal effect on QT prolongation is occurs ~8h after ingestion. Uncommon features include left bundle branch block, supraventricular tachycardia, and torsade de pointes.

Features of the 'serotonin syndrome' may occur in severe poisoning. These include hyperpyrexia, muscle rigidity, and elevation of serum creatine kinase activity.

Management

- Maintain a clear airway and adequate ventilation if consciousness is impaired.
- Consider oral activated charcoal (50g) in adults who have ingested >3mg/kg body weight within 1h.
- Observe asymptomatic patients for at least 6h. Patients with ECG abnormalities should be observed until these resolve. Monitor pulse, BP, temperature, level of consciousness, and cardiac rhythm. Assess QRS and QTc durations. If these are prolonged, administer sodium bicarbonate. Monitor ECG and pulse oximetry.
- Correct hypotension by fluid challenge and raising the foot of the bed. Beta adrenergic agonists such as dobutamine may benefit. The dose of inotrope should be titrated against BP.
- Control convulsions with IV diazepam (5–10 mg in adults) or lorazepam (2–4 mg in adults).
- If metabolic acidosis persists despite correction of hypoxia and adequate fluid resuscitation correct with 250mL of 1.26% sodium bicarbonate IV.
- Ventricular arrhythmias are best treated with IV amiodarone (5mg/kg over 30–60min) or IV disopyramide (2mg/kg over 5min). Avoid lidocaine or mexiletine since they may exacerbate convulsions.
- Haemodialysis or haemofiltration may be required for cases of acute renal failure or severe hyperkalaemia.

Theophylline

Intoxication can be deliberate or iatrogenic due to the low therapeutic index of theophylline.

Presentation

- The features of acute ingestion reflect the local irritant GI effects of theophylline, i.e. nausea, vomiting, abdominal cramps, and diarrhoea. GI bleeding is also well recognized.
- Features of systemic toxicity include cardiac arrhythmias, hypotension, and seizures.

Complications

- Acid–base disturbance: an initial respiratory alkalosis which gives way to a 2° metabolic acidosis.
- Marked hypokalaemia is common.
- Theophylline-induced fits carry a high mortality (up to 30%) and usually reflect serum theophylline levels of >50mg/L (0.28mmol/L).

Management

- ***Gastric lavage*** should be attempted if seen within 1h of ingestion. Multiple-dose activated charcoal should also be given both to prevent further absorption and to enhance systemic clearance (50–100g stat then 50g 4 hourly), although this may not be practical in the presence of severe N&V.
- Take ***blood*** for U&E and theophylline level.
- ***Hypokalaemia*** should be corrected aggressively with IV supplements (40–60mmol/h may be needed).
- Record a ***12-lead ECG*** and then monitor ECG continuously for arrhythmias.
- Verapamil (10mg IV) and propranolol (2–5mg IV) are useful for treating supraventricular and ventricular ***tachyarrhythmias*** respectively. Lidocaine appears to have little effect on ventricular ectopy and should be avoided.
- ***GI bleeding*** should be managed in the usual way (📖 p.224). Avoid cimetidine which substantially inhibits theophylline metabolism (ranitidine is safe, e.g. 50mg IV tds).
- ***Seizures*** should be controlled with diazepam (10mg IV prn).
- ***Haemoperfusion*** (charcoal or resin) should be considered in severe overdoses particularly those with recurrent seizure activity or intractable vomiting. The latter represents direct stimulation of the area postrema and generally responds poorly to antiemetics, e.g. metoclopramide and prochlorperazine but ondansetron is effective (4–8 mg IV).

Tricyclic antidepressants

First-generation agents (e.g. amitriptyline, imipramine, and desipramine) are the most likely to cause lethal intoxication. The newer second-generation tricylics (e.g. lofepramine) and tetracylics are generally much safer in overdose.

Presentation

- Anticholinergic features are prominent early on with dry mouth, dilated pupils, blurred vision, sinus tachycardia, urinary retention, myoclonic jerking, agitation, and hallucinations.
- Cardiac arrhythmias from a quinidine-like effect on the heart, profound hypotension, convulsions, and coma follow.

Complications

- Severe toxicity causes coma with respiratory depression, hypoxia, and a metabolic acidosis.
- Neurological signs include a temporary loss of oculocephalic and oculovestibular reflexes, long tract signs, and internuclear ophthalmoplegia.
- Hypothermia, skin blistering (cf. barbiturates), and rhabdomyolysis are also reported.

Prognostic features

- Death may follow ingestion of as little as 1000mg of a tricyclic.
- Prolongation of the QRS >100ms suggests significant intoxication with a high risk of convulsion; a QRS >160ms is generally seen before ventricular arrhythmias develop. Patients with ischaemic heart disease (especially post MI) and conduction defects are particularly at risk.

Management

- Patients with CNS depression should be monitored closely, preferably on an ITU or high-dependency area.
- Gastric lavage should be attempted if seen within 1h of ingestion. Activated charcoal should be given orally (50g).
- Record a 12-lead ECG and monitor for up to 48h.
- Respiratory failure may require intubation and ventilation.
- Alkalinization with boluses of 50mmol IV 8.4 % sodium bicarbonate aiming for an arterial pH of 7.45–7.55 is the initial treatment for patients with prolonged QRS duration, metabolic acidosis, hypotension or arrhythmias.
- Severe hypotension may be treated with IV glucagon or vasopressors, e.g. noradrenaline (see 🕮 p.315).
- Control seizures with diazepam (5–10mg IV).
- Arrhythmias that do not compromise cardiac output do not need treatment. If BP is failing then correct acidosis or hypoxia before giving antiarrhythmics. Most class I antiarrhythmic agents are ineffective. Magnesium sulphate is used for unresponsive ventricular dysrhythmias.
- Tricyclic coma may last 24–48h. In many patients, recovery is marked by profound agitation and florid visual and auditory hallucination. Sedation may be necessary.

Valproate

- An anticonvulsant used in the treatment of tonic–clonic seizures, particularly in 1° generalized epilepsy, generalized absence and myoclonic seizures.
- Most patients experience mild drowsiness. In severe cases unconsciousness may occur if >200mg/kg body weight of valproate has been ingested. Doses of <5000mg in adults are unlikely to cause toxicity. Fatalities have been reported after ingestion of >20g.
- Toxic effects are frequently associated with blood concentrations >100mg/L. The time to peak plasma concentration depends on the formulation. It is 1–2h for liquid or plain tablets and 3–8h for enteric-coated tablets. In therapeutic doses, the half-life of valproate is 8–14h. In overdose, the half-life may be prolonged to >20h.
- Drowsiness is the commonest feature. Hypotension, nausea, vomiting, diarrhoea and abdominal pain may also occur. In more severe poisoning myoclonic movements, seizures, coma with respiratory and circulatory failure may occur. Cerebral oedema may develop at 12–72h post ingestion. Haemorrhagic pancreatitis can also occur. Diplopia and nystagmus are rarely seen. Metabolic abnormalities include metabolic acidosis, hypernatraemia, hypoglycaemia, hyperammonaemia, and hypocalcaemia.
- Observe for at least 12h after ingestion.
- Monitor pulse, BP and conscious level at least hourly. Check blood glucose, U&Es, LFTs and amylase. Check ABGs and ammonia in severely poisoned patients.
- Consider the use of naloxone in patients with reduced level of consciousness. Although rapid improvement has been reported in moderately severe toxicity.
- Correct hypotension by raising the foot of the bed and by giving an appropriate fluid challenge. Where hypotension is thought mainly due to ↓systemic vascular resistance, drugs with alpha-adrenergic activity such as noradrenaline or high dose dopamine (10–30mcg/kg/min) may be beneficial. The dose of inotrope should be titrated against BP.
- Consider giving L-carnitine to patients who have taken a massive valproate overdose and have hyperammonaemia or hepatotoxicity.

Chapter 15

Practical procedures

Arterial blood sampling

- An arterial blood sample is used to measure the arterial oxygen tension (P_aO_2), carbon dioxide tension (P_aCO_2), pH and bicarbonate/ base excess levels, and Hb saturation (S_aO_2).
- Familiarize yourself with the location and the use of the blood gas machine. Arterial blood is obtained either by percutaneous needle puncture or from an indwelling arterial line.
- ***Radial artery:*** more accessible and more comfortable for the patient; best palpated between the bony head of the distal radius and the tendon of the flexor carpi radialis with the wrist dorsiflexed. The Allen test is used to identify impaired collateral circulation in the hand (a contraindication to radial artery puncture): The patient's hand is held high with the fist clenched and both the radial and ulnar arteries compressed. The hand is lowered, the fist is opened and the pressure from the ulnar artery is released. Colour should return to the hand within 5sec.
- ***Brachial artery:*** best palpated medial to the biceps tendon in the antecubital fossa with the arm is extended and the palm facing up. The needle is inserted just above the elbow crease.
- ***Femoral artery:*** best palpated just below the midpoint of the inguinal ligament, with the leg extended. The needle is inserted below the inguinal ligament at a 90° angle.
- The chosen puncture site should be cleaned. Local anaesthetic should be infiltrated (not into the artery). Use one hand to palpate the artery and the other hand to advance the heparin-coated syringe and needle (22–25G) at 60–90° angle to the skin with gentle aspiration. A flush of bright red blood indicates successful puncture. Remove about 2–3mL of blood, withdraw the needle and ask an assistant to apply pressure to the puncture site for 5–15min. Air bubbles should be removed. The sample is placed on ice and analyzed within 15min (to reduce O_2 consumption by WBC).
- ***Complications*** include persistent bleeding, bruising, injury to the blood vessel and local thrombosis.

Arterial line insertion 1

Indications

- Continuous monitoring of arterial BP in critically ill patients with haemodynamic instability
- Repeated arterial blood sampling.

Contraindications

- Coagulopatghy
- Raynaud's phenomenon
- Thromboangiitis obliterans
- Advanced atherosclerosis
- End arteries such as the brachial artery should be avoided.

Initial measures

- Locate a palpable artery (e.g. radial or femoral).
- Assess ulnar blood flow using Allen test before inserting radial line (see 📖 p.736).
- Position the hand in moderate dorsiflexion with the palm facing up (to bring the artery closer to the skin).
- The site should be cleaned with a sterile preparation solution and draped appropriately.
- Use sterile gloves.
- Use local anaesthetic (1% lidocaine) in a conscious patient.

Over-the-wire technique (Fig. 15.1)

- Palpate the artery with the nondominant hand (1–2cm from the wrist between the bony head of the distal radius and the flexor carpi radialis tendon).
- The catheter and needle are advanced towards the artery at a 30–45° angle (Fig. 15.1a) until blood return is seen (Fig. 15.1b).
- The catheter and needle are then advanced through the vessel a few mm further (Fig. 15.1c).
- The needle is removed (Fig. 15.1d).
- Catheter is slowly withdrawn until pulsatile blood flow is seen (Fig. 15.1e).
- When pulsatile blood flow is seen, the wire is advanced into the vessel (Fig. 15.1f).
- The catheter is advanced further into the vessel ***over the wire*** (Fig. 15.1g).
- While placing pressure over the artery, the wire is removed (Fig. 15.1h) and the catheter is connected to a transduction system.
- Secure the catheter in place using suture or tape.
- Check perfusion to the hand after insertion of the arterial line and at frequent intervals.
- The line should be removed if there are any signs of vascular compromise or as early as possible after it is no longer needed.

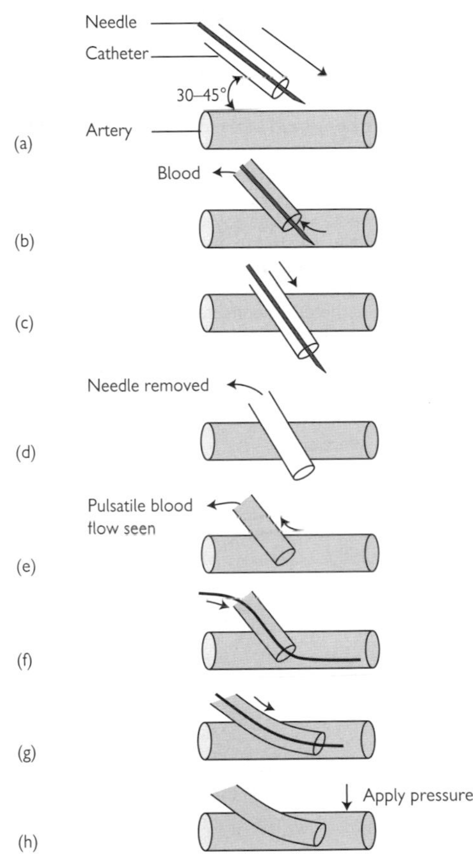

Fig. 15.1 Arterial line insertion: over-the-wire technique.

Arterial line insertion 2

Over-the-needle technique (Fig. 15.2)

Locate and palpate the artery with the nondominant hand (1–2 cm from the wrist between the bony head of the distal radius and the flexor carpi radialis tendon)

- The catheter and needle are advanced towards the artery at a 30–45° angle (Fig. 15.2a) until blood return is seen (Fig. 15.2b).
- The catheter and needle are then advanced slightly further and the catheter/needle angle is lowered to 10–15° (Fig. 15.2c).
- The catheter is advanced ***over the needle*** into the vessel (Fig. 15.2d).
- Proximal pressure is applied to the artery, needle is removed (Fig. 15.2e) and the catheter is connected to the transduction system.
- Secure the catheter in place using suture or tape.
- Check perfusion to the hand after insertion of the arterial line and at frequent intervals.

Complications

- Local and systemic infection.
- Bleeding, haematoma, bruising.
- Vascular complications: blood vessel injury, pseudoaneurysm, thromboembolism, and vasospasm.
- Arterial spasm may occur after multiple unsuccessful attempts at arterial catheterization. If this occurs use an alternative site.
- There may be difficulty in passing wire or catheter despite the return of pulsatile blood. Adjustment of the angle, withdrawal of the needle or a slight advance, may be helpful.

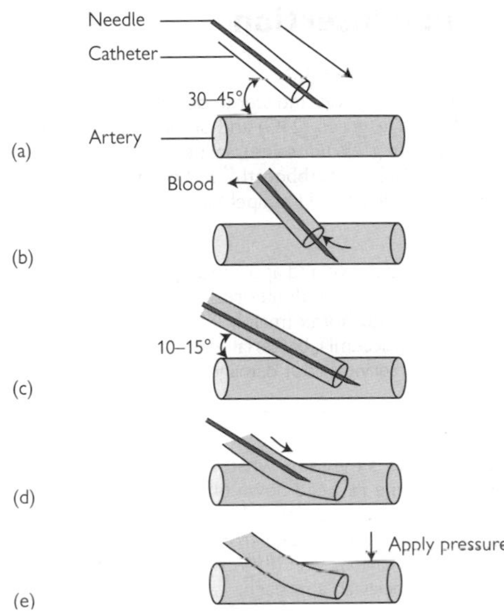

Fig. 15.2 Arterial line insertion: over-the-needle technique.

Central line insertion

You will need the following:

- Sterile dressing pack, gloves and sterile occlusive dressing
- 5- and 10-mL syringe, green (21G) and orange (25G) needles.
- Local anaesthetic (e.g. 2% lidocaine), saline flush.
- Central line (e.g. 16G long Abbocath® or Seldinger catheter).
- Silk suture and needle, No. 11 scalpel blade.

Risks

- Arterial puncture (remove and apply local pressure)
- Pneumothorax (insert chest drain or aspirate if required)
- Haemothorax or chylothorax (mainly left subclavian lines)
- Infection (local, septicaemia, bacterial endocarditis)
- Brachial plexus or cervical root damage (infiltration with LA)
- Arrhythmias.

General procedure

- The basic technique is the same whatever vein is cannulated.
- Lie the patient supine (± head-down tilt).
- Turn the patient's head away from the side you wish to use.
- Clean the skin with chlorhexidine: from the angle of the jaw to the clavicle for internal jugular vein (IJV) cannulation and from the midline to axilla for the subclavian approach.
- Use the drapes to isolate the sterile field.
- Flush the lumen of the central line with saline.
- Identify your landmarks (see 🕮 Figs. 15.3, p.745 and 15.4, p.746).
- Infiltrate skin and subcutaneous tissue with local anaesthetic.
- Have the introducer needle and Seldinger guidewire within easy reach so that you can reach them with one hand without having to release your other hand. Your fingers may be distorting the anatomy slightly making access to the vein easier and if released it may prove difficult to relocate the vein.
- With the introducer needle in the vein, check that you can aspirate blood freely. Use the hand that was on the pulse to immobilize the needle relative to the skin.
- Remove the syringe and pass the guidewire into the vein; it should pass freely. If there is resistance, remove the wire, check that the needle is still within the lumen, and try again.
- Remove the needle leaving the wire within the vein and use a sterile swab to maintain gentle pressure over the site of venepuncture to prevent excessive bleeding.
- With a No. 11 blade make a nick in the skin where the wire enters, to facilitate dilatation of the subcutaneous tissues. Pass the dilator over the wire and remove, leaving wire *in situ*.
- Pass the central line over the wire into the vein. Remove the guidewire, flush the lumen with fresh saline, and close to air.
- Suture the line in place and cover the skin penetration site with a sterile occlusive dressing.
- Measuring the CVP, see Box 15.1.

Box 15.1 Measuring the CVP—tips and pitfalls

- When asked to see a patient at night on the wards with an abnormal CVP reading, it is a good habit to always re-check the zero and the reading yourself.
- Always do measurements with the mid-axillary point as the zero reference. Sitting the patient up will drop the central filling pressure (pooling in the veins).
- Fill the manometer line, being careful not to soak the cotton ball stop. If this gets wet it limits the free-fall of saline or glucose in the manometer line.
- Look at the rate and character of the venous pressure. It should fall to its value quickly and swing with respiration.
- If it fails to fall quickly consider whether the line is open (i.e. saline running in), blocked with blood clot, positional (up against vessel wall; ask patient to take some deep breaths), arterial blood (blood tracks back up the line). Raise the whole dripstand (if you are strong), and make sure that the level falls. If it falls when the whole stand is elevated it may be that the CVP is very high.
- It is easier, and safer, to cannulate a central vein with the patient supine or head down. There is an ↑risk of air embolus if the patient is semi-recumbent.

Internal jugular vein cannulation

The IJV runs just posterolateral to the carotid artery within the carotid sheath and lies medial to the SCM in the upper part of the neck, between the 2 heads of SCM in its medial portion and enters the subclavian vein near the medial border of the anterior scalene muscle (see Fig. 15.3a). There are 3 basic approaches to IJV cannulation: medial to sternocleidomastoid (SCM), between the 2 heads of SCM, or lateral to SCM. The approach used varies and depends on the experience of the operator and the institution.

- Locate the carotid artery between the sternal and clavicular heads of SCM at the level of the thyroid cartilage; the IJV lies just lateral and parallel to it.
- Keeping the fingers of one hand on the carotid pulsation, infiltrate the skin with LA thoroughly, aiming just lateral to this and ensuring that you are not in a vein.
- Ideally, first locate the vein with a blue or green needle. Advance the needle at 45° to the skin, with gentle negative suction on the syringe, aiming for the ipsilateral nipple, lateral to the pulse.
- If you fail to find the vein, withdraw the needle slowly, maintaining negative suction on the syringe (you may have inadvertently transfixed the vein). Aim slightly more medially and try again.
- Once you have identified the position of the vein, change to the syringe with the introducer needle, cannulate the vein, and pass the guidewire into the vein (Fig. 15.3).

Tips and pitfalls

- Venous blood is dark, and arterial blood is pulsatile and bright red!
- Once you locate the vein, change to the syringe with the introducer needle, taking care not to release your fingers from the pulse; they may be distorting the anatomy slightly making access to the vein easier and if released it may prove difficult to relocate the vein.
- The guidewire should pass freely down the needle and into the vein. With the left IJV approach, there are several acute bends that need to be negotiated. If the guidewire keeps passing down the wrong route, ask your assistant to hold the patient's arms out at 90° to the bed, or even above the patient's head, to coax the guidewire down the correct path.
- For patients who are intubated or requiring respiratory support it may be difficult to access the head of the bed. The anterior approach may be easier (see Fig. 15.3b) and may be done from the side of the bed (the left-side of the bed for right-handed operators, using the left hand to locate the pulse and the right to cannulate the vein).
- The IJV may also be readily cannulated with a long Abbocath®. No guidewire is necessary, but, as a result, misplacement is commoner than with the Seldinger technique.
- When using an Abbocath®, on cannulating the vein, remember to advance the sheath and needle a few mm to allow the tip of the plastic sheath (~1mm behind the tip of the bevelled needle) to enter the vein. Holding the needle stationary, advance the sheath over it into the vein.
- Arrange for a CXR to confirm the position of the line.

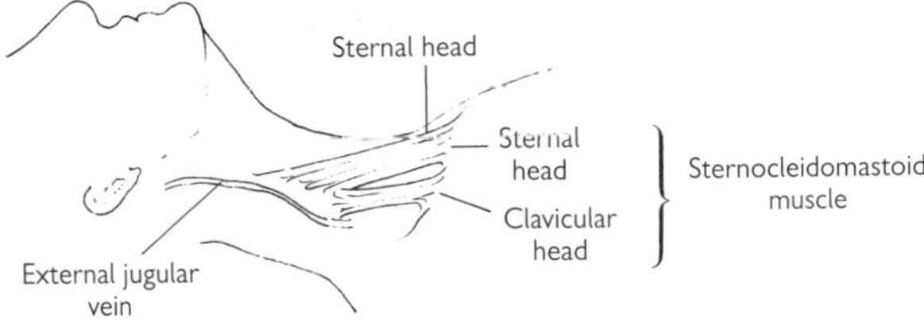

(a) Surface anatomy of external and internal jugular veins

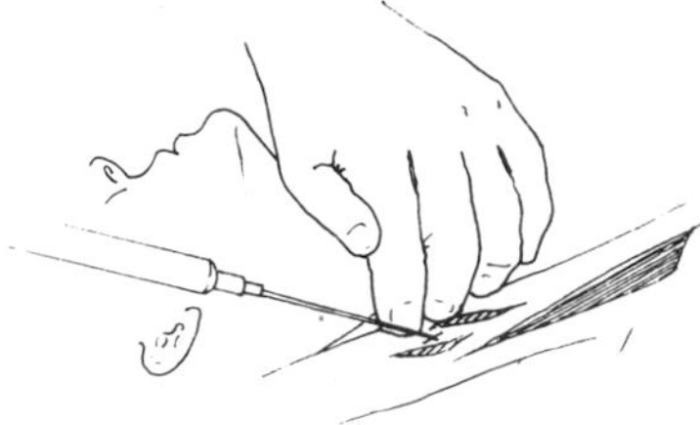

(b) Anterior approach: the chin is in the midline and the skin puncture is over the sternal head of SCM muscle

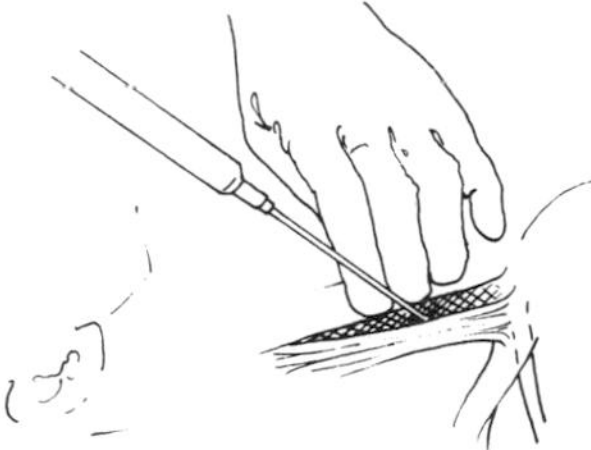

(c) Central approach: the chin is turned away and the skin puncture is between the two heads of SCM muscle

Fig. 15.3 Internal jugular vein cannulation.

Subclavian vein cannulation

The axillary vein becomes the subclavian vein (SCV) at the lateral border of the 1st rib and extends for 3–4cm just deep to the clavicle. It is joined by the ipsilateral IJV to become the brachiocephalic vein behind the sternoclavicular joint. The subclavian artery and brachial plexus lie posteriorly, separated from the vein by the scalenus anterior muscle. The phrenic nerve and the internal mammary artery lie behind the medial portion of the SCV and, on the left, lies the thoracic duct.

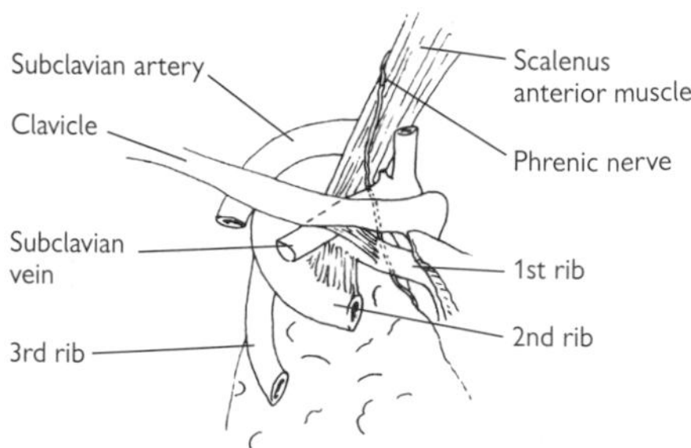

Fig. 15.4 The subclavian vein and surrounding structures.

- Select the point 1cm below the junction of the medial 1/3 and middle 1/3 of the clavicle. If possible place a bag of saline between the scapulae to extend the spine.
- Clean the skin with iodine or chlorhexidine.
- Infiltrate skin and subcutaneous tissue and periosteum of the inferior border of the clavicle with local anaesthetic up to the hilt of the green (21G) needle, ensuring that it is not in a vein.
- Insert the introducer needle with a 10-mL syringe, guiding gently under the clavicle. It is safest to initially hit the clavicle, and 'walk' the needle under it until the inferior border is just cleared. In this way you keep the needle as superficial to the dome of the pleura as possible. Once it has skimmed underneath the clavicle, advance it slowly towards the contralateral sternoclavicular joint, aspirating as you advance. This technique minimizes the risk of pneumothorax, with high success.
- Once the venous blood is obtained, rotate the bevel of the needle towards the heart. This encourages the guidewire to pass down the brachiocephalic rather than up the IJV.
- The wire should pass easily into the vein. If there is difficulty, try advancing during the inspiratory and expiratory phases of the respiratory cycle.
- Once the guidewire is in place, remove the introducer needle, and make a small incision in the skin near the wire to allow the dilator to pass over the wire. When removing the dilator, note the direction that

it faces; it should be slightly curved downwards. If it is slightly curved upwards, then it is likely that the wire has passed up into the IJV. When this happens it is safer to remove the wire and start again.

- After removing the dilator pass the central venous catheter over the guidewire, remove the guidewire, and secure.
- A CXR is mandatory after subclavian line insertion to exclude a pneumothorax and to confirm satisfactory placement of the line, especially if fluoroscopy was not employed.

Ultrasound (US)-guided central venous catheterization 1

Traditional central venous catheterization methods rely on anatomical landmarks to predict vein position. However, the relationship between such landmarks and vein position varies significantly in 'normal' individuals. Failure and complication rates using landmark methods are significant and therefore serious complications may occur. Recent advances in portable US equipment have now made it possible to insert central venous catheters under 2D US guidance.

Advantages of this technique include:
- Identification of actual and relative vein position
- Identification of anatomical variations
- Confirmation of target vein patency.

Guidelines from the National Institute for Health and Clinical Excellence (NICE, September 2002) state: '*Two-dimensional imaging ultrasound guidance is recommended as the preferred method for insertion of central venous catheters into the internal-jugular vein (IJV) in adults and children in elective situations*'. However, training and equipment availability render such recommendations effectively useless in the UK at present.

Equipment/personnel needed
- Standard Seldinger-type kit or whatever is locally available.
- An assistant is essential.
- US equipment:
  - Screen: displays 2D US image of anatomical structures.
  - Sheaths: dedicated, sterile sheaths of PVC or latex long enough to cover probe and connecting cable (a rubber band secures the sheath to the probe).
  - Probe: transducer which emits and receives US information to be processed for display. Marked with arrow or notch for orientation.
  - Power: battery or mains.
  - Sterile gel: transmits US and provides good interface between patient and probe.

Preparation
Perform a preliminary non-sterile scan to access each internal jugular vein for patency and size.

Patient
Sterile precautions should be taken with patient's head turned slightly away from the cannulation site. Head-down tilt (if tolerated) or leg elevation to increase filling and size of the internal jugular vein. Ensure adequate drapes to maintain a sterile field.

Excessive head rotation or extension may decrease the diameter of the vein.

US equipment

- Ensure that the display can be seen.
- Sheath is opened (operator) and gel squirted in (assistant). *A generous amount of gel ensures good contact and air-free coupling between probe tip and sheath. Too little may compromise image quality.*
- Probe and connecting cable are lowered into sheath (assistant) which is then unrolled along them (operator).
- Rubber band secures sheath to probe.
- Sheath over probe tip is smoothed out (wrinkles will degrade image quality).
- Apply liberal amounts of gel to the sheathed probe tip for good US transmission and ↑ patient comfort during movement.

US-guided central venous catheterization 2

Scanning

The most popular scanning orientation for IJV central catheter placement is the transverse plane:

- Apply probe tip *gently* to neck lateral to the carotid pulse at the cricoid level or in the sternomastoid-clavicular triangle
- Keep probe perpendicular at all times with the tip flat against the skin
- Orientate the probe so that movement to the left ensures that the display looks to the left (and vice versa). Probes are usually marked to help orientation. By convention the mark should be to the patient's right (transverse plane) or to the head (longitudinal scan). The marked side appears on the screen as a bright dot
- If the vessels are not immediately visible, keep the probe perpendicular and gently glide medially or laterally until found.

When moving the probe watch the screen—not your hands.

After identification of the IJV

- Position probe so that IJV is shown at the display's horizontal midpoint.
- Keep probe immobile.
- Direct needle (bevel towards probe) caudally under the marked midpoint of the probe tip at approximately 60° to the skin.
- The needle bevel faces the probe to help direct the guidewire down the IJV later.
- Advance the needle towards IJV.

Needle passage causes a 'wavefront' of tissue compression. This is used to judge the progress of the needle and position. Absence of visible tissue reaction indicates incorrect needle placement. Just before vessel entry 'tenting' of the vein is usually observed.

One of the most difficult aspects to learn initially, is the steep needle angulation required, but this ensures that the needle enters the IJV in the US beam and takes the shortest and most direct route through the tissues.

Needle pressure may oppose vein walls resulting in vein transfixion. Slow withdrawal of the needle with continuous aspiration can help result in lumen access.

Pass the guidewire into the jugular vein in the usual fashion.

Re-angling the needle from 60° to a shallower angle, e.g. 45°, may help guidewire feeding. Scanning the vein in the longitudinal plane may demonstrate the catheter in the vessel but after securing and dressing the CVC, an XR should still be obtained to confirm the CVC position, and exclude pneumothorax.

The most common error in measurement of central venous pressure, particularly in CVP lines which have been in place for some time, is due to partial or complete line blockade. With the manometer connected, ensure that the line is free flowing, minor blockages can be removed by squeezing the rubber bung, with the line proximal being obliterated by acute angulation (i.e. bend the tube proximal). Measure the CVP at the mid-axillary line with the patient supine. CVP falls with upright or semi upright recumbency, regardless of the reference point. If the CVP is high, lift the stand that holds the manometer so that the apparent CVP falls by 10cm or so, and replace the CVP stand to ground level. If the saline or manometer reading rises to the same level, then the CVP reading is accurate. In other words, one ensures that the CVP manometer level both falls to and rises to the same level.

Pulmonary artery catheterization 1

Indications

PA catheters (Swan–Ganz catheters) allow direct measurement of a number of haemodynamic parameters that aid clinical decision-making in critically ill patients (evaluate right and left ventricular function, guide treatment, and provide prognostic information). The catheter itself has no therapeutic benefit and there have been a number of studies showing ↑mortality (and morbidity) with their use. Consider inserting a PA catheter in any critically ill patient, after discussion with an experienced physician, if the measurements will influence decisions on therapy (and not just to reassure yourself). Careful and frequent clinical assessment of the patient should always accompany measurements and PA catheterization should not delay treatment of the patient.

General indications (not a comprehensive list) include:

- Management of complicated MI
- Assessment and management of shock
- Assessment and management of respiratory distress (cardiogenic vs non-cardiogenic pulmonary oedema)
- Evaluating effects of treatment in unstable patients (e.g. inotropes, vasodilators, mechanical ventilation, etc.)
- Delivering therapy (e.g. thrombolysis for PE, epoprostenol for pulmonary hypertension, etc.)
- Assessment of fluid requirements in critically ill patients.

Equipment required

- Full resuscitation facilities should be available and the patient's ECG should be continuously monitored.
- Bag of heparinized saline for flushing the catheter and transducer set for pressure monitoring. (Check that your assistant is experienced in setting up the transducer system ***before*** you start.)
- 8F introducer kit (prepackaged kits contain the introducer sheath and all the equipment required for central venous cannulation).
- PA catheter: commonly a triple lumen catheter, that allows simultaneous measurement of RA pressure (proximal port) and PA pressure (distal port) and incorporates a thermistor for measurement of cardiac output by thermodilution. Check your catheter before you start.
- Fluoroscopy is preferable, though not essential.

General technique

- Do not attempt this unless you are experienced.
- Observe strict aseptic technique using sterile drapes, etc.
- Insert the introducer sheath (at least 8F in size) into either the IJV or SCV in the standard way. Flush the sheath with saline and secure to the skin with sutures.
- Do not attach the plastic sterile expandable sheath to the introducer yet but keep it sterile for use later once the catheter is in position (the catheter is easier to manipulate without the plastic covering).

- Flush all the lumens of the PA catheter and attach the distal lumen to the pressure transducer. Check the transducer is zeroed (conventionally to the mid-axillary point). Check the integrity of the balloon by inflating it with the syringe provided (2mL air) and then deflate the balloon.
- The procedure is detailed on 📖 p.754 and p.756.

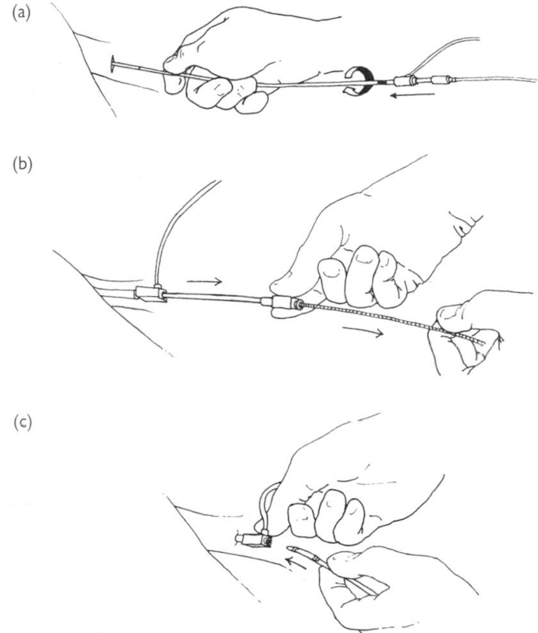

Fig. 15.5 Pulmonary artery catheterization. (a) The sheath and dilator are advanced into the vein over the guidewire. A twisting motion makes insertion easier. (b) The guidewire and dilator are then removed. The sheath has a haemostatic valve at the end preventing leakage of blood. (c) The PA catheter is then inserted through the introducer sheath into the vein.

Pulmonary artery catheterization 2

Insertion technique

- Flush all the lumens of the PA catheter and attach the distal lumen to the pressure transducer. Check the transducer is zeroed (conventionally to the mid-axillary point). Check the integrity of the balloon by inflating it with the syringe provided (~2mL air) and then deflate the balloon.
- Pass the tip of the PA catheter through the plastic sheath, keeping the sheath compressed. The catheter is easier to manipulate without the sheath over it; once in position, extend the sheath over the catheter to keep it sterile.
- With the balloon deflated, advance the tip of the catheter to approx. 10–15cm from the right IJV or SCV, 15–20cm from the left (the markings on the side of the catheter are at 10-cm intervals: 2 lines = 20cm). Check that the pressure tracing is typical of the right atrial pressure (see Fig. 15.6 and Box 15.2).
- Inflate the balloon and advance the catheter gently. The flow of blood will carry the balloon (and catheter) across the tricuspid valve, through the right ventricle, and into the pulmonary artery.
- Watch the ECG tracing closely whilst the catheter is advanced. The catheter commonly triggers runs of VT when crossing the tricuspid valve and through the RV. The VT is usually self-limiting, but should not be ignored. Deflate the balloon, pull back, and try again.
- If >15cm of catheter is advanced into the RV without the tip entering the PA, this suggests the catheter is coiling in the RV. Deflate the balloon, withdraw the catheter into the RA, reinflate the balloon and try again using clockwise torque while advancing in the ventricle, or flushing the catheter with cold saline to stiffen the plastic. If this fails repeatedly, try under fluoroscopic guidance.
- As the tip passes into a distal branch of the PA, the balloon will impact and not pass further, the wedge position and the pressure tracing will change (see Fig. 15.6).
- Deflate the balloon and check that a typical PA tracing is obtained. If not, try flushing the catheter lumen, and, if that fails, withdraw the catheter until the tip is within the PA and begin again.
- Reinflate the balloon slowly. If the PCWP is seen before the balloon is fully inflated, it suggests the tip has migrated further into the artery. Deflate the balloon and withdraw the catheter 1–2cm and try again.
- If the pressure tracing flattens and then continues to rise, you have 'overwedged'. Deflate the balloon, pull back the catheter 1–2cm, and start again.
- When a stable position has been achieved, extend the plastic sheath over the catheter and secure it to the introducer sheath. Clean any blood from the skin insertion site with antiseptic and secure a coil of the PA catheter to the patient's chest to avoid inadvertent removal.
- Obtain a CXR to check the position of the catheter. The tip of the catheter should ideally be no more than 3–5cm from the midline.

Box 15.2 Normal values of right heart pressures and flows

Right atrial pressure	0–8mmHg
Right ventricle	
Systolic	15–30mmHg
End diastolic	0–8mmHg
Pulmonary artery	
Systolic/diastolic	15–30/4–12mmHg
Mean	9–16mmHg
Pulmonary capillary wedge pressure	2–10mmHg
Cardiac index	2.8–4.2L/min/m^2)

(see 📖 p.326 for haemodynamic formulae)

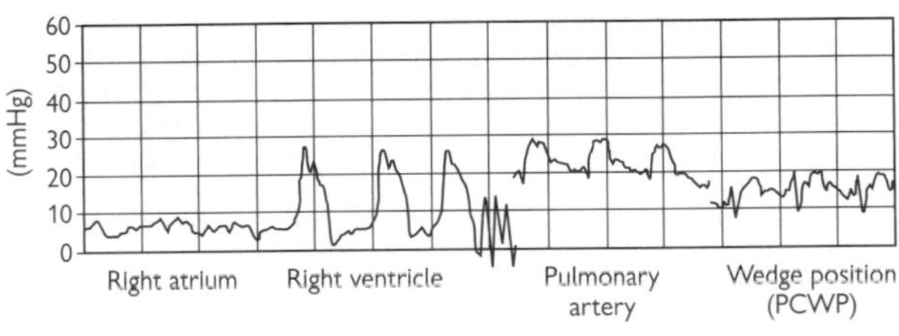

Fig. 15.6 Pressure tracings during pulmonary artery catheterization.

Pulmonary artery catheterization 3

Tips and pitfalls

- Never withdraw the catheter with the balloon inflated.
- Never advance the catheter with the balloon deflated.
- Never inject liquid into the balloon.
- Never leave the catheter with the balloon inflated as pulmonary infarction may occur.
- The plastic of the catheter softens with time at body temperature and the tip of the catheter may migrate further into the PA branch. If the pressure tracing with the balloon deflated is 'partially wedged' (and flushing the catheter does not improve this), withdraw the catheter 1–2cm and reposition.
- Sometimes it is impossible to obtain a wedged trace. In this situation one has to use the PA diastolic pressure as a guide. In health there is ~2–4mmHg difference between PA diastolic pressure and PCWP. Any condition which causes pulmonary hypertension (e.g. severe lung disease, ARDS, long-standing valvular disease) will alter this relationship.
- *Valvular lesions, VSDs, prosthetic valves, and pacemakers*: if these are present then seek advice from a cardiologist. The risk of SBE may be sufficiently great that the placement of a PA catheter may be more detrimental than beneficial.
- PEEP (see 📖 p.781). Measurement and interpretation if PCWP in patients on PEEP depends on the position of the catheter. Ensure the catheter is below the level of the left atrium on a lateral CXR. Removing PEEP during measurement causes marked fluctuations in haemodynamics and oxygenation and the pressures do not reflect the state once back on the ventilator.

Complications

- ***Arrhythmias:*** watch the ECG tracing closely whilst the catheter is advanced. The catheter commonly triggers runs of VT when crossing the tricuspid valve and through the RV. If this happens, deflate the balloon, pull back, and try again. The VT is usually self-limiting, but should not be ignored.
- ***Pulmonary artery rupture:*** (~0.2% in one series): damage may occur if the balloon is overinflated in a small branch. Risk factors include mitral valve disease (large v wave confused with poor wedging), pulmonary hypertension, multiple inflations, or hyperinflations of balloon. Haemoptysis is an early sign. It is safer to follow PA diastolic pressures if these correlate with the PCWP.
- ***Pulmonary infarction.***
- ***Knots:*** usually occur at the time of initial placement in patients where there has been difficulty in traversing the RV. Signs include loss of pressure tracing, persistent ectopy, and resistance to catheter manipulation. If this is suspected or has occurred, stop manipulation and seek expert help.

- ***Infection:*** risks increase with length of time the catheter is left *in situ*. Pressure transducer may occasionally be a source of infection. Remove the catheter and introducer and replace only if necessary.
- ***Other complications:*** complications associated with central line insertion, thrombosis and embolism, balloon rupture, intracardiac damage.

Indications for temporary pacing

1 Following acute MI

- Asystole
- Symptomatic complete heart block (CHB) (any territory)
- Symptomatic 2° heart block (any territory)
- Trifascicular block:
  - Alternating LBBB and RBBB
  - 1st -degree heart block + RBBB + LAD
  - New RBBB and left posterior hemiblock
  - LBBB and long PR interval
- After anterior MI:
  - Asymptomatic CHB
  - Asymptomatic 2nd-degree (Mobitz II) block
- Symptomatic sinus bradycardia unresponsive to atropine
- Recurrent VT for atrial or ventricular overdrive pacing.

2 Unrelated to MI

- Symptomatic sinus or junctional bradycardia unresponsive to atropine (e.g. carotid sinus hypersensitivity)
- Symptomatic 2° heart block or sinus arrest
- Symptomatic CHB
- Torsades de pointes tachycardia
- Recurrent VT for atrial or ventricular overdrive pacing
- Bradycardia-dependent tachycardia
- Drug overdose (e.g. verapamil, β-blockers, digoxin)
- Permanent pacemaker box change in a patient who is pacing dependent.

3 Before general anaesthesia

- The same principles as for acute MI (see earlier)
- Sinoatrial disease, 2° (Wenckebach) heart block only need prophylactic pacing if there are symptoms of syncope or pre-syncope
- CHB.

Transvenous temporary pacing

- The technique of temporary pacing is described on 📖 p.760.
- The most commonly used pacing mode and the mode of choice for life-threatening bradyarrhythmias is ventricular demand pacing (VVI) with a single bipolar wire positioned in the right ventricle: (see 📖 p.760 for an explanation of common pacing modes).
- In critically ill patients with impaired cardiac pump function and symptomatic bradycardia (especially with right ventricular infarction), cardiac output may be ↑ by up to 20% by maintaining AV synchrony. This requires 2 pacing leads, 1 atrial and 1 ventricular, and a dual pacing box.

Epicardial temporary pacing

Following cardiac surgery, patients may have *epicardial wires* (attached to the pericardial surface of the heart) left in for up to 1 week in case of postoperative heart block or bradyarrhythmia. These may be used in the same way as the more familiar transvenous pacing wires, but the threshold may be higher.

AV sequential pacing

In critically ill patients with impaired cardiac pump function and symptomatic bradycardia (especially with right ventricular infarction), cardiac output may be ↑ by up to 20% by maintaining AV synchrony. This requires 2 pacing leads, 1 atrial and 1 ventricular, and a dual pacing box.

Patients most likely to benefit from AV sequential pacing

- Acute MI (especially RV infarction)
- 'Stiff' left ventricle: (aortic stenosis, HCM, hypertensive heart disease, amyloidosis)
- Low cardiac output states (cardiomyopathy)
- Recurrent atrial arrhythmias.

Temporary cardiac pacing: ventricular pacing

- ***Cannulate a central vein:*** the wire is easiest to manipulate via the RIJ approach but is more comfortable for the patient via the right SCV. The LIJ approach is best avoided as there are many acute bends to negotiate and a stable position is difficult to achieve. Avoid the left subclavicular area as this is the preferred area for permanent pacemaker insertion and should be kept 'virgin' if possible. The femoral vein may be used but the risk of DVT and infection is high.
- ***Insert a sheath*** (similar to that for PA catheterization) through which the pacing wire can be fed. Pacing wires are commonly 5F or 6F and a sheath at least one size larger is necessary. Most commercially available pacing wires are pre-packed with an introducer needle and plastic cannula similar to an Abbocath® which may be used to position the pacing wire. However, the cannula does not have a haemostatic seal. The plastic cannula may be removed from the vein, leaving the bare wire entering the skin, once a stable position has been achieved. This reduces the risk of wire displacement but also makes repositioning of the wire more difficult should this be necessary, and the infection risk is higher.
- Pass the wire through the sterile plastic cover that accompanies the introducer sheath and advance into the upper right atrium (see Fig. 15.7) but do not unfurl the cover yet. The wire is much easier to manipulate with gloved hands without the additional hindrance of the plastic cover.
- Advance the wire with the tip pointing towards the right ventricle; it may cross the tricuspid valve easily. If it fails to cross, point the tip to the lateral wall of the atrium and form a loop. Rotate the wire and the loop should fall across the tricuspid valve into the ventricle.
- Advance and rotate the wire so that the tip points inferiorly as close to the tip of the right ventricle (laterally) as possible.
- If the wire does not rotate down to the apex easily, it may be because you are in the coronary sinus rather than in the right ventricle. (The tip of the wire points to the left shoulder.) Withdraw the wire and re-cross the tricuspid valve.
- Leave some slack in the wire; the final appearance should be like the outline of a sock with the 'heel' in the right atrium, the 'arch' over the tricuspid and the 'big toe' at the tip of the right ventricle.
- Connect the wire to the pacing box and check the threshold. Ventricular pacing thresholds should be <1.0V, but threshold up to 1.5V is acceptable if another stable position cannot be achieved.
- Check for positional stability. With the box pacing at a rate higher than the intrinsic heart rate, ask the patient to take some deep breaths, cough forcefully, and sniff. Watch for failure of capture, and if so reposition the wire.
- Set the output to 3V and the box on 'demand'. If the patient is in sinus rhythm and has an adequate BP set the box rate to just below the patient's rate. If there is CHB or bradycardia set the rate at 70–80/min.

- Cover the wire with the plastic sheath and suture sheath and wire securely to the skin. Loop the rest of the wire and fix to the patient's skin with adhesive dressing.
- When the patient returns to the ward, obtain a CXR to confirm satisfactory positioning of the wire and to exclude a pneumothorax.

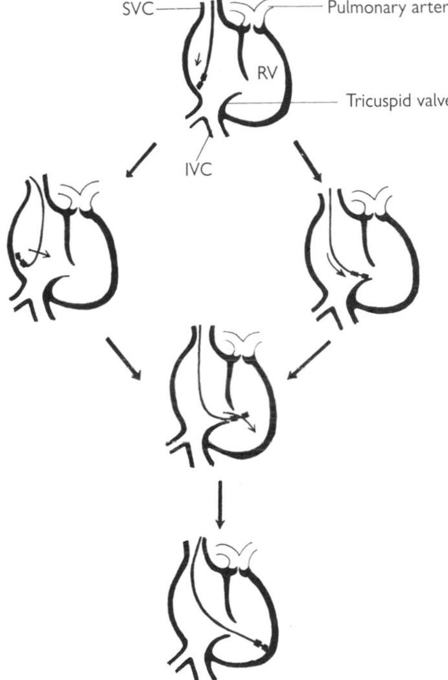

Fig. 15.7 Insertion of a ventricular pacing wire.

Temporary cardiac pacing: atrial pacing

See Fig. 15.8.

- The technique of inserting an atrial temporary wire is similar to that of ventricular pacing (see 📖 p.760 and Box 15.3).
- Advance the atrial wire until the 'J' is reformed in the right atrium.
- Rotate the wire and withdraw slightly to position the tip in the right atrial appendage. Aim for a threshold of <1.5V.
- If atrial wires are not available, a ventricular pacing wire may be manipulated into a similar position or passed into the coronary sinus for left atrial pacing.

Box 15.3 Checklist for pacing wire insertion

- Check the screening equipment and defibrillator work.
- Check the type of pacing wire: atrial wires have a pre-formed 'J' that allows easy placement in the atrium or appendage and is very difficult to manipulate into a satisfactory position in the ventricle.
- Ventricular pacing wires have a more open, gentle 'J'.
- Check the pacing box (single vs. dual or sequential pacing box) and leads to attach to the wire(s). Familiarize yourself with the controls on the box: you may need to connect up in a hurry if the patient's intrinsic rhythm slows further.

Remember to don the lead apron before wearing the sterile gown, mask, and gloves.

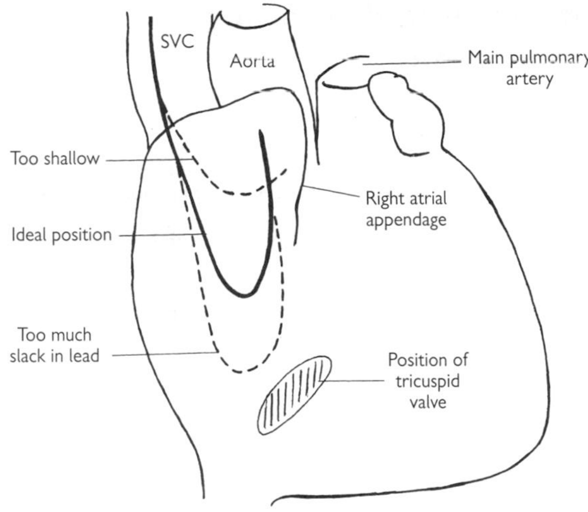

Fig. 15.8 Positioning an atrial wire for atrial pacing.

Temporary cardiac pacing: complications

See Box 15.4.

Ventricular ectopics or VT

- Non-sustained VT is common as the wire crosses the tricuspid valve (especially in patients receiving an isoprenaline infusion) and does not require treatment.
- Try to avoid long runs of VT and if necessary withdraw the wire into the atrium and wait until the rhythm has settled.
- If ectopics persist after the wire is positioned, try adjusting the amount of slack in the wire in the region of the tricuspid valve (either more or less).
- Pacing the RV outflow tract can provoke runs of VT.

Failure to pace and/or sense

- It is difficult to get low pacing thresholds (<1.0V) in patients with extensive MI (especially of the inferior wall), cardiomyopathy, or who have received class I antiarrhythmic drugs. Accept a slightly higher value if the position is otherwise stable and satisfactory.
- If the position of the wire appears satisfactory and yet the pacing thresholds are high, the wire may be in a left hepatic vein. Pull the wire back into the atrium and try again, looking specifically for the ventricular ectopics as the wire crosses the tricuspid valve.
- The pacing threshold commonly doubles in the first few days due to endocardial oedema.
- If the pacemaker suddenly fails, the most common reason is usually wire displacement:
  - Increase the pacing output of the box.
  - Check all the connections of the wire and the battery of the box.
  - Try moving the patient to the left lateral position until arrangements can be made to reposition the wire.

Perforation

- A pericardial rub may be present in the absence of perforation (esp. post MI).
- ***Presentation:*** pericardial chest pain, increasing breathlessness, falling BP, enlarged cardiac silhouette on CXR, signs of cardiac tamponade, left diaphragmatic pacing at low output.
- ***Management:***
  - If there are signs of cardiac tamponade arrange for urgent Echo and pericardial drainage (see 🕮 p.766).
  - Reposition the wire.
  - Monitor the patient carefully with repeat Echos to detect incipient cardiac tamponade.

Diaphragmatic pacing

- High output pacing (10V), even with satisfactory position of the ventricular lead may cause pacing of the left hemidiaphragm. At low voltages this suggests perforation (see 'Perforation').

- Right hemidiaphragm pacing may be seen with atrial pacing and stimulation of the right phrenic nerve.
- Reposition the wire if symptomatic (painful twitching, dyspnoea).

Box 15.4 Complications of temporary pacing

- Complications associated with central line insertion
- Ventricular ectopics
- Non-sustained VT
- Perforation
- Pericarditis
- Diaphragmatic pacing
- Infection
- Pneumothorax
- Cardiac tamponade.

Pericardial aspiration 1

Equipment

Establish peripheral venous access and check that full facilities for resuscitation are available. Pre-prepared pericardiocentesis sets may be available. You will need:

- Trolley as for central line insertion, with iodine or chlorhexidine for skin, dressing pack, sterile drapes, local anaesthetic (lidocaine 2%), syringes (including a 50mL), needles (25G and 22G), No. 11 blade, and silk sutures
- Pericardiocentesis needle (15cm, 18G) or similar Wallace cannula
- J-guidewire (≥80cm, 0.035 inch diameter)
- Dilators (up to 7Fr)
- Pigtail catheter (≥60cm with multiple sideholes, a large Seldinger-type CVP line can be used if no pigtail is available)
- Drainage bag and connectors
- Facilities for fluoroscopy or echocardiographic screening.

Technique (Fig. 15.9)

- Position the patient at ~30°. This allows the effusion to pool inferiorly within the pericardium.
- Sedate the patient lightly with midazolam and fentanyl if necessary. Use with caution as this may drop the BP in patients already compromised by the effusion.
- Put on sterile gown and gloves, clean the skin from mid-chest to mid-abdomen and the sterile drapes on the patient.
- Infiltrate the skin and subcutaneous tissues with local anaesthetic starting 1–1.5cm below the xiphisternum and just to the left of midline, aiming for the left shoulder and staying as close to the inferior border of the rib cartilages as possible.
- The pericardiocentesis needle is introduced into the angle between the xiphisternum and the left costal margin angled at >30°. Advance slowly aspirating gently and then injecting more lignocaine every few mm, aiming for the left shoulder.
- As the parietal pericardium is pierced, you may feel a 'give' and fluid will be aspirated. Remove the syringe and introduce the guidewire through the needle.
- Check the position of the guidewire by screening. It should loop within the cardiac silhouette only and not advance into the SVC or pulmonary artery.
- Remove the needle leaving the wire in place. Enlarge the skin incision slightly using the blade and dilate the track.
- Insert the pigtail over the wire into the pericardial space and remove the wire.
- Take specimens for microscopy, culture (and inoculate a sample into blood culture bottles), cytology and haematocrit if blood stained (a FBC tube; ask the haematologists to run on the Coulter counter for rapid estimation of Hb).

- Aspirate to dryness watching the patient carefully. Symptoms and haemodynamics (tachycardia) often start to improve with removal of as little as 100mL of pericardial fluid.
- If the fluid is heavily blood stained, withdraw fluid cautiously; if the pigtail is in the right ventricle, withdrawal of blood may cause cardiovascular collapse. Arrange for urgent Hb/haematocrit.
- Leave on free drainage and attached to the drainage bag.
- Suture the pigtail to the skin securely and cover with a sterile occlusive dressing.

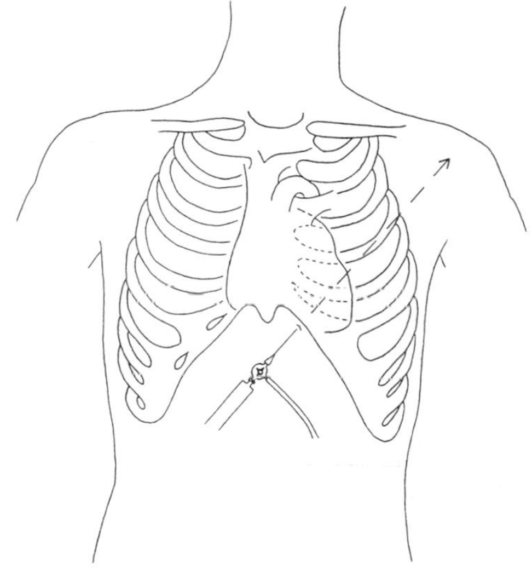

Fig. 15.9 Pericardial aspiration.

Pericardial aspiration 2

Aftercare

- Closely observe the patient for recurrent tamponade (obstruction of drain) and repeat Echo.
- Discontinue anticoagulants.
- Remove the drain after 24h or when the drainage stops.
- Consider the need for surgery (drainage, biopsy or pericardial window) or specific therapy (chemotherapy if malignant effusion, antimicrobials if bacterial, dialysis if renal failure, etc.).

See Box 15.5 for complications of pericardiocentesis.

Tips and pitfalls

If the needle touches the heart's epicardial surface, you may feel a 'ticking' sensation transmitted down the needle: withdraw the needle a few mm, angulate the needle more superficially, and try cautiously again, aspirating as you advance.

If you do not enter the effusion

- Withdraw the needle slightly and advance again, aiming slightly deeper, but still towards the left shoulder.
- If this fails, try again aiming more medially (midclavicular point or even suprasternal notch).
- Consider trying the apical approach (starting laterally at cardiac apex and aiming for right shoulder), if Echo confirms sufficient fluid at the cardiac apex.

Difficulty in inserting the pigtail

- This may be because of insufficient dilatation of the tract.
- Hold the wire tort (by gentle traction) while pushing the catheter; take care not to pull the wire out of the pericardium.

Haemorrhagic effusion vs. blood

- Compare the Hb of the pericardial fluid to venous blood Hb.
- Place some of the fluid in a clean container; blood will clot whereas haemorrhagic effusion will not as the 'whipping' action of the heart tends to defibrinate it.
- Confirm the position of the needle by first withdrawing some fluid and then injecting 10–20mL of contrast; using fluoroscopy, see if the contrast stays within the cardiac silhouette.
- Alternatively, if using Echo guidance, inject 5–10mL saline into the needle looking for 'microbubble contrast' in the cavity containing the needle tip. Injecting 20mL saline rapidly into a peripheral vein will produce 'contrast' in the right atrium and ventricle and may allow them to be distinguised from the pericardial space.
- Connect a pressure line to the needle; a characteristic waveform will confirm penetration of the right ventricle (see 🕮 Fig. 15.6, p.755).

Box 15.5 Complications of pericardiocentesis

- Penetration of a cardiac chamber (usually right ventricle)
- Laceration of an epicardial vessel
- Arrhythmia (atrial arrhythmias as the wire is advanced, ventricular arrhythmias if the RV is penetrated)
- Pneumothorax
- Perforation of abdominal viscus (liver, stomach, colon)
- Ascending infection.

DC cardioversion 1

Relative contraindications

- Digoxin toxicity
- Electrolyte disturbance (↓Na^+, ↓K^+, ↓Ca^{2+}, ↓Mg^{2+}, acidosis)
- Inadequate anticoagulation and chronic AF.

Checklist for DC cardioversion

• Defibrillator	Check this is functioning with a fully equipped arrest trolley to hand in case of arrest.
• Informed consent	(Unless life-threatening emergency.)
• 12-lead ECG	AF, flutter, SVT, VT, signs of ischaemia or digoxin. If ventricular rate is slow have an external (transcutaneous) pacing system nearby in case of asystole.
• Nil by mouth	For at least 4h.
• Anticoagulation	Does the patient require anticoagulants? Is the INR >2.0? (Has it been so for >3 weeks?).
• Potassium	Check this is >3.5mmol/L.
• Digoxin	Check there are no features of digoxin toxicity function and recent digoxin level are normal. If there are frequent ventricular ectopics, give IV Mg^{2+} 8mmol.
• Thyroid function	Treat thyrotoxicosis or myxoedema first.
• IV access	Peripheral venous cannula.
• Sedation	Short general anaesthesia (propofol) is preferable to sedation with benzodiazepine and fentanyl. Bag the patient with 100% O_2.
• Select energy	See Box 15.7.
• Synchronization	Check this is selected on the defibrillator for all shocks (unless the patient is in VF or haemodynamically unstable). Adjust the ECG gain so that the machine is only sensing QRS complexes and not P or T waves.
• Paddle placement	Most centres now use 'hands-free' adhesive paddles for DC cardioversion. Some continue with the traditional hand-held paddles. Conductive gel pads should be placed between right of the sternum and the other to the left of the left nipple (ant.-mid-axillary line), Alternatively, place one anteriorly just left of the sternum, and one posteriorly to the left of midline. There is some evidence that the AP position is superior for AF.
• Cardioversion	Check no one is in contact with the patient or with the metal bed. Ensure your own legs are clear of the bed! Apply firm pressure on the paddles if using the handheld device.

- Unsuccessful — Double the energy level and repeat up to 360J. Consider changing paddle position (see 'Paddle placement'). If prolonged sinus pause or ventricular arrhythmia during an elective procedure, stop.
- When complete, repeat ECG. Place in recovery position until awake. Monitor for 2–4h and ensure effects of sedation have passed. Patients should be accompanied home by friend or relative if being discharged.

Box 15.6 Complications of DC cardioversion

- Asystole/bradycardias
- Ventricular fibrillation
- Thromboembolism
- Transient hypotension
- Skin burns
- Aspiration pneumonitis.

Box 15.7 Suggested initial energies for DC shock for elective cardioversion

• Sustained VT	200J	Synchronized.
• AF	50–100J	Synchronized.
• Atrial flutter	50J	Synchronized.
• Other SVTs	50J	Synchronized.

- If the initial shock is unsuccessful, increase the energy (50, 100, 200, 360J) and repeat.
- If still unsuccessful consider changing paddle position and try 360J again. It is inappropriate to persist further with elective DC cardioversion.

DC cardioversion 2

Notes

Anticoagulation

The risk of thromboembolism in patients with chronic AF and dilated cardiomyopathy is 0–7% depending on the underlying risk factors.

Increased risk

- Prior embolic event
- Mechanical heart valve
- Mitral stenosis
- Dilated left atrium.

Low risk

- Age <60 years
- No heart disease
- Recent onset AF (<3 days).

Anticoagulate patients at risk with warfarin for at least 3–4 weeks. For recent onset AF (1–3 days), anticoagulate with IV heparin for at least 12–24h and, if possible, exclude intracardiac thrombus with a transoesophageal Echo prior to DC shock. If there is thrombus, anticoagulate with warfarin as described earlier. For emergency cardioversion of AF (<24h), heparinize prior to shock.

The risk of systemic embolism with cardioversion of atrial flutter and other tachyarrhythmias is very low, provided there is no ventricular thrombus, since the coordinated atrial activity prevents formation of clot. Routine anticoagulation with warfarin is not necessary but we would recommend heparin before DC shock as the atria are often rendered mechanically stationary for several hours after shock even though there is coordinate electrical depolarization.

After successful cardioversion, if the patient is on warfarin, continue anticoagulation for at least 3–4 weeks. Consider indefinite anticoagulation if there is intrinsic cardiac disease (e.g. mitral stenosis) or recurrent AF.

Special situations

Pregnancy DC shock during pregnancy appears to be safe. Auscultate the fetal heart before and after cardioversion and if possible, fetal ECG should be monitored.

Pacemakers There is a danger of damage to the pacemaker generator box or the junction at the tip of the pacing wire(s) and endocardium. Position the paddles in the anteroposterior position as this is theoretically safer. Facilities for back-up pacing (external or transvenous) should be available. Check the pacemaker post cardioversion—both early and late problems have been reported.

Intra-aortic balloon counterpulsation 1

Indications

- Cardiogenic shock post MI
- Acute severe mitral regurgitation
- Acute ventricular septal defect
- Preoperative (ostial left coronary stenosis)
- Weaning from cardiopulmonary bypass.

Rarely

- Treatment of ventricular arrhythmias post MI
- Unstable angina (as a bridge to CABG).

Contraindications

- Aortic regurgitation
- Dilated cardiomyopathy
- Aortic dissection
- Severe aorto-iliac atheroma
- Bleeding diathesis.

Complications

- Aortic dissection
- Thrombocytopenia
- Arterial perforation
- Peripheral embolism
- Limb ischaemia
- Balloon rupture.

Principle

The device consists of a catheter with a balloon (40mL size) at its tip which is positioned in the descending thoracic aorta. The balloon inflation/deflation is synchronized to the ECG. The balloon should inflate just after the dicrotic notch (in diastole), thereby increasing pressure in the aortic root and increasing coronary perfusion. The balloon deflates just before ventricular systole, thereby decreasing afterload and improving left ventricular performance (see Fig. 15.10).

Counterpulsation has many beneficial effects on the circulation:

- ↑ in coronary perfusion in diastole
- Reduced LV end-diastolic pressure
- Reduced myocardial O_2 consumption
- ↑cerebral and peripheral blood flow.

The IAB cannot assist the patient in asystole or VF; it requires a minimum cardiac index of 1.2–1.4L/min/m^2, often necessitating additional inotropes.

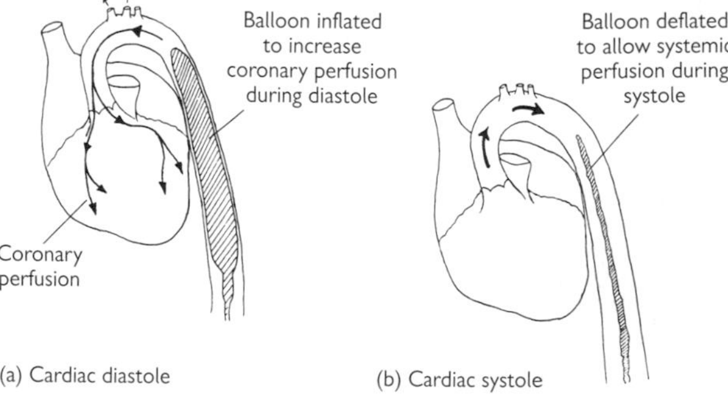

Fig. 15.10 Intra-aortic balloon counterpulsation.

Intra-aortic balloon counterpulsation 2

Technique

Balloon insertion

Previous experience is essential. Formerly, a cut-down to the femoral artery was required, but newer balloons come equipped with a sheath which may be introduced percutaneously. Using fluoroscopy, the balloon is positioned in the descending thoracic aorta with the tip just below the origin of the left subclavian artery. Fully anti-coagulate the patient with iv heparin. Some units routinely give iv antibiotics (flucloxacillin) to cover against *Staph.* infection.

Triggering and timing

The balloon pump may be triggered either from the patient's ECG (R wave) or from the arterial pressure waveform. Slide switches on the pump allow precise timing of inflation and deflation during the cardiac cycle. Set the pump to 1:2 to allow you to see the effects of augmentation on alternate beats.

Trouble-shooting

- Seek help from an expert! There is usually an on-call cardiac perfusionist or technician, senior cardiac physician or surgeon.
- Counterpulsation is inefficient with heart rates over 130/min. Consider anti-arrhythmics or 1:2 augmentation instead.
- Triggering and timing: For ECG triggering, select a lead with most pronounced R wave; ensure that the pump is set to trigger from ECG not pressure; permanent pacemakers may interfere with triggering-select lead with negative and smallest pacing artefact. Alternatively, set the pump to be triggered from the external pacing device. A good arterial waveform is required for pressure triggering; the timing will vary slightly depending on the location of the arterial line (slightly earlier for radial artery line, cf. femoral artery line). Be guided by the haemodynamic effects of balloon inflation and deflation rather than the precise value of delay.
- Limb ischaemia: Exacerbated by poor cardiac output, adrenaline, noradrenaline and peripheral vascular disease. Wean off and remove the balloon (see below).
- Thrombocytopenia: Commonly seen; does not require transfusion unless there is overt bleeding and returns to normal once the balloon is removed. Consider epoprostenol infusion if platelet counts fall below 100×10^9/L.

IABP removal

- The patient may be progressively weaned by gradually reducing the counterpulsation ratio (1 : 2, 1 : 4, 1 : 8, etc.) and/or reducing the balloon volume and checking that the patient remains haemodynamically stable.
- Stop the heparin infusion and wait for the ACT (activated clotting time) to fall <150s (APTT <1.5 normal).
- Using a 50ml syringe, have an assistant apply negative pressure to the balloon.
- Pull the balloon down until it abuts the sheath; do not attempt to pull the balloon into the sheath.
- Withdraw both balloon and sheath and apply firm pressure on the femoral puncture site for at least 30 minutes or until the bleeding is controlled.

Principles of respiratory support

The aim of therapy is to relieve hypoxia and maintain or restore a normal P_aCO_2 for the individual. Relative indications for mechanical ventilation are discussed in the appropriate chapters. This section discusses some of the principles involved.

Oxygen therapy

- O_2 should be administered by a system that delivers a defined percentage, between 28% and 100% according to the patient's requirements (e.g. via fixed percentage delivery masks such as Ventimask Mk IV).
- A Hudson mask or nasal cannulae give very variable F_iO_2 depending on flow rate and the patient's breathing pattern.
- Nasal prongs only deliver at F_iO_2 of 30% at flows of 2L/min, and become less efficient at higher flow rates (>35% at 3L/min with little further increase with increasing flow). Higher flow rates require humidification.
- A properly positioned, high-flow O_2 mask, using O_2 at 6L/min, can provide an F_iO_2 of 60%.
- Combining nasal prongs and a high flow mask can achieve an F_iO_2 of >80–90%.
- In practice it is rarely possible to consistently deliver >60% unless using CPAP or ventilation.
- When sudden deterioration in oxygenation occurs check the delivery system for empty cylinders, disconnected tubing, etc.

Indications

- Type I or II respiratory failure
- Bronchial asthma
- Acute MI
- Sickle cell crisis
- Carbon monoxide poisoning
- Cluster headaches.

Complications

- Tracheobronchitis occurs with prolonged inhalation of ≥80% O_2. It causes retrosternal pain, cough, and dyspnoea.
- Parenchymal lung damage from O_2occurs with F_iO_2 >60% for >48h without intermittent air breathing periods.

Monitoring oxygen therapy

- O_2 therapy should be assessed continuous oximetry and intermittent ABGs.
- Oximetry is an invaluable aid, but has limitations. In some situations (e.g. Guillain–Barré syndrome) falling oximetry is a very late marker of impending respiratory failure, and CO_2 accumulation (e.g. in COPD) is clearly not monitored by oximetry. A S_aO_2 of 93% correlates with a P_aO_2 of 8kPa, and below 92% the P_aO_2 may fall disproportionately quickly.

Lung expansion techniques

- Periodic 'sighs' are a normal part of breathing and reverse microatelectasis. Lung expansion techniques are indicated for patients who cannot or will not take periodic large breaths (e.g. post-abdominal or chest surgery, neuromuscular chest wall weakness).
- Postoperative techniques used commonly by physiotherapists include incentive spirometry, coached maximal inspiration with cough, postural drainage, and chest percussion.
- Volume-generating devices such as '***the Bird***' are triggered by the patient initiating inspiration, and deliver a pre-set tidal volume to augment the patient's breath. Liaise with your physiotherapist.
- Pressure-generating techniques (such as CPAP, NIPPV, and BiPAP) have the advantage that even if a leak develops around the mask, the ventilator is able to 'compensate' to provide the prescribed positive pressure (see following sections).
- For both volume and pressure generating techniques, the patients must be able to protect their airway and generate enough effort to trigger the machine.

Continuous positive airways pressure (CPAP)

- CPAP provides a constant positive pressure throughout the respiratory cycle.
- It acts to splint open collapsing alveoli which may be full of fluid (or a collapsing upper airway in obstructive sleep apnoea), increases functional residual capacity (FRC) and compliance, such that the work of breathing is reduced and gas exchange is improved.
- It allows a higher F_iO_2 (approaching 80–100%) to be administered, cf. standard O_2 delivery masks.
- CPAP should usually be commenced after liaison with anaesthetists; in a patient for active management it should usually be started on the ITU.
- A standard starting pressure is 5cmH_2O.

Indications

- Pulmonary oedema.
- Acute respiratory failure (e.g. 2° to infection), where simple face mask O_2 is insufficient.
- Acute respiratory failure where ventilation is inappropriate.
- Weaning from the ventilator.
- Obstructive sleep apnoea (OSA).
- Patient needs to:
  - Be awake and alert
  - Be able to protect the airway
  - Possess adequate respiratory muscle strength
  - Be haemodynamically stable.

Mechanical ventilation

Negative pressure ventilation (NPV)

- This works by 'sucking' out the chest wall and is used in chronic hypoventilation (e.g. polio, kyphoscoliosis, or muscle disease). Expiration is passive.
- These techniques do not require tracheal intubation. However, access to the patient for nursing care is difficult.

Intermittent positive pressure ventilation (IPPV)

Indications

Deteriorating gas exchange due to a potentially reversible cause of respiratory failure.

- Pneumonia
- Head injury
- Exacerbation of COPD
- Cerebral hypoxia
- Massive atelectasis (e.g. post cardiac arrest)
- Respiratory muscle weakness
- Intracranial bleed
- Myaesthenia gravis
- Raised ICP
- Acute infective polyneuritis
- Major trauma or burns

Ventilation of the ill patient on the ITU is via either an ET tube or a tracheostomy. If ventilation is anticipated to be needed for >1 week, consider a tracheostomy.

There are 2 basic types of ventilator.

- ***Pressure cycled ventilators*** deliver gas into the lungs until a prescribed pressure is reached, when inspiratory flow stops and, after a short pause, expiration occurs by passive recoil. This has the advantage of reducing the peak airway pressures without impairing cardiac performance in situations such as ARDS. However, if the airway pressures increase or compliance decreases the tidal volume will fall, so patients need to be monitored closely to avoid hypoventilation.
- ***Volume cycled ventilators*** deliver a preset tidal volume into the lungs over a predetermined inspiratory time (usually ~30% of the breathing cycle), hold the breath in the lungs (for ~10% of the cycle), and then allow passive expiration as the lungs recoil.

Nasal ventilation

- Nasal intermittent positive pressure ventilation (NIPPV) delivers a positive pressure for a prescribed inspiratory time, when triggered by the patient initiating a breath, allowing the patient to exhale to atmospheric pressure.
- The positive pressure is supplied by a small machine via a tight-fitting nasal mask.
- It is generally used as a method of home nocturnal ventilation for patients with severe musculoskeletal chest wall disease (e.g. kyphoscoliosis) or with obstructive sleep apnoea (OSA).
- It has also been used with modest success as an alternative to formal ventilation via ETT in patients where positive *expiratory* pressure is not desirable, e.g. acute asthma, COPD with CO_2 retention, and as a weaning aid in those in whom separation from a ventilator is proving difficult.
- The system is relatively easy to set up by experienced personnel, but some patients take to it better than others. It should not be commenced by inexperienced personnel.

Positive pressure ventilation

Continuous mandatory ventilation (CMV)

- CMV acts on a preset cycle to deliver a given number of breaths per minute of a set volume. The duration of the cycle determines the breath frequency.
- The *minute volume* is calculated by (tidal volume x frequency).
- The relative proportions of time spent in inspiration and expiration (I:E ratio) is normally set at 1:2, but may be altered, e.g. in acute asthma, where air trapping is a problem, a longer expiratory time is needed (see 📖 p.182); in ARDS, where the lung compliance is low, a longer inspiratory time is beneficial (inverse ratio ventilation, see 📖 p.200).
- The patients should be fully sedated. Patients capable of spontaneous breaths who are ventilated on CMV can get 'stacking' of breaths, where the ventilator working on its preset cycle may give a breath on top of one which the patient has just taken, leading to over-inflation of the lungs, a high peak inspiratory pressure, and the risk of pneumothorax.
- Prolonged use of this mode will result in atrophy of the respiratory muscles; this may prove difficult in subsequent 'weaning', especially in combination with a proximal myopathy from steroids, e.g. in acute asthma.
- Ventilation may either be terminated abruptly or by gradual transfer of the ventilatory workload from the machine to the patient ('weaning').

Synchronized intermittent mandatory ventilation (SIMV)

- SIMV modes allow the patient to breath spontaneously and be effectively ventilated and allows gradual transfer of the work of breathing on to the patient. This may be appropriate when weaning the patient whose respiratory muscles have wasted. It is inappropriate in acutely ill patients (e.g. acute severe asthma, ARDS); CMV with sedation reduces O_2 requirement and respiratory drive and allows more effective ventilation.
- Exact details of the methods of synchronization vary between machines, but all act in a similar manner: the patient breathes spontaneously through the ventilator circuit. The ventilator is usually preset to ensure that the patient has a minimum number of breaths per minute, and if the number of spontaneous breaths falls below the preset level then a breath is delivered by the machine.
- Most SIMV modes of ventilation provide some form of positive pressure support to the patient's spontaneous breaths to reduce the work of breathing and ensure effective ventilation (see 'Pressure support').

Pressure support

- Positive pressure is added during inspiration to relieve part or all of the work of breathing.
- This may be done in conjunction with an SIMV mode of ventilation, or as a means of supporting entirely spontaneous patient-triggered ventilation during the process of weaning.

- It allows the patients to determine their own respiratory rate, and should ensure adequate inflation of the lungs and oxygenation. It is, however, only suitable for those whose lung function is reasonably adequate and who are not confused or exhausted.

Positive end-expiratory pressure (PEEP)

- PEEP is a preset pressure added to the end of expiration only, to maintain the lung volume, prevent airway or alveolar collapse, and open up atelectic or fluid-filled lung (e.g. in ARDS or cardiogenic pulmonary oedema).
- It can significantly improve oxygenation by making more of the lung available for gas exchange. However, the trade-off is an increase in intrathoracic pressure which can significantly decrease venous return and hence cardiac output. There is also an ↑risk of pneumothorax.
- 'Auto-PEEP' is seen if the patient's lungs do not fully empty before the next inflation (e.g. asthma).
- In general PEEP should be kept at a level of 5–10cmH_2O where required, and the level adjusted in 2–3cmH_2O intervals every 20–30min according to a balance between oxygenation and cardiac performance.
- Measurement and interpretation if PCWP in patients on PEEP depends on the position of the catheter. PCWP will always reflect pulmonary venous pressures if they are greater than PEEP. If the catheter is in an apical vessel where the PCWP is normally lower due to the effects of gravity, the pressure measured may be the alveolar (PEEP) pressure rather than the true PCWP; in a dependent area the pressures are more accurate. Removing PEEP during measurement alters haemodynamics and oxygenation and the pressures do not reflect the state once back on the ventilator.

Percutaneous cricothyrotomy

Indications

- To bypass upper airway obstruction (e.g. trauma, infections, neoplasms, postoperative, burns and corrosives) when oral or nasotracheal intubation is contraindicated.
- In situations when ET intubations fail (e.g. massive nasopharyngeal haemorrhage, structural deformities, obstruction due to foreign bodies, etc.)

Percutaneous cricothyrotomy using the Seldinger technique is quicker, may be performed by non-surgeons at the bedside, and is safer, see Fig. 15.11. After anaesthetizing the area, a needle is used to puncture the cricothyroid membrane and through this a guidewire is introduced into the trachea. Over this a series of dilators and the tracheostomy tube can be safely positioned.

Complications of cricothyrotomy

- Haemorrhage
- Subglottic stenosis
- Hoarseness
- laryngotracheal-cutaneous fistula.

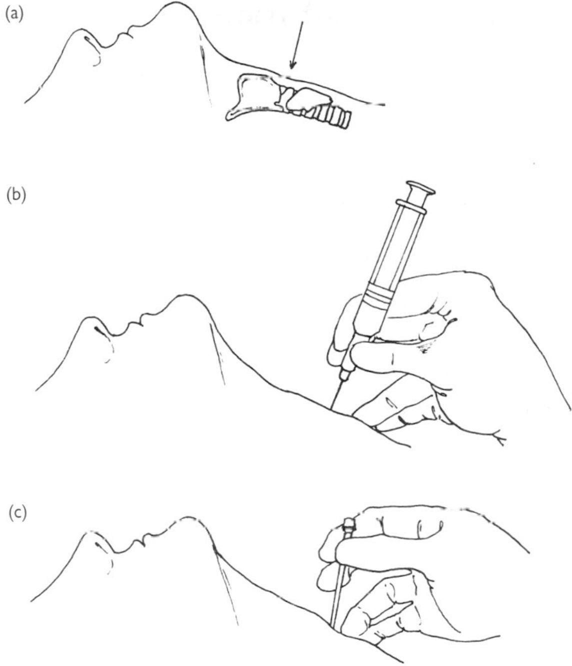

Fig. 15.11 Needle cricothyroidotomy.

Endotracheal intubation

This is the best method for providing and maintaining a clear airway for ventilation, protection against aspiration, and suctioning and clearing lower respiratory tract secretions. The most common indication for urgent intubation by a physician is cardiac arrest. This is not a technique for the inexperienced: the description given here is not intended as a substitute for practice under supervision of a skilled anaesthetist.

You will need

- Laryngoscope, usually with a curved blade (Macintosh)
- ETT (8–9mm internal diameter for ♂ and 7–8mm for ♀) and appropriate adaptors
- Syringe for cuff inflation and clamp to prevent air escaping from the cuff once inflated
- Scissors and tape or bandage to secure the tube
- Lubricating jelly (e.g. K-Y® jelly)
- Suction apparatus with rigid (Yankauer) and long flexible catheters.

Potential problems during intubation

- Certain anatomical variations (e.g. receding mandible, short neck, prominent incisors, high arched palate) as well as stiff neck or trismus may make intubation complicated; summon experienced help.
- Vomiting: suction if necessary. Cricoid pressure may be useful.
- Cervical spine injury: immobilize the head and neck in line with the body and try not to extend the head during intubation.
- Facial burns or trauma may make orotracheal intubation impossible. Consider cricothyrotomy (see 🕮 p.782).

Procedure

- Place the patient with the neck slightly flexed and the head extended. Take care if cervical injury is suspected.
- Cricoid pressure: The oesophagus can be occluded by compressing the cricoid cartilage posteriorly against the body of C6. This prevents passive regurgitation into the trachea but not active vomiting. Ask your assistant to maintain pressure until the tube is in place and the cuff inflated.
- Pre-oxygenate the patient by hyperventilation with ≥85% O_2 for 15–30sec. Suction throat to clear the airway.
- With the laryngoscope in your left hand, insert the blade on right side of mouth. Advance to base of tongue, identifying the tonsillar fossa and the uvula. Push the blade to the left moving the tongue over. Advance the blade until the epiglottis comes into view.
- Insert the blade tip between the base of the tongue and the epiglottis and pull the whole blade (and larynx) upwards along the line of the handle of the laryngoscope to expose the vocal cords. Brief suction may be necessary to clear the view.
- Insert the ETT between the vocal cords and advance it until the cuff is just below the cords and no further. Inflate the cuff with air.

- If the cords cannot be seen, do not poke at the epiglottis hoping for success, call for more skilled help and revert to basic airway management.
- Intubation must not take longer than 30sec; if there is any doubt about the position, remove the tube, reoxygenate, and try again.
- With the tube in place, listen to the chest during inflation to check that ***both*** sides of the chest inflate. If the tube is in the oesophagus, chest expansion will be minimal though the stomach may inflate.
- Tie the ETT in place to prevent it from slipping up or down the airway. Ventilate with high concentration O_2.

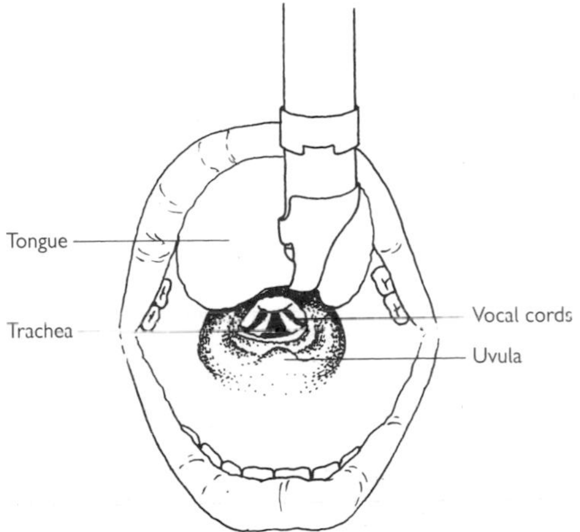

Fig. 15.12 Landmarks for endotracheal intubation.

Aspiration of a pneumothorax

If the pneumothorax is <75% and the patient is haemodynamically stable, it is reasonable to attempt aspiration of the pneumothorax in the first instance (📖 p.204).

You will need the following:

- 10-mL and 50-mL syringe with green (18G) and orange (25G) needles
- Dressing pack (swabs, sterile drapes, antiseptic) and sterile gloves
- 19G Venflon® or alternative cannula
- Local anaesthetic (e.g. 2% lidocaine)
- 3-way tap.

Procedure

- 1 assistant is required.
- Sit patient up, propped against pillows with hand behind his/her head; ensure you are comfortable and on a similar level.
- Select the space to aspirate, the 2nd intercostal space in the mid-clavicular line. Confirm with CXR that you are aspirating the correct side (a surprisingly common cause of disasters is aspirating the normal side).
- Clean the skin and use aseptic technique.
- Connect a 50-mL syringe to a 3-way tap in readiness, with the line which will be connected to the patient turned 'off' so that no air will enter the pleural cavity on connecting the apparatus.
- Infiltrate 5–10mL of lidocaine from skin to pleura, just above the upper border of the rib in the space you are using. Confirm the presence of air by aspirating approximately 5mL via a green needle.
- Insert a 16G or larger IV cannula into the pneumothorax, preferably whilst aspirating the cannula with a syringe, so that entry into the pleural space is confirmed. Allow the tip of the cannula to enter the space by approximately 1cm.
- Ask the patient to hold their breath and remove the needle. Swiftly connect the 3-way tap. Aspirate 50mL of air/fluid and void it through the other lumen of the tap. Repeat.
- Aspiration should be stopped when resistance to suction is felt, the patient coughs excessively, or ≥2.5L of air has been aspirated.
- Withdraw the cannula and cover the site with a dressing plaster (e.g. Elastoplast® or Band-aid®)
- Check post procedure CXR. If there is significant residual pneumothorax insert a chest drain.

Aspiration of a pleural effusion

The basic procedure is similar to that for a pneumothorax—the site is different: 1 or 2 intercostal spaces posteriorly below the level at which dullness is detected. Ideally all cases should have an USS first to confirm the level of the effusion and ensure that the diaphragm is not higher than anticipated due to underlying pulmonary collapse.

- Position the patient leaning forward over the back of a chair or table. Clean the skin and infiltrate with local anaesthetic as described for a pneumothorax aspiration.
- Insert the cannula and aspirate the effusion with a 50-mL syringe, voiding it through the 3-way tap. Repeat until resistance is felt and the tap is dry.
- Check a post-procedure CXR.

Insertion of a chest drain 1

You will need the following:

- Dressing pack (sterile gauze, gloves, drapes, povidone-iodine)
- Local anaesthetic (~20mL 1% lidocaine), 10-mL syringe, green (18G) and orange (25G) needles
- Scalpel and No. 11 blade for skin incision; 2 packs silk sutures (1–0)
- 2 forceps (Kelly clamps), scissors, needle holder (often pre-packaged as a 'chest drain set')
- Where possible, use the new Seldinger-type chest tubes—especially for pneumothorax
- Chest tubes—a selection of 24, 28, 32, and 36Fr
- Chest drainage bottles, with sterile water for underwater seal
- 1 assistant.

Procedure

- Position the patient leaning forward over the back of a chair or table. If possible, premedicate the patient with an appropriate amount of opiate ~30min before.
- Mark the space to be drained in the mid-axillary line; usually the 5th intercostal space for pneumothorax, below the level of the fluid for an effusion. Clean the skin.
- Select the chest tube: small (24Fr) for air alone, medium (28Fr) for serous fluid, or large (32–36Fr) for blood/pus. Remove the trocar. Check that the underwater seal bottles are ready.
- Infiltrate the skin with 15–20mL of lidocaine 1%. Make a short subcutaneous tunnel for the chest tube before it enters the pleural space (see Fig. 15.13). Anaesthetize the periosteum on the top of the rib. Check that you can aspirate air/fluid from the pleural space.
- Make a horizontal 2-cm incision in the anaesthetized skin of the rib space. Use the forceps to blunt-dissect through the fat and intercostal muscles to make a track large enough for your gloved finger down to the pleural space. Stay close to the upper border of the rib to avoid the neurovascular bundle.
- Check the length of the tube against the patient's chest to confirm how much needs to be inserted into the patient's chest. Aim to get the tip to the apex for a pneumothorax; keep the lowermost hole as low as possible (>2cm into the chest) to drain pleural fluid.
- Insert two sutures across the incision (or a purse-string, see Fig. 15.13). These will gently tighten around the tube once inserted to create an airtight seal but do not knot—these sutures will be used to close the wound after drain removal.
- Remove the trocar. Clamp the end of the tube with the forceps and gently introduce the tube into the pleural space. Rotating the forceps 180° directs the tube to the apex (see Fig. 15.13). Condensation in the tube (or fluid) confirms the tube is within the pleural space. Check that all the holes are within the thorax and connect to underwater seal. Tape these to the skin.
- Gently tighten the skin sutures but do not knot. The drain should be secured with several other stitches and copious amounts of adhesive tape. They are very vulnerable to accidental traction.

Wrap adhesive tape around the join between the drain and the connecting tubing.

- Prescribe adequate analgesia for the patient for when the local anaesthetic wears off.
- Arrange for a CXR to check the position of the drain.
- Do not drain off >1L of pleural fluid/24h to avoid re-expansion pulmonary oedema.

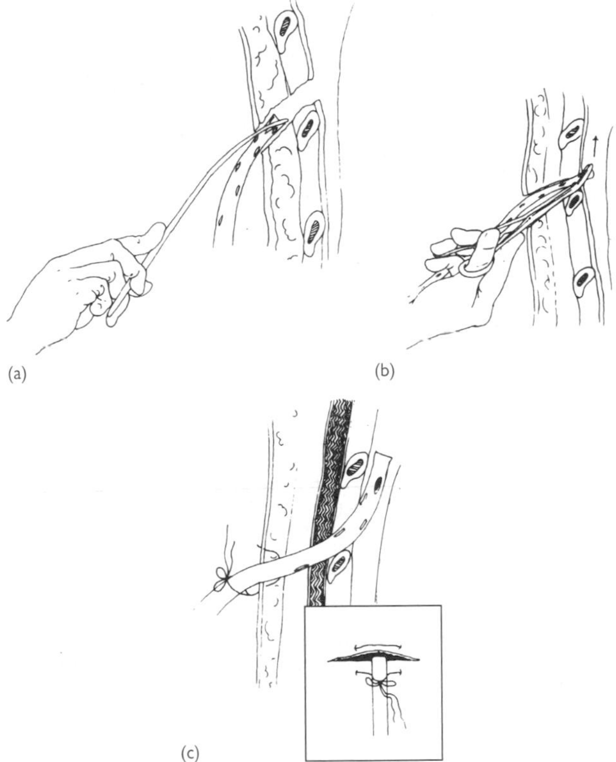

Fig. 15.13 Insertion of a chest drain.

Insertion of a chest drain 2

Tips and pitfalls

- The chest drain should only be left in place while air or fluid continue to drain. The risk of ascending infection increases with time. Prophylactic antibiotics are not usually indicated.

Malpositioned tube

- Obtain a CXR (and then daily) to check the position of the drain and examine the lung fields.
- If the drain is too far out, there will be an air leak and the patient may develop subcutaneous emphysema. Ideally, remove the drain and replace with a new drain at a new site; the risk of ascending infection is high if the 'non-sterile' portion of the tube is just pushed into the chest.
- If the drain is too far in, it may be uncomfortable for the patient and impinge on vital structures (e.g. thoracic aorta). Pull the tube out the appropriate distance and re-suture.

Obstructed tube

- Check the water column in the chest drain bottle swings with respiration. This stops if tube is obstructed.
- Check the drains and tubing are free of bends and kinks.
- Blood clots or fibrin may block the tube.
- If the lung is still collapsed on CXR, replace the chest drain with a new tube at a new site.

Lung fails to re-expand

- This is either due to an obstructed system or persistent air leak (e.g. tracheobronchial fistula).
- If the chest drain continues to bubble, apply suction to the drain to help expand the lung. Consider inserting further drains or surgical repair of leak. If the chest drain is obstructed (described earlier), replace the drain.

Removing the chest drain

- ***Do not*** clamp the chest drain.
- Remove the dressings and release the sutures holding the drain in place. Leave the skin incision sutures (purse-string) in position to close the wound once the drain is removed.
- Remove the drain in a gentle motion, either in inspiration or in expiration with Valsalva.
- Tighten the skin sutures. These should be removed after 3–4 days and a fresh dressing applied.
- Any residual pneumothorax should be treated depending on the patient's symptoms.

Complications

- Bleeding (intercostal vessels, laceration of lung, spleen, liver)
- Pulmonary oedema (too rapid lung expansion)
- Empyema
- Subcutaneous emphysema
- Residual pneumothorax or effusion (malpositioned or obstructed chest drain).

Ascitic tap (paracentesis)

Indications

- Diagnose or exclude spontaneous bacterial peritonitis
- To obtain ascites for measurement of protein, albumin, or amylase (pancreatic ascites)
- Ascitic cytology may require 100mL fluid
- Stain and culture for AFBs; lymphocyte >500 cells/mm^3)
- To drain cirrhotic or malignant ascites.

Relative contraindications

- Previous abdominal surgery increase risk of perforation
- Severe coagulopathy (platelets <20,000, INR>4.0)
- Massive hepatomegaly or splenomegaly (avoid same side).

Ascitic tap

- Lie patient supine, and tilted slightly to one side.
- Select the site for paracentesis (e.g. on horizontal line across umbilicus, and 4cm lateral to a line passing to mid-inguinal point). Clean the area with chlorhexidine. Avoid scars.
- Use a 20-mL syringe with a 18G (green) needle. In obese patients use a longer needle (e.g. 18G Abbocath®). Infiltrate the area with local anaesthetic. Insert the needle slowly into the abdomen whilst aspirating until fluid is obtained.
- Inoculate 5mL of the fluid into each bottle of a set of blood culture bottles and send 5mL in a sterile bottle for microscopy and protein determination. Add 2mL ascites to EDTA tube and send to haematology for cell count.
- Remove and apply a sterile plaster over the puncture site.

Total paracentesis

Daily small volume paracentesis is time-consuming, unnecessary, and increases the risk of infection and ascitic leakage. The risk of infection is high if a peritoneal drain is left *in situ* in cirrhotic ascites. It is safer to drain the ascites to dryness.

The rate of fluid drainage can be fast, and it is generally safe to drain >10L of ascites over 1–2h. During the first 3–6h of paracentesis, there is a significant increase in cardiac output, a decrease in systemic vascular resistance, and a modest fall in mean arterial pressure (by 5–10mmHg). Tense ascites increases the right atrial pressure (RAP), which falls acutely following paracentesis.

- To avoid the catheter blocking due to omentum plugging the end, use a catheter with side-holes.
- If a conventional cannula is used with holes fashioned in the side, you can attach it to a 'drip set' (IV fluid 'giving set') which has been modified by removal of the reservoir, but retention of the luer locking device, and rate control mechanism.
- Position the patient supine and tilted to one side. Clean, and infiltrate the site with 2% lidocaine as for ascitic tap.
- Insert the cannula (attached to a 20-mL syringe), aspirating as one advances the cannula. When ascitic fluid is obtained, advance the needle 3–4cm more, and then advance the plastic cannula into the abdomen and attach the drainage system.
- Strap the introducer to the abdominal wall with sticking plaster. It is not necessary to suture the cannula in place since it will be removed within 3–4h.
- Drain the ascites as rapidly as possible.
- When the ascites stops draining or slows down, move the patient from side to side, and lie towards the drainage site.
- When complete, remove the catheter, apply plaster, lie the patient with the drainage site uppermost for at least 4h.
- Replace albumin with an infusion of 20% albumin to give 8g of albumin for every litre of ascites removed.

Insertion of Sengstaken–Blakemore tube

The Sengstaken–Blakemore tube is inserted to control variceal bleeding when endoscopic therapy or IV terlipressin have failed. It should not be used as primary therapy since it is unpleasant, and increases the risk of oesophageal ulceration and aspiration.

Seek experienced or specialist help early. Balloon tamponade is a temporary procedure to prevent exsanguination.

Procedure

- It is assumed that the patient is undergoing resuscitation, and has received IV terlipressin. To reduce the risk of aspiration the patient should ideally be intubated and ventilated.
- The Sengstaken tube should be stored in the fridge (to maximize stiffness) and removed just before use. Familiarize yourself with the ports before insertion. Check the integrity of the balloons before you insert the tube.
- Place an endoscope protection mouthguard in place (to prevent biting of the tube). Cover the end of the tube with lubricating jelly, and, with the patient in the left semi-prone position, push the tube down, asking the patient to swallow (if conscious). If the tube curls up in the mouth, try again.
- Insert at least 50–60cm, making sure that the tube is not coiled up in the back of the mouth. Inflate the gastric balloon with 250mL water. Clamp the balloon channel. Then gently pull back on the tube until the gastric balloon abuts the gastro-oesophageal junction (resistance felt), then pull further until the patient is beginning to be tugged by pulling. Note the position at the edge of the mouth piece (mark with pen), and attach with sticking plaster to the side of the face.
- ***Tip:*** if the above fails place the tube through the mouthguard to the back of the throat, and then follow with an endoscope. The endoscope will push the tube down the oesophagus, and can be retroverted to directly visualize the gastric balloon being filled, before being removed.
- In general, the oesophageal balloon should ***never*** be used. Virtually all bleeding varices occur at the oesophagogastric junction and are controlled using the gastric balloon.
- Do ***not*** leave the balloon inflated for >12h since this increases the risk of oesophageal ulceration.
- Obtain a CXR to check the position of the tube.
- The gastric channel should be aspirated continuously.

Percutaneous liver biopsy

This should only be done by experienced doctors.

Procedure

Patients should be warning of risk of bleeding, pneumothorax, gall-bladder puncture, failed biopsy, and shoulder-tip pain, which may last several hours. The mortality is ~1:10,000.

Relative contraindications

- Prothrombin time >3sec prolonged.
- Platelet count is $<80 \times 10^9$/L or bleeding diathesis.
- Ascites.
- Liver cancer (risk of tumour seeding).

Pre-medicate the patient with analgesia (e.g. 30–60mg dihydrocodeine) before the procedure. The patient lies supine with their right hand behind their head. Always carry out the liver biopsy under US guidance, especially if the liver is small and cirrhotic. The skin is cleaned, local anaesthetic infiltrated down to the liver capsule, and a liver biopsy needle is inserted when the breath is held in expiration. The biopsy itself takes about 5–10sec and may cause shoulder-tip pain.

A plugged biopsy can be performed when the prothrombin time is up to 6sec prolonged with a platelet count of $>40{,}000\text{mm}^3$. The biopsy is done through a sheath and the tract embolized using Gelfoam® to prevent bleeding.

Transjugular liver biopsy

This liver biopsy is taken through the hepatic vein, with 2° bleeding occurring into the circulation. It is not without risk, as the hepatic capsule may be punctured leading to bleeding. It is used for patients in whom a prolonged PT or low platelet count precludes a normal liver biopsy.

A large introducer is placed into the IJV. A catheter is introduced through this and manipulated into the hepatic vein. The catheter is removed leaving a guidewire *in situ*. A metal transjugular biopsy needle is passed over the wire and advanced into the hepatic vein. One has to avoid being too peripheral (risk of capsular puncture). The wire is removed, and the needle advanced whilst suction is applied. A biopsy is obtained by the 'Menghini' technique. The biopsies obtained are smaller and more fragmented than those obtained by conventional techniques.

Transjugular intrahepatic portosystemic shunt (TIPS)

Indications

- Uncontrolled bleeding of oesophageal or gastric varices
- Diuretic resistant ascites
- Hepatic hydrothorax.

Principle

To decrease the portal pressure acutely, a shunt is placed between a hepatic vein and portal vein tributary. Blood then flows from the high pres sure portal system to the lower pressure hepatic venous system which drains into the IVC.

It is carried out in specialist centres and is technically quite difficult. It does not require a general anaesthetic, and it does not hinder future liver transplantation.

Method

The internal jugular vein is catheterized, and a cannula passed through the right atrium into the IVC, and into a hepatic vein. The portal vein is localized by USS, and a metal transjugular biopsy needle pushed through the liver from the hepatic vein into a portal vein tributary (usually right portal vein). A wire is then passed into the portal vein and the metal needle withdrawn, leaving the wire joining the hepatic vein and portal vein. An expandable stent is then passed over the wire. A typical stent size is 8–12mm.

Complications

- Immediate mortality is ~3%, usually from a capsular puncture and bleeding. 4-6 week mortality in patients treated by TIPSS for uncontrolled haemorrhage is up to 50% (from cirrhosis).
- Hepatic encephalopathy occurs in 20%.
- Failure to reduce portal pressure may occur if there are large extrahepatic shunts. These may need to be embolized.

Peritoneal dialysis (PD)

Rarely used but does not require vascular access or anticoagulation. A clearance rate of ~10mL/min may be achieved.

It requires:

- PD catheter (inserted under local anaesthetic)
- Intact peritoneal cavity free of infection, herniae, adhesions.

Complications

Peritonitis occurs at 0.8 episode per patient per year.

Assessment

- Features of peritonitis are: cloudy PD bag (99%), abdominal pain (95%), and abdominal tenderness (80%).
- Other features include: fever (33%), N&V (30%), leucocytosis (25%), diarrhoea or constipation (15%).
- Investigations: PD effluent cell count (peritonitis if >100 neutrophils/mm^3), culture PD fluid (inoculate a blood culture bottle), Gram stain PD fluid, FBC (for leucocytosis), blood cultures.

Management

- All patients require antibiotics, but may not require admission. The antibiotics used depends on Gram stain and culture results. A typical protocol would be ciprofloxacin or vancomycin, plus metronidazole. Patients with high fever with leucocytosis, and/or who are systemically unwell warrant IV antibiotics.
- Gram-negative infection, in particular *Pseudomonas*, is associated with more severe infection.
- Peritonitis can lead to development of an ileus.
- Patients may lose up to 25g protein/day in severe cases and should receive adequate nutritional support.
- If the infection is resistant to treatment, consider removal of Tenckhoff catheter and atypical organisms (e.g. fungi).
- Consider underlying GI pathology especially if multibacterial, Gram-negative organisms, or other symptoms.

Other problems

Mild cases of fluid overload may respond to hypertonic exchanges (6.36% or 4.25% glucose), fluid restriction (1L/day), and large doses of diuretics (e.g. furosemide 500mg bd).

Other problems include poor exchanges, malposition of the catheter, omental blocking, fibrin deposition, and hyperglycaemia.

Intermittent haemodialysis

A blood flow of 250–300mL/min is needed across the dialysis membrane and leads to a clearance of 20mL/min.

- ***Vascular access*** Vascular access may be obtained using an AV shunt involving the radial artery, or more commonly by using a Vascath which uses venous rather than arterial blood.
- ***Anticoagulation*** Heparin is normally used. If contraindicated, e.g. recent haemorrhage, then prostacyclin may be used, but may cause hypotension and abdominal cramps.
- ***Haemodynamic stability*** Patients with multiorgan failure commonly develop hypotension during haemodialysis. This may be ameliorated by high sodium dialysate, and priming the circuit with 4.5% human albumin solution.

Complications of haemodialysis

Hypotension

Usually occurs within the first 15min of commencing dialysis. It probably involves activation of circulating inflammatory cells by the membrane, osmotic shifts, and possibly loss of fluid. *Treatment*: cautious fluid replacement and inotropes (watch for pulmonary oedema if over-transfused).

Dialysis disequilibrium

This occurs during the initial dialysis especially in patients with marked uraemia, and is more common in patients with pre-existing neurological disease. *Clinical features*: headache, N&V, fits, cerebral oedema. *Treatment*: treat cerebral oedema as on 📖 p.380. Short and slow initial dialyses may prevent this.

Dialyser reaction

This is caused by an IgE or complement response against the ethylene oxide (sterilizing agent) or the cellulose component. Use of 'biocompatible' membranes, e.g. polysulfone, polyacrylonitrile (PAN), or dialysers sterilized by steam or γ-irradiation may prevent further reactions.

Haemofiltration

Continuous arteriovenous haemofiltration (CAVH) implies bulk solute transport across a membrane and replacement. Haemodiafiltration (CAVHD) involves the pumping of dialysate across the other side of the membrane. For both, arterial blood (driven by arterial pressure) is continuously filtered at a relatively low flow rate (50–100mL/min). Continuous venovenous haemofiltration involves pumping blood from a venous access to the dialysis membrane (150–200mL/min) (CVVH or CVVHD). The equivalent GFR obtained by these are approximately 15–30mL/min. These are used most commonly on ITU. Both of these methods cause less haemodynamic instability, and are particularly useful in patients with multiorgan failure.

Plasmapheresis

A therapy directed towards removal of circulating high molecular weight compounds not removed by dialysis. Particularly used in the removal of antibodies, or lipoproteins.

Indications

- Myasthenia gravis
- Guillain–Barré syndrome
- Goodpasture's syndrome
- TTP
- HUS
- Severe hyperlipidaemia
- Multisystem vasculitis
- Hyperviscosity syndrome (e.g. Waldenstrom's macroglobulinaemia)
- HLA antibody removal.

Method

Requires central venous access with a large bore, dual lumen cannula. Usually 5 treatment sessions are given on consecutive days. Plasma is removed and replaced with, typically, 2U FFP, 3L 4.5% albumin. IV calcium (10mL 10% calcium gluconate) should be given with the FFP. Febrile reactions may occur as with other blood products. Plasmapheresis has no effect on the underlying rate of antibody production, but is a useful treatment in acute situations such as Goodpasture's and myasthenia gravis.

- For HUS and TTP one must use FFP ***only*** (preferably cryodepleted), usually a minimum of 3L/day (see 🕮 p.598).
- For hyperviscosity syndrome, a centrifugation system is required rather than a plasma filter (see 🕮 p.616).
- For lipopheresis there may be severe reactions if the patient is on an ACEI.
- An alternative to plasmapheresis is immunoabsorption in which 2 columns are used in parallel. This may be used in the removal of HLA antibodies, anti-GBM disease, or multisystem vasculitis.

Renal biopsy

Indications (see Box 15.8)

Biopsy is now performed using real-time US guidance by trained doctors.

Contraindications

- Bleeding diathesis—unless correctable prior to biopsy
- Solitary functioning kidney
- Uncontrolled hypertension, i.e. DBP >100mmHg
- Urinary tract obstruction
- Small kidneys, since it is unlikely to be helpful.

Prior to biopsy

- Check Hb, clotting screen, G&S serum.
- Ensure IVU or US has been carried out to determine presence and size of 2 kidneys.
- Consent patient. >1% risk of bleeding requiring transfusion.

Technique

- The biopsy is taken with the patient prone on the bed with pillows under abdomen. The lower pole of either kidney is visualized by US. A trucut biopsy is taken from lower renal pole under sterile conditions with local anaesthesia. The biopsy is taken with the patient holding their breath at the end of inspiration (displaces kidney inferiorly). Following biopsy they should have bed rest for 24h to minimize risk of bleeding, and the BP and pulse monitored half-hourly for 2h, 1-hourly for 4h, then 4-hourly for 18h.
- Send renal biopsy tissue for light microscopy, immunofluorescence, EM and Special stains (e.g. Congo red).

Complications

- Bleeding: microscopic haematuria is usual; macroscopic haematuria in 5–10%; bleeding requiring transfusion in 1%.
- Formation of an intrarenal AV fistula may occur.
- Severe loin pain suggests bleeding.
- Pneumothorax and ileus are rare.

Renal transplant biopsy

Indications

- Decline in transplant function
- 1° non-function post transplant.

Procedure

Biopsy may be taken from either upper or lower pole. Some centres find FNAB useful in diagnosis of transplant rejection.

Box 15.8 Indications for renal biopsy

- Cause is unknown
- Heavy proteinuria (>2g/day)
- Features of systemic disease
- Active urinary sediment
- Immune-mediated ARF
- Prolonged renal failure (>2 weeks)
- Suspected interstitial nephritis (drug induced).

pH_i determination (gastric tonometer)

Patients in shock have reduced splanchnic perfusion and O_2 delivery. The resulting mucosal ischaemia may be difficult to diagnose clinically until it presents as GI bleeding or the sepsis syndrome. The earliest change detectable following an ischaemic insult to the gut is a fall in intramucosal pH. Gastric mucosal pH parallels the changes in pH in other portions of the GI tract and monitoring this allows detection of gut ischaemia early.

A tonometer is essentially an NG-tube with a second lumen leading to a balloon which lies within the mucosal folds of the stomach. The balloon is inflated with 0.9% saline for 30–90min. This allows CO_2 from the mucosa to diffuse into the saline and equilibrate. The saline is then removed and analysed for pCO_2 with simultaneous arterial blood [HCO_3^-] measurement. pH_i is then calculated using a modification of the Henderson–Hasselbalch equation.

Joint aspiration

Many synovial joints can be safely aspirated by an experienced operator. Knee effusions are common and aseptic aspiration can be safely performed in the Emergency Department. The risk of inducing a septic arthritis is <1 in 10,000 aspirations, but certain rules should be followed.

- Anatomical landmarks are identified
- The skin is cleaned with alcohol or iodine
- Local anaesthetic is applied to the area
- A no touch technique is essential.

Indications for synovial fluid aspiration in casualty

- Suspected septic arthritis
- Suspected crystal arthritis
- Suspected haemarthrosis
- Relief of symptoms by removal of effusion in degenerative arthritis.

Contraindications to joint aspiration

- Overlying sepsis
- Bleeding diathesis.

Knee joint

Patient lies with knee slightly flexed and supported. The joint space behind the patella either medially or laterally is palpated, the skin cleaned, and a needle (18G, green) inserted horizontally between the patella and femur using a no-touch technique. There is a slight resistance as the needle goes through the synovial membrane. Aspirate on the syringe until fluid is obtained.

Elbow joint

Flex the elbow to 90° and pass the needle between the proximal head of the radius (locate by rotating patients hand) and the lateral epicondyle; or the needle can be passed posteriorly between the lateral epicondyla and the olecranon.

Ankle joint

Plantarflex the foot slightly, palpate the joint margin between extensor hallucis longus (lateral) and tibialis anterior (medial) tendons just above tip of medial malleolus.

When synovial fluid is obtained:

- Note the colour and assess viscosity
- Microscopy for cell count and crystals (Table 15.1)
- Gram stain and culture
- Synovial fluid glucose (↓cf. blood glucose in sepsis).

Table 15.1 Synovial fluid analysis

Condition	Viscosity	Opacity	Leucocyte count (per mm^3)
Normal	High	Clear	<200
Osteoarthritis	High	Clear	1000 (<50% PMN)
Rheumatoid	Low	Cloudy	1–50 000 PMN
Crystal	Low	Cloudy	5–50 000 PMN
Sepsis	Low	Cloudy	10–100 00 0 PMN

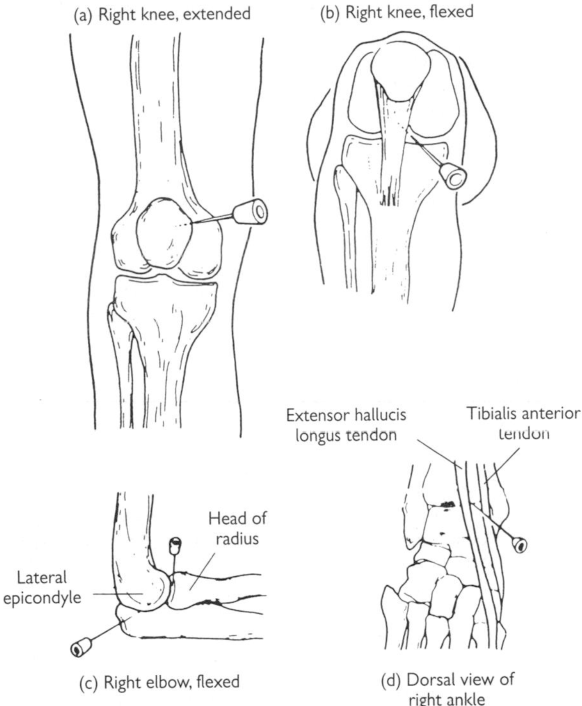

Fig. 15.14 Approaches used for joint aspiration (after Crawley M (1974). *Br Hosp Med* **11**: 747–55).

Intracranial pressure monitoring

Indications

- Cerebral trauma (GCS ≤8, compression of basal cistern on CT, midline shift >0.5mm on CT, non-surgical raised ICP
- Acute liver failure (Grade 4 coma with signs of raised ICP)
- Metabolic diseases with raised ICP (e.g. Reye's syndrome)
- Postoperative oedema (after neurosurgery)
- After intracranial haemorrhage (SAH or intracerebral).

ICP monitoring should be started before 2° brain injury in patients who are at risk of sudden rises in ICP and where it would influence management of the patient. These patients may be effectively managed in District Hospitals.

Contraindications

- Uncorrectable coagulopathy
- Local infection near placement site or meningitis
- Septicaemia.

Method

- There are several types of devices available (subdural, extradural, parenchymal, or intraventricular); parenchymal and intraventricular monitors carry a high risk.
- There are pre-packaged kits available (e.g. the Codman® subdural bolt). This monitor is inserted in the pre-frontal region and the kit contains the necessary screws for creating a burr-hole, spinal needles to perforate the dura, etc.
- The ICP waveform obtained is a dynamic recording that looks similar to a pulse waveform, and is due to pulsations of the cerebral blood vessels within the confined space of the cranium, together with the effects of respiration.
- Cerebral perfusion pressure = mean arterial pressure – ICP.
- The normal resting mean ICP measured in a supine patient is <10mmHg (<1.3kPa).
- The level which requires treatment depends to some extent on the disease: in benign intracranial hypertension values of >40mmHg may not be associated with neurological symptoms; but in patients with cerebral trauma treatment should be initiated when ICP is >25mmHg.
- There are several types of pressure waves described of which the most significant are '*A waves*'—sustained increases of the ICP lasting 10–20min up to 50–100mmHg (6–13kPa). These are associated with a poor prognosis.
- The readings of the ICP monitors should always be accompanied by careful neurological examination.
- Treatment of raised ICP is discussed on 📖 p.372.

Complications

- Infection (up to 5%)
- Bleeding (local, subdural, extradural, or intracerebral)
- CSF leak
- Seizures
- Misreading of ICP pressures.

Lumbar puncture 1

Contraindications

- Raised ICP (falling level of consciousness with falling pulse, rising BP, vomiting, focal signs, papilloedema). A CT scan should be carried out prior to LP to exclude an obstructed CSF system or SOL (see 📖 p.372).
- Coagulopathy or ↓platelets (<50 × 10^9/L).

You will need the following:

- Spinal needles and manometer for measuring the opening CSF pressure
- Dressing pack (gauze, drapes, antiseptic, gloves, plaster)
- Local anaesthetic (e.g. 2% lidocaine), 3 sterile bottles for collecting CSF, and glucose bottle.

Procedure

Give antibiotics first if suspected meningitis (see 📖 p.355).

- Explain the procedure to the patient.
- Position the patient. This is crucial to success. Lie patient on their left side if you are right handed or their right side if you are left handed, with back on edge of bed, fully flexed (knees to chin), with a folded pillow between their legs, keeping the back perpendicular to the bed. Flexion separates the interspaces.
- The safest site for LP is the L4–L5 interspace (the spinal cord ends at L1–L2). An imaginary line drawn between the iliac crests intersects the spine at the L4 process or L4–L5 space exactly. Mark the L4,5 intervertebral space.
- Clean the skin and place the sterile drapes over the patient.
- Inject and anaesthetize the deep structures with 2% lignocaine.
- Insert the spinal needle (stilette in place) in the midline, aiming slightly cranially (towards umbilicus), horizontal to the bed. Do not advance the needle without the stylet in place.
- You will feel the resistance of the spinal ligaments, and then the dura, followed by a 'give' as the needle enters the subarachnoid space. Replace the stylet before advancing.
- Measure CSF pressure with manometer and 3-way tap. Normal opening pressure is 7–20cm CSF. CSF pressure is ↑ with anxiety, SAH, infection, space-occupying lesion, benign intracranial hypertension, CCF.
- Collect 0.5–1.5mL fluid in 3 serially numbered bottles incl. a glucose bottle.
- Send specimens promptly for microscopy, culture, protein, glucose (with a simultaneous plasma sample for comparison), and where appropriate, virology, syphilis serology, cytology for malignancy, AFB, oligoclonal bands (multiple sclerosis), cryptococcal antigen, India ink stains, and fungal culture.
- Remove needle and place a plaster over the site.
- Patient should lie flat for at least 6h and have hourly neurological observation and BP measurement.

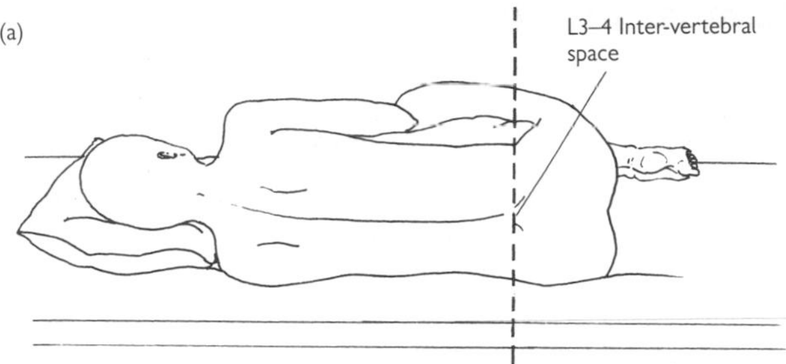

Position the patient so that the line joining the iliac crests is perpendicular to the bed.

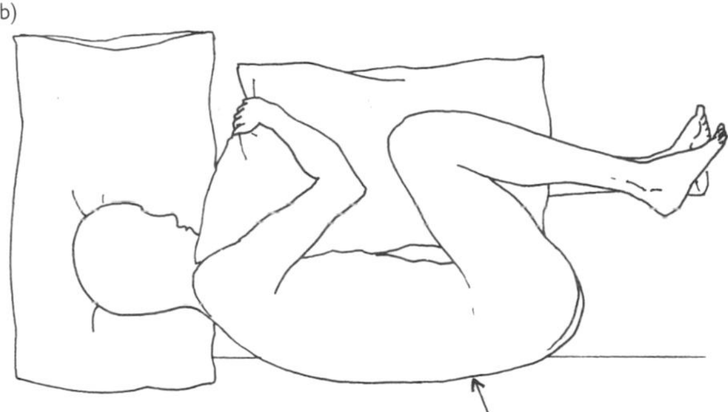

Ask the patient to curl up with a pillow between the knees to open the interspace. Point the needle cranially and advance gently.

Fig. 15.15 Lumbar puncture.

Lumbar puncture 2

Complications of lumbar puncture

- ***Headache*** Common (up to 25%). Typically present when the patient is upright and better when supine. May last for days. Thought to be due to CSF depletion from a persistent leak from the LP site. Prevented by using finer spinal needles, keep the patient supine for 6–12h post LP, and encourage fluids. Treat with analgesia, fluids, and reassurance.
- ***Trauma to nerve roots*** Rarer but seen if the needle does not stay in the midline. The patient experiences sharp pains or parasthesiae down the leg. Withdraw the needle and if the symptoms persist, stop the procedure and seek expert help.
- ***Bleeding*** Minor bleeding may occur with a 'traumatic tap' when a small spinal vein is nicked. The CSF appears bloody (see 'CSF analysis') but the bleeding stops spontaneously and does not require specific therapy. Coagulopathy, severe liver disease, or thrombocytopenia carries the risk of subarachnoid/subdural bleeding and paralysis.
- ***Coning*** Herniation of cerebellar tonsils with compression of the medulla is very rare unless the patient has raised ICP. Always get a CT brain scan prior to LP and review this yourself if possible. Mortality is high, but the patient may respond to standard measures for treating this (see 📖 p.372).
- ***Infection*** Rare if proper sterile technique used.

CSF analysis

- **Normal values:**
  - Lymphocytes <4/mm^3; polymorphs 0mm^3
  - Protein <0.4g/L
  - Glucose >2.2mmol/L (or >70% pl. glucose)
  - Opening pressure <20 cm CSF.
- ***A bloody tap*** is indicated by progressively fewer red cells in successive bottles, no yellowing of CSF (xanthochromia). The true WBC count may be estimated by:

  True CSF WBC =CSF WBC – (Blood WBC × CSF RBC)/blood RBC

  If the patient's blood count is normal, subtract approx. 1 white cell for every 1000 RBC). To estimate the true protein level subtract 10mg/L for every 1000 RBCs/mm^3 (be sure to do the count and protein estimation on the same bottle.
- ***Subarachnoid haemorrhage:*** (see 📖 p.384) xanthochromia (yellowing of CSF). Red cells in equal numbers in all bottles. The RBCs will excite an inflammatory response (increasing CSF WCC), most marked after 48h.
- ***Very high CSF protein:*** a marked increase in CSF protein: acoustic neuroma and spinal tumours; Guillain–Barré syndrome (see 📖 p.426).

Table 15.2 CSF Analysis

	Bacterial	**Viral**	**TB meningitis**
Appearance	Turbid	Clear	Clear
Cells (mm^3)	5–2000	5–500	5–1000
Main cell type	Neutrophil	Lymphocyte	Lymphocyte
Glucose (mM)	Very low	Normal	Low
Protein (g/L)	Often >1.0	0.5–0.9	Often >1.0
Other tests	Gram stain	PCR	Ziehl–Niehlson
	Bacterial Ag		Fluorescent test PCR

Needlestick injuries

Occupational exposures to bloodborne viruses (BBVs) in healthcare workers can be divided into 2 groups: percutaneous (needlestick) and mucocutaneous (through broken skin or via splashes into the eyes). High-risk body fluids include: blood, pleural fluid, peritoneal fluid, pericardial fluid, synovial fluid, amniotic fluid, human breast milk, cerebrospinal fluid, saliva (in dentistry), semen, vaginal secretions, and unfixed tissues and organs as well as vomit, faeces and urine when contaminated with blood.

The major pathogens associated with needlestick injuries and mucocutaneous exposures are:
- Hepatitis B virus (HBV)
- Hepatitis C virus (HCV)
- Human immunodeficiency virus (HIV).

Occupational exposures to BBVs can be caused by certain work practices such as:
- Not properly disposing of used needles
- Recapping needles
- Not using protective equipments e.g. eye protection.

Prevention

Assume that every patient is potentially infected with a blood-borne infection. The same precautions should be taken for every patient and every procedure.
- Cover skin cuts and abrasions with waterproof dressings.
- Never recap needles or pass sharps hand-to-hand.
- Always dispose of used needles promptly in sharps disposal.
- Never leave sharps to be cleared up by others.
- Use eye protection. Ordinary spectacles offer inadequate protection. Use safety glasses which fit over spectacles.
- Double gloving: In case of needlestick, 80% of the visible blood can be removed by latex in a surgical glove. With double gloving, the inner glove will remove a further 80% of the remaining blood on the needle.

Management of exposure incidents

- If the mouth or eyes are involved, wash thoroughly with water.
- If skin is punctured, let the wound bleed and wash it with soap or chlorhexidine and running water. Avoid scrubbing or sucking.
- Report to Occupational Health department to arrange immediate assessment or, if out of hours, attend the A&E department in accordance with the local policy.

Assessment of the risk of BBVs transmission

Estimated seroconversion risks are:
- ***HBV:*** 30% for percutaneous exposure of a non-immune individual to HBsAg and HBeAg positive source.
- ***HCV:*** 1.9% for percutaneous exposure to HCV infected blood with detectable HCV RNA.
- ***HIV:*** 0.3% for percutaneous exposure to HIV infected blood.

Factors increasing the risk following injury include:

- Percutaneous injury is higher risk than mucous membrane or broken skin exposure
- Injury with a device directly from a source patient's artery/vein
- Injury from hollow bore and wide gauge needle
- Deep injury
- Visible blood on the device
- High HIV viral load, or HBeAg in the source patient.
- Staff member inadequately immunized against hepatitis B.

Approaching source patients for blood-borne virus testing

- Due to the sensitivity of the issue, source patient should not be approached by the exposed member of staff.
- Occupational health (or A&E if out of hours) will arrange this test in accordance with local policies.

Post-exposure prophylaxis (PEP) for HIV

Risk assessment and follow up is carried out by occupational health (A&E out of hours). If indicated, PEP with should be started within an hour. However, it can be started up to 2 weeks after exposure (see 📖 p.513).

PEP for HBV

If the patient has been vaccinated at least twice with HB vaccine, and is known to be a responder (anti-HBS >10IU/ml), they should be given a booster injection, with a 2nd dose 1 month later. For patients who have not been vaccinated or are known to be non-responders, they should be given an immediate injection of hepatitis B immunoglobulin (HBIG) and commence an accelerated course of HB vaccination, or have a booster dose if previously immunised.

PEP for HCV

Although there is no vaccine or effective PEP against hepatitis C, evidence suggests that early treatment with high-dose interferon can result in viral clearance in >90% of recently infected individuals. This emphasizes the importance of close and timely follow-up of exposed workers. Therefore, all exposed to HCV should be tested for HCV antibodies at the time of exposure and at 6–12 weeks and at 26 weeks.

Chapter 16

Differential diagnosis of common presentations

Introduction

It is often said that 80% of the diagnosis depends on a good history. The differential diagnosis formed from the history, can then be narrowed down by physical examination and investigations.

The history of the presenting complaint is a key component of establishing a diagnosis, and should be divided into 3 subsections to ensure that the most crucial points in the history are dealt with at an early stage:

About the symptom

I.e. what, where (including radiation), when (onset, duration, course), how bad (severity), exacerbating/relieving factors etc.

About the most relevant organ system

(e.g. questions relating to the respiratory and cardiovascular systems for a patient presenting with breathlessness). It is important to ask about the most relevant organ systems and common 'associated symptoms' during the initial history rather than during the systemic enquiry. See 📖 'Systemic enquiry, p.815 for summary of most important questions.

Risk factors

Go through your list of differential diagnoses for the presenting complaint (see below) and ask questions about the various differentials and risk factors that increase the likelihood of their development. For example, if a patient presents with diarrhoea, the list of differential diagnoses includes infection. Therefore risk factors such as contacts, food history, recent travel, etc. should be addressed.

The following pages will outline relatively short/memorable lists of differential diagnoses for the most common presenting symptoms. These lists are not comprehensive, but are a good starting point. Each list of differential diagnoses can be used as a guide to for asking the important questions about each differential and the risk factors.

See the appropriate sections in the rest of his book for further information on the clinical signs and the specific investigations needed to exclude or confirm a diagnosis.

Systemic enquiry

General questions

Fever, sweats, fatigue, malaise, loss of appetite, weight loss, lumps.

Cardiovascular

Chest pain, palpitation, breathlessness (exertional, at rest, orthopnoea, paroxysmal nocturnal dyspnoea), ankle swelling, dizziness.

Respiratory

Wheeze, breathlessness, cough, sputum, haemoptysis, chest pain, calf pain/swelling.

Gastrointestinal

Loss of appetite/weight, nausea/vomiting, dysphagia, indigestion/heartburn, abdominal pain, change of bowel habit (diarrhoea or constipation), bloating, blood/mucus PR, melaena or haemetemesis, jaundice, pruritus, dark urine, pale stool.

Urogential

Urinary frequency, urgency, dysuria, haematuria, loin pain, vaginal/penile discharge, periods/sexual problems.

Neurological

Cognitive impairment or reduced consciousness (from collateral history), visual disturbance, hearing loss, speech/ swallowing problems, headache, neck/back pain, weakness, paraesthesia, balance/co-ordination problems, bowel/bladder control.

Rheumatological

Morning stiffness, joint pain/swelling/stiffness, deformity, malaise/fatigue/weight loss, arthralgia, myalgia, rash, raynaud's phenomenon, hair loss, red or sore or dry eyes, dry mouth, oral ulcers, gential ulcers.

Diabetes and endocrine

Polyuria, polydipsia, fatigue, weight loss, neck swelling or tenderness, tremor, heat/cold intolerance, sweating, changes in hair, skin, voice, face, hands or feet appearance, pigmentation.

Ear, nose, throat

Ear pain/discharge, nasal discharge/crusting, sore throat.

Abdominal pain 1

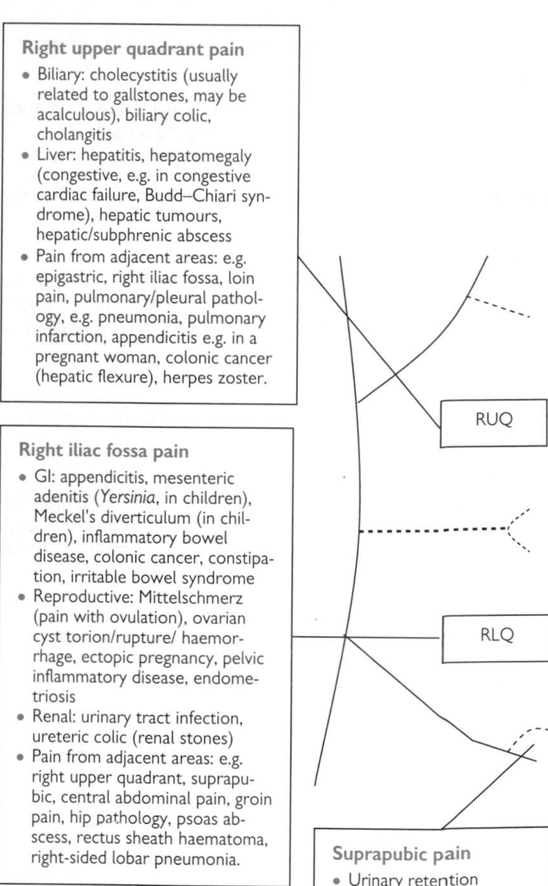

Right upper quadrant pain
• Biliary: cholecystitis (usually related to gallstones, may be acalculous), biliary colic, cholangitis
• Liver: hepatitis, hepatomegaly (congestive, e.g. in congestive cardiac failure, Budd–Chiari syndrome), hepatic tumours, hepatic/subphrenic abscess
• Pain from adjacent areas: e.g. epigastric, right iliac fossa, loin pain, pulmonary/pleural pathology, e.g. pneumonia, pulmonary infarction, appendicitis e.g. in a pregnant woman, colonic cancer (hepatic flexure), herpes zoster.
RUQ
Right iliac fossa pain
• GI: appendicitis, mesenteric adenitis (*Yersinia*, in children), Meckel's diverticulum (in children), inflammatory bowel disease, colonic cancer, constipation, irritable bowel syndrome
• Reproductive: Mittelschmerz (pain with ovulation), ovarian cyst torion/rupture/ haemorrhage, ectopic pregnancy, pelvic inflammatory disease, endometriosis
• Renal: urinary tract infection, ureteric colic (renal stones)
• Pain from adjacent areas: e.g. right upper quadrant, suprapubic, central abdominal pain, groin pain, hip pathology, psoas abscess, rectus sheath haematoma, right-sided lobar pneumonia.
RLQ
Suprapubic pain
• Urinary retention
• Cystitis
• Pain from adjacent areas: e.g. right iliac fossa and left iliac fossa.

Fig. 16.1 Causes of regional abdominal pain.

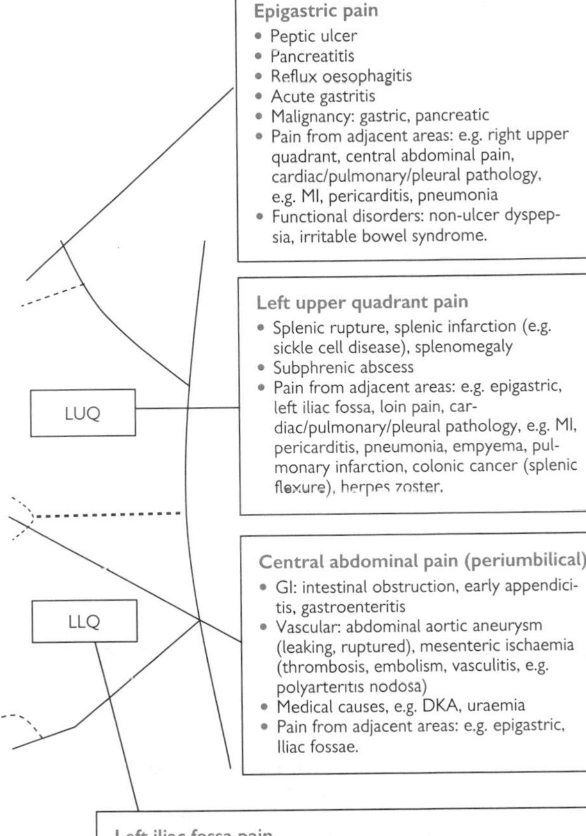

Epigastric pain
• Peptic ulcer
• Pancreatitis
• Reflux oesophagitis
• Acute gastritis
• Malignancy: gastric, pancreatic
• Pain from adjacent areas: e.g. right upper quadrant, central abdominal pain, cardiac/pulmonary/pleural pathology, e.g. MI, pericarditis, pneumonia
• Functional disorders: non-ulcer dyspepsia, irritable bowel syndrome.
Left upper quadrant pain
• Splenic rupture, splenic infarction (e.g. sickle cell disease), splenomegaly
• Subphrenic abscess
• Pain from adjacent areas: e.g. epigastric, left iliac fossa, loin pain, cardiac/pulmonary/pleural pathology, e.g. MI, pericarditis, pneumonia, empyema, pulmonary infarction, colonic cancer (splenic flexure), herpes zoster.
LUQ
Central abdominal pain (periumbilical)
• GI: intestinal obstruction, early appendicitis, gastroenteritis
• Vascular: abdominal aortic aneurysm (leaking, ruptured), mesenteric ischaemia (thrombosis, embolism, vasculitis, e.g. polyarteritis nodosa)
• Medical causes, e.g. DKA, uraemia
• Pain from adjacent areas: e.g. epigastric, Iliac fossae.
LLQ

Left iliac fossa pain

- GI: diverticulitis, IBD, colonic cancer, constipation, irritable bowel syndrome
- Reproductive: Mittelschmerz (pain with ovulation), ovarian cyst tortion/rupture/haemorrhage, ectopic pregnancy, salpingitis/pelvic inflammatory disease, endometriosis
- Renal pain: urinary tract infection, ureteric colic (renal stones)
- Pain from adjacent areas: e.g. left upper quadrant, suprapubic, central abdominal, hip pathology, psoas abscess, rectus sheath haematoma, left-sided lobar pneumonia.

Fig. 16.1 *(Contd).*

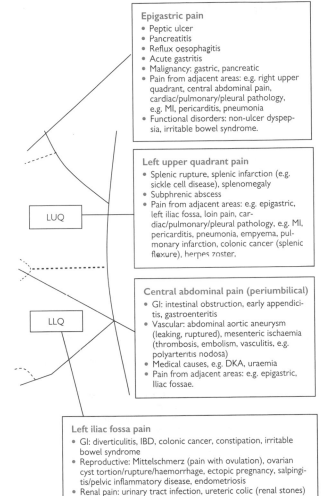

Abdominal pain 2

Loin pain

- Infection: urinary tract infection (pyelonephritis), perinephric abscess/ pyonephrosis
- Obstruction: in the lumen, e.g. stones, tumour, blood clots; in the wall e.g. stricture (ureteric/urethral); pressure from the outside, e.g. prostatic/pelvic mass, retroperitoneal fibrosis
- Other: renal carcinoma, renal vein thrombosis, polycystic kidney disease, pain from vertebral column.

Groin pain

- Renal stones (pain radiating from loin to groin)
- Testicular pain, e.g. torsion, epididymo-orchitis (pain radiating from scrotum to groin). Hernia (inguinal), hip or pelvic pathology e.g. fracture.

Diffuse abdominal pain

- Gastroenteritis
- Peritonitis
- Intestinal obstruction
- IBD
- Mesenteric ischaemia
- Medical causes
- Irritable bowel syndrome.

Medical causes

Most causes of abdominal pain are surgical. However, occasionally there may be a 'medical cause' of abdominal pain:

- Cardiovascular/respiratory: MI, pneumonia, Bornholm's disease (Cosackie B virus infection)
- Metabolic: DKA, Addisonian crisis, hypercalcaemia, uraemia, porphyria, pheochromocytoma, lead poisoning
- Neurological: herpes zoster
- Haematological: sickle cell crisis, retroperitoneal haemorrhage (e.g. anticoagulants), lymphadenopathy
- Inflammatory: vasculitis (e.g. Henoch–Schönlein purpura, polyarteritis nodosa), familial Mediterranean fever
- Infections: intestinal parasites, TB, malaria, typhoid fever
- Irritable bowel syndrome.

Abdominal pain (referred)

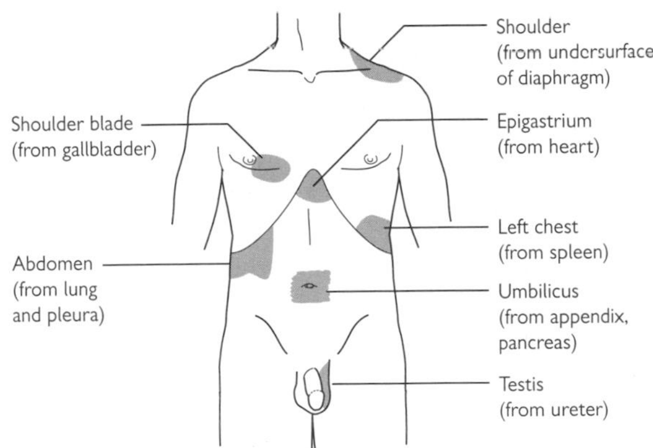

Fig. 16.2 Common sites of referred pain.

Abdominal distension

- Fat (obesity)
- Fluid (ascites, fluid in the obstructed intestine)
- Flatus (intestinal obstruction)
- Faeces
- Fetus
- Giant organomegaly (e.g. an ovarian cystadenoma, lymphoma)
- Small bowel: adhesions, herniae, Crohn's disease, gallstone ileus, foreign body, tumour, tuberculosis
- Large bowel: cancer, volvulus, diverticulitis, faeces.

Back pain

All patients

- Strenuous activity, muscle spasm, trauma, fractures
- Infection: TB or bacterial osteomyelitis of vertebra, disciitis
- Malignancy: metastasis, multiple myeloma, malignant lumbosacral plexopathy (with colorectal and gynaecologic tumours, sarcomas, lymphomas)
- Spinal cord compression
- Infection: epidural abscesses (IV users, vertebral osteomyelitis, haematogenous spread): common pathogens: *Staphylococcus aureus, Mycobacterium tuberculosis*
- Malignancy: myeloma, metastases (vertebral, spinal cord)
- Inflammatory: rheumatoid arthritis, sarcoidosis, or tophaceous gout
- Other: haematomas (bleeding disorders, anticoagulant therapy), arteriovenous malformation

Younger patients (≤40 year)

- Prolapsed disc, ankylosing spondylitis, spondylolisthesis.

Older patients (≥40 year)

- Osteoarthritis, spinal stenosis and spinal claudication
- Osteoporotic fractures, Paget's disease of bone.

Blackouts

Cardiovascular (due to transient reduction in blood flow to the brain)

- Arrhythmia: bradycardia (heart block), tachycardia
- Outflow obstruction: aortic stenosis, hypertrophic obstructive cardiomyopathy, PE, pulmonary stenosis
- Postural hypotension: hypovolaemia, autonomic neuropathy (e.g. diabetes mellitus), antihypertensive medications (e.g. ACEIs)
- MI, aortic dissection and any other condition that may cause a sudden reduction in cardiac output.

Neurological

- Epilepsy, stroke/transient ischaemic attack (rarely).

Neurocardiogenic (vasovagal) syncope and carotid sinus hypersensitivity

Vasovagal syncope may be induced by prolonged standing, cough, micturition, venipuncture, heat exposure, or painful stimuli. There may be no identifiable cause especially in the elderly. Blackouts due to carotid sinus hypersensitivity may be produced by head turning, tight-fitting collars, or shaving.

Metabolic

- Hypoglycaemia (see 📖 p.528)

Breathlessness/dyspnoea

The causes of breathlessness are best classified according to rapidity of onset. However, although the onset gives a significant clue, the following lists are not mutually exclusive.

Acute (seconds)

- PE
- Pneumothorax
- Foreign body
- Anaphylaxis
- Anxiety.

Subacute (minutes–hours)

- Acute left ventricular failure (pulmonary oedema)
- Asthma exacerbation
- COPD exacerbation
- Pneumonia (bacterial, viral, fungal, TB)
- Metabolic acidosis.

Chronic (days–weeks)

- Anaemia
- Thyrotoxicosis
- Recurrent pulmonary emboli
- Cardiac disease (chronic cardiac failure, arrhythmias, valvular heart disease)
- Asthma
- COPD
- Non-resolving pneumonia
- Bronchiectasis
- Lung cancer
- Interstitial lung disease/pulmonary fibrosis (cryptogenic, connective tissue diseases, drugs, environmental/occupational lung disease)
- Pulmonary hypertension
- Pleural effusion
- Neuromuscular disorders, chest wall deformities.

Chest pain

Some causes of chest pain

Chest wall

- Ribs: fracture or neoplasm
- Intercostal muscle: spasm, inflammation (Bornholm's disease)
- Costochondritis
- Herpes zoster
- Thoracic vertebral pain
- Thoracic nerve root pain.

Pleura

- Pleurisy (infectious, neoplastic, vasculitic, irritative).

Lung vasculature

- Pulmonary infarction
- Pulmonary hypertension.

Mediastinal structures

- Lymph nodes (lymphoma, cancer)
- Oesophagitis
- Aortic dissection
- Tracheobronchitis
- Pericarditis
- Myocardial pain (angina, ACS).

Extra thoracic

- Cervical arthritis
- Subdiaphragmatic disease (e.g. hepatitis, splenic infarction, pancreatitis, peptic ulcer, gallstones)
- Migraine.

Chest pain (pleuritic)

- PE
- Pneumothorax
- Pneumonia
- Pericarditis
- Serositis/connective tissue disease
- Malignancy involving pleura
- Pathology under the diaphragm
- Musculoskeletal.

Collapse

See Blackouts, 📖 p.820

Confusion

- Hypoglycaemia
- Hypoxia: cardiac arrest, shock (hypovolaemic, septic), respiratory failure
- Vascular: intracranial haemorrhage/infarction
- Infection: extracranial (most commonly urinary tract infection and pneumonia in the elderly); intracranial (meningitis, encephalitis)
- Inflammation (cerebral vasculitis)
- Trauma (head injury)
- Tumour (↑intracranial pressure)
- Toxic: drugs e.g. opiates, alcohol, anxiolytics, antidepressants
- Metabolic: liver failure, renal failure, electrolyte (Na^+, K^+, Ca^{2+}, Mg^{2+}) disturbances, endocrinopathies e.g. myxoedema coma, vitamin deficiencies (e.g. thiamine, B12), hypothermia
- Post-ictal.

Constipation

- Drugs: opiates, anticholinergics (tricyclics, phenothiazines), iron tablets
- Immobility, old age
- GI/surgical:
- Intestinal obstruction (strictures, IBD, cancers, diverticulosis, pelvic mass e.g. fibroids)
- Pseudo-obstruction in scleroderma
- Anorectal disease (fissure, stricture, rectal prolapse)
- Postoperative
- Endocrine: hypothyroidism, hypercalcaemia, hypokalaemia, porphyria, lead poisoning
- Neurological/neuromuscular: autonomic neuropathy, spinal/pelvic nerve injury, Hirschsprung's disease, Chagas' disease.

Cough

- Upper respiratory tract infection
- All lung diseases:
  - Asthma, COPD, pulmonary emboli, infection (viral/bacterial/fungal/ TB pneumonia), bronchiectasis, malignancy, interstitial lung disease, sarcoidosis, pneumoconiosis
- Other causes:
  - Post-nasal drip
  - Gastro-oesophageal reflux disease
  - ACEIs
  - Cardiac failure
  - Psychogenic.

Cutaneous manifestations of internal malignancy

1. Cutaneous malignancy with frequent internal spread

- Melanoma
- Scar-related squamous cell carcinoma (e.g. mucosal surfaces, old scars)
- Mycosis fungoides
- Kaposi sarcoma.

2. Internal malignancy with cutaneous spread

- Breast carcinoma
- Leukaemia and lymphoma cutis
- Misc (occ. seen with GI, GU, and lung malignancy).

3. Pigmentation changes

- Hyperpigmentation (esp. with melanoma)
- Acanthosis nigricans (esp. gastric cancer)
- Sign of Leser–Trélat (rapid appearance of multiple seborrhoeic keratoses)
- Peutz–Jeghers syndrome
- Jaundice (biliary tract tumours, pancreas, liver metastases from other tunours)
- Purpura (e.g. leukaemia).

4. Flushing and facial erythema

- Carcinoid
- Mastocytosis
- Pheochromocytoma
- Cushing's disease.

5. Specific skin signs sometimes associated with malignancy

- Dermatomyositis in adults
- Bullous disease in adults (pemphigus and pemphigoid)
- Bowen's disease on non-sun-exposed areas
- Arsenic keratosis of palms and soles
- Paget's disease of nipple
- Basel cell naevus syndrome
- Acquired icthyosis (lymphomas)
- Exfoliative erythrodermatitis.

Diarrhoea

Infection

- ***Viral:*** adenovirus, astrovirus, calciviruses (norovirus and related viruses), rotavirus
- ***Bacterial:*** *Campylobacter*, *Salmonella*, *Shigella*, Haemorrhagic *E. coli*, *Clostridium difficile*, *Yersinia enterocolitica*, *C. perfringens*, *Vibrio cholerae*, *Vibrio parahaemolyticus*
- ***Parasites:*** cryptosporidia, *Giardia*, *Entamoeba histolytica*
- ***AIDS:*** AIDS enteropathy, cryptosporidia, microsporidia, CMV)
- IBD
- Malabsorption: small intestine disease/resection, biliary or pancreatic disease
- Medication: laxatives, antibiotics
- Overflow diarrhoea: 2° to constipation
- Endocrine: thyrotoxicosis, VIPomas.

Note: *Staphylococcus aureus* and *Bacillus cereus* mainly present with vomiting 1–6h after ingestion of prepared food e.g. salad, dairy, meat (*S. aureus*) and rice and meat (*B. cereus*)

Diarrhoea (bloody)

- Infective colitis: *Campylobàcter*, haemorrhagic *Escherichia coli*, *Salmonella*, *Shigella*, *Entamoeba histolytica*, CMV in the immunocompromised
- IBD
- Ischaemic colitis
- Diverticulitis
- Malignancy.

Dysphagia

1. Mechanical obstruction of oesophagus

- Congenital stricture
- Corrosive stricture
- Foreign body
- Carcinoma of oesophagus or stomach
- External compression (e.g. aortic aneurysm)
- Oesophageal divertula or pouch
- Reflux oesophagitis with stricture.

2. Dyspagia 2° to pain

- Pharyngitis
- Laryngitis.

3. Neurologic dysfunction of oesophagus

- Bulbar paralysis
- Syphilis
- Lead poisoning
- Tetanus
- Rabies
- Parkinson's disease
- Botulism
- Myasthenia gravis
- Achalasia
- Plummer–Vinson syndrome
- Hysteria.

Falls

- Sensory (visual, hearing, proprioception) impairment
- Gait/balance problem
- Muscle weakness/rigidity
- Urinary incontinence/frequency/urgency
- Medications: psychotropic, opiates
- Cognitive impairment
- Home hazards (especially in elderly).

Fever

- Infection: abscesses (e.g. subphrenic, liver, pelvis), bacterial: infective endocarditis, pneumonia, urinary tract infection, biliary infection, osteomyelitis, TB, brucellosis, viral (e.g. HIV, CMV, EBV), malaria etc.
- Inflammation/connective tissue disease: e.g. rheumatoid arthritis, SLE, sarcoidosis, vasculitides, polymyalgia rheumatica
- Malignancy: lymphomas, leukaemia, renal cell, hepatocellular or pancreatic carcinoma
- Metabolic: thyrotoxicosis
- Drugs: e.g. antibiotics, allopurinol, phenytoin, interferon
- Neutoleptic malignant syndrome, malignant hyperthermia, serotonin syndrome
- Familial Mediterranean fever, familial periodic fever.

Fever in a traveller

- Hepatitis A
- Malaria
- Dengue
- Typhoid
- Leptospirosis
- Haemorrhagic fevers
- Long incubation: malaria, typhoid, TB , brucellosis, leishmaniasis, amoebic abscess.

Fits

- Vascular: haemorrhage, infarction, cortical venous thrombosis, vascular malformation
- Trauma: head injury
- Tumours
- Toxic: alcohol, drugs, lead, carbon monoxide
- Metabolic: hypoxia, hypoglycaemia, electrolyte disturbances (↑ or ↓ Na^+, K^+, Ca^{2+}, Mg^{2+}), renal/hepatic failure, endocrine disorders (e.g. myxoedema), vitamin deficiency
- Infection: meningitis, encephalitis, abscess, TB, cysticercosis, HIV
- Inflammation: multiple sclerosis, vasculitis, SLE, sarcoidosis
- Malignant hypertension.

Haematemesis and melaena

- Peptic ulcer (gastric/duodenal)
- Gastritis/gastric erosions, duodenitis, oesophagitis
- Gastro-oesophageal varices
- Mallory–Weiss tear
- Medications: NSAIDs, anticoagulants, steroids, thrombolytics
- Oesophageal/gastric cancer
- ***Rarely:*** bleeding disorders (thrombocytopenia, haemophilia), hereditary haemorrhagic telangiectasia, Dieulafoy gastric vascular abnormality, aortoduodenal fistulae, angiodysplasia, leiomyoma, Meckel's diverticulum, pseudoxanthoma elasticum.

Haematuria

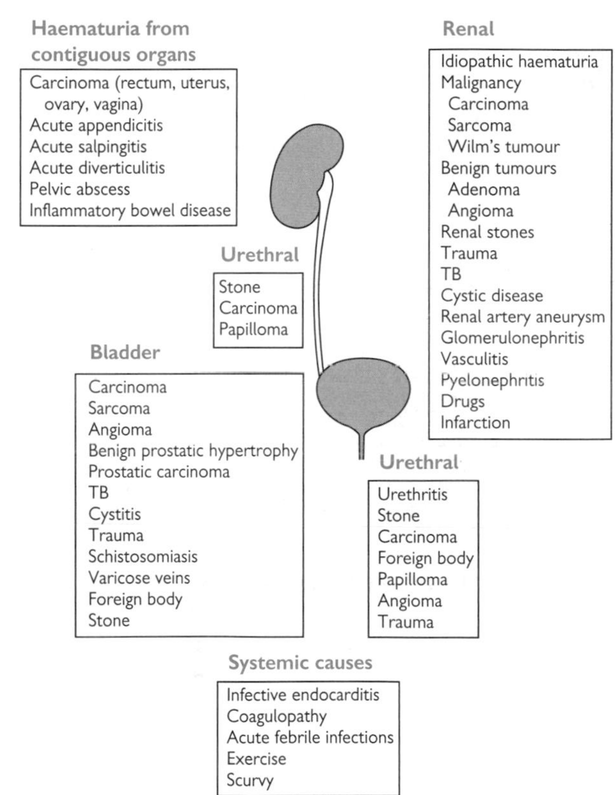
Haematuria from contiguous organs
Carcinoma (rectum, uterus, ovary, vagina)
Acute appendicitis
Acute salpingitis
Acute diverticulitis
Pelvic abscess
Inflammatory bowel disease
Renal
Idiopathic haematuria
Malignancy
Carcinoma
Sarcoma
Wilm's tumour
Benign tumours
Adenoma
Angioma
Renal stones
Trauma
TB
Cystic disease
Renal artery aneurysm
Glomerulonephritis
Vasculitis
Pyelonephritis
Drugs
Infarction
Urethral
Stone
Carcinoma
Papilloma
Bladder
Carcinoma
Sarcoma
Angioma
Benign prostatic hypertrophy
Prostatic carcinoma
TB
Cystitis
Trauma
Schistosomiasis
Varicose veins
Foreign body
Stone
Urethral
Urethritis
Stone
Carcinoma
Foreign body
Papilloma
Angioma
Trauma
Systemic causes
Infective endocarditis
Coagulopathy
Acute febrile infections
Exercise
Scurvy

Fig. 16.3 Causes of haematuria.

Haemoptysis

NB: nasal or upper respiratory tract and GI bleeding may be confused with haemoptysis

1. Infectious

- Acute bronchitis
- Pneumonia
- Bronchiectasis
- Lung abscess
- Mycobacterial infection
- Fungal infection (histoplasmosis, coccidiomycosis, aspergillosis)
- Parasites (paragonimiasis, schistosomiasis, ascariasis, amoebiasis, echinococcus, strongyloidiasis, etc.).

2. Neoplastic

- Bronchogenic carcinoma
- Bronchial adenoma
- Metastatic deposits.

3. Traumatic

- Lung contusion
- Bronchial rupture
- Post-endotracheal intubation.

4. Vascular

- Pulmonary infarction
- Pulmonary vasculitis
- Arteriovenous fistula.

5. Cardiovascular

- Pulmonary oedema.

6. Parenchymal

- Diffuse interstitial fibrosis
- Systemic diseases and vasculitis (Wegener's, rheumatoid arthritis, SLE, Goodpasture's, etc.)
- Sarcoidosis.

Headache

Serious causes to exclude

- Head injury
- Meningitis/encephalitis
- Vascular: haemorrhage (subarachnoid, intracranial), cerebral venous thrombosis, pituitary apoplexy
- Dissection (carotid/vertebral artery)
- Acute angle closure glaucoma
- Giant cell arteritis
- Other causes: malignant hypertension, drugs (e.g. GTN, calcium channel antagonists), infections (bacterial, viral illnesses etc.), electrolyte imbalances (e.g. hyponatraemia), hyperviscosity syndromes (e.g. polycythaemia), reduced ICP (e.g. post lumbar puncture), migraine, migrainous neuralgia

Hemiparesis

- Vascular: infarction, haemorrhage
- Infection: brain abscess from local (e.g. middle ear, sinuses) or distant (e.g. lung) infections, in the immunocompromised: TB, toxoplasmosis, progressive multifocal leucoencephalopathy
- Inflammation: demyelination, cerebral vasculitis
- Trauma: extradural or subdural haemorrhage (a history of trauma may not be apparent in the latter)
- Tumours: 1° (e.g. meningioma, glioma), metastases, lymphoma
- Metabolic: hypoglycaemia (transient)
- Other causes of transient hemiparesis: epileptic seizures (Todd's paralysis), migraine.

Hoarseness

1. Traumatic
- Foreign body
- External injury to larynx
- Voice abuse ('singer's nodules')
- Irritant gases (tobacco and other smoke)
- Aspiration (acid, alcohol).

2. Infectious
- Viral
- Diptheria
- Syphilis
- Leprosy.

3. Idiopathic
- Sarcoidosis
- Lupus erythematosus
- Cricoarytenoid ankylosis in rheumatoid arthritis.

4. Neurological
- Recurrent laryngeal palsy
- Bulbar palsy
- Myasthenia gravis.

5. Other
- Weakness
- Myxoedema
- Acromegaly.

Itching/pruritus

1. Causes of pruritus with visible skin disease

Rashes with excoriation
- Eczematous diseases (atopic, contact dermatitis, stasis dermatitis, anogenital pruritus, seborrheic dermatitis)
- Scabies
- Dermatitis herpetiformis
- Psoriasis
- Superficial fungal disease (esp. feet and intertriginous areas)
- Pinworm infestation (perianal)
- Psychogenic causes.

Rashes with little or no excoriation
- Urticaria
- Erythema multiforme
- Lichen planus
- Drug reactions
- Pityriasis rosea
- Urticaria pigmentosa (mastocytosis)
- Pruritic papules of pregnancy.

2. Causes of pruritus without visible skin disease

Associated with internal disease
- Uraemia
- Liver disease (billiary cirrhosis, obstructive jaundice)
- Lymohoma
- Polycythemia
- Pregnancy
- Misc: (e.g. occasionally seen with diabetes mellitus, thyroid disease, parathyroid disease, iron deficiency, internal malignancy, etc.).

Not associated with internal disease
- Pediculosis pubis
- Pinworm infestation
- Xerosis
- Psychogenis.

Joint pain/swelling

Single joint

- Infection: septic arthritis (staphylococci, gonococci, Gram –ve bacilli, TB, Lyme disease)
- Trauma, haemarthrosis (haemophilia)
- Gout/pseudogout
- Rheumatoid arthritis, osteoarthritis
- Seronegative arthritides (reactive arthritis, enteropathic arthritis (IBD, Whipple's disease), ankylosing spondylitis, psoriatic arthritis)
- Systemic: SLE, Sjögren's syndrome, sarcoidosis, Behçet's disease, vasculitides
- Malignancy.

Multiple joints

- Infection: disseminated septic arthritis (e.g. staphylococcal, gonococcal), viral (e.g. enteroviruses, EBV, HIV, hepatitis B, mumps, rubella), rheumatic fever, Lyme disease, TB
- Gout/pseudogout
- Rheumatoid arthritis, osteoarthritis (generalized)
- Seronegative arthritis: (reactive/Reiter's, enteropathic (Whipple's, IBD), ankylosing spondylitis, psoriatic arthritis)
- Systemic diseases: SLE, sarcoid, Sjögren's, Behçet's, primary vasculitides, polymyalgia rheumatica
- Other: haemochromatosis, sickle cell, malignancy (hypertrophic pulmonary osteoarthropathy).

Leg swelling

Bilateral

- Cardiac failure
- Liver failure
- Other causes of hypoalbuminaemia (malnutrition, malabsorption, nephrotic syndrome, protein-losing enteropathy)
- Renal failure
- Hypothyroidism
- Iatrogenic: oestrogens, calcium channel blockers, 'glitazones', NSAID, fluid overload
- Venous insufficiency: acute (prolonged sitting), chronic venous obstruction, e.g. pelvic mass, pregnancy, inferior vena cava/bilateral iliac vein obstruction.

Unilateral

- *Acute*
- DVT
- Cellulitis
- Compartment syndrome, trauma
- Baker's cyst rupture.

Chronic

- Varicose veins
- Lymphoedema (non-pitting): primary, lymph node involvement (radiotherapy, infection (filariasis), malignant infiltration, excision)
- Immobility.

Melaena

See Haematemesis and melaena, 📖 p.827.

Muscle weakness

1. Congenital
- Muscular dystrophies: (limb-girdle, facioscapulohumoral, Duchenne, myotonic)
- Glycogen storage diseases
- Inherited spinal muscular atrophies.

2. Infectious
- Viral (e.g. influenza)
- Bacterial (e.g. TB, syphilis)
- Parasites (e.g. trichinosis, toxoplasmosis, trypanosomiasis).

3. Toxic
- Alcohol
- Heavy metals (e.g. mercury, lead, arsenic)
- Corticosteroids
- Organophosphates
- Drugs (vincristine, doxorubicin, heroin)
- Botulism.

4. Traumatic
- Exercise
- Injury
- Seizure.

5. Metabolic
- Hyper- or hypo-thyroidism
- Hypokalaemia
- Hypophosphataemia
- Hypocalcaemia
- Hypomagnesaemia
- Hypoglycaemia
- Diabetes mellitus
- Cushing's disease
- Addison's disease
- Hyperparathyroidism
- Hyperaldosteronism
- Acromegaly
- Malnutrition.

6. Vascular insufficiency

7. Immune/idiopathic
- Myasthenia gravis
- Scleroderma
- SLE
- PAN
- RhA
- Polymyalgia rheumatica
- Sarcoidosis
- Polymyositis/ dermatomyositis.

8. Neoplastic
- Carcinomatous myopathy
- Eaton–Lambert syndrome
- Carcinoid myopathy.

Nausea

See Vomiting, 🕮 p.837.

Palpitations

- Fever, dehydration, exercise, anaemia, pregnancy
- Drugs (caffeine, nicotine, salbutamol, anticholinergics, vasodilators, cocaine)
- Cardiac: any arrhythmia (e.g. AF, extrasystoles, supraventricular tachycardia, ventricular tachycardia), valvular disease, cardiomyopathy, septal defects, atrial myxoma
- Endocrine: thyrotoxicosis, pheochromocytomas, hypoglycaemia, mastocytosis
- Psychiatric: panic attacks, generalized anxiety disorder.

Seizures

See Fits, 🕮 p.827.

Tremor

Table 16.1 Characteristics of tremor

Tremor type	Characteristics	Seen in
Simple tremor		
Essential, familial or senile tremor	Not present at rest (except in head)	Persons with family history Fatigue Advanced age Stimulants Fever Thyrotoxicosis
Parkinsonism	Present in hands at complete rest Associated with rigidity; ↓associative movements, small steppage gait, mask-like facies	Parkinsonism of all types
Cerebellar tremor	Worse with motion and associated with cerebellar signs	MS, Wilson's disease, heriditary ataxia
Chorea	Jerky, irregular, sudden movements, intermittent fidgeting	Acute rheumatic fever (Sydenham's chorea) Huntington's chorea
Athetosis	Upper limbs predominate Slow, sinuous, writhing movements	Cerebral palsy Drugs
Myoclonus	Sudden jerks of single muscles or groups	Epilepsy Encephalitis Hyponatraemia Hyperosmolar state Some degenerative CNS diseases
Tetanic spasms	Sustained contractions of single muscles or muscle groups	Tetanus Spasticity
Hemiballismus	Flinging movements of arm and leg on one side	Infarction of the subthalamic nucleus

Unconsciousness/reduced consciousness

- Hypoglycaemia
- Hypoxia: cardiac arrest, shock (hypovolaemic, septic), respiratory failure
- Vascular: intracranial haemorrhage/infarction
- Infection: meningitis, encephalitis
- Inflammation (cerebral vasculitis)
- Trauma (head injury)
- Tumour (↑ICP)
- Toxic: drugs e.g. opiates, alcohol, anxiolytics, antidepressants
- Metabolic: liver failure, renal failure, electrolyte (Na^+, K^+, Ca^{2+}, Mg^{2+}) disturbances, endocrinopathies e.g. myxoedema coma, vitamin deficiencies (e.g. thiamine, B12), hypothermia
- Epilepsy (post-ictal).

Vomiting

- Drugs, poisoning, alcohol
- Abdominal pathology (GI, hepatic, gynaecological)
- Metabolic/endocrine: DKA, Addisonian crisis, hypercalcaemia, uraemia, pregnancy
- ↑ICP (infection, space-occupying lesion, benign intracranial hypertension)
- Acute labyrinthitis
- Acute angle closure glaucoma.

Weak legs

Spastic paraparesis

- Inflammation: demyelination, transverse myelitis (post-infectious, e.g. viral infections, *Mycoplasma*), vasculitides, sarcoidosis, SLE
- Infection: epidural abscess, tuberculous abscess, HIV, HTLV-1 (tropical spastic paraparesis), syphilis
- Trauma: vertebral fractures/dislocation, disc protrusion (usually spontaneous rather than traumatic)
- Tumours: vertebral metastases, intrinsic cord tumours (ependymoma, glioma, metastases), extrinsic tumours (neurofibroma, meningioma), parasigittal meningioma
- Metabolic: vitamin B12 deficiency (subacute combined degeneration)
- Degenerative: of the spine (spondylosis with cord compression), in the cord: motor neuron disease
- Congenital: hereditary spastic paraparesis, Friedreich's ataxia
- Other: syringomyelia
- Flaccid paraparesis
- Polyneuropathies
- Myopathies
- Anterior spinal artery syndrome (spinal cord infarction).

Wheeze

- Angio-oedema/anaphylaxis
- Asthma
- Bronchitis
- Bronchiectasis
- Cardiac wheeze (pulmonary oedema)
- Cancer (lung)
- Carcinoid syndrome
- Pulmonary eosinophilia.

Appendix

Generic listings of national and international guidelines

- Royal College of Physicians listing of national guidelines: ☞ http://www.rcplondon.ac.uk/college/ceeu/search/
- The National Guideline Clearinghouse™, a resource for evidence-based clinical practice guidelines: ☞ http://www.guideline.gov/
- Nice Guidelines: ☞ http://www.nice.org.uk/ ☞ http://www.evidence.nhs.uk/search.aspx?t=guidelines&AspxAutoDetectCookieSupport=1
- Scottish Intercollegiate Guidelines Network (SIGN): ☞ http://www.sign.ac.uk/

By Specialty

Cardiac

- European Society of cardiology: ☞ http://www.escardio.org/guidelines-surveys/esc-guidelines/Pages/GuidelinesList.aspx
- American Heart and American Cardiology College: ☞ http://www.americanheart.org/presenter.jhtml?identifier=3004542

Critical Care

☞ http://www.learnicu.org/Quick_Links/Pages/default.aspx

Dermatology

- British Association of Dermatologists: ☞ http://www.bad.org.uk/site/622/default.aspx

Drugs and toxicology

- Clinical toxicology database of the National Poisons Information Service: ☞ http://www.toxbase.org/

Endocrine

- The Endocrine Society: ☞ http://www.endo-society.org/guidelines/Current-Clinical-Practice-Guidelines.cfm
- American Association of Clinical Endocrinologists: ☞ http://www.aace.com/pub/guidelines/

Gastroenterology and Hepatology

- British Society of Gastroenterology: ☞ http://www.bsg.org.uk/clinical/general/guidelines.html
- European Association for Study of the Liver (EASL): ☞ http://www.easl.ch/easl_cpg.asp
- American Association for Study of Liver Disease (AASLD): ☞ http://www.aasld.org/practiceguidelines/Pages/default.aspx

Haematology

- British Committee for Standards in Haematology (BCSH): ☞ http://www.bcshguidelines.com/guidelinesMENU.asp

HIV

British HIV Association: ☞ http://www.bhiva.org/cms1191540.asp

Infectious diseases

- Health Protection Agency (UK): http://www.hpa.org.uk/
- Infectious Disease Society of America: http://www.idsociety.org/Content.aspx?id=9088
- Surviving Sepsis: http://www.survivingsepsis.org/node/156

Neurological

- American Academy of Neurology: http://www.aan.com/go/practice/guidelines

Nutrition

http://www.espen.org/espenguidelines.html

Renal

- The Renal Association: http://www.renal.org/pages/pages/guidelines/current.php

Respiratory

- British Thoracic Society: http://www.brit-thoracic.org.uk/
- American Thoracic Society: http://www.thoracic.org/sections/publications/statements/index.html

Rheumatological

British Society of Rheumatology:
http://www.rheumatology.org.uk/guidelines
American College of Rheumatology: management guidelines:
http://www.rheumatology.org/publications/guidelines/index.asp?aud=mem

Reference intervals

Biochemistry (always consult your local laboratory)

Table A1

Substance	Reference interval
ACTH	<80ng/litre
Alanine aminotransferase (ALT)	5–35IU/litre
Albumin	35–50g/litre
Aldosterone[1]	100–500pmol/litre
Alkaline phosphatase	30–300IU/litre (adults)
α-fetoprotein	<10kU/litre
Amylase	0–180 Somogyi U/dl
Angiotensin II[1]	5–35pmol/litre
Antidiuretic hormone (ADH)	0.9–4.6pmol/litre
Aspartate transaminase (AST)	5–35IU/litre
Bicarbonate	24–30mmol/litre
Bilirubin	3–17μmol/litre (0.25–1.5mg/dl)
Calcitonin	<0.1μg/litre
Calcium (ionized)	1.0–1.25mmol/litre
Calcium (total)	2.12–2.65mmol/litre
Chloride	95–105mmol/litre
[2] Cholesterol	3.9–5.5mmol/litre
LDL cholesterol	1.55–4.4mmol/litre
HDL cholesterol	0.9–1.93mmol/litre
Cortisol am	450–700nmol/litre
midnight	80–280nmol/litre
Creatine kinase (CK)	Men 25–195IU/litre
	Women 25–170 IU/litre
Creatinine	70–≤130μmol/litre
C-reactive protein (CRP)	0–10
Ferritin	12–200μg/litre
Folate	5–6.3 nmol/litre (2.1–2.8μg/L)
γ-glutamyl transpeptidase (γ-GT)	Men 11–51IU/litre
	Women 7–33IU/litre
Glucose (fasting)	3.5–5.5mmol/litre
Glycosylated haemoglobin (HbA_1C)	5–8%
Growth hormone	<20mU/litre
Iron	Men 14–31μmol/litre
	Women 7–33IU/litre
Lactate dehydrogenase (LDH)	70–250IU/litre
Magnesium	0.75–1.05mmol/litre

Substance	Reference interval
Osmolality	278–305mosmol/kg
Parathyroid hormone (PTH)	<0.8–8.5pmol/litre
Phosphate (inorganic)	0.8–1.45mmol/litre
Potassium (K^+)	3.5–5.0mmol/litre
Prolactin	Men <450 U/L; Women<600U/L
Prostate specific antigen (PSA)	0–4ng/ml
Protein (total)	60–80g/litre
Red cell folate	0.36–1.44μmol/L (160–640μg/L)
Renin (erect/recumbent)[1]	2.8–4.5/1.1–2.7pmol/ml/h
Sodium (Na^+)	135–145mmol/litre
Thyroid stimulating hormone (TSH)	0.3–3.8mU/litre
Thyroxine (T4)	70–140nmol/litre
Thyroxine (free)	10.0–26.0pmol/litre
Triglyceride (fasting)	0.55–1.90mmol/litre
Tri-iodothyronine (T3)	1.2–3.0nmol/litre
Urea	2.5–6.7mmol/litre
Urate	Men 0.21–0.48mmol/litre Women 0.15–0.39mmol/litre
Vitamin B_{12}	0.13–0.68nmol/litre (>150ng/litre)

[1] The sample requires special handling: contact the lab.

Urine

Table A2

Substance	Reference interval
Adrenaline	0.03–0.10μmol/24h
Cortisol (free)	≤280nmol/24h
Dopamine	0.65–2.70μmol/24h
Hydroxyindole acetic acid (HIAA)	16–73μmol/24h
Hydroxymethylmandelic acid (HMMA, VMA)	16–48μmol/24h
Metanephrines	0.03–0.69μmol/mmol creatinine
Noradrenaline	0.12–0.5μmol/24h
Osmolality	350–1000mosmol/kg
Phosphate (inorganic)	15–50mmol/24h
Potassium	14–120mmol/24h
Sodium	100–250mmol/24h

Cerebrospinal fluid

See p.808.

Hematology

Table A3

Measurement		Reference interval
WBC (white blood cells)		$3.2–11.0 \times 10^9$ /L
RBC (red blood cells)	Men	$4.5–6.5 \times 10^{12}$ /L
	Women	$3.9–5.6 \times 1^{12}$ /L
Haemoglobin (Hb)	Men	13.5–18.0g/dl
	Women	11.5–16.0g/dl
Haematocrit (HCT) or packed cell volume (PCV)	Men	0.4–0.54 l/L
	Women	0.37–0.47l/L
Mean cell volume (MCV)		82–98fl
Mean cell haemoglobin (MCH)		26.7–33.0pg
Mean cell haemoglobin concentration (MCHC)		31.4–35.0g/dl
Platelet count		$120–400 \times 10^9$ /L
Neutrophils	%	40–75%
	Abs. no.	$1.9–7.7 \times 10^9$ /L
Monocytes	%	3.0–11.0%
	Abs. no.	$0.1–0.9 \times 10^9$ /L
Eosinophils	%	0.0–7.0 %
	Abs. no.	$0.0–0.4 \times 10^9$ /L
Basophils	%	0.0–1.0 %
	Abs. no.	$0.2–0.8 \times 10^9$ /L
Lymphocytes	%	20–45%
	Abs. no.	$1.3–3.5 \times 10^9$ /L
Reticulocyte count[1]		0.8–2.0% ($25–100 \times 10^9$ /L)
Erythrocyte sedimentation rate (ESR)		depends on age (& ↑ in anaemia)
	Men	~ (age in years)–2
	Women	~ (age in years+ 10)–2
Prothrombin time (PT)-factors II, VII, and X		10–14 seconds
Activated partial thromboplastin time (APTT)-factors VIII, IX, XI, and XII		35–45 seconds

[1] Only use percentages if red cell count is normal; otherwise use absolute value.

Guidelines on oral anti-coagulation

Table A4

International normalized ratio (INR)	Clinical condition
2.0–3.0	Treatment of DVT, PE, TIAs; chronic AF.
3.0–4.5	Recurrent DVTs and PEs; arterial grafts and arterial disease (including MI); prosthetic cardiac valves.

Acid Base Balance

Acid-base balance

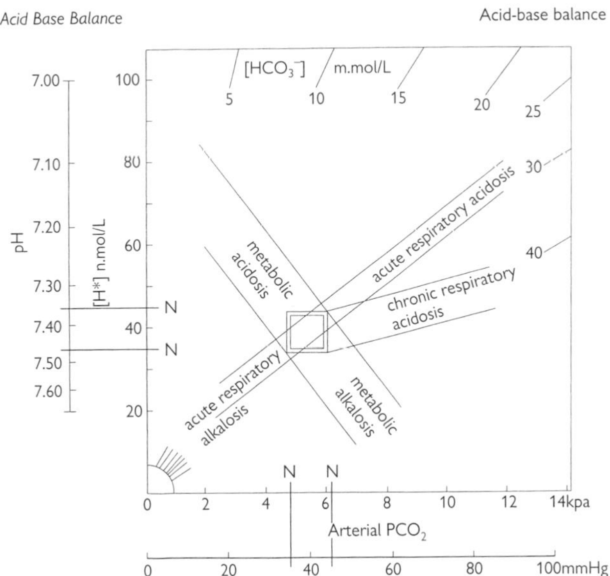

Fig. A1 Acid base nomogram in the interpretation of arterial blood gases (after Flenley DC (1971) *Lancet* **1**: 270–3).

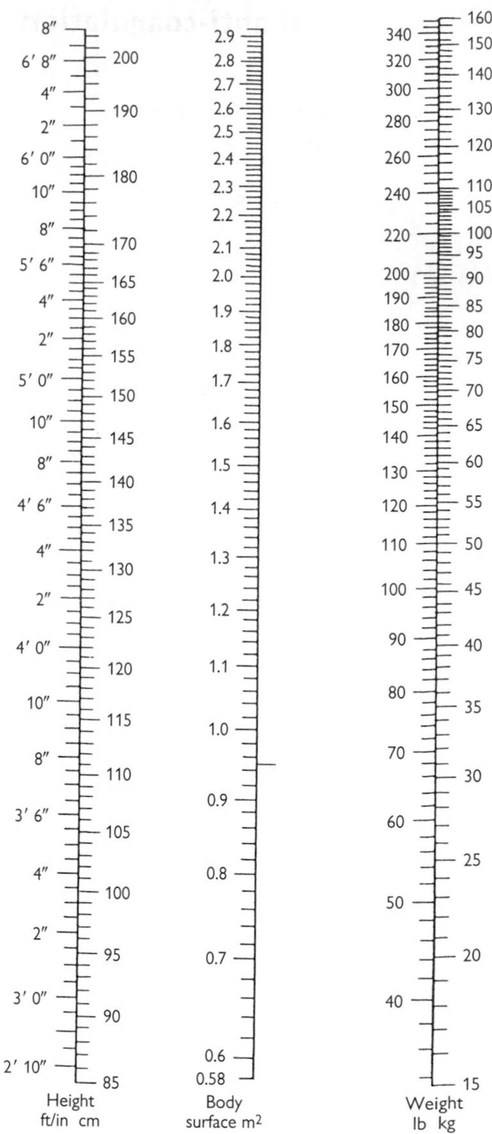

Fig. A2 Nomogram for body size.

Useful contacts

Liver units

Royal Free Hospital, London	0207 794 0500
Addenbrookes Hospital, Cambridge	01223 245 151
Freemans Hospital, Newcastle	0191 233 6161
Queen Elizabeth Hospital, Birmingham	0121 472 1311
St James Hospital, Leeds	0113 243 3144
Edinburgh Royal Infirmary, Edinburgh	0131 536 1000
Kings College Hospital, London	0207 737 4000

ODT

Organ donation and transplantation	0117 975 7575

Poisons units

National Poisons Information Service	0844 892 0111

National Teratology unit

Drug & Chemical Exposure in Pregnancy	0844 892 0909

Tropical and infectious diseases

Hospital for Tropical Diseases, London	0207 387 4411
Northwick Park, London	0208 864 3232 (bleep infectious diseases registrar)
Liverpool	0151 705 3100

Anti-venom kits for snakebites

For information on identification and management contact:

Liverpool	0151 705 3100
London	0207 188 0500

Virus reference laboratory

Colindale, London	0208 200 4400

Change in names of certain medicinal substances

Currently both British Approved Names (BANs) and recommended International Non-Proprietary Names (rINNs) are in use in the UK and for some substances these names differ, giving rise to confusion and the risk of medication error. Since 1 December 2003, where the names differ the rINN is the correct name.

Former BAN	New BAN
Acrosoxacin	Rosoxacin
Adrenaline	Epinephrine (INN)*
Amethocaine	Tetracaine
Amoxycillin	Amoxicillin
Amylobarbitone	Amobarbital
Amylobarbitone Sodium	Amobarbital Sodium
Beclomethasone	Beclometasone
Bendrofluazide	Bendroflumethiazide
Benorylate	Benorilate
Benzhexol	Trihexyphenidyl
Benztropine	Benzatropine
Busulphan	Busulfan
Butobarbitone	Butobarbital
Carticaine	Articaine
Cephalexin	Cefalexin
Cephamandole Nafate	Cefamandole Nafate
Cephazolin	Cefazolin
Cephradine	Cefradine
Chloral betaine	Cloral betaine
Chlorbutol	Chlorobutanol
Chlormethiazole	Clomethiazole
Chlorpheniramine	Chlorphenamine
Chlorthalidone	Chlortalidone
Cholecalciferol	Colecalciferol
Cholestyramine	Colestyramine
Clomiphene	Clomifene
Colistin Sulphomethate Sodium	Colistimethate Sodium
Corticotrophin	Corticotropin
Cyclosporin	Ciclosporin
Cysteamine	Mercaptamine
Danthron	Dantron
Desoxymethasone	Desoximetasone
Dexamphetamine	Dexamfetamine
Dibromopropamidine	Dibrompropamidine

* Adrenaline/noradrenaline remains the British Approved Name, however the International Non-proprietary Name is epinephrine/norepinephrine.

Former BAN	New BAN
Dicyclomine	Dicycloverine
Dienoestrol	Dienestrol
Dimethicone (s)	Dimeticone
Dimethyl Sulphoxide	Dimethyl Sulfoxide
Dothiepin	Dosulepin
Doxycycline Hydrochloride (Hemihydrate Hemiethanolate)	Doxycycline Hyclate
Eformoterol	Formoterol
Ethamsylate	Etamsylate
Ethinyloestradiol	Ethinylestradiol
Ethynodiol	Etynodiol
Flumethasone	Flumetasone
Flupenthixol	Flupentixol
Flurandrenolone	Fludroxycortide
Frusemide	Furosemide
Gestronol	Gestonorone
Guaiphenesin	Guaifenesin
Hexachlorophane	Hexachlorophene
Hexamine Hippurate	Methenamine Hippurate
Hydroxyurea	Hydroxycarbamide
Indomethacin	Indometacin
Lignocaine	Lidocaine
Lysuride	Lisuride
Methimazole	Thiamazole
Methotrimeprazine	Levomepromazine
Methyl Cysteine	Mecysteine
Methylene Blue	Methylthioninium Chloride
Mitozantrone	Mitoxantrone
Mustine	Chlormethine
Nicoumalone	Acenocoumarol
Noradrenaline	Norepinephrine (INN)*
Oestradiol	Estradiol
Oestriol	Estriol
Oestrone	Estrone
Oxpentifylline	Pentoxifylline
Phenobarbitone	Phenobarbital
Pipothiazine	Pipotiazine
Polyhexanide	Polihexanide
Potassium Clorazepate	Dipotassium Clorazepate
Pramoxine	Pramocaine
Procaine Penicillin	Procaine Benzylpenicillin
Prothionamide	Protionamide
Quinalbarbitone	Secobarbital
Riboflavine	Riboflavin

Former BAN	New BAN
Salcatonin	Calcitonin (salmon)
Sodium Calciumedetate	Sodium Calcium Edetate
Sodium Cromoglycate	Sodium Cromoglicate
Sodium Ironedetate	Sodium Feredetate
Sodium Picosulphate	Sodium Picosulfate
Sorbitan Monostearate	Sorbitan Stearate
Stibocaptate	Sodium Stibocaptate
Stilboestrol	Diethylstilbestrol
Sulphacetamide	Sulfacetamide
Sulphadiazine	Sulfadiazine
Sulphamethoxazole	Sulfamethoxazole
Sulphapyridine	Sulfapyridine
Sulphasalazine	Sulfasalazine
Sulphathiazole	Sulfathiazole
Sulphinpyrazone	Sulfinpyrazone
Tetracosactrin	Tetracosactide
Thiabendazole	Tiabendazole
Thioguanine	Tioguanine
Thiopentone	Thiopental
Thymoxamine	Moxisylyte
Thyroxine Sodium	Levothyroxine Sodium
Tribavirin	Ribavirin
Trimeprazine	Alimemazine
Urofollitrophin	Urofollitropin

Index

Note: Pages dealing with the management of drug overdose are shown in **bold** type. Main references to drugs with dosages have been included in the index.

C

N

O

P

Q

R

S

T

U

W

Y

Z